Nuclear Medicine Therapy

Cumali Aktolun • Stanley J. Goldsmith

Editors

Nuclear Medicine Therapy

Principles and Clinical Applications

Springer

Editors
Cumali Aktolun
Tirocenter Nuclear Medicine Center
Istanbul, Turkey

Stanley J. Goldsmith
Division of Nuclear Medicine
  and Molecular Imaging
New York-Presbyterian Hospital
Weill College of Medicine
  of Cornell University
NY, USA

ISBN 978-1-4614-4020-8   ISBN 978-1-4614-4021-5 (eBook)
DOI 10.1007/978-1-4614-4021-5
Springer New York Heidelberg Dordrecht London

Library of Congress Control Number: 2012942473

Springer is part of Springer Science+Business Media (www.springer.com)

'To our patients and mentors who have taught us in the past and continue to teach us about life and medicine.'

Cumali Aktolun, MD, MSc
Stanley J. Goldsmith, MD

Foreword

Targeting radioactive molecules to a disease process for imaging is well accepted and has disseminated rapidly. PET/CT with FDG has revolutionized cancer imaging and cancer management in the past two decades. The concept of nuclear medicine therapy (RIT) of cancers and other diseases has been and remains an attractive one.

While radionuclide therapy is well accepted for benign and malignant thyroid diseases, its growth in application to other diseases has been slower. There has been great progress, however, over the past several years. Recent successes of RIT in patients with non-Hodgkin's lymphoma, therapy of bone metastases (especially new data with Radium-223 chloride in metastatic prostate cancer), the use of radiomicrospheres in liver cancers, as well as with radiopeptides and ^{131}I-MIBG therapy of neuroendocrine and other tumors are undeniable. The use of nuclear medicine therapies as an adjuvant to surgery and chemotherapy is showing great promise. The recent approval of Zevalin® for consolidation RIT of lymphoma offers an integrated approach after initial chemotherapy of follicular lymphoma. More challenging are nuclear medicine treatments of disseminated solid tumors. With improvements in radiopharmaceutical delivery to cancers through multistep pre-targeting approaches, new radiopharmaceuticals and combinations with other agents, hope for improved outcomes exists for many of these difficult diseases.

There has been a recognition that the radiobiology of ultra low-dose radiation differs in some cases from what has been classically believed to be the case with some paradoxical instances of increased radiosensitivity of tumors to very low dose rates, possibly due to damage escaping activation of repair mechanisms. In addition, there has been progress in radiation dosimetry and a greater application of patient-specific dosing based on an imaging dose, which antedates a therapy dose. All of these events are occurring in a shifting regulatory environment where outpatient therapies with radiopharmaceuticals are feasible and safe.

The field of nuclear medicine therapy is showing great and continuing successes. Perhaps the underlying reason for this success is the fact that it is likely that nuclear medicine therapy does not hit just a single pathway; rather it hits many. No tumors are absolutely radioresistant. While some tumors are not as radiosensitive as others, all respond to radiation.

A real and emerging paradigm for nuclear medicine therapy includes:

1. A target is identified on a tumor or benign process.
2. A diagnostic radiotracer to target the tumor or process is identified and quantified on nuclear scans.
3. The targeted therapeutic radiopharmaceutical is administered based on patient-specific dosimetry.
4. The patient's response is followed by radionuclide imaging.

The very real possibility that nuclear medicine therapy could totally replace other treatments of cancer is a real one. I recently had the good fortune to meet with many patients that my colleagues and I had treated with ^{131}I-tositumomab alone as the sole and initial therapy of lymphoma over 12 years ago. Many were still doing well, absent any chemotherapy. They were treated with ^{131}I-tositumomab and now their (lack of) disease can be followed with FDG PET.

With all of these advances, practice patterns are being disrupted and the dissemination of these methods requires a highly informed and experienced cadre of practitioners who understand the multiple complexities of radiopharmaceutical therapies. This textbook fills this major unmet need. The book is comprehensive and extends from fundamental radiobiology, to targeting, to disease-specific applications in both malignant and benign diseases, and also deals with the "challenges" associated with nuclear medicine therapy. Despite challenges, the powerful methods of nuclear medicine therapy will prevail.

When Dr. Goldsmith asked me to write this Foreword, I wanted to have a chance to see the book first. He was kind enough to share most of the prepublication manuscript with me. It is well written and over the course of a busy 24 h, I read all of it. The book is that interesting and fills a very large and critical knowledge gap. This book is an essential component of the continued growth of nuclear medicine as a major therapeutic method in both malignant and benign disease. Nuclear medicine treatments are truly patient specific and require targeted therapies. They represent a major benefit to patients in their current form and a great opportunity for scientific research moving forward.

This book by Drs. Aktolun and Goldsmith, with world experts writing each chapter, will accelerate the field of nuclear medicine therapy, help educate a new cadre of experts in nuclear medicine therapy, and help clinicians to better integrate nuclear medicine treatments into their practices.

Baltimore, MD, USA   Richard L. Wahl

Preface

This volume is devoted entirely to the use of nuclear medicine techniques and technology for therapy of malignant and benign diseases. In recent years, the research activity in this area has undergone exponential growth. Several nuclear medicine therapeutic procedures are already "in the clinic," that is, part of routine nuclear medicine practice and included in the training and certification of nuclear medicine physicians. In many other areas, the science and protocols are still evolving. In the judgment of the editors, it is worthwhile to stay abreast of these matters as they progress so that when the procedure is developed to a point where it is approved for clinical use by government regulatory bodies, the scientific foundation, the details of the protocol and the evidence for its efficacy will not be overwhelmingly complex or remote from one's working knowledge.

It is likely that the initial observation of the biologic effects of radiation began with the skin ulceration that developed on Pierre Curie's chest beneath the vial of radium salts that he carried in his vest pocket. The use of radium externally and its emitted radiation subsequently became the foundation of radiation oncology and a component of tumor therapy. It is ironic that one of the most recent agents to appear on the nuclear medicine horizon is the use of soluble radium chloride for the treatment of osseous metastases. One is tempted to say that "we have come full circle" except that it is clear that the circle has not been completed and there is still a great deal to learn and understand.

Many descriptions of the history of nuclear medicine therapy began with de Hevesy's enunciation of the tracer principal and/or Seidlen's report of the affect of Iodine-131 on the clinical course of hyperthyroidism secondary to excess thyroid hormone production in a patient with thyroid carcinoma metastases. From this beginning, Iodine-131 became a standard component in the management of patients with thyroid carcinoma. As other radionuclides became available during and after World War II, Phosphorus-32 found application in the therapy of polycythemia vera. From the appreciation of the tracer principle and the increased understanding of radioactivity and the availability of instrumentation to detect, localize, and quantify radioactive materials within the human body, imaging techniques and the field of nuclear medicine evolved.

Progress was slow but steady. It was assumed that it was "just a question of time" until biomedical scientists and physicians identified other radionuclides that could be used to treat other diseases, usually malignant tumors. This prediction has proven to be correct but the time line has been much longer than would have been predicted.

This book describes the present "state of the art" of what has come to be known as "targeted radionuclide therapy," both in clinical practice and contemporary clinical investigation and trials.

This volume reports on the scientific principles and clinical applications of targeted radionuclide therapy that have a place in modern medicine and the current status of clinical trials of agents under investigation in the therapy of tumors involving virtually every organ system.

The therapeutic agent should be targeted to minimize irradiation of healthy tissues. In general, targeted radionuclide therapy falls into four different approaches. First, the radionuclide itself may be the definitive therapeutic agent such as the use of ^{131}I as sodium iodide for the treatment of thyroid cancer based on the iodine trapping mechanism inherent in thyroid tissue or ^{89}Sr as strontium chloride and ^{32}P as disodium monophosphate for the treatment of painful bone metastases.

Second, there is the use of small molecules such as MIBG to carry ^{131}I into chromaffin tissue tumors and somatostatin receptor ligands like tyrosine octreotide to carry ^{177}Lu or ^{90}Y into neuroendocrine tumors.

Third is the evolving science of radioimmunotherapy where antibodies, monoclonal antibodies, are the vehicles that deliver radiometals to tumors. At the present time, the clinically approved agents use intact antibodies and either ^{131}I or radiometals as the therapeutic agent. The introduction of radiometals as radiation emitters in place of iodine with its well-known chemistry required the development of the science of "linker chemistry."

Until recently, the radiometals utilized in targeted radiation therapy have emitted beta particles but we are now seeing increasing interest in alpha particle emitters including radium-223. The intact antibody itself is being reengineered beyond simply converting a murine derived antibody into a chimeric or humanized version. Studies are under way evaluating bi-specific antibodies, diabodies, and completely novel constructs of components of the original intact antibody.

Lastly, there is the development of radiolabeled microspheres which are introduced into the arterial circulation of tumors providing localized radiation in a manner that differs from both conventional brachytherapy as well as soluble radiolabeled compounds that have an active metabolic process as the basis for their accumulation.

Loco-regional application of radionuclides for therapeutic purposes has recently been a topic of interest. Radiosynovectomy in this respect has been regaining popularity particularly in developed countries due to an ageing population. Pre-targeting using innovative techniques combined with systemic and loco-regional application of radionuclides for therapy of malignant diseases as described in this text will attract considerable interest.

Radionuclide therapy, even in one of its oldest area of application (i.e., radioiodine therapy of hyperthyroidism), is not yet universally standardized.

It is an evolving aspect of Nuclear Medicine while it also attracts considerable interest from other medical disciplines including but not limited to Radiation Oncology, Medical Oncology, Hematology, Diagnostic Radiology, Hepatology, Endocrinology, Rheumatology due to overlapping interests in the technique itself, indications, and clinical use. Hopefully, this text will contribute to much needed standardization of this practice.

This text will help also to solidify the role of Nuclear Medicine in the "healing process." This is of vital importance at a time when the survival of "pure" Nuclear Medicine as a free-standing specialty is being discussed. Radionuclide therapy is an important tool to integrate Nuclear Medicine with other medical disciplines as almost all of the techniques described in this volume require collaboration with at least one other discipline.

An ever increasing number of new PET and SPECT probes will open the way to translate the data obtained from imaging research studies into new therapeutic techniques. The same molecule that targets for imaging can be used for therapy by replacing the gamma photon emitting agent with a particle emitter. Nuclear Medicine is unique in directly translating diagnostic information and techniques to therapeutic methods (drug development). The developments in radionuclide therapy are all very exciting and increasingly complex phenomena—but they are delightful to behold. By reviewing the present state of even the most complex procedure, our readers will be able to monitor future developments as they evolve.

In the meantime, this volume includes comprehensive descriptions of the development and present state-of-the art of the targeted therapeutic radionuclide procedures currently in practice. This book is unique in that it includes all of the Nuclear Medicine therapy methods in a single text. We hope that it is useful to the practitioner, scientist, trainee, and student in this fascinating coming together of medicine and nuclear science.

Istanbul, Turkey   Cumali Aktolun, MD, MSc
NY, USA   Stanley J. Goldsmith, MD

Acknowledgment

We are grateful to our contributors who showed extraordinary effort to comply with the demanding editorial agenda.

Contents

Contributors

Alain S. Abi-Ghanem, MD Department of Radiology, Dana-Farber Cancer Institute/Brigham and Women's Hospital, Harvard Medical School, Boston, MA, USA

Cumali Aktolun, MD, MSc Tirocenter Nuclear Medicine Center, Istanbul, Turkey

Jacques Barbet GIP ARRONAX, Saint-Herblain, France
Oncology Research Center, Nantes University, Nantes, France

Tushar Barot, MD Department of Surgical Oncology and Radiology/Nuclear Medicine, Florida International University College of Medicine, Miami, FL, USA

Chiara Bampo Department of Nuclear Medicine, Fondazione IRCCS Istituto Nazionale Tumori, Milan, Italy

Neil H. Bander, MD Department of Urology, New York-Presbyterian Hospital-Weill Cornell Medical Center, Weill Cornell Medical College, New York, NY, USA

Emilio Bombardieri Department of Nuclear Medicine, Fondazione IRCCS Istituto Nazionale Tumori, Milan, Italy

Jean François Chatal GIP ARRONAX, BP, Cedex, France

Carlo Chiesa Department of Nuclear Medicine, Fondazione IRCCS Istituto Nazionale Tumori, Milan, Italy

Concetta De Cicco Division of Nuclear Medicine, European Institute of Oncology, Milan, Italy

Chaitanya Divgi, MD Department of Radiology, PET/Nuclear Medicine Division, Columbia University, New York, NY, USA

Chiara Maria Grana Division of Nuclear Medicine, European Institute of Oncology, Milan, Italy

Seza A. Gulec, MD, FACS Department of Radiology/Nuclear Medicine, Florida International University College of Medicine, Miami, FL, USA

Robert Howman-Giles, MD, FRACP, DDU Nuclear Medicine and Diagnostic Ultrasound, RPAH Medical Centre, Newtown, NSW, Australia

Sydney Medical School, The University of Sydney, Sydney, NSW, Australia

Francoise Kraeber-Bodéré, MD, PhD Oncology Research Center, Nantes University, Nantes, France

Nuclear Medicine Department, University Hospital and ICO Gauducheau Cancer Institute, Nantes, France

David V. Gold, PhD Center for Molecular Medicine and Immunology and the Garden State Cancer Center, Morris Plains, NJ, USA

David M. Goldenberg, ScD, MD IBC Pharmaceuticals, Inc, and Immunomedics, Inc, Morris Plains, NJ, USA

Garden State Cancer Center, Center for Molecular Medicine and Immunology, Morris Plains, NJ, USA

Stanley J. Goldsmith, MD Division of Nuclear Medicine and Molecular Imaging, New York-Presbyterian Hospital, Weill Cornell Medical Center, Weill Cornell Medical College, NY, USA

David K. Leung, MD, PhD Department of Radiology, PET/Nuclear Medicine Division, Columbia University, New York, NY, USA

Irina Lipai, MS, CNMT Division of Nuclear Medicine and Molecular Imaging, New York Presbyterian Hospital-Weill Cornell Medical Center, Weill Cornell Medical College, New York, NY, USA

Alexander J. McEwan Division of Oncologic Imaging, Department of Oncology, School of Cancer, Engineering and Imaging Sciences, University of Alberta, AB, Canada

Marco Maccauro Department of Nuclear Medicine, Fondazione IRCCS Istituto Nazionale Tumori, Milan, Italy

Andrew Mallia School of Specialization in Nuclear Medicine, University of Milano, Milan, Italy

Maura Massimino Division of Pediatric Oncology, Fondazione IRCCS Istituto Nazionale Tumori, Milan, Italy

Razmik Mirzayans Department of Oncology, Division of Experimental Oncology, University of Alberta, School of Cancer, Engineering and Imaging Sciences, Edmonton, AB, Canada

Gynter Mödder NURAMED, German Centre for Radiosynoviorthesis, Köln, Germany

Renate Mödder-Reese NURAMED, German Centre for Radiosynoviorthesis, Köln, Germany

David Murray, PhD Department of Oncology, Division of Experimental Oncology, Cross Cancer Institute, School of Cancer, Engineering and Imaging Sciences, University of Alberta, AB, Canada

David M. Nanus, MD, PhD Division of Hematology and Oncology, Deane Prostate Health and Research Center, New York-Presbyterian Hospital-Weill Cornell Medical Center, Weill Cornell Medical College, New York, NY, USA

Anastasia Nikolopoulou, PhD Division of Nuclear Medicine and Molecular Imaging, New York Presbyterian Hospital-Weill Cornell Medical Center, Weill Cornell Medical College, New York, NY, USA

Joseph R. Osborne, MD, PhD Division of Nuclear Medicine and Molecular Imaging, New York Presbyterian Hospital-Weill Cornell Medical Center, Weill Cornell Medical College, New York, NY, USA

Giovanni Paganelli Division of Nuclear Medicine, European Institute of Oncology, Milan, Italy

Gabriele Scaramellini Division of ORL Surgery, Fondazione IRCCS Istituto Nazionale Tumori, Milan, Italy

Ettore Seregni Department of Nuclear Medicine, Fondazione IRCCS Istituto Nazionale Tumori, Milan, Italy

Robert M. Sharkey, PhD Center for Molecular Medicine and Immunology and the Garden State Cancer Center, Morris Plains, NJ, USA

Edward B. Silberstein, MD The University Hospital, University of Cincinnati Medical Center, Cincinnati, OH, USA

Rekha Suthar, MD Department of Radiology/Nuclear Medicine, Florida International University College of Medicine, Miami, FL, USA

Scott T. Tagawa, MD Division of Hematology and Oncology, Deane Prostate Health and Research Center, New York-Presbyterian Hospital-Weill Cornell Medical Center, Weill Cornell Medical College, New York, NY, USA

John F. Thompson Sydney Medical School, The University of Sydney, Sydney, NSW, Australia

Melanoma Institute Australia, North Sydney, NSW, Australia

Roger F. Uren, MD, FRACP, DDU Nuclear Medicine and Diagnostic Ultrasound, RPAH Medical Centre, Newtown, NSW, Australia

Sydney Medical School, The University of Sydney, Sydney, NSW, Australia

Muammer Urhan, MD Nuclear Medicine Service, GATA Haydarpasa Teaching Hospital, Kadiköy, Istanbul, Turkey

Shankar Vallabhajosula, PhD Division of Nuclear Medicine and Molecular Imaging, New York-Presbyterian Hospital-Weill Cornell Medical Centre, Weill Cornell Medical College, New York, NY, USA

William A. Wegener, MD, PhD Clinical Research, Immunomedics, Inc., Morris Plains, NJ, USA

Pat B. Zanzonico, PhD Department of Medical Physics, Memorial Sloan-Kettering Cancer Center, New York, NY, USA

Katherine Zukotynski, MD Department of Radiology, Dana-Farber Cancer Institute, Brigham and Women's Hospital, Harvard Medical School, Boston, MA, USA

Part I

Radionuclide Therapy of Malignant Diseases

Radioimmunotherapy of Lymphoma

Stanley J. Goldsmith

Introduction

Lymphoma is a generic term describing a malignant tumor originating in lymphoid tissue. In the United States, Western Europe, and other developed countries, it is the most common hematologic malignancy. At the present time, lymphomas, both Hodgkin's and non-Hodgkin's, represent 5–6% of all malignant tumors (excluding superficial skin cancers) in these countries. In 2008, there were approximately 450,000 men and women living in the United States who had had the diagnosis of non-Hodgkin's lymphoma (NHL); 55% were men. In 2011, it is estimated that 66,000 new cases of NHL were diagnosed in the United States. NHL can occur at any age but the vast majority (almost 90%) of cases will be diagnosed after age 50. Hodgkin's lymphoma can also occur at any age, but it is more common in a younger age group (<30 years old). Consequently, the median age at diagnosis of NHL is 66 years of age with a median survival of 9 years. Many patients respond well to a variety of treatments and in some cases will be cured of the disease. Nevertheless, in 2011, over 19,000 patients in the United States died of the disease [1].

S.J. Goldsmith, M.D. (✉)
Division of Nuclear Medicine and Molecular Imaging,
New York-Presbyterian Hospital, Weill College
of Medicine of Cornell University,
525 East 68th Street, NY 10065, USA
e-mail: sjg2002@med.cornell.edu

Classification of Lymphoma

Lymphoma is a malignancy that arises from lymphocytes and consequently, usually presents with lymph node involvement. Other organs with significant lymphocyte populations such as the spleen, bone marrow, liver, gastrointestinal tract may be involved, but the disease may occur even in the central nervous system and skeleton.

The diagnosis of lymphoma may be made during a routine physical examination at which time the patient has few if any symptoms (low grade, indolent lymphoma) or it may present in a dramatic manner with the seemingly overnight appearance of a mass due to lymphadenopathy (high grade, aggressive lymphoma). Often in retrospect, the patient with a high grade lymphoma has been increasingly debilitated, has experienced unexplained weight loss, fatigue, fevers, night sweats, and discomfort. In addition to pain associated with lymph node enlargement and interference with specific organ function, there may be general debilitation and often an impact on the immune response rendering the patient vulnerable to a variety of infections and other complications. Given the multifaceted nature of the disease; that is, the various clinical courses and variable response to therapy, it is now recognized that there are many varieties of NHL despite the common denominator of having arisen from lymphocytes.

In 1980s, the hematology-oncology communities in the United States and Europe developed a consensus which has become known as the

Working Formulation which differentiated NHL from Hodgkin's lymphoma and divided NHL into four grades (low, intermediate, high, and miscellaneous) related to onset and prognosis. There were further subdivision into 16 different tumor types based on histopathologic features such as size and shape of affected cells. Subsequently, in the mid-1990s, the European and American hematology-oncology community developed the Revised European-American Lymphoma (REAL) Classification based on immunophenotypic and genetic features of NHL. This classification was revised again by the World Health organization (WHO) in 2001 and updated in 2008. There are now many diagnostic categories of lymphoma but approximately 85% of the lymphomas in the United States and Western Europe are B-cell lymphomas including the two most common NHLs: Follicular lymphoma (an indolent, low grade lymphoma) and diffuse large B-cell lymphoma (DLBCL) (an aggressive, high grade lymphoma) [2].

B-cell lymphoma means that the tumor cells are derived from a malignant transformation of B-cells, lymphocytes that in fetal life originate in the bone marrow, spleen, and liver in contrast to T-cells which are derived from thymic tissue. B-cells and T-cells possess different properties and take on different roles in immune system function.

Both normal B-cells and tumors derived from them have in common the frequent expression of similar surface antigens. When an antigen has been characterized by two different antibodies, it is identified as a "cluster of differentiation" and are designated "CD" followed by a number. Many clusters of differentiation have been identified on cells from all tissues and tumors. Although the individual antigens are not characteristic of a specific tumor, there are patterns of expression of these antigens on specific cell types and tumors arising from those cells. For example, the epitope CD 45 is widely expressed on white blood cells but CD 20 appears on the pro-B lymphocyte as it evolves from the stem cell. CD 20 expression increases as the lymphocyte matures but is no longer expressed after full maturity of the normal lymphocyte or its evolution to a plasma cell or the myeloma tumor cells derived from plasma cells. When certain histopathologi-

cal patterns are ambiguous rendering a precise histopathological diagnosis uncertain, immuno-histopathologic CD cell typing can provide defining information.

As stated, the marker CD 20 is expressed in the pro-B-cell stage (as the B-cell evolves from the stem cell precursor) and throughout the life of the mature B-cell but CD 20 is neither present in stem cells nor in plasma cells derived from B-cells. Other surface markers such as CD 19 and CD 22 are also frequently expressed on the differentiated B-cell and the tumors that evolve when these cells undergo malignant transformation.

The antigen CD 20 was of particular interest since it is expressed on many of the most common B cell lymphomas, follicular lymphoma, and DLBCL. DLBCL is the most common NHL, accounting for 40% of the lymphoma diagnosed in adults and it is the most common aggressive, high grade lymphoma. The median age at presentation is 70 years. With treatment, patients survive with a median duration of 10 years. For many years, chemotherapy with cyclophosphamide, hydroxydaunorubicin, oncovin (vincristine), and prednisone (CHOP) or cytoxin, vincristine, and prednisone (CVP) for older patients was frequently the treatment of choice. This regimen includes multiple treatments for several weeks per month over many months with considerable discomfort and toxic side effects [1–3].

Follicular lymphoma is the second most common NHL, and the most common indolent NHL accounting for approximately 22% of NHLs. Currently, it is expected that nearly 14, 000 people will be diagnosed with Follicular NHL annually. The median age at diagnosis of follicular lymphoma is 59 years and the median survival time is 11 years from the time of diagnosis. As stated, indolent lymphomas such as follicular lymphoma may be asymptomatic at the time of diagnosis. Given the toxicity of standard courses of chemotherapy, treatment may be deferred at the time of initial diagnosis. Eventually the patient will become symptomatic or develop objective evidence of progression resulting in a decision to treat. In the past, the great majority (perhaps about 80%) of the patients responded to their initial course of chemotherapy with CHOP or CVP [1–3].

A feature of the clinical course of low grade follicular lymphoma is the so-called "low grade lymphoma paradox"; as mild as the disease may be when initially diagnosed and even when there is a well documented clinical response to chemotherapy, patients will eventually relapse and require an additional round of therapy. A fraction of patients respond when retreated with the same or a similar regimen. Even when relapsed patients respond to retreatment, the duration of response is frequently shorter than the initial disease-free interval. Characteristically, after the third course of treatment, the remission is usually only a few months in duration.

Despite the frequent success in treating low grade follicular lymphoma, this combination of clinical features: large numbers of patients affected, a multifocal disease, frequent relapses with shorter disease-free intervals rendered follicular lymphoma as a worthwhile target for an innovative therapy that is capable of providing targeted antitumor therapy.

DLBCL and low grade follicular lymphoma, therefore, represent a diagnostic category of greatest need in terms of number of individuals affected as well as providing adequate numbers of patients for clinical trials. This is an important component of bringing a therapeutic agent to clinical application, given the complexity and cost of verifying efficacy in these disorders.

Immunotherapy

The REAL and subsequent WHO revision of the classification of NHL made clear that the CD expression on tumor samples provided the best methodology to identify specific tumor types and characteristics. The CD 20 antigen is frequently expressed in both follicular lymphoma and DLBCL. In addition to the relevance of this designation for the precise diagnosis of an NHL, the CD classification identified "a target of opportunity" for the development of specific monoclonal antibodies directed toward the specific antigens expressed on a particular NHL.

Monoclonal antibodies are immunoglobulins, usually IgG, of approximately 160 kDa composed of several polypeptide chains usually characterized as two heavy chains and two light chains in the characteristic "Y" configuration with disulfide linkages binding the stems of the heavy chains as well as the light chains to the arms of the heavy chains. (Fig. 1.1) The terminal portion of the heavy and light chain is the immunorecognition portion.

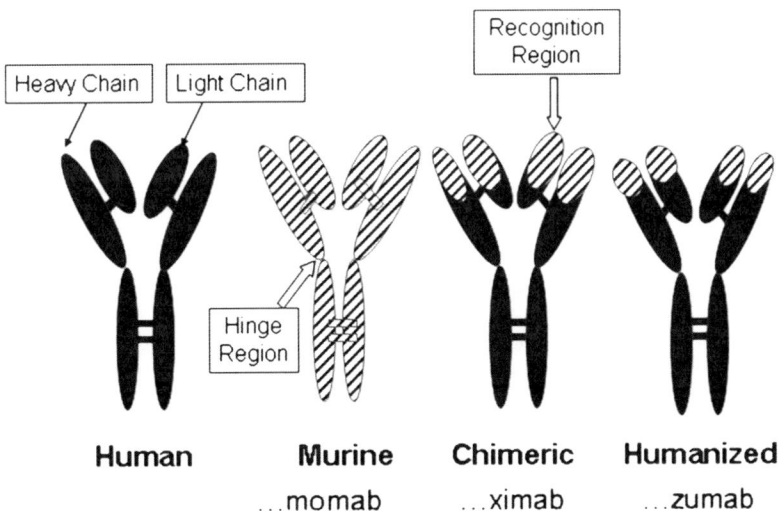

Fig. 1.1 Schematic demonstrating structural similarities and differences amongst human, murine, chimeric and "humanized" IgG molecules. Generic names for monoclonal antibodies end with "mab." Mouse monoclonal antibodies are "-momabs"; chimeric are "-ximabs" and humanized IgGs are "-zumabs." Antibodies to tumor antigens often include "tu"; hence "…tumomab", a murine monoclonal antibody to a tumor antigen; "…tuximab", a chimeric monoclonal antibody to a tumor antigen and "…tuzumab", a humanized monoclonal antibody to a tumor antigen

Immunization of an intact animal results in stimulation of many plasma calls to produce a variety of immunoglobulins with varying degrees of specificity and affinity to the stimulating antigen, summarized in the term "immunoreactivity." In the monoclonal antibody development process, immunoglobulins from isolated hybrid encoded plasma cells are evaluated and selected for their immunoreactivity [4]. Following immunorecognition and binding to an epitope, some immunoglobulin-epitope complexes are internalized whereas others are not. This phenomenon (internalization) is apparently epitope specific and has an influence on the choice of the specific radiolabel, a radiometal vs. radioiodine. Regardless of whether or not the immunoglobulin is internalized, there are several consequences to the immunoglobulin-epitope binding which make possible the use of immunoglobulins as antitumor therapeutic agents. These include: Antibody dependant cell cytolysis, complement dependant cytolysis and antibody-induced apoptosis. These processes represent useful antitumor effects but are dependant upon direct binding to the tumor cell. One of the potential limitations of the immunotherapy approach, therefore, is that although there are usually an abundant number of antigen binding sites on a tumor cell cluster, the immunoglobulin principally affects the cell on which it is bound. Given the vagaries of tumor perfusion, the antibody may not have access to each cell. This limitation tends to impair the effectiveness of immunotherapy for treatment of soft tissue tumors.

Rituximab

After the development of a variety of anti-CD 20 monoclonal antibodies, it was observed that these immunoglobulins had antitumor effects in cell suspensions and other laboratory models. One of these immunoglobulins, ibritumomab, was developed as a chimeric antibody in which the murine IgG backbone of the anti-CD 20 antibody was enzymatically cleaved and replaced with the corresponding portion of a human IgG molecule for the potential treatment of CD 20+ NHL (Fig. 1.1).

This chemical manipulation maintains the immunorecognition portion of the specific murine antibody developed to recognize CD 20 but reduces the likelihood of the patient developing human anti-murine antibodies (HAMA). Development of HAMA would preclude the repeated use of this antisera, primarily because the subsequent HAMA-anti-CD 20 complex would be rapidly eliminated from the circulation without an opportunity to achieve a therapeutic effect. To clarify the sometimes confusing nomenclature, consider that the "ibri-" prefix was cleaved to "ri" and the "mo" component (indicating murine origin) became "xi" (indicating a chimeric structure) according to the custom developed for monoclonal antibody nomenclature. Thus "*ibri* tu *mo* mab" becomes "*ri* tu *xi* mab."

In 1993, a pivotal clinical trial that compared several common chemotherapeutic regimen alone to similar regimen augmented with rituximab infusions was completed [5]. There were greater response rates of longer duration with no additional side effects in the patients who received the monoclonal antibody rituximab in conjunction with chemotherapy. In short order, the addition of rituximab infusions to many different chemotherapeutic regimens became the standard of practice for patients with CD 20+ NHL, including both follicular lymphoma and DLBCL. This was reflected in the regimen terminology which transitioned to CHOP-R or R-CHOP, R-CVP, etc. In addition, it was found that rituximab infusions at regular intervals following the initial chemotherapy course reduced the relapse rate in patients with CD20+ B cell lymphomas (principally follicular lymphoma) and that on occasion, patients with relapsed NHL disease responded to subsequent rituximab infusions. Nevertheless, over time many patients became or were found to be refractory to the chemotherapy-rituximab combination and subsequent rituximab infusions.

Radioimmunotherapy

It is against this background: (1) a relatively large number of patients with follicular, low grade lymphoma who had become refractory to chemotherapy and rituximab; (2) a well-characterized tumor that almost always expressed CD 20 antigen; (3) demonstration that anti-CD 20 monoclonal antibodies were able to target CD 20+ tumor cells and (4) knowledge that lymphoma in general is a relatively radiosensitive tumor—that groups of biomedical scientists began to develop and evaluate radiolabeled anti-CD 20 antibodies. Early in the course of clinical trials, it was appreciated that the principal toxicity, the dose limiting toxicity, was bone marrow suppression, particularly thrombocytopenia. This complication is increasingly manageable with the availability of granulocyte colony stimulating factor (GCSF) and platelet transfusion (and of course, either erythropoietin or packed red blood cell transfusions if necessary). Nevertheless, most clinical trials were designed to evaluate the efficacy of the so-called "nonmyeloablative" protocol which subsequently led to the approval of the two clinical agents, Bexxar® and Zevalin®, in the United States. These agents are currently available for clinical use and the approved protocols are designed to avoid bone marrow ablation or severe damage.

Bexxar® and Zevalin® Nomenclature

It is customary in the scientific literature to use generic names for diagnostic and therapeutic products rather than their proprietary name. Since Bexxar® consists of a combination of tositumomab and ^{131}I-tositumomab administered sequentially and Zevalin® consists of rituximab followed by ^{90}Y-ibritumomab tiuxetan. In this chapter, the "commercial" names, Bexxar® or Zevalin®, are used for convenience and brevity since both the Bexxar® and Zevalin® regimen involve the combination two unlabeled antibody infusions followed by a labeled antibody infusion. In both instances, this sequential infusion of the "cold" antibody followed by the radiolabeled antibody is preceded 1 week earlier by an infusion of the "cold" antibody.

Early in the evolution of radioimmunotherapy, however, there was recognition that since bone marrow transplantation is widely used during the course of other treatment of a variety of tumors including NHL and bone marrow transplantation initially involves effectively destroying the patient's bone marrow, it would seem reasonable to administer larger doses of radioactivity in the hope of eliminating disease even at the expense of the bone marrow which could be salvaged by pretreatment bone marrow or stem cell harvest and subsequent transplantation. This myeloablative approach, however, has been evaluated only in limited investigational studies (to be discussed below).

Physical and Chemical Properties of Radionuclides

By the 1990s, based on the use of iodine-131 [^{131}I] for the treatment of thyroid cancer and hyperthyroidism, there was essentially 50 years of experience with ^{131}I as a radionuclide with a beta particle emission that could provide effective targeted radiation therapy. Accordingly, several of the initial efforts to develop a radiolabeled monoclonal antibody chose ^{131}I as the radionuclide. Proteins including immunoglobulins are readily iodinated and purified with retention of immunoreactivity.

At about the same time, there was a growing interest in the potential for the radiometal Yttrium-90 [^{90}Y] to serve as a radiolabel for therapeutic applications. ^{90}Y had a number of theoretical advantages over ^{131}I: it had a more energetic beta particle with an associated greater range in tissue. It also had a shorter half life and the chemical properties of a metal which meant that once internalized into cells, it remained even if the carrier molecule was subsequently digested.

There has been considerable debate ever since whether or not these differences between the two radiolabels available at that time provide an advantage to one or the other treatment regimen [6–8].

There is evidence that there is a relationship between tumor size and beta emission energy and that low energy is more effective within the zone

Table 1.1 Radionuclides used for radioimmunotherapy of lymphoma

Radionuclide	Physical $T_{1/2}$ (days)	Decay	Particle energy (MeV)	Path length (mm)	γ Energy
^{90}Y	2.7	β	2.3	5.3	None
^{131}I	8.1	β, γ	0.6	0.8	364 keV

Table 1.2 Five clinical trials in the initial evaluation of *Bexxar®* (from Fisher et al. [15])

Trial	Patient population	No. of patients	Median (range)
Phase 1 single center	Relapsed-refractory	42	3 (1–11)
Phase 2 multicenter	Relapsed-refractory	47	4 (1–8)
Randomized phase 2 multicenter	Relapsed-refractory	61	2 (1–4)
Comparative; multicenter	Refractory	60	4 (2–13)
Phase 2 multicenter	Rituximab relapsed-refractory	40	4 (1–11)
Total		250	4 (1–13)

that it irradiates rendering the efficacy dependant upon the distribution of the radiolabel [6]. Moreover, if tumor foci are deposited in sensitive tissue such as bone marrow, there is less irradiation of these surrounding elements when a lower energy beta emitter is used. At one time, it was thought that a shorter physical half-life was advantageous because of the radiobiologic principle "dose rate effectiveness factor" but this is unlikely to be significant when dealing with irradiation rates as slow as encountered with either of these radionuclides.

Furthermore, it is argued by some that a half life similar to the biologic half life of the labeled molecule, in this instance an immunoglobulin, provides the optimal opportunity for tumor irradiation. Of course, the overall product of physical and biologic half life is the effective half life which will always be shorter that the shorter of the two values. Thus, in the instance of ^{131}I labeled to an immunoglobulin whose biologic half life might vary from 1 to 3 weeks, there would be considerable variation in the whole body radiation absorbed dose for any given amount of radiolabeled antibody administered whereas for ^{90}Y, the effective half life of the radiolabeled antibody will always be shorter than the 2.6 day physical half life of ^{90}Y. While there may be small difference in the whole body radiation absorbed dose from patient to patient, these differences will be minor when the physical half life is so short unless there is some other factor affecting the

biodistribution of the radiolabeled product (such as preexisting HAMA or other factors that result in hastened reticuloendothelial extraction of the radiolabeled product from the circulation) [8].

Another difference between ^{131}I and ^{90}Y is that ^{131}I emits both a beta particle and a gamma photon whereas ^{90}Y is a so-called pure beta emitter (Table 1.1). Beta particles are difficult to quantify and image in the event that this is desirable or required to determine or confirm biodistribution. Techniques utilizing Brehmsstrahlung radiation and more recently positron imaging (based on the small component of pair production associated with emission of high energy beta particles) have been described but these techniques have not contributed to the design or execution of clinical studies or practice. More commonly, it has been convenient to use ^{111}In as a substitute for ^{90}Y when it is necessary to evaluate targeting or biodistribution of a ^{90}Y labeled monoclonal antibodies. The combined emissions characteristic of ^{131}I allow for the direct detection and quantification of the radioiodine distribution.

In recent years, another radiometal, Lutetium-177 [^{177}Lu] has become available but has not yet been used in any clinically available radioimmunotherapy regimen for the treatment of NHL. ^{177}Lu has a longer physical half life than ^{90}Y and a lower energy beta emission. Thus, as a generalization, it can be stated that ^{177}Lu has the chemical properties of a radiometal and physical properties closer to ^{131}I than ^{90}Y (Table 1.1).

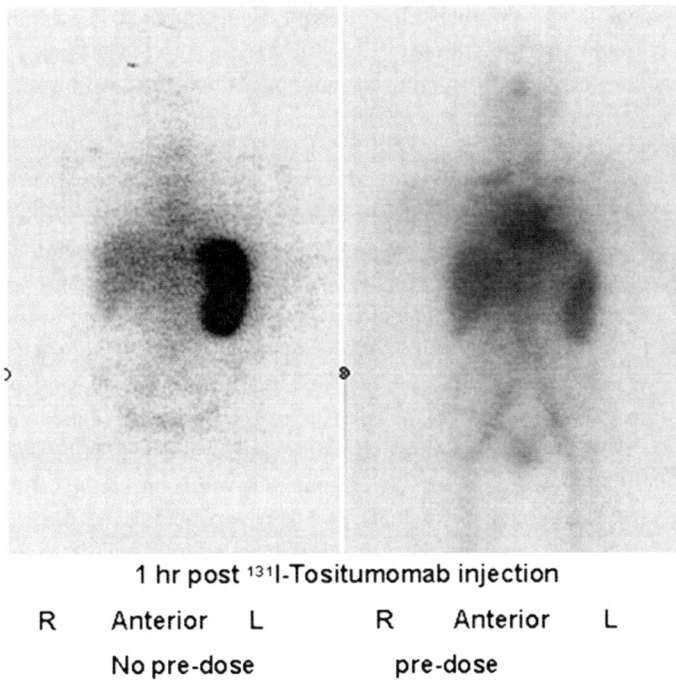

1 hr post ^{131}I-Tositumomab injection

R   Anterior   L   R   Anterior   L

No pre-dose   pre-dose

Fig. 1.2 Anterior whole body scan at 1 h after 131I-tositumomab, without and with prior administration (predose) of unlabeled tositumomab. Without a predose of "cold" antibody, a major portion of the injected radiolabeled antibody is removed by the spleen. When the patient receives a predose of "cold" antibody, a greater fraction of the radiolabeled antibody remains in the circulation. Predosing increases the percent of the administered dose in the tumor. The amount of cold antibody appropriate for this effect depends on the specificity of both the antigen target and the antibody as well as the amount of alternative sites for antibody binding [14]

Despite the differences in the physical properties of the several different radionuclides used in clinical studies to date, there has been no randomized comparison of different beta emitters. Accordingly, the differences in physical properties remain of theoretical interest although these differences do have an impact in the protocol design. For example, if it is necessary or desirable to obtain biodistribution data or to determine Residence Time when using a pure beta emitting radionuclide like ^{90}Y, it is necessary to prepare and administer an ^{111}In labeled version of the antibody of interest prior to or coincidental with the ^{90}Y product.

Role of "Cold Antibody"

When a radiolabeled or nonradiolabeled (naked) antibody is injected into the circulation, it travels through the venous system to the right side of the heart, passes through the pulmonary circulation into the left heart and then it is distributed throughout the arterial system to the capillaries that perfuse the various organs in the body. Even when the plasma is carrying a substance like an antibody, ligand or drug capable of a high affinity interaction, the extraction efficiency is considerably less than 100%. In the instance of a monoclonal antibody against an antigen expressed on a tumor, if the target antigen is not unique to the tumor, the biodistribution of the immunoglobulin will depend in part on the relatively blood flow and tissue distribution. Since there are a large number of B cells in the circulation and the spleen, there is a large extratumoral sink for an antibody that recognizes CD 20. Accordingly, and perhaps somewhat counterintuitive, it is necessary to initially administer unlabeled (cold or naked) antibody to saturate the large number of CD 20 binding sites on cells other than tumor cells (Fig. 1.2). It has been demonstrated that this strategy in fact prolongs the plasma half-life of subsequently infused radiolabeled antibody and increases the amount of subsequently infused radiolabeled antibody. Because of the large CD 20 "sink," it is necessary to administer several hundred milligrams of unlabeled antibody prior to the administration of the labeled antibody regardless of whether it is the ^{131}I-labeled material or the ^{90}Y labeled immunoglobulin. Hence for clinical trials of radiolabeled monoclonal antibodies, the therapies are properly called a regimen consisting of an infusion of cold, unlabeled immunoglobulin followed by the labeled material.

Both Bexxar® and Zevalin® regimens have employed relatively large amounts of "cold" antibody, independent of the tumor burden, in order to prolong plasma levels of the labeled monoclonal antibody to allow continued tumor perfusion and access to the radiolabeled antibody over time. The notion of "individualized" dose selection of both the total antibody dose as well as the administered radiolabeled product was raised early by Press et al. [9]. While this may indeed be an ideal approach, practical issues in terms of production of a uniform radiopharmaceutical renders this concept as an unlikely to be realized.

Clinical Applications

Early Clinical Studies: ^{131}I-Lym-1

Prior to the delineation of clusters of differentiation which provided a specific classification system for cell surface antigens in general, and tumor cells including lymphoma in particular, two monoclonal antibodies, Lym-1 and Lym-2, were developed. These antibodies of murine origin were reactive with membrane antigens on cells of B-cell lineage and tumors derived from these cells. In cell suspensions and immunohistopathologic sections from a variety of lymphoma tissue, it was demonstrated that there were significant number of binding sites on the cell surfaces of these tissue samples and virtually no binding to T cell lymphocytes, T-cell lymphomas or other soft tissue tumors. These antibodies identified 40% (Lym-1) to 80% (Lym-2) of the B-cell lymphoma samples and were specific for B-cell lymphoma with the exception that they bound Hodgkin's tissue also [10].

The group at the University of California, Davis in Sacramento, headed by Drs. Gerald DeNardo and Sally DeNardo, radioiodinated the Lym-1 antibody and determined that predosing with unlabeled antibody prolonged blood clearance and increased tumor uptake of the radiolabeled antibody. Subsequently, they administered the antibody combination using incremental doses of ^{131}I-labeled antibody to a small group of patients with considerable tumor burdens. One of these patients, a 67-year-old woman with Richter's transformation of chronic lymphatic leukemia had massive lymphadenopathy at multiple sites and appeared to be refractory to chemotherapy. She responded to what in retrospect appears to have been relatively small doses of ^{131}I-Lym-1 and survived for 2 years before dying from an infection. In a summary published in 1997, they reported their experience with the treatment of 58 patients, 31 of whom received 60 mCi or less of the ^{131}I-labeled antibody [10]. In 17 of these patients, a partial or complete remission was observed. In a subsequent protocol to determine a maximum tolerated dose (MTD), of 24 patients who received doses from 40 to 100 mCi/m^2, 13 patients had a decrease in tumor size. Myelosuppression was observed and thrombocytopenia was the most frequent dose-limiting toxicity.

Development and Assessment of Current Practice

Bexxar® [^{131}I-Tositumomab and Tositumomab]

Clinical indications and efficacy: In reports dating to the early 1990s, the group at the University of Michigan developed the details of an effective protocol for the use of an anti-CD 20 murine monoclonal antibody, tositumomab, that had been prepared by Coulter, Inc (San Diego, CA)

[11–14]. Although they were working initially with suboptimal doses of unlabeled antibody as well as the radio-iodinated version, they demonstrated an antitumor response. In addition, they realized that response was related to the amount of activity targeted and that the response was more related to the whole body radiation absorbed dose than to the amount of radioactivity administered on a body weight or body surface area basis. From these early clinical trials, the present protocol for Bexxar® administration evolved. The procedure protocol to determine the patient specific dose of ^{131}I-tositumomab is described in detail in a recent review [8].

Limited Availability of Lymphoma Radioimmunotherapy

At the present time, Bexxar® is available only in the United States and Canada whereas Zevalin® is available in Europe and the Middle East as well as the United States. Apparently, availability of production facilities and transportation issues as well as the need for the manufacturer/distributor to provide marketing and educational support has interfered up to this time with wider distribution of Bexxar® as well as Zevalin®.

Initially, Bexxar® was approved by the FDA for the treatment of patients who were refractory or had relapsed following chemotherapy including rituximab.

After completion of early clinical trials using Bexxar® to determine the dose to be administered and demonstrate safety and efficacy, Phase 3 trials were conducted initially in patients with considerable tumor burdens who had relapsed following chemotherapy at least twice [15]. Some of the patients, in fact, had undergone three or more previous courses of chemotherapy. Two hundred and twenty-six of the 250 patients (90%) had Stage III or IV disease; 46% had bone marrow involvement and 61% of the patients had bulky tumors (diameter greater than 5 cm). The overall response rate (ORR) was 56% and the median duration of response was 12.9 months

with a range from 10.9 to 17.3 months. A complete response (CR) was seen in 30% of the patients with a minimum duration of response of 28.3 months and a median duration of response of almost 5 years (58.4 months). Many patients were still in remission beyond 5 years when the results were reported [15].

Despite these impressive results, by the time these studies were complete rituximab as a component of chemotherapy regimens had become the new standard of practice. Accordingly, it was necessary to evaluate the efficacy of the Bexxar® regimen in patients who had become refractory (unresponsive) to rituximab infusions. The median number of prior chemotherapies was 4. Thirty-five patients in this category were treated with Bexxar® according to the established protocol based on whole body radiation absorbed dose adjusted for platelet count. The ORR was 65% (with a 95% confidence limit of 45–79%) and the CR was 29% (15–46% CI). Even more impressive, the duration of response in the ORR was 25 months (4+ to 36 months, CI) and it had not been reached in the CR group with a median duration of follow-up of 26 months. Among follicular grade 1 or 2 patients with tumors ≤7 cm ($n=21$), the OR and CR rates were 86 and 57% [16] (Fig. 1.3).

Given the excellent results that were initially achieved with Bexxar® in heavily pretreated patients, it occurred to several teams to develop protocols that offered Bexxar® therapy earlier in the course of their disease. In patients who had only failed chemotherapy once, Bexxar® performed even better. This encouraged a number of investigators to evaluate the efficacy of Bexxar® as a component of so-called first-line therapy, either as the sole therapeutic or as a component of the initial therapy regimen in combination with chemotherapy [17, 18].

When Bexxar was used as a component of the initial regimen following Fludarabine for 3 cycles in 76 patients with stage III or IV follicular lymphoma, the ORR was 97 and 76% of the patients had a complete response (CR). The minimal progression-free survival (PFS) was 27 months and the median PFS was determined to be greater than 48 months although it had not been reached

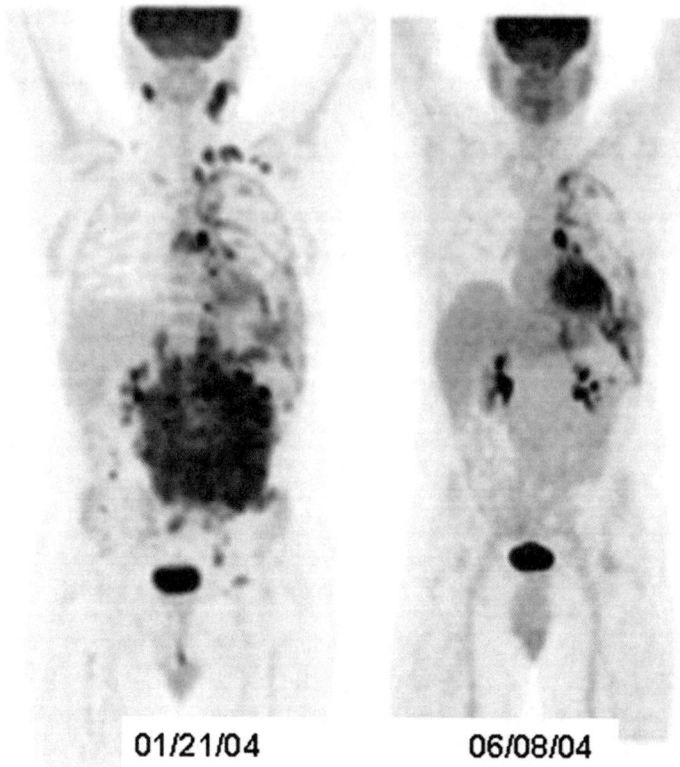

01/21/04   06/08/04

Fig. 1.3 ^{18}F-fluorodeoxy glucose PET maximum intensity projection (MIP) images of a 49-year-old man with documented diffuse large cell lymphoma with a very large abdominal lymphomatous mass as well as multiple sites of smaller lymph node involvement in the neck, chest and abdomen. Patient was initially diagnosed 11 years earlier and underwent treatment with six cycles of CHOP. Relapsed 5 years later at which time he was treated with DICE chemotherapy and rituximab. In January 2004, patient relapsed and was referred for treatment with the Bexxar® regimen. Patient's symptoms subsided over several weeks. Repeat FDG imaging in June 2004 show clearing of tumor metabolic activity consistent with a complete response. Because of involvement of his left hemi-thorax pleura and recurrent effusions, he had previously undergone pleurectomy. Foci of FDG activity from granulation tissue persist in the left pleura. Diffuse large cell lymphoma is not the usual basis for referral for anti-CD20 radioimmunotherapy but the biopsy confirmed expression of CD20 and both the patient and the referring physician were reluctant to retreat with standard chemotherapy

after 58 months of follow-up. In contrast to patients who had received no immunosuppressive therapy, HAMA formation was observed in only 6% of the patients [17, 18].

A multicenter group evaluated the efficacy of Bexxar® in what is essentially a consolidation protocol several weeks after completion of a course of CVP. In 76 patients with CD 20+ NHL, the ORR was 96%, the CR was 76% and the median time to progression (TTP) was not reached after 6 years of follow-up. In other words, although some relapses did occur over time, most of the patients remained in remission [19].

One of the frequently expressed concerns is apprehension about the utility of subsequent therapy in the event of patient relapse. Dosik et al. evaluated the effects of subsequent chemotherapy in 44 of 68 patients who had previously received *Bexxar®* therapy and either failed to respond or relapsed following a response to *Bexxar®* RIT [20]. The median values for the absolute neutrophil count and hemoglobin at the time of disease recurrence were not significantly different from preradioimmunotherapy values. The median platelet value had a modest decrease from 190,000 cells per microliter to 130,000.

The relapsed patients received a variety of cytotoxic chemotherapy regimen and many were provided with stem cell transplantation. At the time of the report, 50% of the patients completed a subsequent course of treatment and responded or were still receiving treatment. Eighteen patients who were severely ill prior to radioimmunotherapy and continued to have progressive disease failed to respond to repeat chemotherapy also. These findings demonstrate that the bone marrow does recover from the radiation exposure from *Bexxar®* radioimmunotherapy. Furthermore, the bone marrow matrix is receptive to stem cell transplantation. Many patients with progressive disease after *Bexxar®* treatment are able to receive subsequent cytotoxic chemotherapy including anthracyclines, platinum, or fludarabine, immunotherapy alone or in combination as well as stem cell transplantation [20]. The subsequent clinical course is similar to patients with similar disease burdens and therapeutic histories who never received Bexxar® radioimmunotherapy.

Zevalin® (⁹⁰Y-Ibritumomab and Rituximab)

The procedure protocol to determine the patient specific dose of ^{90}Y-ibritumomab tiuxetan is described in detail in a recent review [8].

Clinical Indications and efficacy: In 2004, Witzig summarized the various clinical trials involving major steps in the development and subsequent FDA approval of Zevalin® [21]. There were two phase I trials of ^{90}Y-ibritumomab tiuxetan conducted to evaluate the toxicity profile and the maximum tolerated single dose that could be administered to outpatients without the use of stem cells or prophylactic growth factors. In the first trial, cold ibritumomab was used prior to ibritumomab tiuxetan; the second trial used the human chimeric antibody rituximab which is the composition of the subsequently defined Zevalin® protocol. The phase I trials determined that in patients with a platelet count $\geq 150 \times 10^3$ platelets/ mL (150,000), intravenous rituximab 250 mg/m² on days 1 and 8, and 0.4 mCi/kg of intravenous

^{90}Y-ibritumomab tiuxetan on day 8 was safe and effective and did not require stem cell rescue. A 0.3 mCi/kg dose was shown to be safe for patients with a baseline platelet count of 100,000–149,000. Adverse events were primarily hematologic. There was no normal organ toxicity. The Zevalin® protocol includes pretreatment with rituximab 1 week prior to infusion of a repeat rituximab infusion followed by the ^{90}Y-labeled ibritumomab tiuxetan. The initial randomized controlled trial of Zevalin® radioimmunotherapy vs. rituximab immunotherapy for patients with relapsed or refractory low-grade, follicular or transformed B-cell NHL was reported in 2002. The ORR was 80% for 73 patients treated with Zevalin® vs. 56% in 70 patients who received rituximab weekly for 4 weeks [22]. The CR was 30% vs. 16% and there were an additional 4% unconfirmed CRs in each group. The Duration of Response for Zevalin® was 14.2 months compared to 12.1 months for rituximab immunotherapy alone. None of the patients had previously received rituximab. Reversible myelosuppression was observed in the Zevalin® group. Subsequently, there was an additional report evaluating Zevalin® treatment in 57 patients who had not responded to rituximab or who relapsed following rituximab therapy in less than 6 months [23]. The ORR was 74 with 15% CR. The TTP was 8.7 months for the responders. The incidence of grade 4 neutropenia was 35%, thrombocytopenia 9% and anemia 4%. These findings became the basis for the initial approval of Zevalin® as the first radioimmunotherapeutic agent approved in the United States by the FDA f or the treatment of CD20+ follicular low grade lymphoma.

Emmanouilides et al. evaluated the response to Zevalin® therapy in 211 patients in a multicenter trial when it was used after the first relapse compared to patients who had had two or more prior therapies and relapses. 63 patients received Zevalin® after one relapse and 148 patients (70%) had relapsed at least twice. Demographics of the two groups were otherwise similar except that there was higher rate of bone marrow involvement in the group who had had multiple bouts of therapy and relapse. Overall, patients who received Zevalin® after a single relapse responded

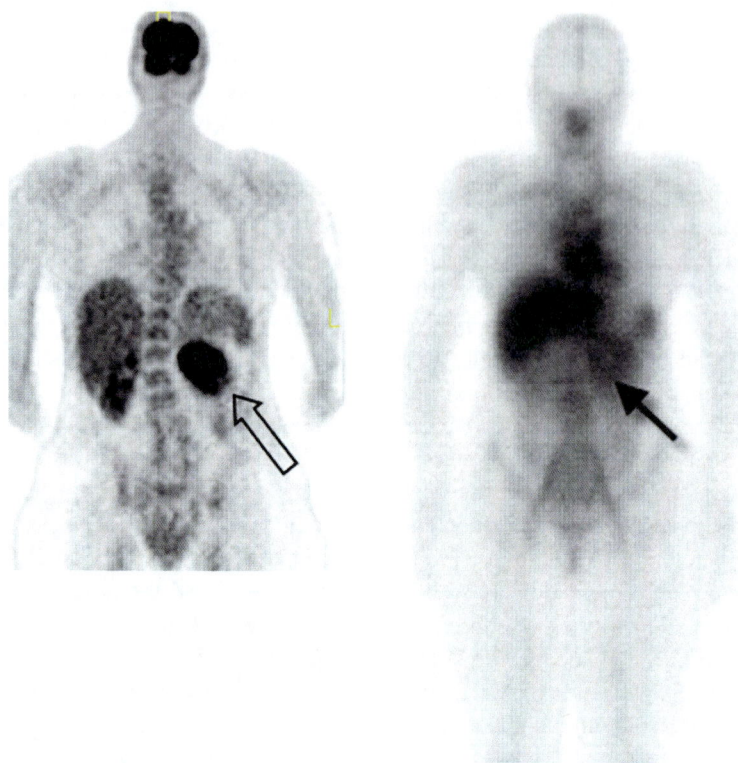

Fig. 1.4 ^{18}F-fluoro deoxy glucose PET coronal projection (left) of a 54-year-old woman who was diagnosed with Follicular non-Hodgkin's lymphoma 5 years earlier; treated with traditional CHOP regimen with a complete response. Clinical relapse after 4½ years; received multiple infusions of rituximab with no response. [18]FDG PET imaging 2 weeks prior to referral for radioimmunotherapy. Whole body planar image 48 h after ^{111}In-ibritumomab tiuxetan infusion as initial component of Zevalin® regimen. Patient was predosed with rituximab infusion as per protocol and subsequently received ^{90}Y-ibritumomab tiuxetan infusion. ^{111}In-ibritumomab imaging is not required for nonmyeloablative therapy in Europe and elsewhere and is no longer required in the United States. Nevertheless, it is a valuable tool to document the pattern of biodistribution. In this instance, there is good correlation of ^{111}In-ibritumomab accumulation in the previously demonstrated FDG avid abdominal mass

better than patients with multiple relapses. 51% of the follicular lymphoma patients and 49% of the entire group of patients including patients with transformed B-cell NHL responded to Zevalin® after their first relapse with a median TTP of 15.4 months and 12.6 months respectively vs. 28% CR regardless of the NHL diagnosis and a TTP of 9.2 and 7.9 months respectively if the patients had relapsed more than once [24] (Fig. 1.4).

Data from several clinical trials involving subsequent treatment of patients with disease progression following Zevalin® radioimmunotherapy were summarized by Ansell et al. [25]. Subsequent therapy varied from site to site and included chemotherapy such as CHOP, CVP, and other aggressive chemotherapeutic protocols, radiation therapy, bioimmunotherapy, or autologous stem cell transplantation (ASCT). An ORR of 53% was obtained in patients receiving chemotherapy. Ansell et al. compared the hematologic toxicity to retreatment with chemotherapy in 59 patients previously treated with Zevalin® to a control group of 60 age, gender, and histopathologically matched patients who had not received Zevalin® [25]. There was no significant difference between the Zevalin® and control group in terms of grade 4 cytopenia, neutropenic fever, number of hospitalizations for complications or requirement for GCSF or platelet transfusion. The recent course of Zevalin® with the attendant radiation exposure of marrow and transient depression of hematologic indices did not interfere with subsequent efforts to harvest stem cells. An adequate collection of stem cells was obtained in 7 of 8 patients who received growth factor mobilization in preparation for autotransplantation. In the eighth patient, direct bone marrow sampling was necessary. In all 8 patients, the subsequent transplant was successful with development of satisfactory blood indices. In another study, successful transplantation was reported in 9 patients who had received Zevalin®, a median of 13.3 months previously.

A 0.3 mCi/kg dose was shown to be safe for patients with a baseline platelet count of 100,000–149,000. Adverse events were primarily hematologic. There was no normal organ toxicity. The ORR was 67% for all NHL patients and 82% in patients with low-grade NHLs. A subsequent phase III trial randomized 143 patients to either rituximab or ibritumomab tiuxetan. The ORR was 80% with the ^{90}Y-ibritumomab tiuxetan protocol vs. 56% for rituximab alone ($p=0.002$). Since the nonradioactive monoclonal antibody had become a key element in management of patients with NHL, another trial evaluated Zevalin® in 54 rituximab refractory patients. An ORR of 74% was found in these rituximab-refractory patients. Another trial evaluated 30 patients in order to evaluate whether the reduced dose of 0.3 mCi/kg ^{90}Y-ibritumomab tiuxetan in patients with platelet counts <150,000 (but at least 100,000 platelets) was as effective as the 0.4 mCi/kg dose is in patients with platelets ≥150,000. The ORR was 83% [22].

In summary, these data demonstrate that Zevalin® is an effective therapy with an ORR of approximately 80% and a CR of approximately 30% in patients who are refractory to unlabeled antiCD20 immunotherapy and chemotherapy, or have relapsed following these therapies. In the CR subgroup, there is an impressive duration of response. These results have been obtained with manageable hematologic toxicity. The concern that patients treated with Zevalin® will have severe marrow impairment rendering them ineligible for further therapy is not substantiated by the results of several studies comparing retreatment with chemotherapy, stem cell mobilization and successful autotransplantation of Zevalin® treated patients to otherwise matched control groups [25].

As stated, the basis for the initial FDA approval of the Zevalin® protocol in the United States and subsequently throughout the European Union, are the studies that show a definite improvement in the ORR and CR in patients who were refractory to rituximab in terms of relief from disease activity or who had relapsed despite rituximab therapy alone or in conjunction with chemotherapy. In 2009, a multicenter Phase III trial was published that demonstrated the efficacy of the Rituxin regimen as consolidation therapy after patients responded (CR or PR) to first-line therapy with a variety of chemotherapeutic agents including CHOP, fludarabine alone or in combination with rituxin. These patients were randomized to one of two groups: either the Control group who received no additional therapy or the consolidation group which involved the Zevalin® regimen (rituxin 250 mg/m^2) on day minus 7 followed 7 days later by repeat rituxin infusion and 14.8 MBq/kg of ^{90}Y-ibritumomab tiuxetan. The demographic and clinical details of the two groups were remarkably similar but the results in terms of PFS were striking. The median TTP was 36.5 months for the group who received Zevalin® vs. 13.3 months for the control group. These findings had a p value of <0.0001. The results were even more impressive when the data was segregated on the basis of whether the patient had been categorized as a CR or PR prior to the Consolidation therapy. CR patients had a median PFS of 53.9 months compared to the controls with a PFS of 29.5 months. The PR patients had a PFS of 29.3 months if they received the consolidation protocol and only 6.2 months if they had no further therapy (control group) [26]. These are really striking results and they support the conclusion that even patients with a good response to the initial therapeutic regimen will do better for a much longer period if they receive radioimmunotherapy even while in remission.

Issues Relevant to Both Bexxar® and Zevalin®

Despite the overall excellent results achieved with Bexxar® and Zevalin®, hematologists and oncologists with clinical responsibilities for patient management have not utilized radioimmunotherapy as frequently as might be expected. In a national survey, it was confirmed that hematologists and oncologists overall continue to harbor concern that the bone marrow radiation exposure associated with radioimmunotherapy compromises the bone marrow and puts the patient at greater risk of adverse hematologic consequences when the need arises for subsequent chemotherapy [27]. Nuclear medicine physicians appear also to be somewhat reluctant to embrace radioimmunotherapy because of the perceived complexity of the procedure including the need to coordinate infusions and patient follow-up [28].

The question frequently arises as which of the two therapeutic regimen is superior. There has been no direct, side by side, randomized study of the relative efficacy of these agents. The group at Johns Hopkins analyzed their experience in 38 patients but reported results at only 12 weeks of follow-up. 20 received Zevalin® and 18 received Bexxar® [29]. Twenty-six of 38 patients received the full dose of the particular regimen (platelet count ≥150,000); 12 received attenuated doses. There was no statistically significant difference between the two groups but it would be difficult to ascertain a difference between two relatively effective therapies when the groups studied were so small. The ORR at 12 weeks was 47% and the CR 13% which are lower values than observed in other reports but the period of follow-up may have been too brief for this purpose also. Nevertheless, not surprisingly, the overall survival was better amongst patients who responded to either regimen (ORR vs. less than a partial response). Grade 3 or 4 thrombocytopenia was observed in 57 and 56% for Zevalin® and Bexxar® respectively. The percent decline in platelets was 79% (±17%) following Zevalin® vs. 63% (±28%) for Bexxar® ($p=0.04$). The ANC nadir for Zevalin® was 36 days±9 vs. 46±14 days ($p=0.01$) for Bexxar® [29].

As summarized in this chapter, there are now abundant reports of statistically impressive ORRs and CRs in patients with CD+NHL, both follicular lymphoma and DLBCLD. These regimens were initially used in standard of therapy-refractory patients, that is patients who had failed chemotherapy repeatedly even if in combination with rituximab and remain either symptomatic or had evidence of impending clinical deterioration. In addition, both regimens have been employed as Consolidation Therapy; that is administered following an initial response to whatever chemotherapeutic agent chosen for initial control of the symptoms and the disease itself. Despite the excellent results reported in the medical literature, the issue of physician reluctance to utilize either Bexxar® or Zevalin® remains a concern to those involved in delivering these apparently effective therapeutics [27, 28].

Clinical Protocols

For both Bexxar® and Zevalin® nonmyeloablative regimens, there are several requirements for eligibility. These include histopathologic confirmation of CD 20 expression on the tumor sample obtained at the time of diagnosis as well as any subsequent tumor tissue that might have become available. Patients should have had a relatively recent (within 2–3 months) bone marrow biopsy to confirm that there is less than 25% bone marrow involvement. Twenty-five percent or greater percent bone marrow involvement results in unacceptable incidence of Grade 4 hematological toxicity. The approved use of these agents is for a so-called "nonmyeloablative" regimen. Although when available, harvested stem cells have been successfully implanted in patients who have had myeloablative doses of radiolabeled antibodies, neither Bexxar® nor Zevalin® are currently approved for that indication and insurance companies and government will not approve reimbursement for that indication.

Both Bexxar® and Zevalin® dose determination is based upon the patients platelet count with full dose (to be defined) for patients with platelets greater than 150,000 cells/mL and somewhat attenuated doses for patients with platelet counts between 100,000 and 150,000.

In the Zevalin® protocol, the full ^{90}Y-ibritumomab tiuxetan dose for patients 150,000 platelets/ml is 0.4 mCi/kg (30 MBq/kg) and 0.3 mCi/kg (22.5 MBq/kg) for patients with platelets between 100,000 and 149,000/mL [21–23]. One week prior to the administration of the ^{90}Y-ibritumomab tiuxetan dose, the patient receives an infusion of 450 mg of rituximab. This infusion is part of the Zevalin® protocol regardless of whether or not the patient will also receive an imaging dose of ^{111}In-ibritumomab tiuxetan. The 450 mg infusion of rituximab is repeated on the day of the ^{90}Y-ibritumomab tiuxetan infusion (0.4 mCi/kg) if platelets exceed 150,00; 0.3 mCi of platelets are below 150,000 but greater than 100,000/mL.

Bexxar® Clinical Protocol

Prior to beginning protocol
Meet patient in consultation
- Confirm diagnosis and request to treat
- Review clinical history and pertinent physical findings (if any)
  - Including age, height, and weight
  - Confirm histopathology report documenting CD 20+ lymphoma
  - Confirm recent bone marrow biopsy (interval flexible; 6–12 weeks at most)
  - Confirm most recent CBC, specifically ANC >3500; platelets >100,000
- Review protocol with patient
- Address radiation safety issues and concerns
- Obtain consent for radioimmunotherapy
- Prescribe SSKI; three drops three times a day; begin at least 24 h prior to first dose of ^{131}I-labeled tositumomab; continue for at least 1 week post treatment dose
Day protocol begins
- Review above details of bone marrow biopsy, WBC count, platelet count
- Administer Tylenol® and Benadryl®; begin IV saline infusion (keep open drip); utilize 22 micron Millipore® filter; three way stopcock to allow access to infusion without interruption of infusion
- Pharmacist brings "cold" and labeled monoclonal antibody preparation to room temperature
- Physician or nurse confirm good IV access and flow
- "Cold" infusion begins
  - Vital signs (heart rate; blood pressure) are monitored

- Following completion of "cold" infusion, shielded pump with ^{131}I-labeled tositumomab is brought to infusion area. IV access confirmed; all valve positions confirmed (open to pump infusion); connect to 3-way stopcock
- ^{131}I-labeled tositumomab infusion begins at rate 90 ml/min; usually completed in 20 min
- Confirm delivery of radiolabeled antibody with survey meter
- Observe patient for 30–60 min
- Obtain whole body scan, anterior and posterior projections
Patient Returns at 48 h after initial infusion
- Obtain whole body scan, anterior and posterior projections
- Perform preliminary dosimetry calculation; order therapy dose
Patient returns at 96–120 h
- Obtain whole body scan, anterior and posterior projections
- Complete dosimetry calculations and determination of dose to be administered
Day of radioimmunotherapy infusion
- Prepare dose to be administered
- Begin IV infusion as on Day 0
- Following: "cold" tositumomab infusion, infuse ^{131}I-labeled tositumomab
- Monitor patient for 30–60 min
- Obtain radiation flux at surface and 1 m with survey meter
- Complete calculation of Radiation Safety Guidelines
Discharge patient with guidance re: weekly CBC including platelet count

Bexxar® dosing is based upon whole body radiation absorbed dose as it was demonstrated that both efficacy and toxicity correlated better with the whole body radiation absorbed dose than with dosing based upon mCi/kg (or MBq/kg) [15, 17, 18, 20]. The procedure to determine the ^{131}I-tositumomab dose to be administered in the Bexxar protocol is described in detail in a recent review [8]. It involves administration of a relatively small amount (5–6 mCi) of ^{131}I-tositumomab after infusion of 450 mg of "cold" tositumomab. A whole body scan is performed within an hour or two and the geometric mean of the anterior and posterior projections is determined to establish the 100% value. This is followed at approximately 48 h and again at 96–120 h. The geometric means of each pair of whole body scans is calculated and expressed as a percent of the initial value. From these values, the Residence Time can be determined using either a computer program provided by the distributor or performing a semilog plot vs. time. By convention, the residence time is the 37% intercept of the semilog plot. All of the calculations of the product of activity and residence time which would result in a whole body radiation absorbed dose of 75 cGy have been predetermined. The nuclear medicine physician is provided with a table of activity time values for various patient weights. The activity time value divided by the residence time yields the dose to be administered. If it is preferred to limit the whole body radiation absorbed dose to 65 cGy (because of a platelet count less than 150,000), the ^{131}I-tositumomab dose is reduced by 65/75 or approximately 87% of the dose that would deliver 75 cGy.

When Zevalin was initially introduced in the United States, a 5–6 mCi dose of ^{111}In-ibritumomab was administered after the infusion of rituximab 1 week prior to the therapeutic infusion. A whole body scan is performed at approximately 48 h to confirm biodistribution. During clinical trials, the whole body scan of the ^{111}In-ibritumomab was performed in order to determine the organ radiation absorbed dose. An instance of abnormal biodistribution was observed during these trials. Consequently, FDA approval continued to require this procedure until recently. The EU Regulatory Agency did not require this imaging component; thus there was no need for the ^{111}In-ibritumomab infusion in the EU and other regions. Currently, this is no longer obligatory in the United States but as of this writing, the ^{111}In-ibritumomab continues to be available albeit optional. However, since rituximab has some antitumor effects, in both the United States and Europe, the initial rituximab infusion 1 week prior to the repeat rituximab and ^{90}Y-ibritumomab tiuxetan continues to be a component of the Zevalin® protocol. It is not clear that this prior infusion of "cold" tositumomab in the Bexxar® protocol or of rituximab in the Zevalin® protocol has any positive impact on the overall clinical response. Moreover, whereas it has been demonstrated the predosing with "cold" antibody increases the plasma biologic half life of the labeled therapeutic dose, thereby increasing the quantity available to the tumor cells, it has been speculated that a non-patient-specific dose based upon tumor burden may decrease the total fraction of the dose delivered to the tumor. It has been suggested that there might be advantages to predosing with an antibody to one anti-B cell CD followed by administration of a labeled monoclonal antibody directed toward a different CD [30].

Zevalin® Clinical Protocol

Prior to beginning protocol
Meet patient in consultation
- Confirm diagnosis and request to treat
- Review clinical history and pertinent physical findings (if any)
  - Including age, height, and weight
  - Confirm histopathology report documenting CD 20+ lymphoma
  - Confirm recent bone marrow biopsy (interval flexible; 6–12 weeks at most)
  - Confirm most recent CBC, specifically ANC >3500; platelets >100,000
- Review protocol with patient

(continued)

(continued)

- Address radiation safety issues and concerns
- Obtain consent for radioimmunotherapy
- Coordinate with referring physician and/or infusion service as to whether "cold" infusion of rituximab is to be administer in office, infusion area or nuclear medicine

Day protocol begins

- Review above details of bone marrow biopsy, WBC count, platelet count
- Based on whether "cold" infusion is to be administered in Nuclear medicine or elsewhere, Tylenol® and Benadryl® are administered; begin IV saline infusion (keep open drip); utilize 22 micron Millipore® filter; three way stopcock to allow access to infusion without interruption of infusion
- "Cold" monoclonal antibody preparation at room temperature is infused
- Vital signs (heart rate; blood pressure) are monitored
- Following completion of "cold" infusion, patient is moved to Nuclear Medicine Infusion area; IV access is confirmed or restarted
- If ¹¹¹In is to be infused, connect appropriately shielded syringe to IV access; administer ¹¹¹In labeled Ibritumomab tiuxetan by slow infusion (mechanical or manual)

Radiation Safety

The radionuclide component of Bexxar® is ¹³¹I, which emits both a beta particle and a gamma photon. Gamma photons have greater penetrability in tissue and hence are more readily detected externally. The gamma emission makes possible imaging and quantitation but the penetrating radiation also results in exposure of medical personnel and family members of the patient following release from the medical facility.

During the infusion of the therapeutic dose, portable shielding should be available and interposed between the patient and medical personnel. During dose escalation trials in which patients received 25–129 mCi [1–5 GBq] of ¹³¹I-tositumomab to deliver 30–75 cGy total body dose, 26 family members from 22 different patients were provided monitoring devices that were worn for up to 17 days. The measured radiation absorbed dose values were from 17 to 409 mrem, well below the 500 mrem limit applicable to members of the general public [31]. In another study with administered quantities of ¹³¹I-tositumomab in a similar range, the median radiation absorbed dose was 150 mrem. Prior to release, patients are given a detailed printout providing guidance on the duration and proximity to others that would minimize exposure (Fig. 1.4). This guidance is based upon patient specific variables such as the administered dose, the measured emission from the patient at the body surface and at 1 m as well as the biologic turnover rate obtained from the dosimetry calculations.

Harwood et al. monitored the whole body radiation exposure of 20 healthcare workers, radiopharmacists, nuclear medicine technologists, nurses and physicians at four institutions for 2–4.5 years involving 300 administrations of ¹³¹I-tositumomab [32]. The additional mean radiation exposure/month per healthcare worker involved in administering Bexxar® therapy was 5.8 mrem.

The therapeutic radionuclide in the Zevalin® regimen is ⁹⁰Y, a pure beta emitter without a gamma emission. Brehmsstrahlung radiation is produced as the beta particle looses energy as it reacts with its environment. It is readily detectable externally and consequently also presents potential radiation exposure of nearby personnel. The exposure as a consequence of Brehmsstrahlung emission is far below the allowable exposure and not hazardous to medical personnel or family members. Patients, nevertheless, should be reassured and provided with instruction about intimacy and contact with family and friends [33]. In general, patients are advised to avoid transmission of body fluids (saliva, blood, urine, seminal fluid and stool).

Evolution of Radioimmunotherapy and Alternatives to Current Practice

[131]I-Rituximab

Bexxar® and Zevalin® were approved by the FDA in the United States in 2002. Shortly thereafter, Zevalin became available® in Western Europe and more recently in Israel and Eastern European nations. In many other areas, it remains unavailable. In Perth, Australia, the inability to obtain either Bexxar® or Zevalin® led a group led by Professor Harvey Turner to develop an initiative of their own. As stated earlier, rituximab, the murine–human chimeric anti-CD 20 monoclonal antibody, is widely available and is used as a immunotherapeutic alone or in conjunction with a variety of chemotherapeutic regimen and is also the unlabeled component of the Zevalin® regimen. Accordingly, Turner et al. undertook to label the readily available rituximab with [131]I [34]. Since immunoglobulins, like other proteins, are more conveniently radio-iodinated (as opposed to covalently linking a chelating moiety and subsequently radiolabeling with a radiometal like ^{90}Y or ^{177}Lu), they performed in-house labeling with ^{131}I using the Chloramine-T® method and subsequently purifying the labeled product. This practice under the auspices of qualified physicians and pharmacy personnel is authorized by the local regulatory authorities.

To their credit, the Perth group recognized that the comparatively long physical half-life of ^{131}I could result in significant variation in the whole body radiation absorbed doses in patients receiving therapeutic doses of the ^{131}I-labeled rituximab because of the variable biologic half-life of the labeled antibody. To control the total body radiation absorbed dose, they designed a protocol for this "hybrid radio-immunotherapeutic" which uses the unlabeled antibody in the Zevalin® protocol as the "cold" antibody component and labeling this "cold" antibody with ^{131}I, the radionuclide used in the Bexxar® regimen, similar to the protocol used in determining Bexxar® doses [34]. With this hybrid regimen, the safety and efficacy of the ^{131}I-rituximab and rituximab was

demonstrated in 91 patients. 86% of the patients had follicular NHL, 7% had mucosal-associated lymphoid tissue (MALT) and 8% had small lymphocytic lymphoma. The ORR was 76% and the CR was 53%. Median PFS for all patients was 23 months. Median overall survival exceeded 4 years. Grade 4 thrombocytopenia was observed in 4% and neutropenia in 16% at 6–7 weeks. This protocol and careful observation of the clinical response is on-going.

Anti-CD 22 (^{90}Y-Epratuzumab)

Although CD 20 is frequently expressed on the two most common B-cell NHLs (follicular low-grade lymphoma and DLBCL), other CDs are commonly expressed also. Goldenberg et al. elected to evaluate the potential utility of an anti-CD 22 antibody. This domain had previously been characterized as LL2. Initially, the murine anti-CD 22 was iodinated. In contrast to the anti-CD 20 monoclonal antibody, the antibody-CD 22 complex is internalized after binding resulting in intracellular metabolism of the complex with release of soluble iodinated products. Accordingly, the group pursued development of a reliable linker moiety which would allow the use of a radiometal such as ^{90}Y for therapeutic purposes and ^{111}In for imaging, biodistribution and dosimetry calculations. They demonstrated that a modified DTPA moiety, DOTA (1, 4, 7, 10-tetra aza cyclododecane-*N*,*N'*,*N''*,*N'''*-tetra acetic acid) chelated radiometals effectively and provided a stable molecule with minimal release of the radiometal resulting in an excellent safety profile in terms of intratumoral retention of radioactivity and virtually no free radiometal with subsequent reticulo-endothelial bone marrow localization. In addition, since it was speculated that fractionated dose administration would allow for a greater total dose of radioactivity to be administered and subsequently delivered to tumor cells, it was decided to alter the immunoglobulin to produce a humanized version (named Epratuzumab) in order to reduce the likelihood of developing anti-antibody antibodies (HAMA) which would be expected with repeated administrations of murine antibody [30]. Epratuzumab was shown to be effective as a "cold" antibody in patients with indolent NHL [34].

In a study of fractionated ^{90}Y-epratuzumab as a radiotherapeutic agent, patients were divided into two groups: patients who had previously received high dose chemotherapy requiring ASCT and patients who had not had prior ASCT [31]. All patients received a pretherapy imaging dose of ^{111}In-epratuzumab. Plasma kinetics of the ^{111}In- and ^{90}Y-labeled version of the antibody were similar; 70% of the confirmed lesions were identified on ^{111}In scintigraphy. Heavily pretreated patients received 5 mCi/kg (185 MBq/kg) of ^{90}Y-Epratuzumab and patients who had not undergone ASCT received 10 mCi/kg (370 MBq/kg). Six weeks later if the hematologic depression had recovered, patients received additional 5 mCi/kg ^{90}Y-epratuzumab infusions. Hematologic toxicity was manageable with the usual supportive measures. Tumor radiation absorbed doses were calculated. Many tumors in patients with indolent and patients with aggressive disease responded [35].

Subsequently, a single center study was performed using once weekly infusions of 5 mCi (or185 MBq)/kg of ^{90}Y-Epratuzumab [36]. Only minor toxicity was observed after three infusions but a fourth was not tolerated with 2 of 3 patients experiencing dose-limiting toxicity. In 16 patients, the ORR was 62%. Amongst patients with indolent NHL, the ORR was 75% and in patients with aggressive disease, the ORR was 50%. CR was achieved in 25% of the patients. In this group, the event-free survival was from 14 to 41 months. Half of the patients experienced a long duration of response than they had following their previous therapy.

In 2010, a multicenter fractionated dose escalation (Phase I/II) study of ^{90}Y-Epratuzumab was reported. Sixty-four patients with relapsed or refractory NHL were evaluated including 17 patients who had undergone prior ASCT. At total cumulative doses up to 45 mCi (1,665 MBq)/m^2, grade 3 or 4 hematologic toxicity was observed but was manageable in patients with less than 25% bone marrow involvement. Hence, going forward, unless ASCT were available, patients with >25% bone marrow involvement would not be eligible for radioimmunotherapy with this agent—not dissimilar to eligibility criteria for Bexxar® and Zevalin®. The ORR for 61 patients was 62% with a median PFS of 9.5 months. Forty-eight percent of the patients achieved CRs. Patients who had not progressed prior to the protocol to the point where they had required therapy necessitating ASCT had an ORR of 71 with 55% CR even if they had been refractory to their previous anti-CD 20 containing therapy.

For patients with indolent follicular lymphoma, the ORR was 100% with CR of 92% and a PFS of 18.3 months. The authors propose additional trials identifying 20 mCi/m^2×2, 1 week apart as a tolerable dose level with impressive results. Since patients who were refractory to anti-CD 20 protocols responded to this anti-CD 22 radiolabeled monoclonal antibody, they suggest that it might be possible and efficacious to utilize combinations of anti-CD 20 and anti-CD 22 antibodies [37, 38].

Myeloablative Clinical Trials

Since it is not uncommon for many patients with a variety of malignant tumors including NHL, multiple myeloma and the leukemias to undergo stem cell harvesting followed by intensive chemotherapy and ASCT, it is somewhat surprising that, in general, the notion of ASCT as a component of high-dose radioimmunotherapy has not been pursued more vigorously or by more medical centers involved in the management of patients with life threatening malignancies. Nevertheless, a few studies deserve review.

^{131}I-Tositumomab and Tositumomab

Oliver Press and his colleagues at the University of Washington and the Fred Hutchinson Cancer Research Center in Seattle noted that although nonmyeloablative radioimmunotherapy achieved objective responses in a variety of hematologic malignancies, there was a steep dose–response curve and concluded that higher, myeloablative radioimmunotherapy followed by ASCT might be beneficial to patients who appeared to be refractory to more conservative therapy [39–41]. In 1998, they provided a long term follow-up report on a group of 29 patients who has received high doses of ^{131}I-tositumomab accompanied by unlabeled tositumomab to provide optimal biodistribution. Organ radiation absorbed doses were calculated since there was concern that although ASCT and other measures would provide support for the hematologic toxicity, it was necessary to identify and avoid if possible secondary organ toxicity.

Doses of the ^{131}I-tositumomab range from 280 to 785 mCi (10.4–29 GBq). Major responses were observed in 25 patients (86%); CR in 23 (79%) complete responses (CRs; 79%). At a median follow-up of 42 months, the overall survival was 68% and the PFS was 42%. Fourteen of the initial group of 29 patients remain asymptomatic without interval therapy and the duration of this apparently disease-free interval was from 27 to 87 months. Two patients experienced cardiopulmonary insufficiency but responded to supportive measures. The radiation absorbed dose to their lungs was calculated to be $\geq$27 Gy. The only late toxicity was elevated TSH which is readily manageable. There were no instances of myelodysplasia [41].

Several conclusions can be drawn from this data. First, myeloablative therapy is effective, and it is likely more effective with a longer disease-free interval than nonmyeloablative therapy. Second, with the availability of ASCT, the hematologic consequences of this approach are manageable. Third, it is likely that relatively detailed organ dosimtery would be a necessary component of myeloablative therapy so as to avoid secondary organ life-threatening toxicity [40, 41].

[90]Y-Ibritumomab and Rituximab

A dose escalation and preliminary efficacy study using essentially the Zevalin® protocol except that organ dosimetry was determined from the initial ^{111}In-ibritumomab tiuxetan whole body images in order to determine a subsequent dose of ^{90}Y-ibritumomab tiuxetan that would not exceed 1,000 cGy to the highest normal organ. ^{90}Y-ibritumomab tiuxetan doses in the order of 37–105 mCi were subsequently administered to 31 patients; 12 with the diagnosis of follicular lymphoma, 14 with DLBCL, and 5 with Mantle cell lymphoma. The median number of prior chemotherapy treatments was two. Ten days following the ^{90}Y-ibritumomab tiuxetan, the patients received high dose eptoposide followed by cyclophosphomide. ASCT was performed 2 days following completion of the chemotherapy component and approximately 14 days after the ^{90}Y-ibritumomab tiuxetan infusion [42]. With a median follow-up of 22 months, there was an estimated 2 year overall survival rate of 92% and relapse-free survival of 78%. There were 2 deaths and 5 relapses.

More recently, another clinical trial was initiated in the European Institute of Oncology in Milan, Italy. Although the results of the trial have not yet been reported, as with the above study, individual organ dosimetry was performed in order to avoid delivering excessive potentially toxic or lethal radiation absorbed doses to organs that cannot be replaced as conveniently as bone marrow. In 2 patients, the investigators observed abnormal biodistribution with increased hepatic extraction that would have resulted in a radiation absorbed dose to the liver far in excess of the 20 Gy limit that had been set as an upper safe limit. The presence of HAMA was subsequently identified in one of the patients and is probably the basis for the rapid and increased hepatic extraction. In the other patient, no basis for the abnormal localization could be identified [43]. This report confirms the important role of organ dosimetry in the event the field of radioimmunotherapy moves on to myeloablative protocols. It also calls into question the decision by the EU regulators and more recently by the FDA that it is not necessary to administer the ^{111}In-component of the Zevalin® protocol or to perform whole body scans of the ^{111}In-ibritumomab tiuxetan biodistribution. In nonmyeloablative protocols using ^{90}Y doses of 0.3–0.4 mCi/kg, abnormal biodistribution is likely not going to result in organ toxicity, neither is it going to allow tumor irradiation at the levels prescribed or expected in Zevalin® therapy.

Summary

Bexxar® and *Zevalin*® are approved by regulatory agencies, government and private health insurance companies in the United States and Canada for the treatment of patients with follicular, low grade NHL. They produce significant improvement and at times eliminate evidence of lymphoma completely (complete response) for many months to several years. Patients with partial responses may also remain symptom-free for long periods of time and depending upon the criteria used to evaluate the response may actually have had complete elimination of lymphoma but inadequate CT resolution. In this regard, the recent availability of ^{18}F-Fluorodeoxyglucone PET/CT is apt to make evaluation of responses more reliable.

Radioimmunotherapy regimens were initially approved for the treatment of low grade, CD 20+ NHL patients who had relapsed or were refractory to previous treatment. Excellent results have been obtained also when these agents have been used earlier in the course of disease management for example as part of initial treatment. ORRs of over 80% to almost 100% have been observed in various studies. In addition, high grade DLBCLs which are CD 20+ have shown excellent response to the anti-CD 20 radiolabeled monoclonal antibodies.

In recent years, other innovative solutions such as ^{131}I-rituximab therapy and novel immunoglobulins directed to CDs other than CD 20 have had impressive results and deserve more attention.

The role of other immunoglobulins, the possible role of combinations of immunoglobulins as well as combinations of radionuclides is still to be explored.

Despite the considerable successes to date, many patients have been denied access to these regimen as well as the newer experimental modalities because of lack of enthusiasm which is a result of the lack of understanding of the features, safety and merits of radioimmunotherapy—even for the treatment of NHL, an application that has had the most success when given an opportunity to treat disease and relieve suffering.

Future Directions

Several potential future directions are possible, some of which have been alluded to throughout the text. These include:

- Greater utilization of Bexxar® and Zevalin®
- Development and utilization of immunoglobulins to CDs other than CD 20.
- Investigation of combinations of immunoglobulins.
- Evaluation of other potential radionuclides, viz., ^{177}Lu, alpha particle emitters.
- Investigation of combination of radionuclides.
- Myeloablative protocols.
- Alternative antibody constructs:
  - Bispecific antibodies.
  - Antibody fragments, diabodies, etc.

Hopefully, future volumes integrating the experience and practice of radioimmunotherapy will see some of these potential "future directions" realized.

Acknowledgments   The author expresses gratitude and appreciation to the staff of the Division of Nuclear Medicine & Molecular Imaging in the Department of Radiology at the New York Presbyterian Hospital/Weill Cornell Medical Center for their support and assistance in the clinical investigations and clinical practice of radioimmunotherapy of non-Hodgkin's Lymphoma. In particular, I am grateful to Morton Coleman, MD, Shankar Vallabhajosula, PhD, John Leonard, MD, and Vasilios Avlonitis, RPh, for their support during the period in which we worked together to understand and improve the principles and practice of radioimmunotherapy and to make this therapy available to patients with non-Hodgkin's lymphoma.

References

1. Cancer statistics, NHL SEER Fact Sheets. National Cancer Institute, 2012, USNIH. www.cancer.gov.
2. Shipp MA, Mauch PM, Harris NL. Non-Hodgkin's lymphomas. In: DeVita VT, Hellman S, Rosenberg

SA, editors. Cancer, principles and practice of oncology. 5th ed. Philadelphia: Lippincott-Raven; 1997. p. 2165–219.

3. Fisher RI, Gaynor ER, Dahlberg S, Oken MM, Grogan TM, Mize EM, Glick JH, Coltman Jr CA, Miller TP. Comparison of a standard regimen (CHOP) with three intensive chemotherapy regimens for advanced non-Hodgkin's lymphoma. N Engl J Med. 1993;328: 1002–6.

4. Kohler G, Milstein C. Continuous cultures of fused cells secreting antibody of predefined specificity. Nature. 1975;256:495–7.

5. Davis TA, Grillo-López AJ, White CA, et al. Rituximab anti-CD20 monoclonal antibody therapy in non-Hodgkin's lymphoma: safety and efficacy of re-treatment. J Clin Oncol. 2000;18:3135–43.

6. O'Donoghue JA, Bardies M, Wheldon TE. Relationships between tumor size and curability for uniformly targeted therapy with beta-emitting radionuclides. J Nucl Med. 1995;36:1902–9.

7. Leonard JP, Siegel JA, Goldsmith SJ. Comparative physical and pharmacologic characteristics of iodine-131 and yttrium-90: implications for radioimmunotherapy for patients with non-Hodgkin's lymphoma. Cancer Invest. 2003;21:241–52.

8. Goldsmith SJ. Radioimmunotherapy of lymphoma: Bexxar and Zevalin. Semin Nucl Med. 2010;40: 122–35.

9. Press OW, Eary JF, Appelbaum FR, Martin PJ, Badger CC, Nelp WB, Glenn S, Butchko G, Fisher D, Porter B, Matthews DC, Fisher LD, Bernstein ID. Radiolabeled-antibody therapy of B-cell lymphoma with autologous bone marrow support. N Engl J Med. 1993;329:1219–24.

10. DeNardo GL, DeNardo SJ. Treatment of B-lymphocyte malignancies with ^{131}I-Lym-1 and ^{67}Cu-2IT-BAT-Lym-1 and opportunities for improvement. In: Goldenberg DM, editor. Cancer therapy with radiolabeled antibodies. Boca Raton: CRC; 1995. p. 217–27.

11. Kaminski MS, Fig LM, Zasadny KR, Koral KF, DelRosario RB, Francis IR, Hanson CA, Normolle DP, Mudgett E, Liu CP. Imaging, dosimetry, and radioimmunotherapy with iodine 131-labeled anti-CD37 antibody in B-cell lymphoma. J Clin Oncol. 1992;10:1696–711.

12. Kaminski MS, Zasadny KR, Francis IR, Milik AW, Ross CW, Moon SD, Crawford SM, Burgess JM, Petry NA, Butchko GM, Glenn SD, Wahl RL. Radioimmunotherapy of B-cell lymphoma with [^{131}I] anti-B1 (anti-CD20) antibody. N Engl J Med. 1993;329:459–65.

13. Kaminski MS, Zelenetz AD, Press OW, Saleh M, Leonard J, Fehrenbacher LT, Lister A, Stagg RJ, Tidmarsh GF, Kroll S, Wahl RL, Knox SJ, Vose JM. Pivotal study of iodine I 131 tositumomab for chemotherapy-refractory low-grade or transformed low-grade B-cell non-Hodgkin's lymphomas. J Clin Oncol. 2001;93:3918–28.

14. Wahl RL. Tositumomab and ^{131}I therapy in non-Hodgkin's lymphoma. J Nucl Med. 2002;46:128S–40.

15. Fisher RI, Kaminski MS, Wahl RL, Knox SJ, Zelenetz AD, Vose JM, Leonard JP, Kroll S, Goldsmith SJ, Coleman M. Tositumomab and iodine-131 tositumomab produces durable complete remissions in a subset of heavily pretreated patients with low-grade and transformed non-Hodgkin's lymphomas. J Clin Oncol. 2005;23:7565–73.

16. Horning SJ, Younes A, Jain V, Kroll S, Lucas J, Podoloff D, Goris M. Efficacy and safety of tositumomab and iodine-131 tositumomab (bexxar) in B-cell lymphoma, progressive after rituximab. J Clin Oncol. 2005;23:712–9.

17. Leonard JP, Coleman M, Kostakoglu L, Chadburn A, Cesarman E, Furman RR, Schuster MW, Niesvitsky R, Muss D, Fiore J, Kroll S, Tidmarsh G, Vallabhajosula S, Goldsmith SJ. Abbreviated chemotherapy with fludarabine followed by tositumomab and iodine I-131 tositumomab for untreated follicular lymphoma. J Clin Oncol. 2005;23:5696–704.

18. Kaminski MS, Tuck M, Estes J, Kolstad A, Ross CW, Zasadny K, Regan D, Kison P, Fisher S, Kroll S, Wahl RL. ^{131}I-tositumomabtherapy as initial treatment for follicular lymphoma. N Eng J Med. 2005;352:441–9.

19. Link BK, Martin P, Kaminski MS, Goldsmith SJ, Coleman M, Leonard JP. Cyclophosphomide, vincristine and prednisone followed by tositumomab and I-131 tositumomab in patients with untreated low-grade follicular lymphoma: eight year follow-up of a multicenter phase II trial. J Clin Oncol. 2010;28:3035–41.

20. Dosik AD, Coleman M, Kostakoglu L, Furman RR, Fiore JM, Muss D, Niesvizky R, Shore T, Schister MW, Stewart P, Vallabhajosula S, Goldsmith SJ, Leonard JP. Subsequent therapy can be administered after tositumomab and iodine I-131 tositumomab for non-Hodgkin's lymphoma. Cancer. 2006;106:616–22.

21. Witzig TE. Yttrium-90-ibritumomab tiuxetan radioimmunotherapy: a new treatment approach for B-cell non-Hodgkin's lymphoma. Drugs Today (Barc). 2004;40:111–9.

22. Witzig TE, Gordon LI, Cabanillas F, Czuczman MS, Emmanouilides C, Joyce R, Pohlman BL, Bartlett NL, Wiseman GA, Padre N, Grillo-Lopez A, Multani P, White CA. Randomized controlled trial of Yttrium-90-labeled ibritumomab tiuxetan radioimmunotherapy versus rituximab immunotherapy for patients with relapsed or refractory low-grade, follicular, or transformed B-cell non-Hodgkin's lymphoma. J Clin Oncol. 2002;20:2453–63.

23. Witzig TE, Flinn IW, Gordon LI, Emmanouilides C, Czuczman MS, Saleh MN, Cripe L, Wiseman GA, Olejnik T, Multani PS, White CA. Treatment with ibritumomab tiuxetan radioimmunotherapy in patients with rituximab refractory follicular non-Hodgkin's lymphoma. J Clin Oncol. 2002;20:3262–9.

24. Emmanouilides C, Witzig TE, Gordon LI, Vo K, Wiseman GA, Flinn IW, Darif M, Schilder RJ, Molina A. Treatment with yttrium 90 ibritumomab tiuxetan at early relapse is safe and effective in patients with previously treated B-cell non-Hodgkin's lymphoma. Leuk Lymphoma. 2006;47:629–36.

25. Ansell SM, Schilder RJ, Pieslor PC, Gordon LI, Emmanouilides C, Vo K, Czuczman MS, Witzig TE, Theuer C, Molina A. Antilymphoma treatments given subsequent to Yttrium 90 ibritumomab tiuxetan are feasible in patients with progressive non-Hodgkin's lymphoma: a review of the literature. Clin Lymphoma. 2004;5:202–4.

26. Morschhauser F, Radford J, Van Hoof A, Vitolo U, Soubeyran P, Tilly H, Huijgens PC, Kolstad A, d'Amore F, Gonzalez Diaz M, Petrini M, Sebban C, Zinzani PL, van Oers MH, van Putten W, Bischof-Delaloye A, Rohatiner A, Salles G, Kuhlmann J, Hagenbeek A. Phase III trial of consolidation therapy with Yttrium-90-ibritumomab tiuxetan compared with no additional therapy after first remission in advanced follicular lymphoma. J Clin Oncol. 2008;26:5156–64.

27. Schaefer NG, Ma J, Huang P, Buchanan J, Wahl RL. Radioimmunotherapy in non-Hodgkin lymphoma: opinions of U.S. Medical Oncologists and Hematologists. J Nucl Med. 2010;51:987–94.

28. Schaefer NG, Huang P, Buchanan JW, Wahl RL. Radioimmunotherapy in non-Hodgkin lymphoma: opinions of nuclear medicine physicians and radiation oncologists. J Nucl Med. 2011;52:830–8.

29. Jacene HA, Filice R, Kasecamp W, Wahl RL. Comparison of ^{90}Y-ibritumomab tiuxetan and ^{131}I-tositumomab in clinical practice. J Nucl Med. 2007;48:1767–76.

30. Sharkey RM, Brenner A, Burton J, et al. Radioimmunotherapy of non-Hodgkin's lymphoma with 90Y-DOTA humanized anti-CD22 IgG (90Y-Epratuzumab): do tumor targeting and dosimetry predict therapeutic response? J Nucl Med. 2003;44:2000–18.

31. Rutar FJ, Augustine SC, Colcher D, Siegel JA, Jacobson DA, Tempero MA, Dukat VJ, Hohenstein MA, Gobar LS, Vose JM. Outpatient treatment with ^{131}I-anti-B1 antibody: radiation exposure to family members. J Nucl Med. 2001;42:907–15.

32. Harwood SJ, Rutar F, Sullivan G, Avlonitis V. Bexxar radioimmunotherapy can be safely administered by healthcare professionals with minimal whole body exposure. J Nucl Med. 2003;44:327P.

33. Wagner HN, Wiseman GA, Marcus CS, Nabi HA, Nagle CE, Fink-Bennett DM, Lamonica DM, Conti PS. Administration guidelines for radioimmunotherapy with ^{90}Y-labled anti-CD20 monoclonal antibody. J Nucl Med. 2002;43:267–72.

34. Leahy MF, Seymour JF, Hicks RJ, Turner JH. Multicenter phase II clinical study of iodine-131–rituximab radioimmunotherapy in relapsed or refractory indolent non-Hodgkin's lymphoma. J Clin Oncol. 2006;24:4418–25.

35. Leonard JP, Coleman M, Matthews JC, et al. Phase I/II trial of Epratuzumab (humanized anti-CD 22 antibody) in indolent non-Hodgkin's lymphoma. J Clin Oncol. 2003;21:3051–9.

36. Linden O, Hindorf C, Cavallin-Stahl E, Wegener WA, Golenberg DM, Horne H, et al. Dose-fractionated radioimmmunotherapy in non-Hodgkin's lymphoma using DOTA-conjugated, 90Y-radiolabeled humanized anti-CD22 monoclonal antibody, Epratuzumab. Clin Cancer Res. 2005;11:5215–22.

37. Morschhauser F, Kraeber-Bodere F, Wegener WA, Harousseau J-L, Petillon M-O, Huglo D, Trumper L, Meller J, Pfreundschuh M, Kirsch CM, Naumann R, Kropp J, Horne H, Teoh N, Le Gouill S, Bodet-Milin C, Chatal J-F, Goldenberg DM. High rates of durable responses with anti-CD22 fractionated radioimmunotherapy: results of a multicenter. Phase I/II study in non-Hodgkin's lymphoma. J Clin Oncol. 2010;28:3709–16.

38. Sharkey RM, Press OW, Goldenberg DM. A re-examination of radioimmunotherapy in the treatment of non-Hodgkin's lymphoma: prospects for dual-targeted antibody/radioantibody therapy. Blood. 2009;113:3891–5.

39. Press OW, Eary JF, Appelbaim FR, Bernstein ID. Treatment of relapsed B cell lymphoma with high dose radioimmunotherapy and bone marrow transplantation. In: Goldenberg DM, editor. Cancer therapy with radiolabeled antibodies. Boca Raton: CRC; 1995. p. 229–37.

40. Liu SY, Eary JF, Petersdorf SH, Martin PJ, Maloney DG, Appelbaum FR, Matthews DC, Bush SA, Durack LD, Fisher DR, Gooley TA, Bernstein ID, Press OW. Follow-up of relapsed B-cell lymphoma patients treated with iodine-131-labeled anti-CD20 antibody and autologous stem-cell rescue. J Clin Oncol. 1998;16:3270–8.

41. Rajendran JG, Gopal AK, Fisher DR, Durack LD, Gooley TA, Press OW. Myeloablative ^{131}I-tositumomab radioimmunotherapy in treating non-Hodgkin's lymphoma: comparison of dosimetry based on whole-body retention and dose to critical organ receiving the highest dose. J Nucl Med. 2008;49:837–44.

42. Nademanee A, Forman S, Molina A, Fung H, Smith D, et al. A phase ½ trial of high-dose etoposide and cyclophosphamide followed by autologous stem cell transplantation in patients with poor-risk or relapsed non-Hodgkin lymphoma. Blood. 2005;106:2896–902.

43. Arico D, Grana CM, Vanazzi A, Ferrari M, Mallia A, Sansovini M, Martinelli G, Paganelli G, Cremonesi M. The role of dosimetry in the high activity ^{90}Y-ibritumomab tiuxetan regimens: two cases of abnormal biodistribution. Cancer Biother Radiopharm. 2009;24:271–5.

Radionuclide Therapy of Leukemias

Alain S. Abi-Ghanem

Introduction

Leukemia is currently the most common fatal cancer in the United States among males younger than 40 years old, whereas bronchopulmonary cancer predominates in men aged 40 years and older. Among females, leukemia is the leading cause of cancer death before age 20 years, breast cancer ranks first at ages 20–59 years, and lung cancer ranks first at ages 60 years and older [1] (Table 2.1). There are 259,889 people living with, or in remission from, leukemia in the US. In 2011, it was estimated that 44,600 new cases of leukemia in the US would be diagnosed (25,320 men and 19,280 women). In total, 21,780 individuals would die from the disease (12,740 men and 9,040 women). In children younger than 14 years old, nearly one-third of the cancers diagnosed are leukemias (particularly acute lymphoblastic leukemia (ALL)) (Table 2.2).

The leukemias are a heterogeneous group of disease. Historically, four major clinical and pathological types have been defined: acute lymphoblastic leukemia (ALL), acute myeloid leukemia (AML), chronic lymphocytic leukemia (CLL), and chronic myelogenous leukemia (CML) (Table 2.3). Acute leukemias are charac-terized by a predominance of blasts and closely related cells in the bone marrow and peripheral blood. Without therapeutic intervention, acute leukemias follow a short and precipitous course marked by anemia, infection, and hemorrhage, and death occurs within 6–12 months. Chronic leukemias are characterized by the proliferation of more mature lymphoid or hematopoietic cells. They have a longer, less devastating clinical course than acute leukemias, but are less responsive to therapeutic intervention.

Despite the substantial morbidity and mortality associated with this diagnosis, leukemia has been transformed from a rapidly fatal disease to one in which palliation is possible in most patients and cure is achievable in many. The overall 5-year relative survival rate for leukemia has nearly quadrupled in the past five decades. From 1960 to 1963, the 5-year relative survival rate among whites with leukemia was 14%, whereas from 1999 to 2006, it was 55.3% (Fig. 2.1).

The ability to correctly diagnose and characterize the disease has advanced. In fact, the third classification of the World Health Organization (WHO) published in 2001 incorporated for the first time genetic information into the diagnostic algorithms, in addition to the morphologic, cytochemical, immunophenotypic, and clinical features. Due to rapidly emerging genetic and biologic information, a revised classification was published in 2008 where a number of "provisional entities" were placed within the major subgroups of diseases. These newly characterized disorders were deemed clinically and/or

A.S. Abi-Ghanem, M.D. (✉)
Department of Radiology, Dana-Farber Cancer Institute/
Brigham and Women's Hospital,
Harvard Medical School, 450 Brookline Avenue,
DL-101, Boston, MA 02115, USA
e-mail: alaina_ghanem@dfci.harvard.edu

C. Aktolun and S.J. Goldsmith (eds.), *Nuclear Medicine Therapy: Principles and Clinical Applications*,
DOI 10.1007/978-1-4614-4021-5_2, © Springer Science+Business Media New York 2013

Table 2.1 Reported deaths for the five leading cancer sites by age and sex, United States, 2007

	All ages	<20	20–39	40–59	60–79	≥80
Male						
	All sites 292,857	All sites 1,124	All sites 4,041	All sites 54,054	All sites 152,231	All sites 81,403
	Lung and bronchus 88,331	Leukemia 365	Leukemia 552	Lung and bronchus 15,174	Lung and bronchus 53,125	Lung and bronchus 19,751
	Prostate 29,093	Brain and ONS 260	Brain and ONS 502	Colorectum 5,434	Colorectum 13,370	Prostate 15,670
	Colorectum 27,005	Bones and joints 92	Colorectum 395	Liver and bile duct 3,944	Prostate 12,187	Colorectum 7,795
	Pancreas 17,132	Other endocrine system 92	Non-Hodgkin lymphoma 301	Pancreas 3,638	Pancreas 9,293	Urinary bladder 4,216
	Leukemia 12,435	Soft tissue 72	Lung and bronchus 268	Esophagus 2,695	Esophagus 5,958	Pancreas 4,084
Female						
	All sites 270,018	All sites 944	All sites 4,639	All sites 50,640	All sites 126,918	All sites 86,873
	Lung and bronchus 70,355	Leukemia 278	Breast 1,094	Breast 11,630	Lung and bronchus 40,187	Lung and bronchus 18,519
	Breast 40,599	Brain and ONS 261	Uterine cervix 468	Lung and bronchus 11,412	Breast 16,900	Colorectum 11,298
	Colorectum 26,216	Other endocrine system 81	Leukemia 393	Colorectum 4,150	Colorectum 10,459	Breast 10,973
	Pancreas 16,985	Bones and joints 80	Colorectum 304	Ovary 3,151	Pancreas 8,211	Pancreas 6,283
	Ovary 14,621	Soft tissue 68	Brain and ONS 300	Pancreas 2,417	Ovary 7,195	Non-Hodgkin lymphoma 4,171

Note: Deaths within each age group do not sum to all ages combined due to the inclusion of unknown ages. "Other and unspecified malignant neoplasm" is excluded from cause of death ranking order

Source: US Mortality Data, 2007, National Center for Health Statistics, Center for Disease Control and Prevention

ONS Other nervous system

Table 2.2 Estimated new cases and deaths of leukemia by sex, United States, 2011[a]

	Estimated new cases			Estimated deaths		
	Both sexes 44,600	Male 25,320	Female 19,280	Both sexes 1,780	Male 12,740	Female 9,040
Acute lymphocytic leukemia	5,730	3,320	2,410	1,420	780	640
Chronic lymphocytic leukemia	14,570	8,520	6,050	4,380	2,660	1,720
Acute myeloid leukemia	12,950	6,830	6,120	9,050	5,440	3,610
Chronic myeloid leukemia	5,150	3,000	2,150	270	100	170
Other leukemias	6,200	3,650	2,550	6,660	3,760	2,900

Source: Estimated new cases are based on 1995–2007 incidence rates from 46 states and the District of Columbia as reported by the North American Association of Central Cancer Registries (NAACCR), representing about 95% of the US population. Estimated deaths are based on data from US Mortality Data, 1969 to 2007, National Center for Health Statistics, Centers for Disease Control and Prevention. © 2011, American Cancer Society, Inc., Surveillance Research
[a]Rounded to the nearest 10

Table 2.3 Approximate US prevalence of the four major types of leukemia as of January 1, 2007

Type	Prevalence
Acute lymphocytic leukemia	57,526
Chronic lymphocytic leukemia	100,760
Acute myeloid leukemia	29,711
Chronic myeloid leukemia	24,800

Source: Surveillance, Epidemiology and End Results (SEER) Program (http://www.seer.cancer.gov). Prevalence database: "US Estimated 32-Year L-D Prevalence Counts on 1/1/2007." National Cancer Institute, DCCPS, Surveillance Research Program, Statistical Research and Applications Branch, updated 30 June 2010

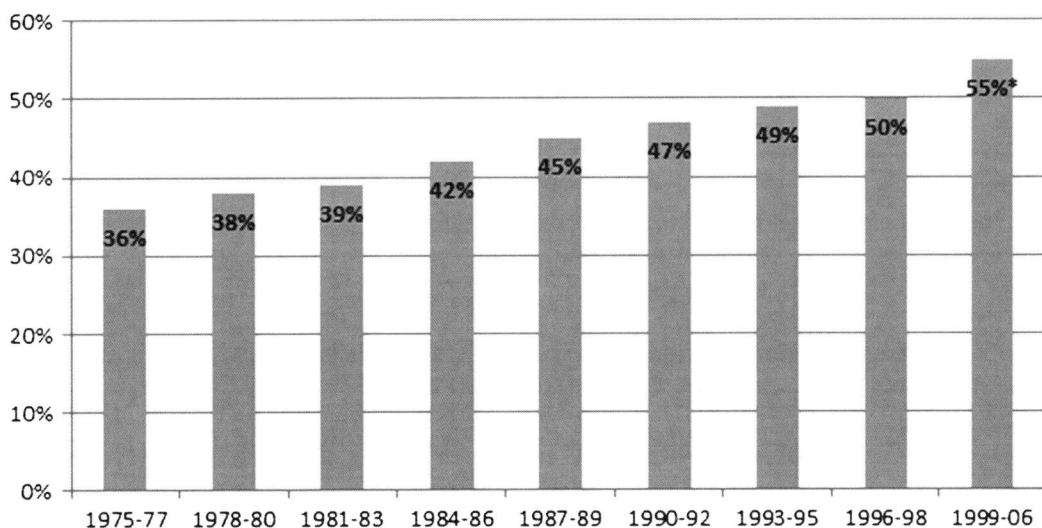

Fig. 2.1 Five-year relative survival rates for all ages, all types of leukemia, 1975–2006. *Source*: SEER (Surveillance, Epidemiology and End Results) Cancer Statistics Review, 1975–2007, National Cancer Institute; 2010. *The difference in rates between 1975–1977 and 1999–2006 is statistically significant ($P < 0.05$)

scientifically important but additional studies were still needed to clarify their significance [2].

Our knowledge of the pathophysiology also has significantly improved and newer classes of therapeutic agents have been developed and used in combination with chemotherapy. These include BCR-ABL tyrosine kinase inhibitors such as imatinib mesylate (Gleevec®), dasatinib (Sprycel®), and nilotinib (Tasigna®); histone deacetylase inhibitors (HDACs) such as vorinostat (Zolinza®); hypomethylating or demethylating agents such as azacitidine (Vidaza®) and decitabine (Dacogen®); immunomodulators such as lenalidomide (Revlimid®) and thalidomide (Thalomid®); monoclonal antibodies; and proteasome inhibitors such as bortezomib (Velcade®). Advanced methods of radiation therapy and stem cell transplant have also become available. Nevertheless, there are many patients with leukemia still dying of their disease or the complications of their antileukemic treatment.

Goal of Radioimmunotherapy

One of the new treatment strategies is based on radioimmunotherapy or the use of monoclonal antibodies labeled with radioactive isotopes. This has emerged in the past two decades as a promising strategy for the treatment of a variety of malignancies, particularly the hematopoietic neoplasms [3–6]. Myeloid leukemia is especially suited for this therapeutic approach since tumor cells are easily accessible in the blood and bone marrow, and myeloid precursors can be identified by differentiation antigens expressed on the cell surface. The killing of tumor cells by monoclonal antibodies is mediated by the immune functions of complement and/or antibody-dependent cellular cytotoxicity, as well as by localized delivery of radiation or toxins that have been conjugated to the immunoglobulin [7, 8].

The goal of radioimmunotherapy is to deliver a large radiation dose to the tumor cells without significantly affecting adjacent normal tissues and organs. The conditions that achieve this goal include rapid tumor uptake of the radioimmunoconjugate with a relatively long effective half-life in the tumor, short effective half-life in the adjacent normal cells and the whole body, and a high tumor-to-normal tissue uptake ratio. In order to increase the effectiveness of radioimmunotherapy, research efforts have concentrated on three different areas: the appropriate selection of a radionuclide specific for therapy, monoclonal antibodies with specific tumor binding and favorable pharmacokinetics, and effective conjugation methods to bind these two components.

Radionuclide Selection

When selecting a specific radionuclide for radionuclide therapy, a number of factors are considered. Besides cost and availability of the radionuclide, tumor size and antigen heterogeneity is considered. Based on the type, range, and energy of the radiations emitted, some radionuclides are better suited for the treatment of microscopic or small-volume disease, whereas others are more appropriate for bulky tumors. The physical half-life should be long enough to permit appropriate radiopharmaceutical preparation and quality control. Depending on tumor pharmacokinetics, a fairly rapid and stable attachment of the radionuclide to the desired chemical species is important. Finally, γ rays, if emitted, are useful for imaging and quantitation. The images obtained aid in biodistribution evaluation and dosimetry calculations [9, 10].

Mechanisms of Radiation Cytotoxicity

Several processes have been implicated as the mechanism by which radiation induces cell death. Radiation is known to induce single- and double-stranded DNA breaks [11], apoptosis [12], and overexpression of p53, leading to delays in the G_1 phase of the cell cycle [13]. Death of cells exposed to α-particles occurs only when the particles traverse the nucleus; high concentrations of α-particles directed at the cytoplasm have no effect on cell proliferation [14].

β-Emitting Radionuclides

A variety of radionuclides have been used for radioimmunotherapy of leukemias, primarily β-emitting radionuclides such as Iodine-131, Yttrium-90, and Rhenium-188 [15]. These radionuclides deposit energy over a relatively long distance (0.8–5.0 mm) allowing irradiation of many cells adjacent to the binding site. This offers the advantage of destroying nearby cells that express limited amounts of the target antigen, or to which the radioimmunoconjugate is not directly bound (crossfire effect). Thus, β-emitters can be effective even if some tumor cells are antigen negative. However, longer range β-rays may target surrounding normal hematopoietic cells and produce nonspecific cytotoxic effects by destroying normal pluripotent stem cells. If the cytotoxic effects are severe, stem cell rescue may be required [16]. These characteristics make β-particle therapy useful in treating bulky tumors or large-volume disease and in selectively irradiating the bone marrow prior to hematopoietic stem cell transplantation. β-Emitting radionuclides with relatively short physical half-lives (less than 10 days) are useful for radioimmunotherapy because the time needed for maximum tumor uptake of the monocloncal antibody is in the same range as the physical half-life. Within the last several years, β-emitting radioimmunotherapy agents such as ^{131}I-tositumomab (Bexxar®) and ^{90}Y-ibritumomab tiuxetan (Zevalin®) have received approval from the Food and Drug Administration (FDA) for the treatment of non-Hodgkin's lymphoma. Finally, some of the β-emitters emit a γ photon as well. These photons are useful to provide in vivo images of antibody biodistribution. γ emission, however, results in normal tissue irradiation.

α-Emitting Radionuclides

Despite the predominant use of β-emitters in radioimmunotherapy trials, investigators have long recognized the potential advantages of α-particle emitters such as Bismuth-213, Actinium-225, and Astatine-211. α-Particles are positively charged helium nuclei with a higher energy (5,000–8,000 keV) than β-particles and shorter range (50–80 μm) in soft tissue. Compared with electrons and β-particles, α-particles exhibit a high density of ionization events along their track [17]. The density of ionizations per unit path length in a material is referred to as the linear energy transfer (LET) of a charged particle. Electrons and β-particles that are emitted by radionuclides generally range in energy from several megaelectron volts (MeV) to as low as several kiloelectron volts (keV), with corresponding LET values ranging from about 0.1 to 1 keV/μm in cells. Auger electrons, which have energies as low as several electron volts are exceptions and have corresponding LET values as high as 25 keV/μm. α-Particles emitted by radionuclides range in energy from 2 to 10 MeV, with initial LET values ranging from 60 to 110 keV/μm. A given tissue-absorbed dose resulting from α-particles, therefore, is likely to yield considerably greater biologic effects than the same absorbed dose delivered by typical electrons or β-particles [18]. In a microdosimetric model using single-cell conditions, Humm demonstrated that one cell-surface decay of the α-emitter [211]At resulted in the same degree of cell killing as approximately 1,000 cell-surface decays of the β-emitter [90]Y [19]. Cell survival studies have shown that cell death may result from as few as one to three α-particle tracks across the nucleus [20–22].

The Principles of RIT in Leukemia

α-Particles are better suited than β-particles for the treatment of microscopic disease since their short range and high energies potentially offer more efficient and specific killing of tumor cells.

α-Emitting radioimmunotherapy has a high probability of nonrepairable DNA double-stranded breaks.

A number of cell-surface antigens have served as targets for radioimmunotherapy, mainly CD33, CD45, and the CD66 antigens.

Promising results have been obtained with [213]Bi- and [225]Ac-labeled HuM195 or lintuzumab.

It follows that α-particles are better suited than β-particles for the treatment of microscopic or small-volume disease since their short range and high energies potentially offer more efficient and specific killing of tumor cells. The deposition of energy over a much shorter range than β-emitters is of interest as targeted cells might be destroyed while neighboring cells are spared. This is advantageous as it avoids bone marrow toxicity [15]. The short half-lives, particularly of bismuth radionuclides, limit the clinical use to diseases in which cancer cells are readily accessible by antibodies. Thus, leukemias are among the best candidates for radioimmunotherapy using α-emitters.

The result of α-emitting radioimmunotherapy is cell-specific targeting with a high probability of nonrepairable DNA double-stranded breaks, because the distance between two strands of DNA is almost the same as the distance between two ionizations of α-particles (2 nm). High-LET radiation also causes more severe chromosomal damage than low-LET radiation, including shattered chromosomes during mitosis and complex chromosomal rearrangements [23]. The cytotoxicity of α-particles may be extremely effective and less dose dependent than that of β-particles, and cell death may occur after a single or a few α-particle emissions [24].

There are more than a hundred α-emitting radioisotopes but only few have been investigated in animal models and humans for potential medical applications [25] (Table 2.4). The majority of these α-emitting radionuclides are produced in nuclear reactors; only a few are cyclotron products. Some radionuclides may be incorporated into a generator system which is subsequently eluted prior to use. The choice of α-emitting radionuclides has to take into account the physical half-life, the duration of elution and compound purification, and the daughter products which could dissociate from the radioimmunoconjugate and be metabolized in a different way to the parent. This is more important if the daughter nuclide is radioactive and has a long physical half-life. The fate of the radionuclide after cell targeting by radioimmunoconjugates may influence the choice of α-emitter. For instance, it has been shown that astatine is

Table 2.4 Physical characteristics of selected α-emitting radionuclides

Isotope	Half-life	Particle(s) emitted	Energy of α-particle (MeV)
^{225}Ac	10 Days	4 α, 2 β	6–8
^{211}At	7.2 h	1 α	6
^{212}Bi	60.6 min	1 α, 1 β	6
^{213}Bi	45.6 min	1 α, 2 β	6
^{212}Pb	10.6 h	1 α, 2 β	7.8
^{223}Ra	11.4 Days	4 α, 2 β	6–7
^{149}Tb	4.2 h	1 α	4

released more rapidly from cells than is bismuth [26]. Finally, many α-emitting radionuclides have multiple emissions including β- and γ-rays. Some of the γ photons emitted are useful for biodistribution and imaging studies.

Actinium-225

^{225}Ac is a radiometal (half-life 10 days) which produces six predominant radionuclide daughters in the decay cascade to stable ^{209}Bi, resulting in the overall emission of five α- and three β-particles, most of which are with high energy (8.38 MeV (α) and 1.42 MeV (β)). ^{225}Ac can be produced by the natural decay of ^{233}U [25] or by accelerator-based methods [27]. Given the relatively long half-life of ^{225}Ac, the multiple α-particle emissions, and the favorable rapid decay chain to stable ^{209}Bi, this radionuclide was recognized as a potential candidate for use in radioimmunotherapy [28]. ^{225}Ac has been proposed as an in vivo generator (nanogenerator) of α-particles [29]. However, the use of ^{225}Ac as a therapeutic radionuclide has been limited by the availability of suitable chelating agents able to stably bind this radionuclide to targeting monoclonal antibody carriers as well as controlling the fate of its daughters [30, 31]. The chelating agent must be able to withstand the recoil energy of α-particles (100–200 keV higher than the binding energy). New opportunities have emerged since two macrocyclic chelates were identified. The first is 1,4,7,10,13,16-hexaazacyclohexadecane hexaacetic acid (HEHA) and the second is 1,4,7,10-tetraazacyclododecane tetraacetic acid (DOTA) [32, 33].

Astatine-211

[211]At is the heaviest radiohalogen nucleus (half-life 7.2 h). It decays through a double-branched pathway with each branch resulting in the production of an α-particle to stable [207]Pb. One route is by α-emission to [207]Bi (42%) followed by electron capture to [207]Pb. The second route is by electron capture to [211]Po (58%) followed by α-emission to [207]Pb [34, 35]. [211]At has several physical properties that make it attractive for radioimmunotherapy. The α-particles produced by the decay of [211]At have an energy of 5.87 MeV (42%) and 7.45 MeV (58%), a high mean LET (97–99 keV/μm), and a short range in soft tissue (55–80 μm), the diameter of few cells. Because of its long half-life, [211]At-labeled conjugates can be used even when the targeting molecule does not gain immediate access to the tumor cells. In addition, the [211]Po daughter emits K X-rays of 77–92 keV allowing external imaging with a γ camera for biodistribution and pharmacokinetic studies [36, 37]. [211]At is produced in a cyclotron by the bombardment of natural bismuth targets with 22–28 MeV α-particles via the [209]Bi(α,2n)[211]At nuclear reaction [38]. Dry distillation procedure is then used for isolation from the cyclotron target [39]. Because of the limited availability of medium-energy cyclotrons with α-particle beams, widespread use of [211]At has been limited. In addition, this radionuclide is less well retained compared to other radiometals such as [205]Bi, [206]Bi, [203]Pb, and ^{111}In after internalization of the antigen–antibody complex [26].

Bismuth-212

[212]Bi is a radiometal (half-life 60.5 min) which decays with a branched pathway through either [208]Tl (36%) or [212]Po (64%) to stable [208]Pb. The decay mode occurs by α- and β-particle emissions. The mean energy of the α-particle is 7.8 MeV and the path length in soft tissue ranges from 40 to 100 μm. [208]Tl produced by the decay of [212]Bi emits a very high energy γ-ray of 2.6 MeV along with other medium-to-high energy γ-particles, requiring heavy shielding to minimize radiation exposure to the staff. Because of the short half-life of 60.5 min, applications involving

i.v. administration of [212]Bi-labeled antibodies are a problem in terms of time required for radiolabeling procedures and the duration of access of the radioimmunoconjugate to the target. All these factors limit the clinical utility of this radioisotope. [212]Bi can be produced from a [224]Ra generator. [224]Ra has a half-life of 3.6 days. Because of high and intermediate γ-emissions in the [224]Ra decay chain, the generator system must be heavily shielded. The generator must also be placed in a trapped or gastight enclosure because of the production of [220]Rn, a radioactive gas, in the decay scheme [40].

Bismuth-213

[213]Bi has similar physical properties than [212]Bi. [213]Bi decays (half-life 45.6 min) through a branched pathway to stable [209]Bi by emitting α- and β-particles. α-Particles contribute to 90.3% of the overall emitted energy with the major energy measuring 8.4 MeV. In addition, a 440-keV γ-photon emission allows tumor imaging as well as biodistribution, pharmacokinetic and dosimetry studies to be performed. Production of [213]Bi for clinical use requires a generator consisting of its parent isotope [225]Ac adsorbed on a cation-exchange resin from which [213]Bi can be eluted using a solution of 0.1 mol/L HCl/0.1 mol/L NaI [41]. The generator is capable of providing clinically useful radionuclides for 10–15 days and requires a minimum amount of shielding. After [213]Bi is eluted from the generator, the isotope is readily conjugated to antibody molecules with bifunctional chelates such as *trans*-cyclohexyldiethylenetriamine pentaacetic acid (CHX-A-DTPA) [42].

Radium-223

[223]Ra (half-life 11.4 days) can be obtained from a generator system using [227]Ac as a parent. [227]Ac has a half-life of 21.8 years. Similar to the previously discussed [225]Ac, five α- and three β-particles are overall emitted in the decay scheme of [223]Ra. This confers an advantage from a therapeutic point of view, but also represents a drawback for stable radiolabeling. Another drawback to its

potential use is that it decays to Radon-219, a gaseous product with unknown biodistribution. In 2004, Henriksen et al. loaded radium and actinium radionuclides into sterically stabilized liposomes coated with folate-F(ab')2 to target tumoral cells expressing folate receptors. Radionuclide loaded liposomes showed excellent stability in serum in vitro [43]. Because of its bone-seeking properties, unconjugated ^{223}Ra is a promising candidate for delivery of high-LET radiation to cancer cells on bone surfaces. Clinical phase I, II, and III studies demonstrated pain relief, reduction in tumor marker levels and improved overall survival in the treatment of skeletal metastases in patients with prostate and breast cancer [44–47].

Terbium-149

^{149}Tb is a radiolanthanide which decays (half-life 4.1 h) by α-emission (3.9 MeV, 17%), positron (β+) emission (4%), and electron capture (79%). Similar to other α-emitting radionuclides, ^{149}Tb appears to be appropriate for the treatment of micrometastases due to the high energy (3.9 MeV), very short path length in normal tissues (28 μm), and high LET (142 keV/μm) of its α-emission. However, the production of ^{149}Tb is difficult, being achieved either by a double reaction ^{142}Nd$(^{12}$C,5$n)^{149}$Dy ^{149}Tb at 70–100 MeV or by bombardment of a sheet of tantalum. The biodistribution and toxicity of its daughters require further assessment because the chemical lanthanide family is known for its bone-seeking properties [48].

Lead-212

^{212}Pb (half-life 10.6 h) is produced from the decay chain of Thorium-228 and can be obtained from a generator of ^{224}Ra. ^{212}Pb can be used as an in vivo generator of ^{212}Bi [49]. The use of ^{212}Pb-labeled immunoconjugates is limited by the destruction of the construct by Auger electrons and by electron capture. The radionuclide has been successfully used in radioimmunotherapy and pretargeted radioimmunotherapy and dem-

onstrated enhanced therapeutic efficacy in combination with chemotherapeutic agents such as gemcitabine and paclitaxel [50].

Target and Targeting Agent Selection

Leukemia is well suited for monoclonal antibody (MAb) therapy due to the accessible differentiation antigens expressed by hematopoietic cells that characterize different stages of maturation. Recent advances in flow cytometry instrumentation and the availability of an expanded range of antibodies and fluorochromes have improved our ability to identify different normal cell populations and recognize phenotypic aberrancies of cell-surface antigens relative to their normal cell counterparts [51]. Leukemias have been shown to express aberrant types or an abundance of cell-surface antigens. In addition to serving as a diagnostic tool as delineated in the 2008 WHO classification [2], a number of these antigens have served as targets for radioimmunotherapy, mainly CD33, CD45, and the CD66 antigens. Studies performed to date have investigated the use of antibodies directed against these surface antigens.

Chimeric and humanized antibodies have been constructed to overcome the weak antitumor activity and the high immunogenicity of many murine MAbs. These types of antibodies are known to retain the binding specificity of the original rodent antibody determined by the variable region but can potentially activate the human immune system through their human constant region [52]. In order to increase the antitumoral effects, monoclonal antibodies have been conjugated to various drugs, bacterial toxins, and radionuclides with encouraging results obtained in all three settings. We will discuss in the following the main surface antigens targeted in leukemias and their respective monoclonal antibodies.

CD25 and Anti-CD25

CD25 or Tac is the α-subunit of the interleukin-2 receptor (IL-2R) which consists of at least three binding subunits: IL-2Rα, IL-2Rβ, and IL-2Rγ.

This receptor is cleaved from the cell surface and can be found in high concentrations in serum. In patients with human T-cell leukemia virus I (HTLV-I)-associated adult T-cell leukemia, IL-2Rα is expressed on virtually all the leukemic cells with an approximate density of 10,000–35,000 receptors/cell [53].

Anti-Tac is a murine MAb that binds to IL-2Rα and prevents its interaction with IL-2. It has been labeled with ^{90}Y and evaluated in a phase I/II trial in patients with adult T-cell leukemia [54].

7G7/B6 is a murine IgG2a MAb directed toward an epitope of the IL-2Rα distinct from the one identified by daclizumab which is a humanized anti-Tac that also recognizes IL-2Rα. This antibody has been labeled with ^{211}At and evaluated in combination with daclizumab in immunodeficient mice injected with human T-cell leukemia cells [55].

CD33 and Anti-CD33

CD33 is a cell-surface glycoprotein found on more than 80% of myeloid leukemic cells and on normal maturing hematopoietic progenitor cells (myelomonocytic and erythroid progenitor cells). Since it is not found on mature granulocytes, lymphoid, or nonhematopoietic cells, an anti-CD33 antibody could selectively eliminate malignant myeloid cells while sparing the normal stem cells [56–58]. However, the utility of CD33 for radioimmunotherapy is limited due to its relatively low concentration on leukemic cell surface resulting in rapid saturation of the antigenic targets. A study by Jilani et al. showed an average of 10,000 molecules/AML cell and 4,400 molecules/CML cell [59]. In addition, a study using ^{131}I-labeled anti-CD33 antibody demonstrated a relatively short retention of the bound antibody in marrow in a mouse model presumably due to rapid internalization, modulation, and degradation [60].

Three anti-CD33 MAbs have been used in the radioimmunotherapy of myeloid leukemias: M195, HuM195, and p67.

M195, a murine monoclonal IgG2a antibody, is derived from a mouse immunized with live human leukemic myeloblasts. The antibody does not

mediate antibody-dependent cellular cytotoxicity and is associated with the formation of human antimouse antibodies (HAMA) [61, 62].

HuM195 or Lintuzumab is a humanized antibody constructed by grafting the complementarity-determining region of M195 onto the constant region and variable framework of a human IgG1 antibody [63]. HuM195 differs from the murine M195 in that it has a higher binding avidity than M195, fixes human complement, and causes in vitro leukemia cell killing by antibody-dependent cell-mediated cytotoxicity [64]. In addition, while significant numbers of patients treated with murine M195 develop HAMA that adversely affect the pharmacokinetics of the antibody and preclude retreatment with it, treatment with HuM195 does not induce a human antihuman antibody (HAHA) response [61, 65, 66]. p67 is a murine IgG1 antibody that was formerly used for radioimmunotherapy.

Gemtuzumab ozogamicin (Mylotarg®) is a recombinant humanized IgG4 anti-CD33 monoclonal antibody conjugated, not to a radioisotope, but to calicheamicin, a potent antitumor antibiotic. After binding to CD33, the antigen–antibody complex is internalized. Calicheamicin dissociates from the antibody in the acidic intracellular environment, then migrates to the nucleus where it binds within the minor groove of DNA and causes double-stranded DNA breaks and subsequent apoptotic cell death. Gemtuzumab ozogamicin is the first anti-CD33 immunoconjugate to be approved by the FDA for the treatment of AML in patients aged 60 years or older with relapsed disease who are not candidates for standard chemotherapy [67].

CD45 and Anti-CD45

CD45 is a cell-surface glycoprotein with tyrosine phosphatase activity. It is known as leukocyte common antigen as it is expressed on virtually all leukocytes, including more than 85% of myeloid and lymphoid leukemic cells. It is not expressed on mature erythrocytes, platelets, and nonhematopoietic cells. CD45 is expressed in a relatively high density on the cell surface (200,000 binding sites/cell). Unlike CD33, it is not internalized or shed after antibody binding [60, 68–70].

BC8 is a murine IgG1 anti-CD45 antibody used for radioimmunotherapy. To date, the anti-CD45 antibody is not being investigated as a single agent. Rather, the immunoconjugate labeled with ^{131}I is being studied as a preparative regimen in combination with busulfan, cyclophosphamide, and total body irradiation prior to allogeneic or autologous stem cell transplant [5, 71, 72].

CD66 and Anti-CD66

CD66a, b, c, and d are glycoproteins expressed on mature myeloid cells but not on leukemia cells. They are expressed at a high density of approximately 200,000 molecules/cell. CD66 can also be found on epithelial or endothelial cells. CD66c is known as nonspecific cross-reacting antigen (NCA). Similar to CD45, CD66 antigens are neither internalized nor shed [73, 74].

BW 250/183 is a murine monoclonal IgG1 antibody directed against CD66c. The antibody also recognizes CD66a and b, and does not have any antileukemic activity as a single agent. Rhenium-188 labeled anti-CD66 antibody has been investigated in Germany as part of a conditioning regimen prior to allogeneic stem cell transplantation [75, 76].

Besides these antigens and antibodies, multiple other targets have been explored for use in radioimmunotherapy of leukemias. A short list of those includes CD5, CD20, CD22, CD23, CD30, CD37, CD52, and HLA-DR.

Immunoconjugate Labeling

The radioimmunoconjugates can be susceptible to catabolism due to the direct effects of radioactive decay or after internalization into a target cell. Therefore, in vivo stability is required in order to maximize delivery of isotope to the tumor and to prevent toxicity. There is a variety of methods used to conjugate radioisotopes to antibodies depending on the nature of the radioisotope.

Radiohalogens

Radiohalogens like [211]At are usually labeled directly to antibodies by incorporation of an aryl carbon–astatine bond into the antibody [34]. This involves astatodemetallation reactions using tin, silicon or mercury precursors in order to create the aryl carbon–astatine bond [39, 77].

Radiometals

Radiometals such as actinium and bismuth, however, require chelation in which one or more atoms in the chelating agent donate pairs of electrons to the foreign metal and the antibody to form covalent bonds (bifunctional chelation). As previously discussed, chelating agents should be able to stably bind radionuclides to targeting monoclonal antibodies and to control the fate of its daughters. In addition, the chelating agent must be able to withstand the recoil energy of α-particles which in some cases is 100–200 keV higher than the binding energy [30, 31, 78]. Chelators derived from DTPA include the cyclic dianhydride derivative [22] and the cyclohexyl-benzyl derivative (CHX-A-DTPA) [42, 79]. CHX-A-DTPA is effective at chelating bismuth to antibodies, resulting in stable constructs that have been used effectively in clinical trials [42]. The macrocyclic ligand 1,4,7,10-DOTA and its derivatives have been used successfully for labeling antibodies with [225]Ac. A two-step procedure was developed in which [225]Ac is first conjugated to DOTA-SCN followed by labeling of this construct to antibody [80]. Another macrocyclic chelate, 4-isothiocyanatobenzyl-1,4,7,10,13,16-hexaazacyclohexadecane hexaacetic acid (HEHA-NCS), was also developed and used to label antibodies with [225]Ac [32, 81]. However, the [225]Ac complex with HEHA demonstrated less stability in vivo than the [225]Ac complex with DOTA. In addition, the monoclonal antibody/antigen systems that were examined using HEHA constructs were noninternalizing immune complexes and the targeted constructs could still release the radioactive daughters systemically contributing to acute radiotoxicity. The [225]Ac complex formed with DOTA was considerably more stable in vivo and the selected antibodies formed internalizing immune complexes with their respective antigen targets [33].

Limitations of α-Emitting Radionuclides

There are several limitations associated with the use of α-emitters in radioimmunotherapy. Once the radionuclide is conjugated to the specific pharmaceutical, release of unbound radionuclides may occur and result in severe toxicities. The complexity of conjugation with either bifunctional chelating agents or attachment to nonactivated aromatic rings is another limitation. In addition, as α-radionuclides decay, bifunctional chelating agent may not appropriately bind daughter radionuclides and thus may ultimately result in the release of the unbound daughter radionuclide. Radiolysis is another limitation of α-decay resulting in the deposition of high radiation within a very small volume. This can result in protein degradation, including protein fragmentation. In the case of monoclonal antibodies, radiolysis may compromise antibody immunoreactivity [35]. McDevitt et al. have suggested the use of ascorbic acid as a radioprotectant agent in the radiolabeling and purification steps of ^{213}Bi-labeled HuM195 [82]. Other significant limitations of α-emitting radionuclides include the lack of commercial availability and unfamiliarity of medical personel with radiation safety measures.

Radiation Protection Related to α-Emitters

α-Particles have very little penetrating power. They can be stopped by a sheet of paper, skin, or a few inches of air. The dead outer layer of the skin absorbs all the α-particles from external radioactive sources. As a result, they do not pose an external radiation hazard [83]. However, α-emitting radionuclides are potentially dangerous when inhaled or ingested. The energy released is deposited in living cells rather than dead tissue as on the skin surface. Multiple studies have

indicated an association between internal exposure of α-emitters and cancer, specifically between exposure to radon gas and lung cancer [84]. As previously discussed, ^{220}Rn is produced in the decay scheme of ^{224}Ra during the production of ^{212}Bi (^{224}Ra/^{212}Bi generator). Special monitoring equipment and facilities may be needed to limit or prevent contamination and airborne release of α-emitting radionuclides during handling and storage.

Radioimmunotherapy with α-Emitters

The translation of radioimmunotherapy with α-particles into the clinical setting has been slow despite the conceptual appeal, in part, because of limited radionuclide availability and the paucity of α-emitters with physical half-lives compatible with clinical use. Clinical literature describing targeted α-particle radiotherapy in human cancer patients is limited to myeloid leukemia, glioma, ovarian cancer, melanoma, non-Hodgkin's lymphoma, and breast and prostate cancer with osseous metastases [44–47] (Table 2.5). These studies have examined radionuclides with short and long half-lives, i.e., ^{211}At (half-life, 7.2 h), ^{213}Bi (half-life, 45.6 min), ^{225}Ac (half-life, 10 days), and ^{223}Ra (half-life, 11.4 days). Absorbed dose estimates for antibodies labeled with long half-life radionuclides require pharmacokinetic information that spans a period of several days. Loss of the radionuclide is determined predominantly by biologic clearance rather than physical decay. In contrast, the pharmacokinetic period relevant for the dosimetry of antibodies labeled with short half-life radionuclides such as ^{213}Bi is measured in minutes and hours rather than days.

The first clinical trial of an α-particle emitter in radiolabeled antibody therapy started in 1996 at Memorial Sloan–Kettering Cancer Center (MSKCC) [85]. The study used ^{213}Bi conjugated to the humanized monoclonal antibody HuM195 also called lintuzumab, specific to CD33 antigen, via the bifunctional chelating agent SCN-CHX-A-DTPA. HuM195 and M195 were conjugated in previous studies to β-emitting radionuclides [61, 86, 87]. When labeled with ^{131}I and ^{90}Y,

Table 2.5 Clinical trials using ^{225}Ac, ^{211}At and ^{213}Bi

Radioisotope	Half-life	Pharmaceutical	Type of malignancy	Summary	References
^{225}Ac	10 Days	Anti-CD33 IgG (HuM195 or lintuzumab)	Acute myeloid leukemia	Ongoing *phase I* trial with 7 patients reported to date. Elimination of peripheral blasts was seen in 3 patients. Greater than 33% dose-related reductions of bone marrow blasts were seen in 4 patients at 4 weeks posttreatment	[91]
^{211}At	7.2 h	Antitenascin IgG (chimeric 81C6)	High grade glioma	*Phase I* trial with 18 patients treated with labeled antibody injected into a surgically created resection cavity. The median survival was 57 weeks; 2 of 14 patients with recurrent glioblastoma multiforme survived for nearly 3 years after treatment	[111]
		MX35 F(ab')2	Ovarian carcinoma	*Phase I* trial with 9 patients treated with labeled antibody injected into the peritoneal cavity. Bone marrow and peritoneal absorbed doses of 0.14 mGy/(MBq/L) and 15.6 mGy/(MBq/L), respectively. No sides effects were seen at the highest activity concentration reached in the study (100 MBq/L). Three patients remained in clinical and CA-125 remission. The maximum tolerated activity (MTD) concentration could not be established because the tolerable absorbed dose to the peritoneum is unknown	[112, 113]
^{213}Bi	45.6 min	Anti-CD33 IgG (HuM195 or lintuzumab)	Myelogenous leukemia (acute or chronic)	*Phase I* completed in 18 patients with no toxicity, substantial decrease in peripheral leukemic cells and bone marrow blasts. No complete remissions were seen. *Phase I/II* in 31 patients after cytoreduction with cytarabine. Significant reductions in marrow blasts were noted at all dose levels. Six of the twenty-five patients who received doses of ≥37 MBq/kg clinically responded to the treatment (two complete remissions (CR), two complete remissions with incomplete platelet recovery (CRp) and two partial remissions (PR)). The response duration ranged between 2 and 12 months with a median of 6 months. The median survival duration among the responders was 13.7 months vs. 4.6 months for all patients	[85, 89, 90]
		Antineurokinin type-1 receptor peptide (DOTAGA-Substance P)	Glioma of World Health Organization (WHO) grades 2–4	Two of twenty patients treated with intracavitary ^{213}Bi (one with glioblastoma and one with oligodendroglioma WHO grade 2). Response was difficult to assess in the first patient due to bulky residual tumor. In the second case, resection of a mass lesion 33 months after α-therapy showed radiation necrosis. There was no signs of tumor recurrence for another 34 months	[114]
		Anti-CD20 IgG (rituximab)	Relapsed/refractory non-Hodgkin lymphoma	*Phase I* study with 9 patients treated to date using activities ranging from 385 to 1,640 MBq. Two patients responded to therapy. Acute toxic side effects were not seen, except two cases of mild leukopenia (grade 1)	[115]
		9.2.27 IgG	Melanoma	*Phase I* study with 16 patients treated with intralesional injection of the labeled antibody. All treated melanoma cells lost their structure. There was near complete cell kill at 450 μCi and above with few remaining viable cell clusters. There was considerable decline in the melanoma-inhibitory-activity serum levels at 2 weeks after treatment	[116]

HuM195 and M195 eliminated large leukemic burdens in patients but produced prolonged myelosuppression requiring hematopoietic stem cell transplantation at high doses. To enhance the potency of native HuM195 yet avoid the crossfire effect of β-emitting constructs, the α-emitting isotope ^{213}Bi was selected.

The aim of the study was to assess the tolerance, pharmacokinetics, and biological activity of ^{213}Bi-HuM195. Eighteen patients with relapsed and refractory AML or chronic myelomonocytic leukemia were treated in a phase I dose-escalation trial. Fourteen patients had AML in relapse, including three who had benefited from a bone marrow transplant, 3 patients had AML refractory to chemotherapy, and one had chronic myelomonocytic leukemia in relapse. Patients received 10.36–37 MBq/kg (0.28–1.0 mCi/kg) of ^{213}Bi-HuM195 in three to seven i.v. infusions in 2–4 days. Five dose levels were employed (10.36, 15.54, 20.72, 25.9, and 37 MBq/kg), yielding total doses of 602–3,515 MBq. Treatment was well tolerated and dose-limiting toxicity was not observed. Transient grade 1 or 2 liver function abnormalities occurred in 6 patients with an onset of 5–14 days following treatment and recovery within 3–14 days. All 17 evaluable patients developed myelosuppression lasting 12–41 days with a medium recovery of 22 days. Dosimetric and biodistribution data were obtained using blood sampling and γ camera imaging. γ Camera imaging centered on the 440-keV photopeak showed localization of ^{213}Bi to expected areas of leukemic involvement, including the bone marrow, liver, and spleen, within 5–10 min after injection. The estimated doses to the bone marrow, liver, and spleen were as much as 40,000 times higher than the doses estimated for kidneys or the whole body. The organ target/whole body ratios of absorbed doses with ^{213}Bi-HuM195 were 1,000-fold higher than the same dose ratios obtained with β-emitting conjugates such as ^{131}I or ^{90}Y [88]. Fourteen of fifteen evaluable patients had reductions in peripheral leukemic cells and 14/18 patients had decreases in the percentage of bone marrow blasts. However, there were no complete remissions. Further analysis revealed that approximately 1 in 2,700 molecules of HuM195 carried

the radiolabel. This was insufficient to deliver one to two atoms of ^{213}Bi to every leukemia cell necessary for their killing, even if optimal antibody targeting was assumed. In addition, the CD33-negative leukemic progenitors would have escaped the cytotoxic effects of the α-particles because of their selectivity, leading to the conclusion that treatment of overt leukemia with ^{213}Bi-HuM195 as a single agent would require extraordinarily high injected activities or higher specific activity, and making α-particle immunotherapy best suited for the treatment of residual disease. The trial was the first proof-of-concept for radioimmunotherapy using α-emitters in humans for a variety of malignancies, particularly those in which small-volume, minimal residual, or micrometastatic disease is present.

Recognizing this "limitation" and in an effort to produce complete remissions, a phase I/II trial was initiated evaluating the effects of ^{213}Bi-HuM195 after partial cytoreduction with cytarabine in 31 patients with newly diagnosed ($n = 13$) or relapsed/refractory ($n = 18$) AML [89, 90]. The patients were treated at MSKCC from April 2001 to June 2006. They first received a nonremittive dose of cytarabine to decrease the leukemic burden (200 mg/m^2 i.v. daily for 5 days). Treatment with ^{213}Bi-HuM195 followed 8 days after at 18.5–46.25 MBq/kg in 1–2 days. Four dose levels were employed (18.5, 27.75, 37, and 46.25 MBq/kg) for those who participated in the phase I portion of the trial (15 patients). The remaining 16 patients received 37 MBq/kg in the phase II portion.

Total administered doses ranged from 1,195 to 4,755 MBq. Nine patients had infusion-related reactions characterized by fever, chills, and rigors, including 1 patient developing bronchospasm. Myelosuppression lasting more than 35 days was dose limiting and the maximum tolerated dose (MTD) of ^{213}Bi-HuM195 following cytarabine was determined to be 37 MBq/kg. Transient grade 3 or 4 liver function abnormalities were seen in 5 patients (16%) with an onset of 3–30 days following treatment (median, 7 days). Two treatment-related deaths occurred in the 21 patients who received the MTD.

Significant reductions in marrow blasts were noted at all dose levels. However, 6 of the 25 patients (24%) who received doses of ≥ 37 MBq/kg clinically responded to the treatment (two complete remissions (CR), two complete remissions with incomplete platelet recovery (CRp), and two partial remissions (PR)) whereas none of the remaining 6 patients who received <37 MBq/kg had a clinical response. This outlined the added benefit of [213]Bi-HuM195 and suggested that cytarabine was not the only cause of remissions. In addition, none of the patients with primary refractory AML or heavily pretreated had a response, indicating the need for effective cytoreduction prior to administering [213]Bi-HuM195 in order to achieve remission. The median response duration ranged between 2 and 12 months with a median of 6 months. The median survival duration among the responders was 13.7 months vs. 4.6 months for all patients. This study demonstrated that sequential treatment with cytarabine and [213]Bi-HuM195 can produce remissions in some patients with advanced myeloid leukemia.

Despite these encouraging results, the authors recognized the persistent obstacles of radioimmunothrapy with [213]Bi, including its short half-life (45.6 min) and the need for an onsite [225]Ac/[213]Bi generator. Therefore, they developed a different strategy, a radioimmunoconjugate using [225]Ac serving as an in vivo nanogenerator (see below). [225]Ac has a half-life of 10 days and, if injected, emits four α-particles in a cascade at or within a cancer cell when coupled to internalizing monoclonal antibodies. In addition, preclinical studies have shown increased potency of [225]Ac constructs compared with [213]Bi containing analogs as well as prolonged survival of animals in several xenograft models [80].

Based on these results, a phase I dose-escalation trial using [225]Ac-HuM195 was initiated in advanced myeloid leukemia [91]. Seven patients with relapsed ($n=3$) or refractory ($n=4$) AML have been reported to date. Three dose levels were employed (0.5, 1, or 2 μCi/kg). There were no acute toxicities related to the infusion. However, myelosuppression, including grade 4

neutropenia and thrombocytopenia, was noted. There was no evidence of radiation nephritis at 10 months when compared with side effects obtained in preclinical studies in which renal tubular damage associated with interstitial fibrosis was seen on nonhuman primates [92]. Antileukemic effects manifested by elimination of peripheral blood blasts were seen in 3 of 6 evaluable patients. In addition, there was greater than 33% dose-related reductions of bone marrow blasts in 4 patients at 4 weeks posttreatment. One patient had 3% bone marrow blasts after therapy. Accrual to this trial continues but the promising results obtained to date confirm the role of α-particle radioimmunotherapy and the efficiency of therapeutic nanogenerator of multiple α-particle emissions within the target cell. Additional studies combining [225]Ac-HuM195 with cytoreductive chemotherapy are planned.

Improving Delivery Methods and Future Orientations

Nanogenerators

The atomic nanogenerator system consists of using a long half-life radionuclide which emits a cascade of α-particles as it decays at or within a cancer cell when coupled to internalizing monoclonal antibodies, thus increasing its capacity of cell killing (Fig. 2.2). [225]Ac has a half-life of 10 days and emits four α-particles in a cascade as it decays to stable [209]Bi. As mentioned earlier, [225]Ac constructs demonstrated increased potency when compared to [213]Bi analogs and specific cell killing at single becquerel (picocurie) levels in vitro. In addition, they induced tumor regression and prolonged survival over controls, without toxicity, in a substantial fraction of animals when injected at kilobecquerels (nanocurie) doses in nude mice [80]. These effects would not have been achieved without overcoming several challenges. Controlling the fate of several radionuclidic progeny represented one of the challenges, including the understanding of their biodistribution, metabolism, and clearance. Finding suitable chelating

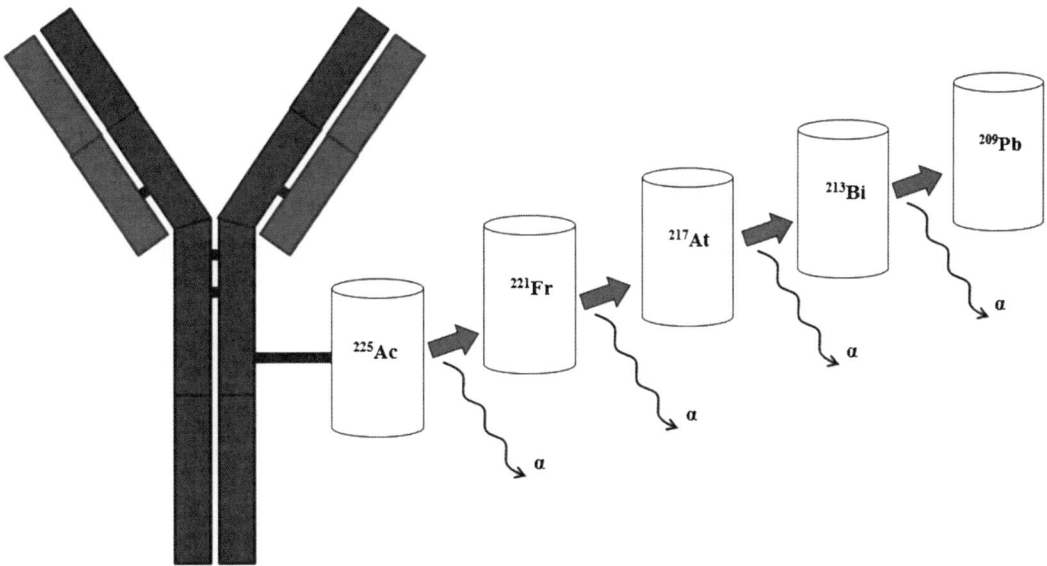

Fig. 2.2 A model showing the multiple emissions generated by the ^{225}Ac-antibody in vivo nanogenerator system

agents that would yield stable ^{225}Ac complexes in vivo was another challenge.

In an effort to overcome these challenges, a series of ligands (1,4,7,10,13,16-hexaazacyclo-hexadecane hexaacetic acid (HEHA); acetate; ethylene diamine tetraacetic acid (EDTA); 1,4,7,10,13-pentaazacyclopentadecane pentaa-cetic acid (PEPA); cyclohexyl diethylenetri-amine pentaacetic acid (CHX-A-DTPA), DTPA) were evaluated for in vivo stability, aiming to find single chelate moieties that bind the parent and the daughters. These efforts proved difficult. Whereas ^{225}Ac-HEHA showed exceptional sta-bility in vivo, the remaining chelators were unstable, likely due to different physical and chemical properties of the daughters [30, 93]. However, when ^{225}Ac-HEHA was bound to monoclonal antibody 201B and injected into mice bearing lung tumor colonies, the slow release of ^{225}Ac from HEHA chelate and the noninternalizing antibody–antigen complex lead to systemic toxicity. ^{225}Ac accumulated predominantly in the liver, spleen, and bone, and ^{213}Bi, the third α-decay daughter, was found to be in excess in the kidney. In addition, ani-mals treated with 1.0 μCi or more of the ^{225}Ac

radioconjugate died of a wasting syndrome within days. Due to these reasons, the use of this system in radioimmunotherapy was com-promised [81].

On a different level, the MSKCC group developed the concept of atomic nanogenerator as it was described above [80] focusing on four principles: (1) stable in vivo chelation to ^{225}Ac; (2) internalization of the ^{225}Ac-antibody construct into the target cell; (3) trapping of the progeny within the target cell; and (4) reduction of the loss of the daughters to nontarget tissues decreasing systemic radiotoxicity. This was successfully achieved using DOTA derivative chelates cou-pled with internalizing IgGs.

Liposomes

Another method to improve retention of the α-emitting daughters of ^{225}Ac consists of engulfing the radioimmunoconjugate in liposomes [94].

As the radionuclides decay inside the lipo-somes, α-particles escape through the liposomal phospholipid membrane because of their high kinetic energy and irradiate the targeted cells.

In addition, daughter atoms can penetrate the phospholipid membrane during their recoil trajectory (80–90 nm). As a reminder, the recoil of the parent nucleus during α-decay can be assimilated to the "kick" of a rifle butt when a bullet goes in the opposite direction. After losing their recoil energy, the newly produced daughter atoms are charged. Consequently, they cannot diffuse freely across the hydrophobic layer of the biphospholipid liposomal membrane. Thus, the probability of daughter retention is greater for larger liposomes assuming homogeneous distribution of the parent radionuclides within the aqueous center of the liposome.

However, when encapsulating ^{225}Ac, Sofou et al. noticed that daughter retention was lower than expected. This was explained by the binding of ^{225}Ac to the phospholipid membrane, instead of uniformly distributing within the liposomal core. To solve this issue, the authors passively entrapped ^{225}Ac constructs in multivesicular liposomes (MUVEL) [95]. MUVELs are large liposomes (greater than 650 nm in diameter) with entrapped smaller lipid vesicles. In this model, ^{225}Ac is engulfed within the small vesicles located in the region of the liposomal core, away from the outer liposomal membrane. In addition, MUVELs were PEGylated. The presence of polyethylene glycol (PEG) at the surface of a liposomal carrier has been shown in a previous study to extend the circulation lifetime of the vehicle [96]. For 30 days, 98% of the encapsulated ^{225}Ac and 17% of the last daughter ^{213}Bi were retained by MUVELs. In a later stage, a monoclonal antibody directed against Her-2/neu, trastuzumab, was labeled with ^{225}Ac-DOTA then conjugated to MUVELs. The immunolabeled MUVELs were then incubated in vitro with human ovarian carcinoma SKOV3-NMP2 cells resulting in greater specific binding and significant internalization (83%) compared to nontargeted liposomes.

This approach has the potential of reducing the fraction of escaped radioactive daughters, and decreasing in consequence their systemic radiotoxicity such as renal toxicity due to ^{213}Bi release in ^{225}Ac-radioimmunotherapy [97, 98]. It has also been suggested for therapy of disseminated peritoneal micrometastases using direct intraperitoneal administration. Nevertheless, immunolabeled MUVELs may become unstable in vivo in the presence of serum proteins, since proteins are known to interact with the lipid membrane of these vehicles in a variety of ways [99, 100]. Research in this field continues to evolve.

Pretargeting

Pretargeting methods of radioimmunotherapy have been developed to reduce radiation doses to normal organs and improve tumor-to-normal organ dose ratios. Pretargeting involves the administration of a "cold" antibody or engineered targeting molecule conjugated to streptavidin, followed by administration of a biotinylated "clearing agent" to remove excess of circulating antibody. In a next stage, radiolabeled biotin is infused at therapeutic doses. The radiolabeled biotin binds specifically to "pretargeted" streptavidin at the tumor site, whereas unbound radiolabeled biotin is rapidly excreted in the urine [101].

Encouraging results were obtained in mouse models xenografted with adult T-cell leukemia and anaplastic large cell lymphoma cells that express CD25 pretargeted with different agents conjugated to streptavidin and treated with ^{213}Bi-DOTA-biotin and ^{90}Y-DOTA-biotin. These results included improved survival in mice treated with ^{213}Bi when compared to controls, longer survival when compared to those treated directly with ^{213}Bi-humanized anti-Tac and cure in a significant number of leukemic (70%) and all lymphoma-xenografted mice [102, 103]. A limitation of the use of avidin and streptavidin clearing agents persists as their immunogenicity may limit their repeated use [104–106]. Several attempts have been made to address this issue such as PEG modification or succinylation of these agents [107, 108].

Carbon Nanotubes

Many of the current targeting molecules suffer from low potency and specificity, weak binding interaction, rapid clearance, and a limited number of target molecules. However, there is currently an increased interest in Medicine in devices constructed from novel nanotechnologies aiming to address these obstacles. One of these technologies consists of single wall carbon nanotubes (CNT) on which multiple molecules may be covalently attached such as fluorochromes, antibodies, chelated radiometals, or other therapeutic effectors, thus giving multiple functions to the resulting nanoconstruct. Works from the MSKCC group have demonstrated lymphoma targeting in vitro and in vivo in a murine model using specific antibodies appended to a soluble nanoscale CNT construct [109].

Prototypes of these constructs were attached to multiple copies of DOTA chelates and radiolabeled with ^{86}Y and ^{111}In. They were then administered to mice and imaged in order to determine the tissue biodistribution and pharmacokinetics. The major sites of accumulation resulting from ^{86}Y-CNT injection were the kidneys, liver, and spleen. Bone accumulation was minimal and excretion was renal. Due to rapid blood clearance ($t_{1/2} < 1$ h), the authors suggested that these constructs may be beneficial in diagnostic applications when labeled with short-lived radionuclides. Further studies, however, are needed to develop and assess this emerging technology [110].

Challenges Associated with RIT of Leukemia

Specific monoclonal antibodies.
Effective conjugation methods.
In vivo stability of the radioimmunoconjugate.
Release of the unbound daughter radionuclide.
Cost and availability of the radionuclide.
Unfamiliarity of medical personnel with radiation safety measures of α-emitters.
Validation trials.

Conclusion

Monoclonal antibodies are reliable therapeutic tools to treat leukemia due to their relatively higher specificity and their reduced toxicity compared to conventional chemotherapeutic drugs. The role of radiolabeled monoclonal antibodies in the treatment of cancer is increasing. A number of cell-surface antigens have served as targets for radioimmunotherapy, mainly CD33, CD45, and the CD66 antigens. Whereas most radioimmunotherapy trials have been performed with β-emitting radionuclides, there has been increased interest in the shorter range higher LET α-particles which allow for more efficient killing of tumor cells. Promising results have been obtained with ^{213}Bi- and ^{225}Ac-labeled HuM195 or lintuzumab.

To date, most preclinical and clinical trials suggest that radioimmunotherapy with α-emitters is better suited than radioimmunotherapy with β-emitters for the treatment of microscopic disease. However, there are persistent challenges associated with this, such as the stability of the radioimmunoconjugate in vivo and the specificity of the monoclonal antibodies to target leukemic cells. New investigations are needed to tackle these challenges as well as to educate medical personnel with radiation safety measures and to identify optimal radioisotopes, dosing regimens, therapeutic strategies, and novel delivery methods of the radioimmunoconjugates using α-emitting radionuclides.

References

1. Jemal A, et al. Cancer statistics, 2010. CA Cancer J Clin. 2010;60(5):277–300.
2. Vardiman JW, et al. The 2008 revision of the World Health Organization (WHO) classification of myeloid neoplasms and acute leukemia: rationale and important changes. Blood. 2009;114(5): 937–51.
3. Kaminski MS, et al. Radioimmunotherapy with iodine (131)I tositumomab for relapsed or refractory B-cell non-Hodgkin lymphoma: updated results and long-term follow-up of the University of Michigan experience. Blood. 2000;96(4):1259–66.

4. Liu SY, et al. Follow-up of relapsed B-cell lymphoma patients treated with iodine-131-labeled anti-CD20 antibody and autologous stem-cell rescue. J Clin Oncol. 1998;16(10):3270–8.

5. Matthews DC, et al. Phase I study of (131) I-anti-CD45 antibody plus cyclophosphamide and total body irradiation for advanced acute leukemia and myelodysplastic syndrome. Blood. 1999;94(4): 1237–47.

6. Witzig TE, et al. Phase I/II trial of IDEC-Y2B8 radioimmunotherapy for treatment of relapsed or refractory CD20(+) B-cell non-Hodgkin's lymphoma. J Clin Oncol. 1999;17(12):3793–803.

7. Grossbard ML, et al. Monoclonal antibody-based therapies of leukemia and lymphoma. Blood. 1992;80(4):863–78.

8. Scheinberg DA. Monoclonal antibodies in the treatment of myelogenous leukemias. Cancer Treat Res. 1993;64:213–32.

9. O'Donoghue JA, Bardies M, Wheldon TE. Relationships between tumor size and curability for uniformly targeted therapy with beta-emitting radionuclides. J Nucl Med. 1995;36(10):1902–9.

10. Siegel JA, Stabin MG. Absorbed fractions for electrons and beta particles in spheres of various sizes. J Nucl Med. 1994;35(1):152–6.

11. Nunez MI, et al. Radiation-induced DNA double-strand break rejoining in human tumour cells. Br J Cancer. 1995;71(2):311–6.

12. Kolesnick RN, Haimovitz-Friedman A, Fuks Z. The sphingomyelin signal transduction pathway mediates apoptosis for tumor necrosis factor, Fas, and ionizing radiation. Biochem Cell Biol. 1994; 72(11–12):471–4.

13. Pandita TK, et al. Ionizing radiation activates the ATM kinase throughout the cell cycle. Oncogene. 2000;19(11):1386–91.

14. Munro TR. The relative radiosensitivity of the nucleus and cytoplasm of Chinese hamster fibroblasts. Radiat Res. 1970;42(3):451–70.

15. Matthews DC, Appelbaum FR. Radioimmunotherapy and hematopoietic cell transplantation. In: Thomas ED, Blume KG, Forman SJ, editors. Thomas' hematopoietic cell transplantation, vol. 1. 3rd ed. Malden: Blackwell; 2004.

16. Appelbaum FR. Antibody-targeted therapy for myeloid leukemia. Semin Hematol. 1999;36 (4 Suppl 6):2–8.

17. Wright HA, et al. Calculations of physical and chemical reactions produced in irradiated water containing DNA. Radiat Prot Dosimetry. 1985;13(1–4):133–6.

18. Mulford DA, Scheinberg DA, Jurcic JG. The promise of targeted {alpha}-particle therapy. J Nucl Med. 2005;46 Suppl 1:199S–204.

19. Humm JL. A microdosimetric model of astatine-211 labeled antibodies for radioimmunotherapy. Int J Radiat Oncol Biol Phys. 1987;13(11):1767–73.

20. Humm JL, Chin LM. A model of cell inactivation by alpha-particle internal emitters. Radiat Res. 1993; 134(2):143–50.

21. Kozak RW, et al. Bismuth-212-labeled anti-Tac monoclonal antibody: alpha-particle-emitting radionuclides as modalities for radioimmunotherapy. Proc Natl Acad Sci U S A. 1986;83(2):474–8.

22. Macklis RM, et al. Radioimmunotherapy with alpha-particle-emitting immunoconjugates. Science. 1988;240(4855):1024–6.

23. Kampf G. Induction of DNA double-strand breaks by ionizing radiation of different quality and their relevance for cell inactivation. Radiobiol Radiother (Berl). 1988;29(6):631–58.

24. Raju MR, et al. Radiobiology of alpha particles: III. Cell inactivation by alpha-particle traversals of the cell nucleus. Radiat Res. 1991;128(2):204–9.

25. McDevitt MR, et al. Radioimmunotherapy with alpha-emitting nuclides. Eur J Nucl Med. 1998;25(9): 1341–51.

26. Yao Z, et al. Comparative cellular catabolism and retention of astatine-, bismuth-, and lead-radiolabeled internalizing monoclonal antibody. J Nucl Med. 2001;42(10):1538–44.

27. Koch L, et al. Production of Ac-225 and application of the Bi-213 daughter in cancer therapy. Czech J Phys. 1999;49:817–22.

28. Geerlings MW, et al. The feasibility of ^{225}Ac as a source of alpha-particles in radioimmunotherapy. Nucl Med Commun. 1993;14(2):121–5.

29. McDevitt MR, Scheinberg DA. Ac-225 and her daughters: the many faces of Shiva. Cell Death Differ. 2002;9(6):593–4.

30. Davis IA, et al. Comparison of 225actinium chelates: tissue distribution and radiotoxicity. Nucl Med Biol. 1999;26(5):581–9.

31. Miederer M, Scheinberg DA, McDevitt MR. Realizing the potential of the actinium-225 radionuclide generator in targeted alpha particle therapy applications. Adv Drug Deliv Rev. 2008;60(12):1371–82.

32. Chappell LL, et al. Synthesis, conjugation, and radiolabeling of a novel bifunctional chelating agent for (225)Ac radioimmunotherapy applications. Bioconjug Chem. 2000;11(4):510–9.

33. McDevitt MR, et al. Design and synthesis of ^{225}Ac radioimmunopharmaceuticals. Appl Radiat Isot. 2002;57(6):841–7.

34. Zalutsky MR, Vaidyanathan G. Astatine-211-labeled radiotherapeutics: an emerging approach to targeted alpha-particle radiotherapy. Curr Pharm Des. 2000;6(14):1433–55.

35. Zalutsky MR, et al. High-level production of alpha-particle-emitting (211)At and preparation of (211) At-labeled antibodies for clinical use. J Nucl Med. 2001;42(10):1508–15.

36. Johnson EL, et al. Quantitation of ^{211}At in small volumes for evaluation of targeted radiotherapy in animal models. Nucl Med Biol. 1995;22(1):45–54.

37. Zalutsky MR, Bigner DD. Radioimmunotherapy with alpha-particle emitting radioimmunoconjugates. Acta Oncol. 1996;35(3):373–9.

38. Larsen RH, Wieland BW, Zalutsky MR. Evaluation of an internal cyclotron target for the production of

[211]At via the [209]Bi (alpha,2n)211 at reaction. Appl Radiat Isot. 1996;47(2):135–43.

39. Zalutsky MR, Narula AS. Astatination of proteins using an N-succinimidyl tri-n-butylstannyl benzoate intermediate. Int J Rad Appl Instrum A. 1988;39(3): 227–32.

40. Atcher RW, Friedman AM, Hines JJ. An improved generator for the production of [212]Pb and [212]Bi from [224]Ra. Int J Rad Appl Instrum A. 1988;39(4): 283–6.

41. McDevitt MR, et al. An [225]Ac/[213]Bi generator system for therapeutic clinical applications: construction and operation. Appl Radiat Isot. 1999;50(5):895–904.

42. Ma D, et al. Rapid preparation of short-lived alpha particle emitting radioimmunopharmaceuticals. Appl Radiat Isot. 2001;55(4):463–70.

43. Henriksen G, et al. Sterically stabilized liposomes as a carrier for alpha-emitting radium and actinium radionuclides. Nucl Med Biol. 2004;31(4):441–9.

44. Bayer-HealthCare. Bayer's investigational compound radium-223 chloride met its primary endpoint of significantly improving overall survival in a phase III trial in patients with castration-resistant prostate cancer that has spread to the bone. 6 June 2011. http://pharma.bayer.com/html/pdf/news_room115. pdf. Last accessed 5 June 2012.

45. Nilsson S, et al. Phase I study of Alpharadin™ ([223]Ra), an alpha-emitting bone-seeking agent in cancer patients with skeletal metastases. Oral presentation, annual congress of the EANM, Helsinki, September 8, 2004. Eur J Nucl Med Mol Imaging. 2004;31(S2):290.

46. Nilsson S, et al. Bone-targeted radium-223 in symptomatic, hormone-refractory prostate cancer: a randomised, multicentre, placebo-controlled phase II study. Lancet Oncol. 2007;8(7):587–94.

47. Nilsson S, et al. First clinical experience with α-emitting radium-223 in the treatment of skeletal metastases. Clin Cancer Res. 2005;11(12):4451–9.

48. Allen BJ, Blagojevic N. Alpha- and beta-emitting radiolanthanides in targeted cancer therapy: the potential role of terbium-149. Nucl Med Commun. 1996;17(1):40–7.

49. Mausner LF, Straub RF, Srivastava SC. The in vivo generator for radioimmunotherapy. J Label Compd Radiopharm. 1989;26(1–12):498–500.

50. Yong K, Brechbiel MW. Towards translation of [212]Pb as a clinical therapeutic; getting the lead in! Dalton Trans. 2011;40(23):6068–76.

51. Craig FE, Foon KA. Flow cytometric immunophenotyping for hematologic neoplasms. Blood. 2008; 111(8):3941–67.

52. Berger M, Shankar V, Vafai A. Therapeutic applications of monoclonal antibodies. Am J Med Sci. 2002;324(1):14–30.

53. Uchiyama T, et al. Interleukin-2 receptor (Tac antigen) expressed on adult T cell leukemia cells. J Clin Invest. 1985;76(2):446–53.

54. Waldmann TA, et al. Radioimmunotherapy of interleukin-2R alpha-expressing adult T-cell leukemia

with yttrium-90-labeled anti-Tac. Blood. 1995; 86(11):4063–75.

55. Zhang Z, et al. Effective treatment of a murine model of adult T-cell leukemia using 211At-7G7/B6 and its combination with unmodified anti-Tac (daclizumab) directed toward CD25. Blood. 2006; 108(3):1007–12.

56. Andrews RG, Torok-Storb B, Bernstein ID. Myeloid-associated differentiation antigens on stem cells and their progeny identified by monoclonal antibodies. Blood. 1983;62(1):124–32.

57. Dinndorf PA, et al. Expression of normal myeloid-associated antigens by acute leukemia cells. Blood. 1986;67(4):1048–53.

58. Griffin JD, et al. A monoclonal antibody reactive with normal and leukemic human myeloid progenitor cells. Leuk Res. 1984;8(4):521–34.

59. Jilani I, et al. Differences in CD33 intensity between various myeloid neoplasms. Am J Clin Pathol. 2002;118(4):560–6.

60. van der Jagt RHC, et al. Localization of radiolabeled antimyeloid antibodies in a human acute leukemia xenograft tumor model. Cancer Res. 1992;52(1): 89–94.

61. Schwartz MA, et al. Dose-escalation trial of M195 labeled with iodine 131 for cytoreduction and marrow ablation in relapsed or refractory myeloid leukemias. J Clin Oncol. 1993;11(2):294–303.

62. Tanimoto M, et al. Restricted expression of an early myeloid and monocytic cell surface antigen defined by monoclonal antibody M195. Leukemia. 1989; 3(5):339–48.

63. Co MS, et al. Chimeric and humanized antibodies with specificity for the CD33 antigen. J Immunol. 1992;148(4):1149–54.

64. Caron PC, et al. Biological and immunological features of humanized M195 (anti-CD33) monoclonal antibodies. Cancer Res. 1992;52(24):6761–7.

65. Caron P, et al. A phase 1B trial of humanized monoclonal antibody M195 (anti-CD33) in myeloid leukemia: specific targeting without immunogenicity. Blood. 1994;83(7):1760–8.

66. Caron PC, Dumont L, Scheinberg DA. Supersaturating infusional humanized anti-CD33 monoclonal antibody HuM195 in myelogenous leukemia. Clin Cancer Res. 1998;4(6):1421–8.

67. Mulford D. Antibody therapy for acute myeloid leukemia. Semin Hematol. 2008;45(2):104–9.

68. Dahlke MH, et al. The biology of CD45 and its use as a therapeutic target. Leuk Lymphoma. 2004;45(2): 229–36.

69. Nakano A, et al. Expression of leukocyte common antigen (CD45) on various human leukemia/lymphoma cell lines. Acta Pathol Jpn. 1990;40(2): 107–15.

70. Press OW, et al. Retention of B-cell-specific monoclonal antibodies by human lymphoma cells. Blood. 1994;83(5):1390–7.

71. Matthews DC, et al. Development of a marrow transplant regimen for acute leukemia using targeted

hematopoietic irradiation delivered by ^{131}I-labeled anti-CD45 antibody, combined with cyclophosphamide and total body irradiation. Blood. 1995;85(4): 1122–31.

72. Pagel JM, et al. ^{131}I-anti-CD45 antibody plus busulfan and cyclophosphamide before allogeneic hematopoietic cell transplantation for treatment of acute myeloid leukemia in first remission. Blood. 2006;107(5):2184–91.

73. Becker W, Goldenberg DM, Wolf F. The use of monoclonal antibodies and antibody fragments in the imaging of infectious lesions. Semin Nucl Med. 1994;24(2):142–53.

74. Gray-Owen SD, Blumberg RS. CEACAM1: contact-dependent control of immunity. Nat Rev Immunol. 2006;6(6):433–46.

75. Bunjes D, et al. Rhenium 188-labeled anti-CD66 (a, b, c, e) monoclonal antibody to intensify the conditioning regimen prior to stem cell transplantation for patients with high-risk acute myeloid leukemia or myelodysplastic syndrome: results of a phase I-II study. Blood. 2001;98(3):565–72.

76. Seitz U, et al. Preparation and evaluation of the rhenium-188-labelled anti-NCA antigen monoclonal antibody BW 250/183 for radioimmunotherapy of leukaemia. Eur J Nucl Med. 1999;26(10): 1265–73.

77. Zalutsky MR, et al. Labeling monoclonal antibodies and F(ab')2 fragments with the alpha-particle-emitting nuclide astatine-211: preservation of immunoreactivity and in vivo localizing capacity. Proc Natl Acad Sci U S A. 1989;86(18):7149–53.

78. Lambrecht RM, Tomiyoshi K, Sekine T. Radionuclide generators. Radiochim Acta. 1997;77(1–2):103–23.

79. Huneke RB, et al. Effective alpha-particle-mediated radioimmunotherapy of murine leukemia. Cancer Res. 1992;52(20):5818–20.

80. McDevitt MR, et al. Tumor therapy with targeted atomic nanogenerators. Science. 2001;294(5546): 1537–40.

81. Kennel SJ, et al. Evaluation of [225]Ac for vascular targeted radioimmunotherapy of lung tumors. Cancer Biother Radiopharm. 2000;15(3):235–44.

82. McDevitt MR, et al. Preparation of alpha-emitting [213]Bi-labeled antibody constructs for clinical use. J Nucl Med. 1999;40(10):1722–7.

83. Cember H, Johnson TE. Introduction to health physics. 4th ed. New York: McGraw-Hill; 2009.

84. Zhou H, et al. Radiation risk to low fluences of alpha particles may be greater than we thought. Proc Natl Acad Sci U S A. 2001;98(25):14410–5.

85. Jurcic JG, et al. Targeted alpha particle immunotherapy for myeloid leukemia. Blood. 2002;100(4): 1233–9.

86. Jurcic JG, et al. Radiolabeled anti-CD33 monoclonal antibody M195 for myeloid leukemias. Cancer Res. 1995;55(23 Suppl):5908s–10.

87. Jurcic JG, et al. Potential for myeloablation with yttrium-90-labeled HuM195 (anti-CD33): a phase

I trial in advanced myeloid leukemias. Blood. 1998; 92(10):613A.

88. Sgouros G, et al. Pharmacokinetics and dosimetry of an alpha-particle emitter labeled antibody: [213]Bi-HuM195 (anti-CD33) in patients with leukemia. J Nucl Med. 1999;40(11):1935–46.

89. Mulford DA, et al. Sequential therapy with cytarabine and Bismuth-213 ([213]Bi)-labeled-HuM195 (anti-CD33) for acute myeloid leukemia (AML). ASH Annu Meet Abstr. 2004;104(11):1790.

90. Rosenblat TL, et al. Sequential cytarabine and alpha-particle immunotherapy with bismuth-213-lintuzumab (HuM195) for acute myeloid leukemia. Clin Cancer Res. 2010;16(21):5303–11.

91. Rosenblat TL, et al. Phase I trial of the targeted alpha-particle nano-generator actinium-225 ([225]Ac)-HuM195 (anti-CD33) in acute myeloid leukemia (AML). ASH Annu Meet Abstr. 2007;110(11):910.

92. Miederer M, et al. Pharmacokinetics, dosimetry, and toxicity of the targetable atomic generator, [225]Ac-HuM195, in nonhuman primates. J Nucl Med. 2004;45(1):129–37.

93. Deal KA, et al. Improved in vivo stability of actinium-225 macrocyclic complexes. J Med Chem. 1999;42(15):2988–92.

94. Sofou S, et al. Engineered liposomes for potential alpha-particle therapy of metastatic cancer. J Nucl Med. 2004;45(2):253–60.

95. Sofou S, et al. Enhanced retention of the alpha-particle-emitting daughters of actinium-225 by liposome carriers. Bioconjug Chem. 2007;18(6):2061–7.

96. Allen C, et al. Controlling the physical behavior and biological performance of liposome formulations through use of surface grafted poly(ethylene glycol). Biosci Rep. 2002;22(2):225–50.

97. Jaggi JS, et al. Efforts to control the errant products of a targeted in vivo generator. Cancer Res. 2005; 65(11):4888–95.

98. Jaggi JS, et al. Renal tubulointerstitial changes after internal irradiation with alpha-particle-emitting actinium daughters. J Am Soc Nephrol. 2005;16(9): 2677–89.

99. Busquets MA, Alsina MA, Haro I. Peptides and liposomes: from biophysical to immunogenic studies. Curr Drug Targets. 2003;4(8):633–42.

100. Sofou S, Sgouros G. Antibody-targeted liposomes in cancer therapy and imaging. Expert Opin Drug Deliv. 2008;5(2):189–204.

101. Axworthy DB, et al. Cure of human carcinoma xenografts by a single dose of pretargeted yttrium-90 with negligible toxicity. Proc Natl Acad Sci U S A. 2000;97(4):1802–7.

102. Zhang M, et al. Pretargeting radioimmunotherapy of a murine model of adult T-cell leukemia with the alpha-emitting radionuclide, bismuth 213. Blood. 2002;100(1):208–16.

103. Zhang M, et al. Pretarget radiotherapy with an anti-CD25 antibody-streptavidin fusion protein was effective in therapy of leukemia/lymphoma

xenografts. Proc Natl Acad Sci U S A. 2003;100(4): 1891–5.

104. Paganelli G, et al. Two-step tumour targetting in ovarian cancer patients using biotinylated monoclonal antibodies and radioactive streptavidin. Eur J Nucl Med. 1992;19(5):322–9.

105. Paganelli G, et al. Three-step monoclonal antibody tumor targeting in carcinoembryonic antigen-positive patients. Cancer Res. 1991;51(21): 5960–6.

106. Paganelli G, Malcovati M, Fazio F. Monoclonal antibody pretargetting techniques for tumour localization: the avidin-biotin system. International workshop on techniques for amplification of tumour targeting. Nucl Med Commun. 1991; 12(3):211–34.

107. Chinol M, et al. Biochemical modifications of avidin improve pharmacokinetics and biodistribution, and reduce immunogenicity. Br J Cancer. 1998;78(2): 189–97.

108. Marshall D, et al. Polyethylene glycol modification of a galactosylated streptavidin clearing agent: effects on immunogenicity and clearance of a biotinylated anti-tumour antibody. Br J Cancer. 1996; 73(5):565–72.

109. McDevitt MR, et al. Tumor targeting with antibody-functionalized, radiolabeled carbon nanotubes. J Nucl Med. 2007;48(7):1180–9.

110. McDevitt MR, et al. PET imaging of soluble yttrium-86-labeled carbon nanotubes in mice. PLoS One. 2007;2(9):e907.

111. Zalutsky MR, et al. Clinical experience with alpha-particle emitting 211At: treatment of recurrent brain tumor patients with 211At-labeled chimeric antitenascin monoclonal antibody 81C6. J Nucl Med. 2008;49(1):30–8.

112. Andersson H, et al. Intraperitoneal alpha-particle radioimmunotherapy of ovarian cancer patients: pharmacokinetics and dosimetry of (211)At-MX35 F(ab')2—a phase I study. J Nucl Med. 2009;50(7):1153–60.

113. Hultborn R, et al. Pharmacokinetics and dosimetry of (211)AT-MX35 F(AB')(2) in therapy of ovarian cancer—preliminary results from an ongoing phase I study. Cancer Biother Radiopharm. 2006;21(4):395.

114. Kneifel S, et al. Local targeting of malignant gliomas by the diffusible peptidic vector 1,4,7,10-tetraazacyclododecane-1-glutaric acid-4,7,10-triacetic acid-substance P. Clin Cancer Res. 2006;12(12):3843–50.

115. Heeger S, et al. Alpha-radioimmunotherapy of B-lineage non-Hodgkin's lymphoma using 213Bi-labelled anti-CD19-and anti-CD20-CHX-A''-DTPA conjugates. Abstr Pap Am Chem Soc. 2003; 225:U261.

116. Allen BJ, et al. Intralesional targeted alpha therapy for metastatic melanoma. Cancer Biol Ther. 2005; 4(12):1318–24.

Radiophosphorus Treatment of Myeloproliferative Neoplasms

3

Edward B. Silberstein, L. Eugene, and S.R. Saenger[†]

Introduction

Sodium ^{32}P-phosphate (actually sodium dihydrogen phosphate; NaH_2PO_4) was the first therapeutic radiopharmaceutical employed in clinical medicine and has been used in numerous clinical settings, virtually all now obsolete except for a few remaining important indications in the treatment of myeloproliferative neoplasia. This chapter will review the history of radiophosphorus in medicine, the dosimetry of ^{32}P-phosphate, and important clinical applications of the radiopharmaceutical, as well as the controversy which arose around its potential for leukemogenesis and the current clinical role for sodium ^{32}P-phosphate.

History

Radiophosphorus, as phosphorus-30 and the radiophosphorus-based radiopharmaceutical sodium phosphate-32, has played a central role in the history of nuclear medicine. After the discovery of spontaneous decay or transmutation of

radioactive elements by Henri Becquerel in 1896, the first artificial transmutations were produced by Ernest Rutherford (1919) who bombarded certain of the lighter atoms, e.g., nitrogen and aluminum, with alpha particles, causing the ejection of protons or neutrons. The very first artificially produced radioisotope, phosphorus-30, was created by Irene Curie and Frederick Joliot in early 1934 by bombarding aluminum (^{27}Al) with alpha particles to produce ^{30}P ($t_{1/2} = 150$ s).

> It was at the beginning of 1934, while working on the emission of these positive electrons that we noticed a fundamental difference between this transmutation and all others so far produced; all the reactions of nuclear chemistry induced were instantaneous phenomena, explosions. But the positive electrons produced by aluminum under the action of a source of alpha rays continue to be emitted for some time after the removal of the source. The number of electrons decreased by half in three minutes [1].

Ernest Lawrence, inventor of the cyclotron, reproduced this French discovery shortly after learning of it and, bombarding 12 elements with deuterons in his cyclotron, produced 12 new radioisotopes, including ^{32}P. The physical properties of ^{32}P (Table 3.1) suggested new therapeutic uses of this radioisotope to the Berkeley investigators [2].

Metabolism of ^{32}P-Orthophosphate

Studies by Ernest Lawrence's brother, John, with ^{32}P indicated that neoplastic tissues have greater uptake and exchange of phosphorus than do

E.B. Silberstein, M.D. (✉)
The University Hospital, University of Cincinnati Medical Center, 234 Goodman Street, Cincinnati, OH 45219, USA
e-mail: silbereb@uchealth.com

L. Eugene • S.R.Saenger
†(Deceased)

Table 3.1 Physical properties of phosphorus-32

Emission	Beta
Mean betas/disintegration	1
Maximum beta energy	1.710 MeV
Mean beta energy	0.6948 MeV
Maximum range in tissue	8 mm
Mean range in tissue	3 mm
Physical half life	14.3 days

Principles of P32 Therapy in Polycythemia Vera

- Intravenous administration preferable
- High uptake in bones and neoplastic tissues
- Mean biological half life of 39.2 ± 4.5 days (70%)
- Incorporation to DNA resulting in apoptosis and cell death
- Prolonging median survival up to 13–16 years

---

normal tissues, although the total phosphorus content of neoplastic and normal tissues is equivalent [3–5]. Within 6–24 h of parenteral administration of ^{32}P-orthophosphate, bone concentrations exceed those of muscle, skin, or fat by a factor of 4–6, increasing to 6–10 after 3 days. Liver and spleen ratios to muscle, fat, or skin are of the same order of magnitude [6, 7].

In addition to the damage to nuclear DNA caused by the beta particle emitted by ^{32}P (as orthophosphate incorporated into DNA and RNA), the decay of ^{32}P in the DNA molecule to ^{32}S is another potential mechanism by which DNA alteration could result in cell apoptosis and death. No acute radiation syndrome has been described as occurring with the dosages of ^{32}P which have been employed to treat myeloproliferative neoplasms. Since the required intravenous dose is 75% of that given orally, the former route is preferable, although there is the potential of high skin irradiation with sloughing if the dose infiltrates subcutaneously.

Dosimetry

Studies of whole blood and plasma retention of ^{32}P in patients with polycythemia vera are consistent with a two compartment model, with biological mean half lives of 1.7 ± 0.7 and 22.5 ± 5.9 days for whole blood and 0.8 ± 0.5 and 20.0 ± 5.1 days for plasma [8]. However, the whole body retention curves are monoexponential with a mean biological half life of 39.2 ± 4.5 days with 70% decaying in the body [7]. The biological half life in the iliac marrow, 9 days, and the sternum, 7 days, are not significantly different.

Dosimetry calculations are complicated by the situation in which two interpenetrating nonequilibrium depositions exist, in trabecular bone and marrow. There is also a small contribution to the marrow dose in trabecular bone by cortical radiophosphate. Furthermore, one should account for the absorbed dose in the Haversian canals of compact bone, central holes about 11–55 μm in radius surrounded by concentric layers of calcified lamellar bone. Haversian canals contain blood cells, capillaries, and osteoblasts [9].

Several decades ago, Spiers et al. calculated a total absorbed dose to marrow in trabecular bone as about 6.49 mGy/MBq or 24 rad/mCi of ^{32}P-phosphate injected, with 2.7 mGy/MBq (10 rad/mCi) coming from trabecular bone, 3.5 mGy/MBq (13 rad/mCi) from marrow, and 0.27 mGy/MBq (1 rad/mCi) from cortical bone [8]. Twenty years later, the Radiation Internal Dose Information Center (RIDIC) quantitated the red marrow dose as 7.6 mGy/MBq (28 rad/mCi) and the bone surface dose as 1.0 mGy/MBq (3.7 rad/mCi) [10], corresponding closely to the data of Spiers et al. [8].

Clinical Uses of ^{32}P-Orthophosphate

The first therapeutic use of ^{32}P occurred when John Lawrence and his research team injected sodium ^{32}P-phosphate into a patient with chronic lymphocytic leukemia in 1936. ^{32}P has been employed in chronic granulocytic leukemia,

Hodgkin's and non-Hodgkin's lymphomas, multiple myeloma, and mycosis fungoides, unfortunately with little clinical effectiveness detected. Pain reduction from osseous metastases and myeloma has been reported with the use of ^{32}P, lasting 3–9 months [11, 12], although newer radiotracers are now in use which have at least equal efficacy and probably less myelosuppression, such as ^{89}Sr and ^{153}Sm-lexidronam. ^{32}P as chromic phosphate has also been employed to treat the arthropathy of hemophilia, as well as malignant pleural and peritoneal effusions, but more effective therapies have also replaced these uses of radiophosphorus.

In 1940, Lawrence described his favorable experience with ^{32}P in five patients with leukemia and two with polycythemia vera [13]. One patient with polycythemia vera who was treated with ^{32}P between 1936 and 1938 was still alive at the time of a memoir that Lawrence authored 42 years later [14]. The ability of ^{32}P therapy to prolong median survival of patients with polycythemia vera up to 13–16 years has been well documented [15–23].

Myeloproliferative Neoplasms

The marrow disorders known as polycythemia vera and essential thrombocythemia were first described in 1892 [24] and 1934 [25], respectively. In 1951, William Dameshek first recognized the significant parallels in the clinical and laboratory manifestations of these disorders (Table 3.2) [26] and grouped them with chronic myeloid leukemia, primary myelofibrosis, and erythroleukemia, first using the term myeloproliferative disorder [27].

The most recent diagnostic criteria for both disorders, produced by the World Health Organization, appear in Tables 3.3 and 3.4 [28]. In evaluating the natural history and efficacy of therapy for these disorders, it is necessary that the correct disease has been treated. Hence, data on these disorders produced prior to the Polycythemia Vera Study Group efforts to establish diagnostic criteria may be suspect [29]. The chronic myeloproliferative disorders have been characterized

Table 3.2 Clinicopathologic commonalities of polycythemia vera and essential thrombocythemia as myeloproliferative neoplasms [26]

- Abnormal multipotent hematopoietic progenitor cell
- Dominance of the abnormal clone over normal clones
- Abnormalities of chromosomes 1, 8, 9, 13, 20
- Marrow hypercellularity and megakaryocytic dysplasia
- Hematopoietic growth factor hypersensitivity
- Resistance to apoptosis
- Growth factor independent (endogenous colony formation)
- Altered production of one or more of the formed elements of the blood
- Thrombosis and hemorrhage
- Myelofibrosis
- Extramedullary hematopoiesis
- Transformation but at low and differing frequencies
- Expression of JAK2 V617F, overexpression of PRV-1 mRNA, and impaired expression or mutation of Mpl, but not in all patients

Table 3.3 WHO diagnostic criteria for polycythemia vera[a] [28]

Major criteria

Hemoglobin > 18.5 g/dL in men or 16.5 g/dL in women or other evidence of increased red blood cell volume

Presence of JAK2 V617F or other functionally similar mutation, e.g., JAK2 exon 12 mutation

Minor criteria

Bone marrow biopsy showing hypercellularity for age with trilineage growth with prominent erythroid, myeloid, and megakaryocytic proliferation

Serum erythropoietin level below the reference range for normal

Endogenous erythroid colony formation in vitro

[a]The diagnosis of polycythemia vera requires the presence of both major criteria and one minor criterion or the presence of the first major criterion together with two minor criteria

based largely on anecdotal reports, as having several hypothetical sequential phases [30, 31]. These include an initially asymptomatic proliferative phase consisting of marked increases in disease-specific intramedullary hematic elements; a "metastatic" phase [31] in which monoclonal expansion of a pluripotential hematic progenitor cell increases greatly in the marrow; a compensated or inactive period; a spent phase with migration to extramedullary sites, often the

Table 3.4 WHO diagnostic criteria for essential thrombocythemia[a] [28]

Criteria
Sustained platelet count $\geq 450 \times 10^9/L$
Bone marrow biopsy showing proliferation mainly of the megakaryocytic lineage with increased numbers of enlarged, mature megakaryocytes
No significant increase or left shift of neutrophil granulopoiesis or erythropoiesis
Not meeting World Health Organization criteria for polycythemia vera, primary myelofibrosis, BCR-ABL1 positive chronic myelogenous leukemia, myelodysplastic syndrome, or other myeloid neoplasm
Demonstration of JAK2 V7617F or other clonal marker, or, in the absence of JAK2 V7617F, no evidence of reactive thrombocytosis

[a]Diagnosis requires meeting all criteria

spleen, liver, and thorax, usually accompanied by myelofibrosis; and then acute leukemia. Since there were insufficient data underlying the formulation of this controversial simplification, this hypothetical sequence is not inevitable. It does reflect, however, an early controversy about the natural history of polycythemia vera and the probability of its malignant transformation to leukemia.

Leukemogenesis and ^{32}P-Phosphate

It was the belief of some of the first physicians to employ ^{32}P-phosphate for polycythemia vera that this radiopharmaceutical prolonged life to such an extent that the natural history of this marrow disease was revealed, and leukemia would result if the patient lived long enough [32–34]. In 1950, evidence was published examining the claim that acute leukemia was a feature of polycythemia vera in the absence of exposure to radiation or chemotherapy. Eighty-three published cases were analyzed where the coexistence of polycythemia vera and leukemia was claimed, but only 30 of these had unequivocal evidence of the diagnosis of polycythemia vera preceding acute leukemia, and 25 of these had been irradiated. Undisputable evidence for the absence of radiotherapy was present in only one patient of the remaining five, and the diagnosis of leukemia was not confirmed

histologically in this patient [35]. In a nonrandomized retrospective study with follow-up of 8–25 years, Modan and Lillienfeld documented in 1965 that the apparent leukemogenic effect of irradiation or ^{32}P was real and not a consequence of prolonged survival, since acute leukemia occurred in 11% of radiation treated patients, but only 1% in non-irradiated patients [36]. A contradictory study appeared in the same year when Halnan and Russell reported that the incidence of ^{32}P-induced leukemia in treated polycythemia patients was negligible [37]. This apparent conflict appears to have been resolved.

The observation was that the mean time to onset of ^{32}P-induced leukemia is 8.5 years, while most of Halnan and Russell's patients were followed for only 5 years [34, 38]. A more recent retrospective review from 1976 suggested that the prevalence of acute leukemia in ^{32}P-treated polycythemic patients was 10–20% [39]. The issue of ^{32}P as a leukemogenic agent was settled by the Polycythemia Vera Study Group PVSG-01 Trial comparing phlebotomy alone, phlebotomy plus chlorambucil, and phlebotomy plus [32]P. The actuarial risk of leukemia at 10 years was: phlebotomy, 1.5%; chlorambucil, 18%; [32]P (as phosphate), 16% [40]. It should be noted that the group in this PVSG trial which had phlebotomy alone was not entirely randomized or analyzed on an "intention to treat" basis, because patients felt to require cytoreductive therapy, e.g., due to high platelet or leukocyte counts especially in elderly patients, and those with vascular risk factors or thrombocytosis were excluded and received another form of therapy, so the true risk of leukemia in this group may have been underestimated [41, 42]. After the 15th year post-treatment, the risk of leukemia appears to decrease, but this could be due to statistical fluctuations in the low residual number of patients [43].

Current Recommended Treatment with ^{32}P-Phosphate

The therapy of polycythemia vera and essential thrombocythemia should be risk-adapted. It has been suggested that patient age >60 years,

Table 3.5 Initial therapeutic approach to polycythemia vera and essential thrombocythemia [46]

Risk categories	Polycythemia vera	Essential thrombocythemia
Low risk: (age <60 and no thrombosis history)	Low dose aspirin *plus* phlebotomy	Low dose aspirin
Low risk with extreme thrombocytosis (platelets >1,000 × 10⁹/uL)	Low dose aspirin if ristocetin cofactor[a] (von Willebrand factor) activity >30% plus phlebotomy	Low dose aspirin if ristocetin cofactor activity >30%
High risk (age >60 years and/or presence of thrombosis history)	Low dose aspirin *plus* phlebotomy *plus* hydroxyurea.	Low dose aspirin *plus* hydroxyurea

[a]This factor can be decreased in patients with very high platelet counts

Table 3.6 European leukemia net definition of resistance/intolerance to hydroxyurea in patients with polycythemia vera [28]

Need for phlebotomy to keep hematocrit <45% after 3 months of at least 2 g/day of hydroxyurea, or

Uncontrolled myeloproliferation (i.e., platelet count >400 × 10⁹/L and WBC count >10 × 10⁹) after 3 months of at least 2 g/day of hydroxyurea, or

Failure to reduce massive[a] splenomegaly by >50% as measured by palpation, or failure to completely relieve symptoms related to splenomegaly after 3 months of at least 2 g/day of hydroxyurea, or

Absolute neutrophil count <1.0 × 10⁹/L, or platelet count <100 × 10⁹/L, or hemoglobin < 10 g/L, at the lowest dose of hydroxyurea required to achieve a complete or partial clinicohematologic response,[b] or

Presence of leg ulcers or other unacceptable hydroxyurea-related nonhematologic toxicities, such as mucocutaneous manifestations, gastrointestinal symptoms, pneumonitis, or fever at any dose of hydroxyurea

[a]Organ extending >10 cm from the costal margin
[b]Complete response is defined as hematocrit <45% without phlebotomy, platelet count ≤400 × 10⁹/L, WBC count ≤10 × 10⁹/L, and no disease-related symptoms. Partial response is defined as hematocrit <45% without phlebotomy or response in three or more of the other criteria

hemoglobin below normal values, and a leukocyte count >15,000/µL are risk factors for survival, since the median survival of patients with both diseases was >20 years in the absence of all three factors, but about 9 years in the presence of two of the three [44, 45].

Therapeutic approaches must be directed at preventing thrombohemorrhagic complications and controlling vasomotor symptoms (e.g., erythromelalgia, headache, lightheadedness, atypical chest pain) and, in polycythemia, severe pruritus. A suggested initial approach to these two neoplasms appears in Table 3.5 [46].

Hydroxyurea is recommended to control platelet and leukocyte counts in high risk patients. There has been some concern about the leukemogenicity of hydroxyurea, but the most recent analyses of available data show no increased risk of leukemic transformation of polycythemia vera or essential thrombocythemia vera at cumulative dosages in

Table 3.7 European leukemia net definition of resistance/intolerance to hydroxyurea in patients with essential thrombocythemia [28]

Platelet count >600 × 10⁹/L after 3 months of at least 2 g/day or hydroxyurea (2.5 gm/day in patients with a body weight >80 kg), or

Platelet count >400 × 10⁹/L and WBC count <2.5 × 10⁹/L at any dose of hydroxyurea, or

Platelet count >400 × 10⁹/L and hemoglobin <10 g/dL at any dose of hydroxyurea, or

Presence of leg ulcers or other unacceptable mucocutaneous manifestations at any dose of hydroxyurea, or

Hydroxyurea-related fever

excess of 1,000 g of this drug [47, 48]. Hydroxyurea failure is defined in Tables 3.6 and 3.7. If this occurs, there are several options including pegylated interferon-alpha-2a, pipobroman, and busulfan for both diseases; anagrelide is also available for essential thrombocythemia [46].

Table 3.8 ^{32}P-Phosphate therapy of polycythemia vera (PV)[a] and essential thrombocythemia (ET) [49]

The radiopharmaceutical is administered intravenously after informed consent
Several successful regimens have been described: 74–111 MBq/m² body surface area (2–3 mCi/m²) with maximum upper activity limit of 185 MBq (5 mCi)
3.7 MBq/kg body weight (0.1 mCi/kg) with maximum upper activity limit of 260 MBq (7 mCi); some investigators recommend a decrease in activity of 25% of patients over 80 years of age
Administration of a fixed lower dose of 111 MBq (3 mCi); in the absence of an adequate response (PV, hematocrit 45% or less ET, platelets <450 × 10⁹/L), retreat in 3 months with a 25% escalation of dosage. Repeat this dosage augmentation every 3 months until the desired response is achieved (maximum dosage for a single administration is 260 MBq (7 mCi))

[a]For polycythemia vera, phlebotomy is performed initially to decrease the hematocrit to 45–47%

Current Role of ^{32}P-Phosphate

For older patients with life expectancy less than 10 years who cannot tolerate the drugs listed above, who have vascular or other serious comorbid risk factors, are difficult to follow, cannot remember, or refuse to take the medications listed above, there remains a consensus that ^{32}P-phosphate retains an important role in treating polycythemia vera and essential thrombocythemia [28, 43, 44, 49]. The guidelines for the administration of intravenous ^{32}P-phosphate to treat polycythemia vera and essential thrombocythemia have changed little since their codification by the Polycythemia Vera Study Group and are reproduced in Table 3.8.

Conclusion

[32]P-phosphate was the first therapeutic radiopharmaceutical employed, with patient studies beginning in 1936, and continues to be an important form of treatment in selected patients with two myeloproliferative neoplasms, polycythemia vera and essential thrombocythemia. Because of its leukemogenic potential, ^{32}P-phosphate is now limited to patients, usually the elderly with vascular and other severe comorbid conditions, who are difficult to follow or who cannot or will not take or tolerate hydroxyurea and the other forms of therapy described above. For such patients, this treatment prolongs life as it does in all patients with these disorders. [15–23]

Possible Areas of Research

There are three methods in use of employing ^{32}P-phosphate to treat polycythemia vera and essential thrombocythemia (Table 3.8). An outcome study comparing these approaches to the use of ^{32}P-phosphate might be helpful in optimizing patient treatment.

Also a study of the natural history of these older patients given ^{32}P would seem to be important, given the longer life span of our population, to determine if the risk of leukemia remains sufficiently high that another form of treatment should be considered under a certain patient age. Since the numbers of such patients are small [50, 51], randomized study of alternate therapies for this age group will be difficult to perform.

References

1. Joliot-Curie I. Artificial production of radioactive elements. In: Nobel lectures, chemistry. Amsterdam: Elsevier; 1966. pp. 1922–1941.
2. Heilbron JL, Seidel RW, Wheaton BR. Lawrence and his laboratory. Berkeley: Berkeley National Laboratory; 1981.
3. Lawrence JH, Scott KG, Tuttle LW. Studies on leukemia with the aid of radioactive phosphorus. Int Clin. 1939;3:33–58.
4. Lawrence JH, Tuttle I, Scott W, et al. Studies on neoplasms with the aid of radioactive phosphorus. I-The total phosphorus metabolism of normal and leukemic mice. J Clin Invest. 1940;19:267–71.
5. Erf LA, Lawrence JH. Clinical studies with the aid of radioactive phosphorus. I. The absorption and distribution of radio-phosphorus in the blood and its

excretion by normal individuals and patients with leukemia. J Clin Invest. 1941;20:567–75.

6. Levenson SM, Adams MA, Rosen H, et al. Studies in phosphorus metabolism in man. J Clin Invest. 1953;32:497–509.

7. Low-Beer BVA, Blais RS, Scofield NE. Estimation of dosage for intravenously administered ^{32}P. Am J Roentgenol. 1952;67:28–41.

8. Spiers FW, Beddoe AH, King SD, et al. The absorbed dose to bone marrow in the treatment of polycythemia by ^{32}P. Br J Radiol. 1976;49:133–40.

9. Akabani G. Absorbed dose calculations in Haversian canals for several beta-emitting radionuclides. J Nucl Med. 1993;34:1361–6.

10. Stabin MG, Stubbs JB, Toohey RE. Radiation dose estimates for radiopharmaceuticals. Oak Ridge Institute for Science and Education, Oak Ridge, TN, 30 April 1996. p. 17.

11. Navarro-Izquierdo AL, Baringo T, Dominguez J, et al. Metabolic curietherapy with P-32 in bone metastases with breast cancer. Rev Esp Oncol. 1980;27:101–8.

12. Lawrence JH, Wasserman LR. Multiple myeloma: a study of 24 patients treated with radioactive isotopes (^{32}P and ^{89}Sr). Ann Intern Med. 1950;33:41–55.

13. Lawrence JH. Nuclear physics and therapy: preliminary report on a new method for the treatment of leukemia and polycythemia. Radiology. 1940;35:51–60.

14. Lawrence JH. Early experiences in Nuclear Medicine. J Nucl Med. 1979;20:561–4.

15. Stroebel CF. Current status of radiophosphorus therapy. Proc Staff Meet Mayo Clin. 1954;29:1–4.

16. Reed C. Polycythemia rubra vera. Med J Aust. 1965;2:654–8.

17. Szur L, Lewis SM. The haematological complications of polycythemia vera patients treated with radioactive phosphorus. Br J Radiol. 1966;39:122–30.

18. Duggan HE. Polycythemia rubra vera and radioactive phosphorus-90 patients. J Can Assoc Radiol. 1966;17:4–9.

19. Watkins PJ, Fairly GH, Scott RB. Treatment of polycythemia vera. Br Med J. 1967;2:664–6.

20. Harmath JB, Ledlie EM. Survival of polycythemia vera patients treated with radioactive phosphorus. Br Med J. 1967;2:146–8.

21. Osgood EE. The case for ^{32}P in treatment of polycythemia vera. Blood. 1968;32:492–9.

22. Campbell A, Emery EW, Godlee JN, et al. Diagnosis and treatment of primary polycythemia. Lancet. 1970;1:1074–7.

23. Wasserman LR. The treatment of polycythemia vera. Semin Hematol. 1976;13:57–78.

24. Vaquez H. Sur une forme speciale de cyanose s'accompagnant d'hyperglobulie excessive et persistante. C R Soc Biol (Paris). 1892;44:384–8.

25. Epstein E, Goedel A. Haemorrhagische thrombocythamie bei vasculare schrumpf-milz. Virchow Archiv Abteilung. 1934;293:233–47.

26. Zhan H, Spivak JL. The diagnosis and management of polycythemia vera, essential thrombocythemia, and primary myelofibrosis in the JAK2 V617F era. Clin Adv Hematol Oncol. 2009;7:334–42.

27. Dameshek W. Some speculations on the myeloproliferative syndromes. Blood. 1951;6:372–5.

28. Barbui T, Barosi G, Birgegard G, et al. Philadelphia-negative classical myeloproliferative neoplasms: Critical concepts and management recommendations from European LeukemiaNet. J Clin Oncol. 2011;29:761–70.

29. Dameshek W. Physiopathology and course of polycythemia as related to therapy. JAMA. 1950;142:790–7.

30. Wasserman LR. Polycythemia vera—its course and treatment; relation to myeloid metaplasia and leukemia. Bull N.Y. Acad Med. 1954;30:343–75.

31. Gilbert HS. Modern treatment strategies in polycythemia vera. Semin Hematol. 2003;40 Suppl 1:26–9.

32. Lawrence JH, Berlin NI, Huff RL. The nature and treatment of polycythemia. Medicine. 1953;32:323–88.

33. Osgood EE. Contrasting incidence of acute monocytic, and granulocytic leukemia in ^{32}P treated patients with polycythemia vera and chronic lymphocytic leukemia. J Lab Clin Med. 1964;64:560–73.

34. Spivak JL. Polycythemia vera: myths, mechanisms and management. Blood. 2002;100:4272–90.

35. Schwartz SO, Ehrlich L. The relationship of polycythemia to leukemia: A critical review. Acta Med Scand. 1950;4:129–47.

36. Modan B, Lillienfeld AM. Polycythemia vera and leukemia—the role of radiation treatment. Medicine. 1965;44:305–44.

37. Halnan KE, Russell MH. Comparison of survival and causes of death in patients managed with and without radiotherapy. Lancet. 1965;1:760–3.

38. Brandt L, Anderson H. Survival and risk of leukemia in polycythemia vera and essential thrombocythaemia treated with oral radiophosphorus: are safer drugs available? Eur J Hematol. 1995;54:21–6.

39. Landaw SA. Acute leukemia in polycythemia vera. Semin Hematol. 1976;13:33–48.

40. Berk PD, Wasserman LR, Fruchtman SM, et al. Treatment of polycythemia vera: a summary of clinical trials conducted by the Polycythemia Vera Study Group. In: Wasserman LR, Berk PD, Berlin NI, editors. Polycythemia vera and the myeloproliferative diseases. Philadelphia, PA: Saunders; 1995. p. 166.

41. Pearson TC, Green AR, Reilly JT, et al. Letter to the editor: Leukemic transformation in polycythemia vera. Blood. 1998;92:1837–42.

42. Najean Y. Response to Pearson et al. Blood. 1998;92:1837–8.

43. Parmentier C. Use and risks of phosphorus-32 in the treatment of polycythemia vera. Eur J Nuc Med Mol Imaging. 2003;30:1413–7.

44. Gangat N, Strand J, Li CY, et al. Leucocytosis in polycythemia vera predicts both inferior survival and leukaemic transformation. Br J Haematol. 2007;138:354–8.

45. Gangat N, Wolanskyj AP. McClure RF et al Risk stratification for survival and leukemic transformation in essential thrombocythemia: A single institution study of 605 patients. Leukemia. 2007;21:270–6.

46. Tefferi A. Polycythemia vera and essential thrombocythemia: 2011 update on diagnosis, risk-stratification, and management. Am J Hematol. 2011;86:293–301.

47. Stock W, Godwin J, et al. Leukemogenic risk of hydroxyurea therapy in polycythemia vera, essential thrombocythemia, and myeloid metaplasia with myelofibrosis. Am J Hematol. 1996;52:42–6.

48. Bjorkholm M, Derolf AR, Hultcrantz M, et al. Treatment-related factors for transformation to acute myeloid leukemia and myelodysplastic syndromes in myeloproliferative neoplasms. J Clin Oncol. 2011;29: 2410–5.

49. Tennvall J, Brans B. EANM procedure guideline for 32P phosphate treatment of myeloproliferative diseases. Eur J Nucl Med Mol Imag. 2007;34: 1324–7.

50. Tefferi A. Personal communication. 27 April 2011.

51. Spivak J. Personal communication. 27 April 2011.

Radionuclide Therapy of Neuroendocrine Tumors

4

Andrew Mallia, Marco Maccauro, Ettore Seregni,
Chiara Bampo, Carlo Chiesa, and Emilio Bombardieri

Introduction

Neuroendocrine tumors (NETs) are a group of tumors which frequently express somatostatin receptors (SSTRs) and represent 1% of all neoplasms that may arise in the body. NETs of the gastro-entero-pancreatic tract (GEP NETs) and tumors of the sympatho-adrenal lineage are the most frequent tumors observed in clinical practice. Improved diagnostic techniques, both functional and anatomical, have resulted in an increased incidence of NETs. The term *neuroendocrine* defines cells that share common characteristics, such as the ability to take up and decarboxylate several amine precursors (APUD system), the absence of axons and synapses, the production of cell type-specific hormonal products and the demonstration of particular histopathological staining [1]. The variation in biological characteristics of these tumors poses considerable problems when deciding the optimal treatment strategies.

They frequently express trans-membrane G-protein-coupled peptide receptors, such as SSTRs, which bind the 14-amino-acid peptide somatostatin and its high-affinity 28-amino-acid precursor. Of the five major subtypes of SSTRs, $SSTR_1$, $SSTR_2$, and $SSTR_5$ are the ones most commonly expressed in NETs even though considerable variation may exist [1, 2]. Neuroendocrine cells set up the so-called diffuse endocrine system.

NETs are classified on the basis of their anatomical and clinical features and include:

1. NETs of the GEP, known as the largest endocrine organ of the body with at least 16 different types of endocrine cells
2. Tumors of the sympatho-adrenal lineage (pheochromocytomas (PCCs), paragangliomas (PGLs), and neuroblastomas)
3. Medullary thyroid carcinoma of the thyroid
4. Pituitary tumors
5. NETs of the lung
6. Multiple neuroendocrine neoplasms (MEN1, MEN 2A, MEN 2B) [1]

Peptide-receptor radionuclide therapy (PRRT) using somatostatin radiolabeled analogues indium-111(^{111}In)-DTPA-octreotide, yttrium-90 (^{90}Y)-DOTA-TOC, lutetium-177 (^{177}Lu) DOTA-TATE, and yttrium-90 (^{90}Y)-DOTA-TATE for GEP NETs and radiolabeled meto-iodo-benzyl-guanidine (MIBG) (iodine-131 (^{131}I)-MIBG) for NETs of the sympatho-adrenal system have shown promising overall tumor response rates. They appear to be well tolerated by patients with very few side-effects reported. Particular attention

A. Mallia
School of Specialization in Nuclear Medicine, University of Milano, Milan, Italy

M. Maccauro • E. Seregni • C. Bampo • C. Chiesa
E. Bombardieri (✉)
Department of Nuclear Medicine,
Fondazione IRCCS Istituto Nazionale Tumori,
Milan, Italy
e-mail: emilio.bombardieri@istitutotumori.mi.it

C. Aktolun and S.J. Goldsmith (eds.), *Nuclear Medicine Therapy: Principles and Clinical Applications*,
DOI 10.1007/978-1-4614-4021-5_4, © Springer Science+Business Media New York 2013

57

to patient selection, pre-therapy preparation, and post-therapy follow-up are essential to ensure optimal treatment efficacy. Various dosimetric calculations are increasingly being employed in PRRT and iodine-131 (^{131}I)-MIBG protocols with the aim of personalizing the therapy for the single patient and the radiopharmaceutical used. The use of more specific somatostatin analogues, combination and locoregional therapies in PRRT, and the administration of higher individual doses for iodine-131 (^{131}I)-MIBG represent the future for the treatment of NETs.

This chapter will focus on the GEP NETs and tumors of the sympatho-adrenal lineage, since they are the most frequent tumors observed in clinical practice. Radionuclide therapy of medullary carcinoma of thyroid is detailed in another chapter. Nuclear medicine therapy of NETs has been employed to treat a good number of patients, and clinical evidence has given us encouraging results with significant objective responses.

Gastro-Entero-Pancreatic Tracts

GEP NETs represent 2% of all gastrointestinal tumors with a clinical incidence of 2.5–5 cases/100,000 per year. They include the serotonin secreting tumors, known as *carcinoids* that are predominantly of enterochromaffin cell origin. Two thirds of carcinoid tumors occur somewhere along the gastrointestinal tract. The small intestine is the most frequent location, followed by the lungs or bronchi, rectum, appendix, and stomach. Bronchial carcinoid tumors account for approximately 1–2% of all lung malignancies in adults and roughly 20–30% of all carcinoid tumors. Carcinoid lung tumors represent the most indolent form of a spectrum of broncho-pulmonary NETs that includes small cell carcinoma of the lung as its most malignant member and several other forms of intermediately aggressive tumors, such as atypical carcinoid. They may be located centrally or peripherally with radiological findings being related to bronchial obstruction since most are centrally located. Peripheral bronchial carcinoids appear as solitary nodules.

Most carcinoid tumors are indolent and slow-growing but a small proportion metastasize and are difficult to manage. They may secrete various bioactive compounds, including serotonin and bradykinin, resulting in the carcinoid syndrome, which includes bronchospasm, diarrhea, skin flushing, and cardiac abnormalities. Treatment is with surgical removal, with poor responses seen to chemotherapeutic agents. Symptomatic relief of carcinoid syndrome from metastatic disease has been achieved by administration of octreotide, which is administered subcutaneously or intra-muscularly.

Pancreatic NETs may be classified as functioning or nonfunctioning, depending on hormone secretion (insulinoma, gastrinoma, VIPoma, glucagonoma, and somatostatinoma). In case of secretion, they display the related syndrome [3].

NETs of Sympatho-Adrenal Lineage

The other important groups of NETs are those of the sympatho-adrenal lineage, including *neuroblastoma*, PCC, and PGLs.

Neuroblastoma is the most common extracranial solid tumor in childhood and the most common cancer in infancy. It is usually localized in one of the adrenal glands but it can also develop in nerve tissues in the neck, chest, abdomen, or pelvis. About 50–60% of children have metastases at the time of diagnosis.

PCCs arise from the cells of the sympathetic nervous system and 90% of tumor masses are located in the adrenal medulla. They can be bilateral and familial, associated with multiple endocrine syndrome type 2 (MEN2 A-B), von Hipple-Lindau disease, and neurofibromatosis type 1.

All extra-adrenal primary tumors are known as *paragangliomas* (PGLs). Approximately 10% of PCCs are malignant and PGLs are known to metastasize more often than adrenal PCCs (approximately 33%).

Rationale for Radionuclide Therapy

Treatment of NETs includes various options based on their biological characteristics: radical or debulking surgery when possible, hormone therapy, chemotherapy, radiotherapy, or palliation of painful metastases. Nuclear medicine therapy with radiopharmaceuticals is based on targeting cancer cells with specific radioactive probes which are able to localize the tumor mass and to deliver high radiation doses to the cancer cells [4]. This is the current concept utilized for radiometabolic therapy using somatostatin radiolabeled analogues for GEP NETs and radiolabeled MIBG for NETs of the sympatho-adrenal system. In the former, the target is the SSTR systems, and in the latter, the target is the pathway of catecholamine synthesis.

In both PRRT and MIBG therapy, the same or very similar radiopharmaceuticals are used for diagnosis and therapy. The diagnostic application, apart from allowing detection and localization of tumor masses, confirms the biological status of the tumor in terms of recognizing the ligand or precursor and thus predicts the feasibility and success of radiometabolic therapy.

Diagnosis of GEP NETs

NETs are relatively slow-growing malignancies and usually are often not diagnosed until the disease is advanced. At diagnosis, 50% of patients show local invasion, lymph node involvement, and/or distant metastases. Functioning tumors are usually detected in earlier stages due to their hormone secretion that cause some characteristic syndromes [5].

The diagnosis of NETs should be based on the following: presence of tumor mass, clinical manifestations, peptide and amine secretion, circulating tumor markers, histopathology, radiological and nuclear medicine imaging. For GEP NETs, the commonest clinical manifestations include obstructive symptoms, such as abdominal pain, nausea and vomiting, syndromes due to hormonal hypersecretion, and symptoms related to the presence of distant metastases. Due to the slow-growing behavior of these tumors, the patient may remain asymptomatic for many years.

Biochemical markers such as serum Chromagranin A (CgA), neuron-specific enolase (NSE), pancreatic peptide (PP), human chorionic gonadotropin (hCG), and 24 h urinary 5-HIAA may aid in the diagnosis of NETs. CgA was found to be the most sensitive marker both for the diagnosis and for the follow-up of NETs [6]. This marker is contained in the secretory dense core granules of most neuroendocrine cells and is elevated with both functioning and nonfunctioning tumors. False-positive results are possible in patients with impaired renal function, chronic atrophic gastritis, treatment with proton-pump inhibitors, pregnancy, and Parkinson disease. Finally hormone provocation tests may be required. An example of this is the secretin test for the diagnosis of a gastrinoma [7].

The histopathological diagnosis allows the clinician to make optimal treatment decisions and may also be of prognostic value. The tissue obtained should be examined macroscopically (tumor size, number, necrosis, invasiveness) and microscopically, including the mitotic index. Immunohistochemical staining for CgA, Synaptophysin, and Ki67 must be undertaken. Staining for hormones such as insulin, gastrin, and SSTRs is optional [8]. Based on the information obtained from the histopathological evaluation, NETs may be classified according to the WHO criteria or the recently proposed ENETS-TNM staging and grading system [8, 9]. WHO classifies the tumors into: well-differentiated NETs (WDNETs), well-differentiated neuroendocrine carcinomas (WDNECs), poorly differentiated neuroendocrine carcinomas (PDNECs), mixed exocrine-endocrine carcinoma (MEEC), and tumor-like lesions (TLL) [9].

Features of Neuroendocrine Tumors

- Slow-growing differentiated tumors
- Most commonly seen in sympatho-adrenal lineage and C-cells of thyroid
- SSTRs, $SSTR_2$, and $SSTR_5$ being the ones most commonly expressed
- Local invasion, lymph node involvement, and/or distant metastases at initial diagnosis in 50%
- Functional imaging with ^{111}In-pentetreotide and ^{68}Ga-DOTA-TATE/NOC/TOC
- ^{131}I-MIBG or ^{123}I-MIBG imaging in some patients
- ^{18}F-FDG imaging in poorly differentiated tumors

Imaging

The radiological diagnosis of NETs can be performed by ultrasonography (US), computed tomography (CT), and magnetic resonance (MR). The sensitivity changes according to the size and the location of the tumors [10]. There is little difference in sensitivity between CT and MRI, although the former is probably superior in localizing the primary tumor and thoracic lesions, whereas the latter is better in characterizing liver lesions [10]. Both show a higher diagnostic value in visualizing lesions greater than 1–2 cm in size. Endoscopic ultrasonography (EUS) is the most sensitive method for diagnosing pancreatic NETs and a mean 90% detection rate has been reported. The sensitivity of EUS for duodenal tumors and lymph node metastases is lower (63%) [11].

The most sensitive imaging modality, particularly for metastatic disease, is functional imaging with radiolabeled SSTR analogues (planar scintigraphy, SPECT, SPECT/CT or PET, PET/CT) that also provide data reflecting the biological status of the tumor. These methods enable the physician to identify the tumor location, the expression of various receptors and radiotracer uptake, and accumulation [12]. As a general rule, if a tumor is imaged by radiolabeled SSTR analogues, it can be treated by radiolabeled SSTR analogues. A high uptake of the radiopharmaceutical indicates high receptor expression, usually associated with good cell differentiation. This feature is the fundamental indication for PRRT. On the other hand, poorly differentiated NETs do not express SSTRs and are not detected by imaging techniques using radiolabeled SSTR analogues.

At present, the most widely used radiolabeled somatostatin analogue for planar and SPECT imaging is indium-111 (^{111}In)-pentetreotide, commercially available as Octreoscan®. This modality depicts mainly well-differentiated tumors. Depending on the tumor type and receptor status, the diagnostic sensitivity is 60–99% and specificity is 85–98% [13, 14]. This sensitiv-

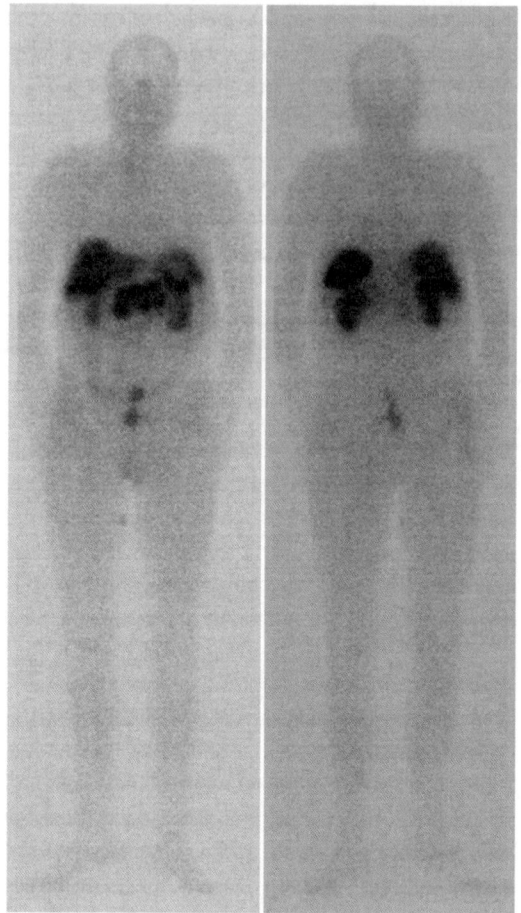

Fig. 4.1 Anterior (*left*) and posterior (*right*) views of an ^{111}In DTPA-octreotide (pentetreotide) scintigraphy showing SSR positive liver and abdominal lymph node metastases

ity is satisfactory for carcinoid tumors, gastrinomas, glucagonomas, and VIPomas but it is lower for insulinomas.

A typical imaging protocol includes planar images at 4–6 h p.i. with planar and SPECT images at 24 h p.i. (Fig. 4.1). The physiological distribution of the radiopharmaceutical in a variety of benign conditions (autoimmune diseases, granulomas, radiation pneumonitis, and bacterial infections) and non-NETs (lymphomas, melanomas, sarcomas, and breast cancer) could interfere with the interpretation of the images

[15]. Other limitations include the limited spatial resolution when dealing with small-sized lesions. These may be partially overcome by fusing SPECT images with images from computed tomography (SPECT/CT) [16].

Recent advances have led to the radiolabeling of somatostatin analogues with positron emitting isotopes such as gallium-68 (^{68}Ga). The most studied radiopharmaceuticals are ^{68}Ga-DOTA-TOC (DOTA-Phe-Tyr$_3$-octretide), ^{68}Ga-DOTA-TATE (DOTA-Tyr$_3$-Thr$_8$-octretide), and ^{68}Ga-DOTA-NOC (DOTA-NaI$_3$-octretide). ^{68}Ga has a half-life of 68.3 min and is produced by a commercially available germanium-68 (^{68}Ge) generator [17]. Compared with ^{111}In pentetreotide SPECT, PET imaging with ^{68}Ga. radiolabeled peptides has several advantages: better spatial resolution, whole-body scanning in a short time, and the added value of fusion imaging using a PET/CT hybrid scanner (Figs. 4.2–4.4). Data suggest that the diagnostic efficacy of ^{68}Ga-somatostatin analogues is higher than that of ^{111}In-pentetreotide especially in the presence of small lesions [18]. A drawback of this modality is that long interval studies cannot be obtained due to the short half-life of ^{68}Ga. This means that with the use of ^{68}Ga radiolabeled somatostatin, it is possible to detect the presence of SSTRs on the membrane surface while it is not possible to document internalization and retention of the radiolabel.

Other PET tracers are fluorine-18 (^{18}F)-DOPA and carbon-11 (^{11}C)-5-HTP. These rely on the ability of neuroendocrine cells to take up and decarboxylate monoamine precursors such as dihydroxyphenylalanine (DOPA) and 5-hydroxytryptophan (5-HTP), the precursor of serotonin, which is a prominent secretory product of NETs. Published results suggest that fluorine-18 (^{18}F)-DOPA can be superior to ^{111}In-pentetreotide but ^{68}Ga labeled peptides remain more sensitive in detecting WDNETs. Haug et al. recommend imaging with ^{68}Ga-DOTA-TATE should be employed as the first choice diagnostic method for NETs. ^{18}F-DOPA could be useful in those

patients with absent SSTR expression and elevated serotonin levels [19].

^{18}F-FDG scanning has gained great importance for tumor staging and treatment response evaluation for a number of tumor types. The method is based on glucose utilization by tumors. Fast-growing tumors, therefore, show high tracer uptake. Due to the low proliferation rate of NETs, ^{18}F-FDG is less suited for NET imaging and is only recommended in cases of poorly differentiated tumors which tend to grow faster. In these cases, FDG accumulation could be considered as a prognostic parameter [20].

Some GEP NETs can be imaged with ^{131}I-MIBG or ^{123}I-MIBG. Nevertheless, the overall diagnostic accuracy of MIBG-SPECT for GEP tumors and medullary carcinoma of the thyroid is lower than that using radiolabeled somatostatin analogues. ^{131}I-MIBG or ^{123}I-MIBG is considered the first choice radiopharmaceuticals to image PCCs, paragangliomas, and neuroblastomas.

Radiolabeled Somatostatin Analogues

The requirements for PRRT therapy include a peptide, a chelator, and a radionuclide. The half-life of somatostatin hormone is very short since it is readily attacked by aminopeptidases and endopeptidases [21]. Various synthetic analogues of somatostatin have been produced that retain a similar biological profile but are more resistant to plasma degradation and therefore have a longer half-life (90 min vs. 2 min) [22]. The first somatostatin analogue available for clinical use was octreotide, a synthetic peptide with a cyclic 8-amino-acid structure, followed by lanreotide, vapreotide, and depreotide. All display a high affinity for SSTR2 and SSTR5, a moderate affinity for SSTR3, and a low affinity for SSTR1. Lanreotide and octreotide also have a moderate affinity for SSTR4. The substitution of phenylalaline at position 3 with a tyrosine residue produced Tyr$_3$-Octreotide (TOC). This substitution increased

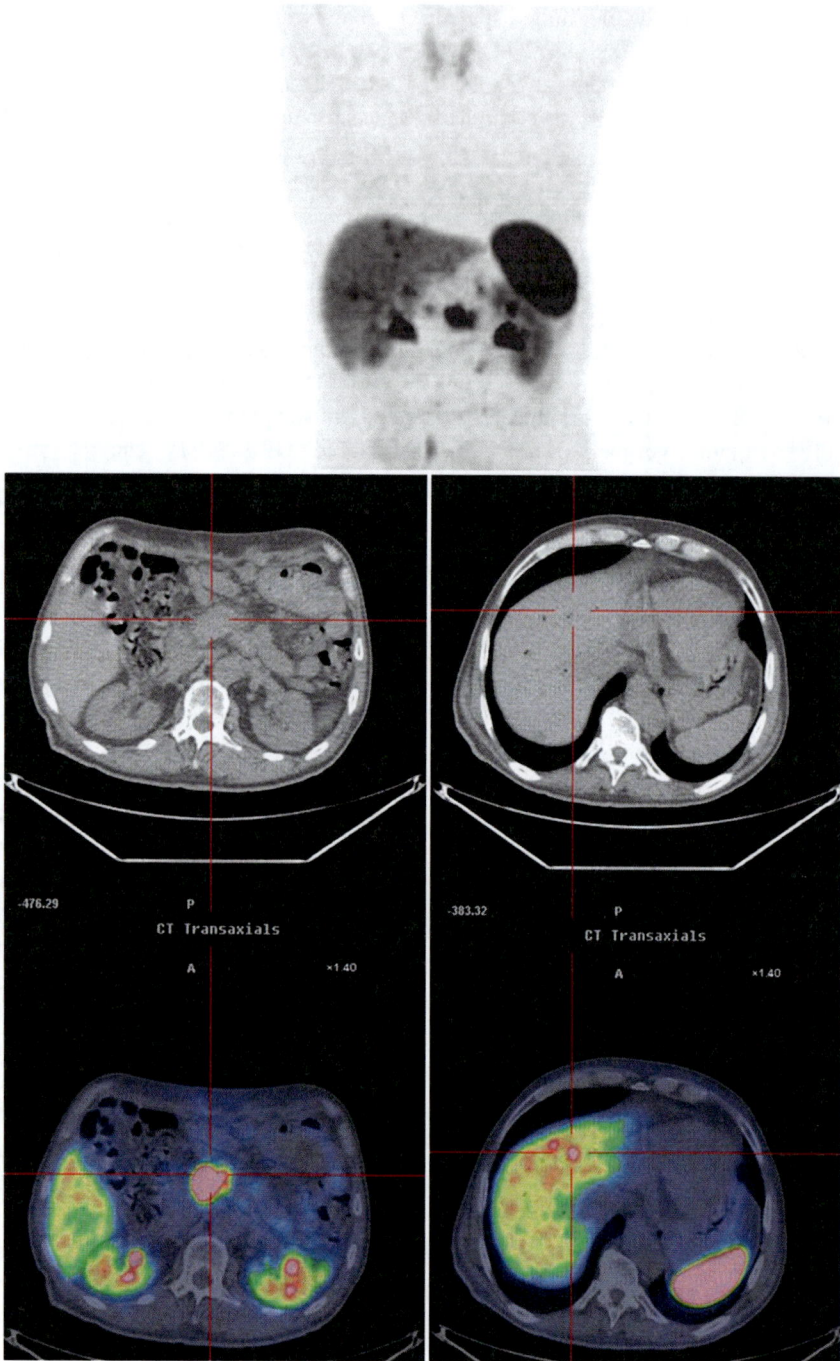

Fig. 4.2 ^{68}Ga-DOTATOC PET/CT showing a pancreatic NET with liver metastases. (By the courtesy of Annibale Versari, MD, Ospedale IRCCS St. Maria Nuova Reggio Emilia (I))

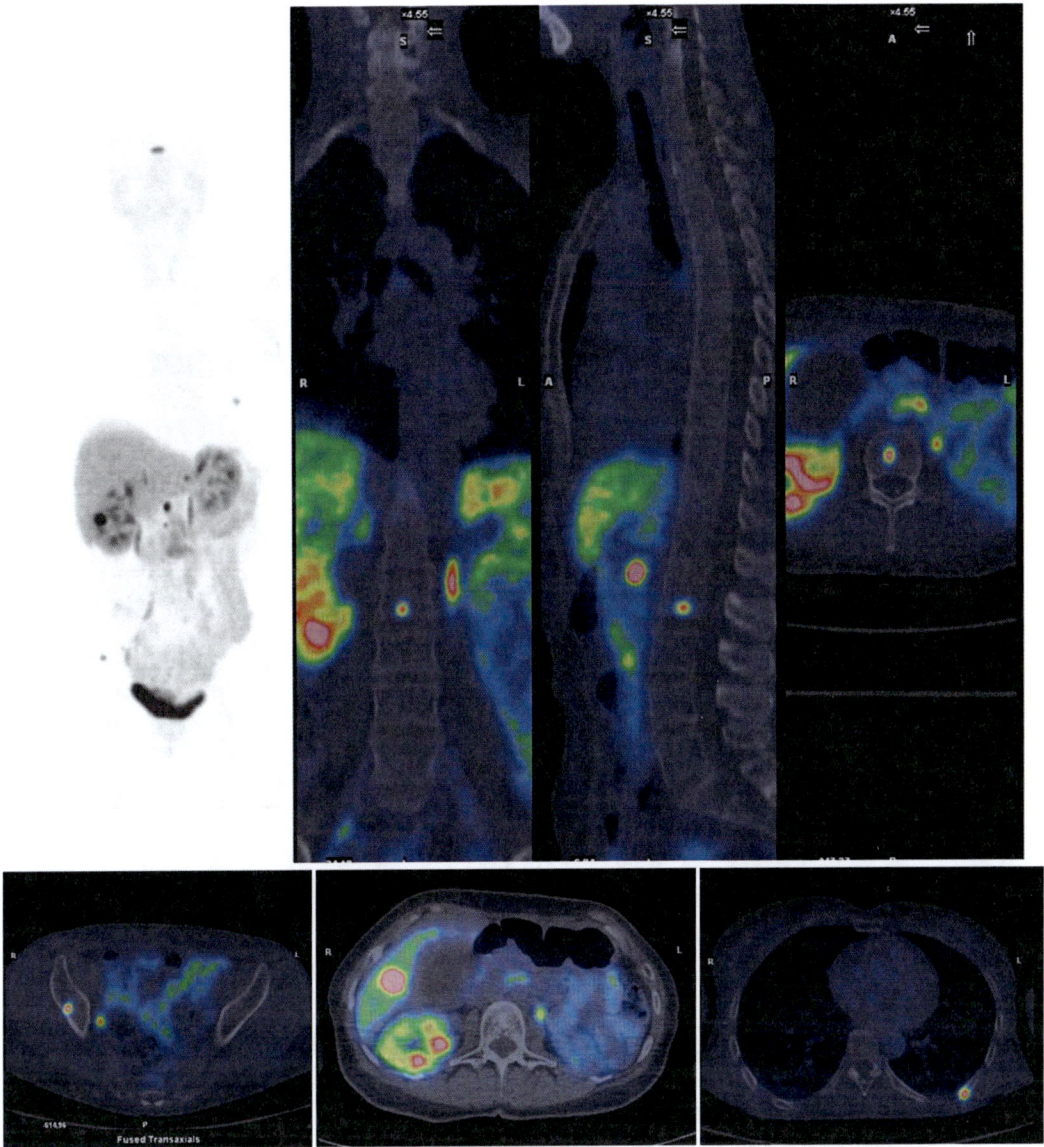

Fig. 4.3 ^{68}Ga-DOTATOC PET/CT showing multiple metastases from a pancreatic NET. (By the courtesy of Annibale Versari, MD, Ospedale IRCCS St. Maria Nuova Reggio Emilia (I))

the affinity toward SSTR2 receptors. Replacing the C-terminal threoninol with threonine results in the synthesis of TATE, which has been shown to have ninefold higher affinity for SSTR2 when compared to octreotide. Similar properties to octreotate have been described for NOC and BOC (BzThi$_3$, Thr$_8$-octreotide) [23, 24].

The somatostatin analogue is linked to a radionuclide by means of a stable connection in the form of a chelator such as diethylene-triamine-penta-acetic acid (DTPA) and tetra-aza-cyclo-dodecane-tetra-acetic acid (DOTA). The chelator affects the ligand-receptor affinity profile and

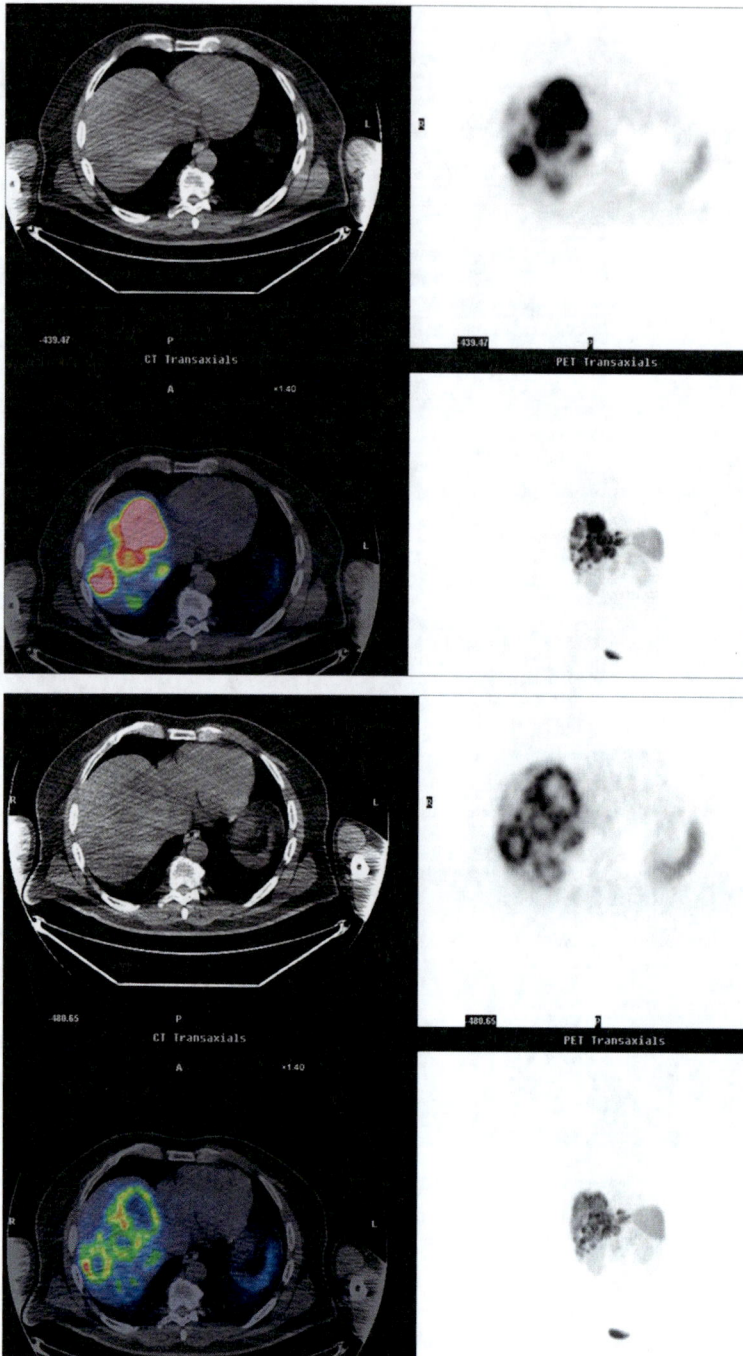

Fig. 4.4 ^{68}Ga-DOTATOC PET/CT in a patient with liver metastases from a neuroendocrine tumor of unknown origin: partial remission of liver lesions following treatment with one cycle of 90-Y-DOTATOC. (By the courtesy of Annibale Versari, MD, Ospedale IRCCS St. Maria Nuova Reggio Emilia (I))

Table 4.1 Physical properties of isotopes used in PRRT and MIBG therapy

Radioisotope	Emission	Half-life (days)	Maximum range (mm)	E_{max} (keV)
^{90}Y	β	2.67	12	2,280
^{177}Lu	$\beta + \Upsilon$	6.68	2	500 (β) 210 (Υ)
^{111}In	Auger + Υ	2.8	<1	0.5–25 (Auger) 171/245 (Υ)
^{131}I	$\beta + \Upsilon$	8.04	4	600 (β) 364 (Υ)

also influences the type of radionuclide, which can be attached to the ligand-receptor complex.

Radiopeptide Therapy

Radionuclides

The radionuclides commonly used for PRRT are indium-111 (^{111}In), yttrium-90 (^{90}Y), and lutetium-177 (^{177}Lu) (Table 4.1). The potential utility of ^{111}In is based on the Auger electron emissions with an E_{max} of 0.5–25 keV. Since Auger electrons travel very short distances (0.02–10 µm), they are effective only if the radiopharmaceutical is internalized into the cell, preferably close to the nucleus [25].

^{90}Y is a pure beta (β) particle emitter of high-energy electrons (maximum energy E_{max} of 2.3 MeV) with a physical half-life of 2.67 days and a maximum range in tissue of approximately 11 mm which results in crossfire involving neighboring cells [26].

^{177}Lu has physical half-life of 6.7 days and emits a shorter range (2 mm), lower energy (0.5 MeV) beta (β) particle making it more suitable for irradiation of smaller tumors. It also emits gamma radiation, which allows imaging to be performed after therapy [27] (Fig. 4.5a, b).

Since the majority of NETs express SSTRs, they are able to bind radiolabeled somatostatin analogues with a high affinity resulting in the formation of a peptide-receptor complex, which is then internalized into the cell. This promotes the retention of the radionuclide into the neoplastic cells and subsequent cell death directly, by causing DNA damage. Indirect cellular damage may also occur through the creation of free radicals or via spread of radiation energy beyond the target cell [25].

Principles of PRRT

- Three essentials: a peptide, a chelator, and a radionuclide
- Chelators: TOC, TATE, NOC
- 90Y: high-energy beta particle emitter, physical half-life 2.67 days
- 177Lu: low-energy short-range beta particle emitter, physical half-life 6.7 days
- 177Lu-DOTA-TATE: currently radiolabeled somatostatin of choice
- PRRT with fixed activities or individual activity based on dosimetry
- Multiple cycles of therapy may be needed for objective response and/or disease stabilization
- Radiotoxicity associated with kidney, bone marrow, and liver
- Future studies with alpha-emitters for intra-cavitary disseminated disease

Indium-111 (^{111}In)-DTPA-Octreotide

This was the first chelated radiolabeled somatostatin analogue used for PRRT in the mid-1990s. Animal studies have shown that high doses of ^{111}In-octreotide can inhibit the growth of liver metastases in rats [28]. Valkema et al. [29] treated 26 patients with GEP NETs tumors with high doses of ^{111}In-DTPA-octreotide, giving a total cumulative dose of more than 20 GBq. Two patients showed a 25–50% reduction in tumor size on CT scan (minor remission, MR) and 15 patients (58%) had stable disease (SD). None, however, had partial remission (PR).

In another study of 26 patients with GEP NETs by Anthony et al. [30], a PR was observed

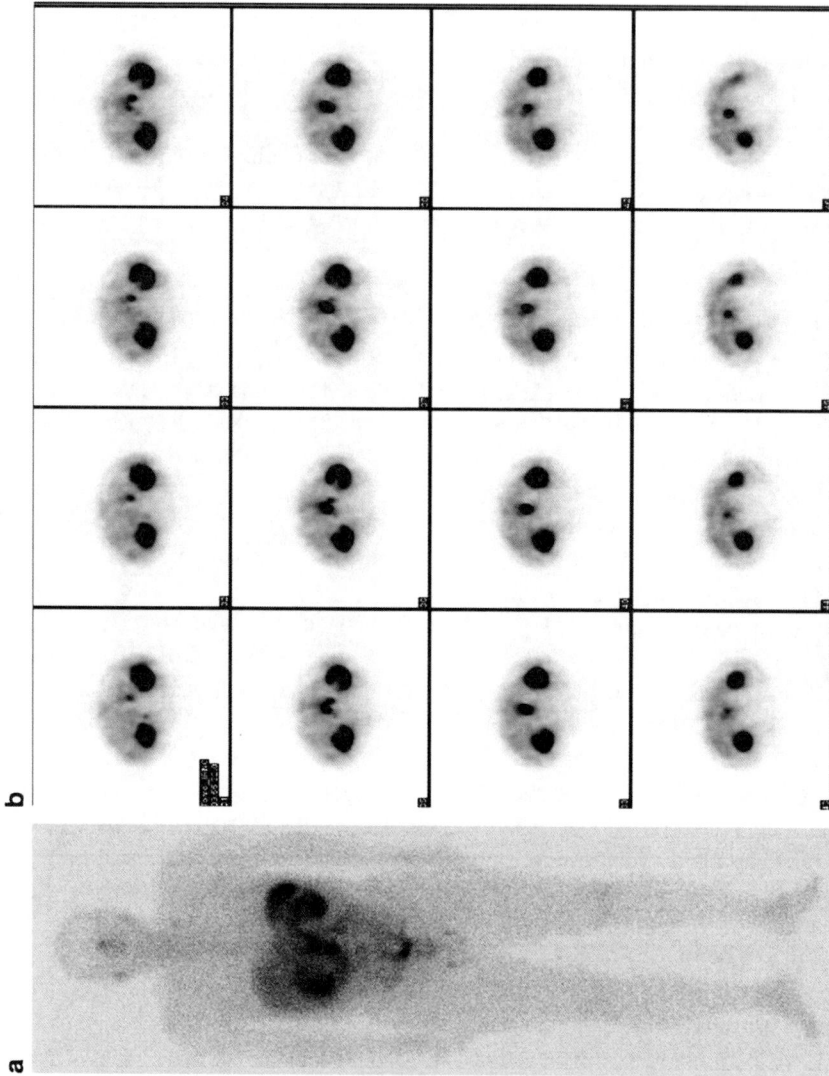

Fig. 4.5 (a) Post-therapy scan 4 days after administration of 5.2 GBq ^{177}Lu-DOTATATE in a patient with abdominal and left supra-clavicular lymph node metastases from a previously operated GEP-NET. (b) Abdominal SPECT images of the same patient following administration of ^{177}Lu-DOTATATE

in 2 patients (8%) and SD in 21 patients (81%). Buscombe et al. [31] treated 12 GEP NET patients with high cumulative activities (upto 36.6 GBq) and reported a PR in 2 patients (17%), SD in 7 patients (58%), and progressive disease (PD) in 3 patients (25%).

Recently Kong et al. [32] combined high doses of ^{111}In-DTPA-Octreotide with 5-fluorouracil (5-FU) chemotherapy in 21 GEP tumor patients. They reported a 67% stabilization rate on CT and stabilization/improvement on scintigraphy in 77% of patients. Gancel et al. followed up 19 patients for 3.8 years after having been treated with 6.6 GBq ^{111}In-DTPA-Octreotide administered in 3-month intervals [33]. One patient showed PR, eight had SD, and the rest were progressive. In all studies, the most common toxicity was due to bone marrow suppression.

All clinical PRRT studies using ^{111}In-DTPA-Octreotide showed encouraging results especially from a clinical and biochemical point of view. The same cannot be said when talking about tumor regression. Some reports suggest that this treatment is more suitable for treatment of micrometastases rather than larger metastases or big tumor masses.

Indications for Targeted Therapy with 131I-MIBG
Inoperable PCC
Inoperable paraganglioma
Inoperable carcinoid tumor
Stage III or IV neuroblastoma
Metastatic/recurrent medullary thyroid carcinoma

^{90}Y-DOTA-TOC

This somatostatin analogue, TOC, with a higher affinity for SSTRs was developed for its high hydrophilicity, simple labeling with ^{111}In and ^{90}Y, and its tight binding to the bifunctional chelator DOTA. The first dosimetric studies by Cremonesi et al. were performed using ^{111}In-DOTA-TOC

since the in vivo behavior was found to be similar to the yttrium labeled peptide [34]. They concluded that therapy with ^{90}Y-DOTA-TOC delivered a short-term total body irradiation with the kidneys being the critical organs. ^{90}Y-DOTA-TOC in vivo stability appeared to be high both in urine and in plasma. Jamar et al. reached similar conclusions after performing accurate dosimetric studies with ^{86}Y-DOTA-TOC [35].

One of the first evaluations was performed by Otte et al. [36], who treated 29 patients with GEP NETs using a dose escalating scheme of four or more cycles of ^{90}Y-DOTATOC up to a cumulative dose of 6.120 ± 1.347 MBq/m^2. Twenty patients had SD, two had PR, four MR, and three had disease progression. Later studies, in 2001–2002, by Waldherr et al. [37, 38] treated patients with GEP NETs with 6 GBq/m^2. In a later study, with 7.4 GBq/m^2, an overall response rate of 24% was obtained.

Bodei et al. [39, 40] published data of a phase 1 study in 21 patients with GEP NETs. The cumulative total doses given in two cycles ranged from 5.9 to 11.1 GBq. Six of 21 patients (29%) had tumor regression with a median duration of response of 9 months. The same group evaluated the objective responses of 141 patients with various types of NETs treated with doses higher than 7.4 GBq of ^{90}Y-DOTA-TOC (cumulative activity 7.4–26.4 GBq) divided into 2–16 cycles. An overall clinical benefit (CR + PR + SD) was observed in 76% of patients with progressive disease and 32% of stable patients showed a response (CR + PR). The range of response duration was between 2 and 59 months.

A multicentre phase 1 study performed in Rotterdam (The Netherlands), Brussels (Belgium), and Tampa (USA) treated 58 patients with escalating doses up to 14.8 GBq/m^2 in 4 cycles or up to 9.3 GBq/m^2 in 1 cycle. Five patients (9%) had PR, 7 (12%) had a MR with a median time to progression of 30 months in patients who had SD, MR, or PR [41].

Various other trials using ^{90}Y-DOTA-TOC were performed in different centers. A general observation can notice that there is a very great variety in the protocols being used. However, in most trials, the best overall response was achieved when ^{90}Y-DOTA-TOC was used in patients with GEP NETs, and when was compared to ^{111}In-DTPA-Octreotide, ^{90}Y-DOTA-TOC resulted so far superior and from 10 to 30% of patients showed an improved therapeutic effectiveness.

^{90}Y-DOTA-Lanreotide

In contrast to labeled octreotide, lanreotide has a greater affinity for SSTR2, 4 and 5. The agent has been used in a multicentre European study (MAURITIUS) in 154 patients with proven progressive disease. Thirty-nine patients had GEP tumors and these were treated with a cumulative dose that ranged from 1.9 to 8.6 GBq of ^{90}Y-DOTA-lanreotide. Eight out of 39 (20%) patients had MR and 44% had SD [42].

^{177}Lu-DOTA-TATE and ^{90}Y-DOTA-TATE

The somatostatin analogue DOTA-Tyr$_3$-octreotate showed improved binding to SSTRs in animal studies [42]. Further studies confirmed that DOTA-Tyr$_3$-octreotate exhibits the highest affinity for SSTR2 receptors. An advantage of using ^{177}Lu-DOTA-TATE is the better tumor kidney, spleen, and liver uptake ratio which allows higher tumor absorbed doses (especially to small tumors) without major effects on the dose-limiting organs. Other advantages include the longer residency time of ^{177}Lu-DOTA-TATE in tumors and the gamma emission of ^{177}Lu, which make it available for scintigraphy/dosimetric studies [43, 44].

Most of the studies using ^{177}Lu-DOTA-TATE have been performed by Kwekkeboom et al. who proposed ^{177}Lu octreotate as the radiolabeled somatostatin of choice for PRRT. In 2003, this group assessed the effects of ^{177}Lu-DOTATATE in 34 patients with GEP tumors. Three months after the end of treatment, a complete remission (CR) was found in 1 patient (3%), PR in 12 (35%), SD in 14 (41%), and PD in 7 (21%) patients [45]. Following this study, they treated 131 patients with GEP tumors with a cumulative dose of 22.2–29.6 GBq of ^{177}Lu-DOTA-TATE, 3 (2%) obtained CR, 32 (26%) PR, 24 (19%) MR, 44 (35%) had SD, and 22 (818%) developed PD [46].

A more extensive study by the same group was published in 2008. The efficacy of ^{177}Lu-DOTA-TATE was evaluated in 310 patients and toxicity was evaluated in 510 patients, each receiving a cumulative radiation dose of 27.8–29.6 GBq in 4 treatment cycles with 6- to 10-week intervals between each cycle. Complete remission was seen in 2%, PR in 28%, and a MR in 16% of patients with an overall objective tumor response rate of 46%. Acute side-effects such as nausea and vomiting occurred after 25 and 10% of administrations, respectively. Subacute WHO hematological toxicity (grade 3 or 4) occurred in 3.6% of treatment cycles. Delayed toxicities included serious liver toxicity in 2 patients and myelodysplastic syndrome in 3 patients [47].

Experiences by Kwekkeboom et al. have lead them to conclude that the two significant factors predicting favorable treatment outcome when using ^{177}Lu-ocreotate were a high patient performance score and high uptake on the pretreatment Octreoscan. An example of disease reduction in a patient treated in our department with four cycles of PRRT is shown in Fig. 4.6.

Data regarding the use of ^{90}Y-DOTA-TATE are emerging from a number of phase 1 trials. Baum et al. [48] reported an objective response rate of 37% (28/75) and disease stabilization in 52% (39/75) of patients.

Clinical Protocols with Radiolabeled Somatostatin Analogues

Since there are no existing randomized clinical trials for both ^{90}Y and ^{177}Lu labeled somatostatin analogs comparing optimal treatment cycle, interval, and cumulative dose, treatment guidelines depend on local expertise, clinical judgment, and according to national legislation and ethical committee approval. The common treatment schemes cited in the literature are given below.

Protocols using ^{90}Y-peptides
1. 4 cycles with 0.9–3.7 GBq/m^2 every 6–9 weeks
2. 3 cycles with 1.1–2.6 GBq every 6–9 weeks
3. 4 cycles with 1.85–5.5 GBq every 6 weeks

Protocols using ^{177}Lu peptides
1. 4 cycles with 3.7–7.4 GBq every 6–12 weeks
2. 4–7 cycles with 3.7–5.2 GBq every 8–12 weeks

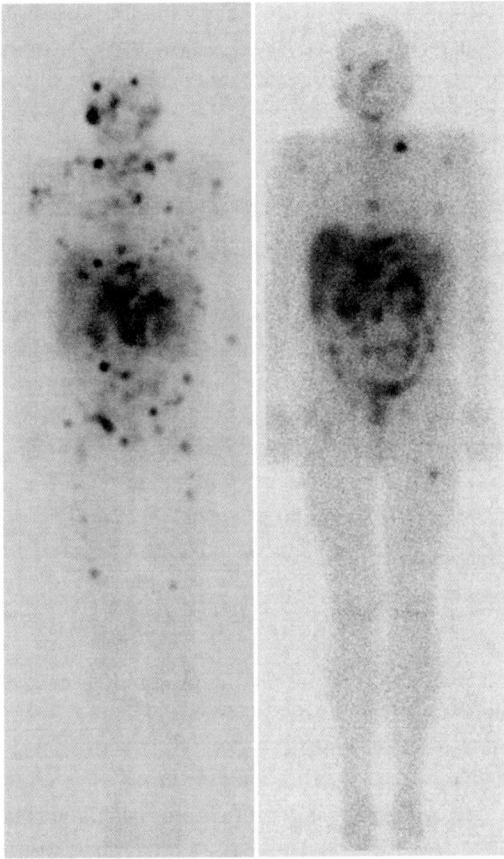

Fig. 4.6 177-Lu post-therapy scans showing a significant reduction of multiple and diffuse metastatic SSR positive lesions (*left*) following three cycles of PRRT (*right*) with ^{177}Lu-DOTATATE in patient with a previously operated GEP-NET

The stage of disease at which PRRT therapy should be started is still being debated and the reports on the relationship between patient survival and PRRT therapy are few. Currently, PRRT is used mainly in patients with metastasized, unresectable NETs and evidence of tumor progression. Several authors currently are proposing PRRT at an earlier stage, in order to increase the effectiveness of the therapy, to avoid the tumor spreading, and to overcome cancer resistance.

Eligibility

According to the Consensus Guidelines for the Standard of Care for Patients with Digestive NETs published by the European Neuroendocrine Tumour Society (ENETS) in 2007, the eligibility criteria for PRRT (based on multidisciplinary discussion) therapy include:

1. Tumor uptake on the Octreoscan being at least as high as the normal liver uptake seen on the planar images
2. Inoperable disease
3. Life expectancy of at least 3–6 months
4. Karnofski Performance Score >50%, or Performance Score (ECOG) <4
5. Signed informed consent

Contraindications

Absolute and relative contraindications include:

1. Pregnancy and lactation
2. Renal impairment (creatinine clearance <40–50 mL/min)
3. Impaired hematological function, Hgb <5 mmol/L (8 g/dL); platelets $<75 \times 10^9$/L; WBC $<2 \times 10^9$/L
4. Severe hepatic impairment, that is, total bilirubin $>3 \times$ upper limit of normal or albumin <30 g/L and pro-thrombin time increased
5. Severe cardiac impairment [49]

In many countries, the patient has to be hospitalized in a special protected ward designed for targeted radionuclide therapy (TRT), with the aim to isolate patients and to collect the radioactive wastes. These requirements vary from region to region and within a specific jurisdiction, individual medical centers may impose additional requirements. Laboratory evaluations should include renal and liver function tests, a full cell blood count and Chromogranin A levels, or other serum markers such as serotonin, gastrin, or NSE if elevated at baseline. If clinically possible long-acting somatostatin analogues should be stopped 6 weeks before PRRT and the patient should be started on short-acting formulations. Amino-acid solutions are given approximately 3 h before PRRT, and are ideally preceded by the infusion of a gastric proton-pump inhibitor and an antiemetic. Dosimetric procedures should be carried out according to local protocols. Upon discharge, written instructions should be given to patients regarding contact with others following the therapy.

Causes for discontinuation of treatment include: evidence of disease progression during the treatment period (based on patient's clinical condition and/or imaging studies) and WHO grade 3 or 4 hematological, renal, or hepatic toxicity.

Follow-Up

The follow-up of patients receiving PRRT therapy consists of laboratory monitoring and imaging studies. A full blood count, renal, and liver function tests should ideally be done 3 and 6 months after therapy and every 6 months thereafter. Basal chromogranin levels are compared with follow-up values. The imaging modality and technique used should be the same as the baseline study (usually CT, MRI, or Octreoscan/PET/CT) and tumor response is defined according to the RECIST criteria [49].

Common Side-Effects

The side-effects of PRRT can be divided into direct side-effects and delayed side-effects. The commonest direct effects include nausea, vomiting, and abdominal pain [25]. Nausea and vomiting are usually radiation induced and also as a result of pretreatment with amino acids. They are easily treated with antiemetic drugs. In certain cases, prophylaxis with corticosteroids may help. It has been reported that 1% of patients receiving PRRT develop a hormonal crisis after therapy due to a release of vasoactive substances from the tumor [50]. Delayed effects concern the functional impairment of the critical organs, that is the kidneys, liver, and the bone marrow (see dosimetry section).

Dosimetric Considerations

The data available showing the utility of dosimetry to avoid under and overtreatment and to standardize the radionuclide therapy is still very limited. This aspect of radionuclide targeted therapy remains inadequately explored and discussed.

Some physicians claim that dosimetry is not necessary since they use fixed activities. On the other hand, many recommend that dosimetry should be used to individualize the therapeutic regimens. The EURATOM Council Directive 97/43 stipulated that in medical exposures for radiotherapeutic purposes, including nuclear medicine "exposures of target volumes shall be individually planned" [51].

Dosimetric estimates are time consuming and require complex methods, including pharmacokinetic, biodistribution, and washout studies of the radiopharmaceutical to be used for therapy. Dosimetry may be carried out in a pretreatment setting as part of the treatment planning or as a peri-treatment modality to help ascertain actual dose distribution. Different approaches can be applied for dosimetry; however, the aim of this text is not to give a detailed account of these methods.

In summary, dosimetry requires blood samples and scintigraphic images, which can be in the form of planar images, SPECT/CT, or even PET/CT images, depending on the radionuclide used. Dose calculation is performed in the framework of the MIRD formalism with commercially available software, such as OLINDA/EXM, currently available for calculation of internal absorbed doses in both organs and tumors [52, 53].

More accurate dosimetric calculations can be achieved if other elements, apart from the mean absorbed doses, are taken into account. These include dose rate and fractionation, voxel dose distribution, actual organ mass, tissue density, and radiosensitivity. Personalized dosimetry requires details that are specific for the individual patient and the specific radiopeptide used.

Experience has shown that the radiopeptides used in PRRT therapy share similar characteristics with ^{111}In-octreotide, that is: fast blood clearance, almost complete excretion through the kidneys, with the "hottest" organs being the spleen, kidneys, and the liver. Uptake in the bone marrow is rarely seen [54]. ^{111}In-octreotide was first proposed as a tracer for dosimetric calculations of ^{90}Y peptides. At present, however, its use is not recommended as it has different kinetics and receptor affinity properties; ^{111}In-DOTA-TOC

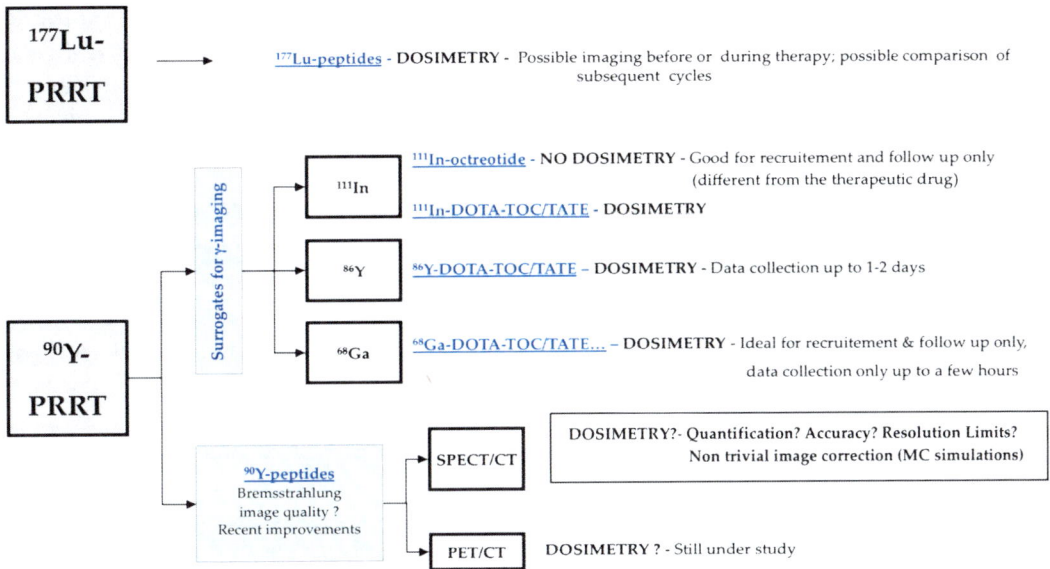

Fig. 4.7 Possible methods for pre and post-therapeutic imaging and adequacy of radiotracers for dosimetry purposes

and ^{111}In-DOTA-TATE are better for this purpose as they have comparable in vivo behavior to the ^{90}Y derivatives.[54] Figure 4.7 shows the possible methods for pre- and post-therapeutic imaging and the adequacy of radiotracers for dosimetry purposes [55].

The lack of gamma emission is a problem when using [90]Y. Two options are available:

1. [90]Y Bremsstrahlung images (Fig. 4.8), even though they are difficult to analyze making the calculation of patient-specific dosimetry very challenging.
2. [90]Y PET obtained by detecting the annihilation photons that occur after internal pair formation in [90]Y. Promising high-resolution biodistribution images by Lhommel et al. [56] after liver SIRT show that this method may, in the near future, become a versatile adjunct for dosimetry in PRRT.

On the other hand, using ^{177}Lu allows dosimetric calculations to be done before therapy or following the first cycle due to its low abundance gamma ray emissions (113 and 208 keV).

Labeling molecules with [86]Y totally preserves the chemical nature of yttrium-90 (^{90}Y) derivatives. [86]Y has a significant positron emission of 33% that allows PET imaging thus providing better spatial resolution and quantitiation.

Disadvantages of [86]Y include: a significant short half-life (14.6 h) when compared to that of [90]Y (64.2 h), high costs, low availability, and an emission of gamma rays which, without correction, may cause an overestimation in the uptake assessment (difficult quantification in bone and red marrow) [57].

Gallium-68 (^{68}Ga) peptides have the advantage of providing high-quality PET images but are not ideal since the half-life of ^{68}Ga is so short. The other problem is that ^{68}Ga labeled peptides may have different affinities for the receptors and physiologic distribution compared to the ^{90}Y therapeutic agent [58].

[90]Y and ^{177}Lu peptides have shown a similar biological half-life for organs and tumors: different uptake depends on the relationship between SSTRs and peptide affinity [54]. This allows similar dosimetric methods to be applied for both ^{90}Y and [177]Lu.

Studies of the various dosimetric data of ^{90}Y and ^{177}Lu peptides published in the literature highlight important similarities:

1. Low whole-body exposure as a result of rapid blood and urinary clearance is observed
2. High kidney absorbed doses making it the dose-limiting organ, followed by the liver and spleen

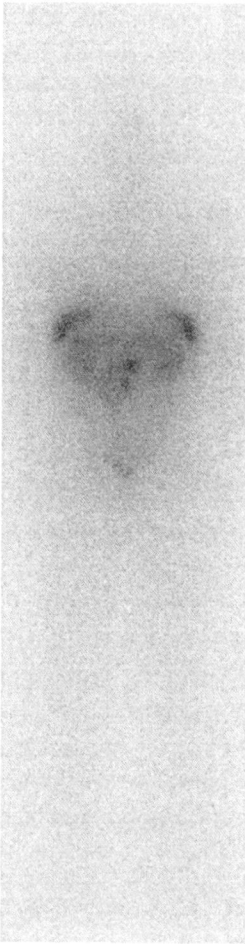

Fig. 4.8 ^{90}Y-Bremsstrahlung image 4 days after treatment with 2.5 GBq ^{90}Y-DOTATATE. Pathological abdominal lymph nodes may be observed

3. Wide intra-patient variation in absorbed doses
4. Higher absorbed doses when using ^{90}Y-peptides when compared to ^{177}Lu-peptides

Renal and Hematologic Toxicities

Particular attention should be given to the kidney and bone marrow dose absorption. Most of the activity is excreted by the kidneys but approximately 2% of the total dose is re-absorbed by the proximal tubular cells, with the scavenger cell megalin being the mediator of uptake, and retained in the interstitium. Radiation nephropathy has been described in several patients. Experience with external beam radiation therapy (EBRT) shows that the risk of developing radiation nephropathy within 5 years in patients receiving a total absorbed dose of 23 Gy is 5%. The risk rises to 50% with an absorbed dose of 28 Gy [59]. It has been suggested that the real threshold for kidney toxicity with internal emitters is higher due to the different kinetics of irradiation exposure. Histological damage with PRRT is similar to that seen with EBRT. The process usually involves thrombotic microangiopathy with subsequent renal failure.

Barone et al. [60] showed that the absorbed dose does not explain the observed renal toxicity but could be accounted for using the elaborate radiobiological parameter biological effective dose (BED), which allows a direct quantitative comparison between EBRT and TRT. Recent studies by Valkema et al. [61] and Barone et al. [60] proposed as a safe cumulative BED, a value of approximately 37 Gy. Bodei et al. [62] propose a maximum BED of 40 Gy. The BED has to be reduced (approximately 28 Gy) when dealing with old, diabetic, and hypertensive patients, and in patients with prior exposure to nephrotoxic chemotherapy or ionizing radiation.

Dosimetric studies stress that kidney protection plays an important role in PRRT. Various methods are used to interfere with the receptor-mediated endocytosis process occurring at the level of the proximal renal tubule helping in order to achieve satisfactory kidney protection. Such methods include coadministration of positively charged basic amino acids and the bovine gelatine containing solutions Gelofusine or albumin fragments. The amino acids L-lysine and L-arginine are most commonly used in the clinical setting resulting in a decrease in renal absorbed dose ranging from 9 to 53% [61]. Common side-effects of these amino acids infusion include nausea, vomiting, and hyperkaliemia.

In spite of the above-mentioned warnings, severe side-effects using these amino acids prior to PRRT therapy have never been observed to date in our department. New approaches, which block the renin–angiotensin–aldosterone system by using the angiotensin-converting enzyme

(ACE) inhibitors and angiotensin II receptor blockers (ARBs), are under study [59].

Even though the observed doses in the bone marrow are usually significantly below the threshold value for toxicity, the bone marrow remains a critical organ during PRRT therapy, particularly in patients with multiple bone involvement and those receiving repeated administrations. Grade 3 or 4 hematological toxicity (especially after ^{90}Y-peptides), myelodisplastic syndromes, and acute myeloid leukemia have been reported [63].

Future Developments of PRRT

The ultimate goal is to develop new somatostatin analogues, which have a high affinity for the different SSTR subtypes resulting in more specific receptor selection. Wild et al. [64] have shown that DOTA-NOC, which was synthesized by further exchanging the amino acid in position 3 of octreotide for labeling with radiometals like ^{68}Ga, ^{111}In, ^{90}Y, and ^{177}Lu, is a somatostatin analogue that displays a high affinity for sstr-2, sstr3, and sstr5. The potential of these radiopeptides is to allow physicians to target a broader range of receptors and a larger spectrum of tumors, both from an imaging and a therapeutic point of view.

Combination of ^{90}Y-DOTA-TATE and ^{177}Lu-DOTA-TATE

Having noted the individual effect of therapies with ^{90}Y and ^{177}Lu labeled somatostatin analogues, and taking into consideration the different properties of both radionuclides, combination treatments with ^{90}Y and ^{177}Lu peptides is being evaluated, especially in tumors with heterogeneous properties. The limiting factor in this case is the combined toxicity which can be caused by the radiolabeled peptides. Data from animal studies have shown that the association of different radioisotopes was more effective in the overall survival of mice.

The combination of ^{90}Y-DOTA-TATE and ^{177}Lu-DOTA-TATE determined a 62% survival rate 150 days after therapy as opposed to the same rate of survival occurring only 88 days after ^{90}Y-DOTA-TATE alone and 96 days after ^{177}Lu-DOTA-TATE alone [65]. Preliminary results in our group on 15 patients treated with four therapeutic cycles alternating 5.55 GBq ^{177}Lu-DOTA-DATE and 2.6 GBq ^{90}Y-DOTA-TATE suggest that the treatment is well tolerated with only rare cases of hematological toxicities, which when occurred, appeared transient and mild. We observed a partial remission in 67% of patients, stable disease in 27%, and tumor progression in 6% of patients. A positive palliative effect of the treatment was also noted [66].

Other Receptors

It is well known that NETs express several other receptor types apart from SSTRs. These include gastrin-releasing peptide (GRP), neurotensin (NT) receptors, glucagon-like peptide-1 (GLIP-1) receptors, cholecystokinin receptors, bombesin and vasoactive intestinal peptide (VIP) receptors [66]. The advantage of knowing these receptors is twofold:

1. Multireceptor PRRT using a combination of radiolabeled compounds improving targeting efficacy and tumor dose.
2. Labeling of different radioligands with isotopes of different ranges to obtain optimal therapy for lesions of different sizes.

Radiosensitization

Radiosensitization using chemotherapy, immunotherapy, and external beam radiation has been evolving over the last few years. Numerous trials have shown the increased efficacy in terms of tumor growth control when combining chemotherapeutic agents together with external beam radiotherapy. Tu et al. [67] demonstrated the concomitant benefit of strontium-89 (^{89}Sr) radionuclide therapy with doxorubicin in patients with painful metastases from prostate carcinoma. Wong et al. [68] have shown that the combination of 5-FU and ^{90}Y labeled peptide is feasible and safe. Also, 5-FU combined with ^{111}In-DTPA-octreotide resulted in symptomatic response in 71% of patients with NETs [68]. Only randomized controlled trials can tell us whether current results may be improved. Van Eijck et al. [69] have also described the use of PRRT as a neo-adjuvant therapy in patients with an initial diagnosis of locally advanced inoperable disease. Other developments include methods of upregulating SSTRs or the possibility of transferring genes encoding SSTRs to receptor negative tumors, thus enabling a more effective therapy.

Locoregional Therapy

In order to overcome one of the major drawbacks of radionuclide therapy, namely bone marrow and kidney toxicity, whilst optimizing the received tumor dose, locoregional radionuclide therapy in patients with liver metastases from NETs has been proposed. Other locoregional therapies include trans-arterial chemoembolization (TACE), trans-arterial embolization (TAE), and radiofrequency ablation. According to available data, all techniques achieve a 50–60% radiological response rate and almost 80% of symptomatic relief for the patients. Limouris et al. [70] used ^{111}In-DTPA-pentetreotide infusions following selective catheterization of the hepatic artery in 17 patients with inoperable SST2 receptor positive liver metastases. They reported that 70.6% of the patients showed some radiological benefit from the treatment with no associated hepatic or renal toxicities. Trials using different isotopes with a particular focus on clinical outcome differences between embolization techniques and surgery are needed.

Targeted Alpha Therapy

The development and safe use of alpha-emitter therapies may offer a new approach for patients with metastatic NETs. The effectiveness of targeted alpha therapy can be explained by the properties of alpha particles. Alpha particles are helium nuclei and are approximately 8,000 times larger than beta(−) particles. Radionuclides that decay

via an alpha-decay pathway release enormous amounts of energy over a very short distance. Typically, the range of alpha particles in tissue is 50–100 μm. They have high linear energy transfer (LET) with a mean energy deposition of 100 keV/μm, providing a more specific tumor cell killing ability without damaging surrounding normal tissues. It is thought that a single alpha particle can kill a cell as it is emitted. Due to these properties, the majority of preclinical and clinical trials have demonstrated that alpha-emitters are ideal for the treatment of smaller tumor burdens, micrometastatic disease, and disseminated disease [71]. During the 58th Annual Meeting of the Society of Nuclear Medicine held in San Antonio, Texas (June 2011), Kratochwil et al. presented a preliminary study which showed the efficacy of bismuth-213 (^{213}Bi)-DOTATOC in targeting NETs and inducing the remission of metastases without causing severe toxicity [72]. Additional alpha-emitter therapy studies are also continuing to determine their efficacy for treating other therapy-resistant cancers.

Diagnosis of Tumors of Sympatho-Adrenal Lineage

Neuroblastomas are very frequent tumors in childhood with an annual incidence of 650 new cases per year in the USA. There is marked variability in clinical behavior ranging from spontaneous regression or differentiation into benign tumors to rapid and progressive fatal disease. The most common symptoms of neuroblastoma include tiredness, loss of appetite, and joint pain. Other signs and symptoms such as abdominal pain, pallor, neurological deficits, and respiratory complications may be present, depending on the location of the primary tumor and presence of metastatic lesions. The most frequent site of location is adrenal gland, but sometimes nerve tissues of other districts are involved [73, 74]. Amplification of the oncogene MYCN is a genetic change frequently observed in neuroblastoma and is an indicator of poor prognosis [75].

PCCs present with tumor mass generally located in the adrenal medulla. The primary tumors of extra-renal origin are described as paragangliomas. PCCs can be also bilateral and familial associated with a genetic multiple endocrine syndrome [76]. Common sites of metastases include lymph nodes, liver, lung, and bones [77]. Signs and symptoms often reflect uncontrolled release of catecholamines. Most patients suffer from hypertension (paroxysmal or sustained), headaches, palpitations, and chest and abdominal pain.

Biochemistry

Upon clinical suspicion of a sympatho-adrenal tumor, a search for the presence of elevated levels of plasma and/or urinary levels of catecholamines and their metabolites (HVA, VMA, and metanephrines) is undertaken. Plasma metanephrine testing has the highest sensitivity (96%) for detecting a PCC, but it has a lower specificity (85%). In comparison, a 24-h urinary collection for catecholamines and metanephrines has a sensitivity of 87.5% and a specificity of 99.7% [73]. A single sample or collected urine test for VMA/HVA is highly accurate in cases of neuroblastomas. As occurs with other NETs, elevated levels of plasma CgA is a highly specific marker for these tumors.

Imaging

Diagnostic imaging examinations for tumor localization currently performed are computed tomography (CT), magnetic resonance imaging (MR), and iodine-123 (^{123}I)-MIBG/iodine-131(^{131}I-MIBG) whole-body scintigraphy. Abdominal CT and MR have a sensitivity of 90–100% and specificity of 70–80% for detection of PCC [78]. Similar values are reported for detection of neuroblastomas (87% sensitivity and 80% specificity). CT is able to differentiate between neuroblastoma and Wilm's tumor, the two main malignant causes of an abdominal mass in childhood [79].

Iodine-labeled MIBG (^{123}I-MIBG or ^{131}I-MIBG) scintigraphy has good sensitivity for the diagnosis of neuroblastoma (93%) and PCC (87.5%) and specificity close to 100% for both

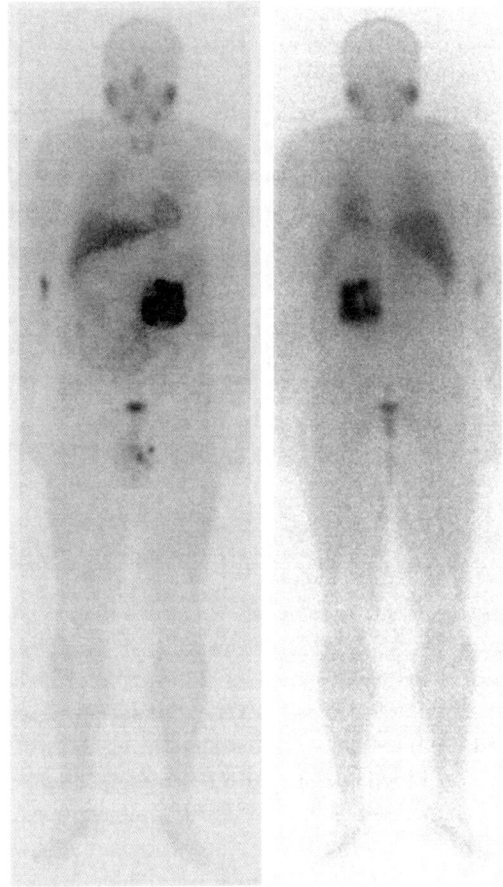

Fig. 4.9 Anterior (*left*) and posterior (*right*) views of an ^{123}I-MIBG scintigraphy in a patient with an inoperable necrotic retroperitoneal paraganglioma. No distant metastases are observed. The patient was subsequently treated with ^{131}I-MIBG

[79]. Diagnostic accuracy is improved by integrating the SPECT images with the CT images. ^{123}I-MIBG is currently considered the radiopharmaceutical of choice due to its better image quality and more favorable dosimetry (Fig. 4.9). If the MIBG scan is negative, fluorine-18 (^{18}F)-FDG PET and fluorine-18 (^{18}F)-DOPA PET may be considered, because these tumors sometimes show a high uptake of glucose and ^{18}F-DOPA PET explores the pathway of catecholamine metabolism. This class of tumors may express SSTRs; therefore, in certain cases, imaging with radiolabeled SSTR analogues should be considered. Clinical evidence demonstrates that the sensitivity of ^{111}In-pentetreotide scintigraphy

or PET with gallium-68 (^{68}Ga)-somatostatin analogues is not superior to MIBG scintigraphy so as to be defined as the first choice imaging modality; however, at present, they can be considered as valid options for diagnosis.

Carcinoids are classified as GEP NETs and tend to express SSTRs. However, since they arise from the cells of chromoaffine origin, they often show intense uptake of MIBG, thus allowing treatment with radiolabeled MIBG. Many of them present with a typical carcinoid syndrome and their diagnostic approaches may involve the above-mentioned modalities [80, 81].

Therapy with Radiolabeled MIBG (^{131}I-MIBG)

Various treatment modalities are available but surgery remains the most effective and first choice therapy especially when dealing with localized disease. Surgical debulking of locally extended tumors or metastases can, in some cases, help to reduce catecholamine secretion. When metastatic disease is present, an aggressive multimodal therapeutic approach including surgery, chemotherapy, external beam radiotherapy, and immunotherapy is usually performed.

^{131}I-MIBG has been used for targeted radiotherapy to treat tumors of neuroectodermal origin since the mid-1980s. At present, it still represents an invaluable therapeutic option either to complement conventional treatment or to replace it when ineffective [82]. In the field of ^{131}I-MIBG therapy, many discussions exist because of a large variation in treatment schedules, response rates, and the lack of randomized controlled studies and potential side-effects [78]. The main difference with PRRT, in which substances bind cell surface receptors, is that the target cell takes up MIBG via a metabolic pathway. Another difference is that MIBG is linked directly to the radionuclide ^{131}I, without any linking moiety.

MIBG is an analkylguanidine resulting from the combination of the benzyl group of bretylium and the guanidine group of guanethidine, the end product being a structural analogue of noradrenaline. MIBG is taken up by the tumor cells derived from the primitive neural crest (via VMA transporters VMAT1 and VMAT2) since these cells maintain certain characteristic features, such as the incorporation of amine precursors and neurosecretory storage granules in the cytoplasm. Unlike noradrenaline, MIBG is not metabolized and is secreted unchanged [83]. ^{131}I is a beta (β) emitting radionuclide with a physical half-life of 8.04 days, maximum energy of 0.61 MeV, and a mean range in tissue of approximately 0.5 mm. It also emits gamma radiation of 364 keV.

Clinical Therapy Protocols with ^{131}I-MIBG

At the first international review of ^{131}I-MIBG therapy, held in Rome in 1991, the results of treating 451 patients with ^{131}I-MIBG therapy were presented (225 neuroblastomas, 127 PCC, 51 carcinoids, 18 MTC). It was agreed that ^{131}I-MIBG therapy induces significant tumor responses in about 30–50% of cases, long-term stabilization of disease in several cases and significant reduction of cathecholamine-related symptoms in almost all patients [84].

Between 1988 and 1999, our group treated 45 patients (22 neuroblastomas, 10 PCC, 3 PGG, 6 MTC, and 4 carcinoids) with ^{131}I-MIBG. Doses ranged from 3.7 to 7.4 GBq in adults and 2.77 to 5.55 GBq in children. The tumor response ranged from 14.3 to 66.6% and stable disease ranged from 33 to 75%. Considering that most patients had been previously treated with other myelotoxic therapies, the overall toxicity was acceptable: the most relevant side-effect was bone marrow toxicity [85].

Loh et al. reviewed 116 patients treated with individual doses of 3.7–7.4 GBq ^{131}I-MIBG before 1997. He concluded that ^{131}I-MIBG induces tumor responses, mostly partial, in 24–45% of the patients among whom disease progression occurred after approximately 2 years [86].

A retrospective analysis of 37 patients receiving ^{131}I-MIBG therapy in a single institution for various indications was performed. They demonstrated that 82% of patients receiving MIBG alone and 84% of those receiving additional therapy had stable disease for a median follow-up period of 32 months [25].

In a summary of cumulative responses to treatment in a total of 23 studies comprising a total of 166 patients, with a wide range of total activities (administered as a series of treatments), there was a complete response based on imaging criteria in 4.2%, a PR in 25.3%, SD in 43.4%, and PD in 22.9%. No tumor response was recorded in 4.2% of patients [87].

Rose et al. [88] in 2003 adapted a high-dose approach by treating 12 patients with a median single dose of 29.6 GBq and a median cumulative dose of 37.6 GBq ^{131}I-MIBG. Three patients had a CR and seven patients had a PR (median follow-up was 3.5 years). The main toxic effects were severe thrombocytopenia and neutropenia, with one patient requiring infusion of stem cells harvested routinely before high-dose treatment.

Castellani et al. [89] recently published the results of low versus intermediate activity regimens in the ^{131}I-MIBG treatment of PCCs at our Institute. One group of 12 patients (between 1990 and 2009) received a fixed dose of 5.55 GBq/session and another group of 16 patients were treated with 9.25–12.95 GBq/session (between 2001 and 2009). They were able to demonstrate that intermediate single session activity decreased the global treatment time by one third, showing similar efficacy and only a moderate increment of toxicity.

Figure 4.10 is an example of partial reduction of MIBG avid lesions following two cycles of ^{131}I-MIBG therapy in a patient with metastatic medullary thyroid carcinoma. As already described for PRRT, since no randomized clinical trials exist for ^{131}I-MIBG therapy, the clinical studies are not easily comparable.

According to the EANM procedure guidelines published in 2008, the indications for ^{131}I-MIBG therapy include:

1. Inoperable PCC
2. Inoperable paraganglioma
3. Inoperable carcinoid tumor
4. Stage III or IV neuroblastoma
5. Metastatic or recurrent medullary thyroid cancer

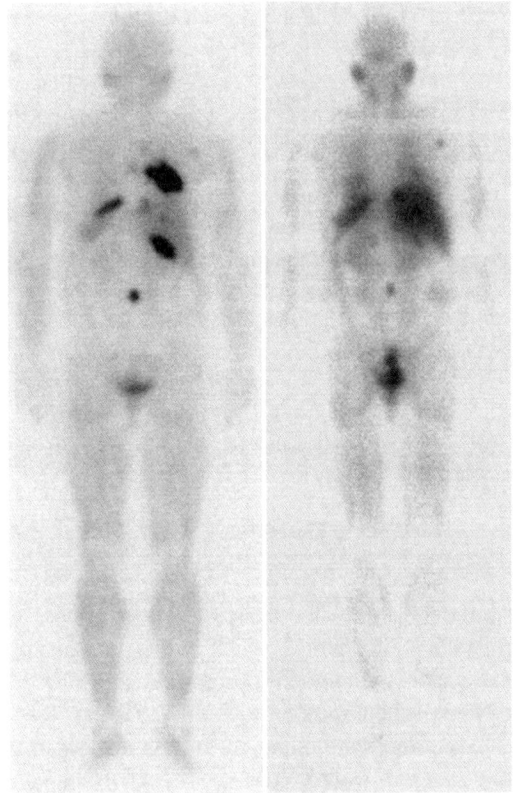

Fig. 4.10 MIBG scintigraphy showing partial reduction of MIBG positive lesions (*left*) following two cycles of ^{131}I-MIBG therapy (*right*) in a patient with metastatic medullary carcinoma

All eligible patients need to have MIBG positive tumors, documented by planar SPECT scintigraphy using ^{123}I-MIBG or ^{131}I-MIBG (in adults). Therefore, patients are selected according to clinical diagnosis, histology, and results of the diagnostic scintigraphy. The contraindications for ^{131}I-therapy are listed in the same guidelines. These include absolute contraindications such as pregnancy and breast-feeding and relative contraindications such as rapidly deteriorating renal function and myelosuppression [83].

Prior to admission, patients should undergo serological and urinary tests such as CBC, renal and liver function tests, catecholamine levels, Chromogranin A, NSE, VMA, HVA, 5-HIAA, and calcitonin levels. Thyroid blocking is essential before administration of ^{131}I-MIBG so as to prevent thyroid irradiation caused by the uptake

Table 4.2 Drug interactions with 131I-MIBG

Drug group	Recommended withdrawal time
Amioderone (antiarrhythmic drug)	Not practical to withdraw
Labetalol (combined alpha/beta blocker)	72 h
Amlodipine (calcium-channel blocker)	48 h
Phenoxybenzamine IV (alpha blocker)	15 days
Salbutamol (beta$_2$ stimulant)	24 h
Chlorpromazine (neuroleptic)	24 h
Haloperidol (neuroleptic)	48 h (1 month for depot)
Promethazine (antihistamine)	24 h
Amitryptiline (tricyclic antidepressant)	48 h
Cocaine (CNS stimulant)	24 h

Table 4.3 Common early and later side-effects of 131I-MIBG therapy

Early effects	Late effects
Milda nausea, flushing	Bome marrow suppression
Vomiting	Hypothyroidism
Hypertensive crisis (rare)	Hepatic disfunction
Renal failure (rare)	

of free [131]I. Oral iodine (capsules or drops) is given to the patient 24–48 h before the therapy starts and is continued for approximately 10–15 days post-therapy.

Since there are a number of medications that have been shown to interfere with MIBG uptake and storage, these might have to be suspended 24–72 h before treatment [90] (Table 4.2). In certain situations, such as patients taking alpha and beta blockers due to catecholamine secreting tumors, the withdrawal of treatment may cause further complications and therefore ^{131}I-MIBG treatment is done without suspension of drug treatment.

^{131}I-MIBG is administered via a slow intravenous infusion (45 min to 4 h) using a lead-shielded infusion pump in order to avoid the release of norepinephrine from storage granules resulting in a hypertensive crisis. In general, single administered doses range between 3.7 and 11.2 GBq. Premedication with steroids, antiemetics, and proton-pump inhibitors may be given. Strict blood pressure monitoring is required during and after the therapy and short-acting alpha and beta blockers should be easily available if needed. A post-therapy whole-body scintigraphy is performed prior to discharge.

Patients are advised to avoid pregnancy for at least 4 months after the treatment is completed. Several treatments may be required at intervals of 3–6 months in order to obtain an objective response. The follow-up usually consists of clinical evaluation, instrumental evaluation with conventional imaging methods (US, X-ray, CT, MRI, radionuclide imaging), and laboratory tests, with particular attention to hematological monitoring and thyroid function tests [83].

The side-effects of ^{131}I-MIBG therapy may be divided into early and late side-effects. The commonest side-effects which may occur at an early stage are nausea and vomiting. Bone marrow toxicity typically appears 4–6 weeks following the completion of therapy and tends to occur with greater frequency in patients with diffuse bone marrow disease, poor renal function, and those previously treated with chemotherapy. Renal failure and a hypertensive crisis are rare acute side-effects which may occur with ^{131}I-MIBG therapy. Delayed side-effects include hypothyroidism and persistent bone marrow suppression (Table 4.3).

Dosimetry

The dose-limiting organ in ^{131}I-MIBG therapy is the bone marrow. It is important not to exceed the maximal allowable bone marrow absorbed dose of 2 Gy for adults and 2.5 Gy for children [91, 92]. Sisson proposed that whole-body dosimetry can be used to represent bone marrow toxicity, assuming that this will be proportional to the uptake and retention of the activity in the body. Whole-body retention relies heavily on kidney function and the uptake in tumor and normal organs [93]. The various dosimetric methods applied make use of planar whole-body scans with or without SPECT or SPECT/CT images using either ^{131}I or [123]I. Whole-body counts from an external counter have also been proposed. Blood samples for derivation of red marrow absorbed doses are not recommended. Monsieur et al. used a combination of pre-therapeutic ^{123}I-MIBG and post-therapeutic ^{131}I-MIBG images. Matthay et al. used a less time consuming method by acquiring whole-body images from day 3 to 7. An advantage of whole-body dosimetry is that the first measurement, if acquired immediately after administration, can be calibrated to the administered activity [93]. Results of various dosimetric studies during ^{131}I-MIBG therapy have shown a wide variation in whole-body and tumor absorbed doses and a discrepancy between whole-body absorbed doses in adults and in children.

Future Developments

The most effective way of using ^{131}I-MIBG therapy has not yet been established. Combination therapies have already been performed with chemotherapeutic agents such as topotecan, cisplatin, vincristine, cyclophosphamide, and carboplatin. The association of topetecan (a topoisomersae I inhibitor) has been studied in order to establish both its effectiveness and correct timing of treatment. Mairs et al. [94] showed that therapy with topotecan after or in concomitance with ^{131}I-MIBG is superior to topotecan administered before, with the bone marrow being the dose-limiting organ.

Combination with hyperbaric therapy, which is thought to increase the production of superoxide radicals, has shown promising results. Bayer et al. demonstrated that corticosteroids can improve NET imaging and therapy. The administration of ^{123}I-MIBG and steroids together increases tumor to background ratio and enhances tumor sensitivity [95].

Increased long-term survival may be achieved with the administration of higher individual doses. This may be achieved by a double infusion with autologous stem cells. A total of 4.0 Gy whole-body dose with stem cell rescue has been given with good tolerance and no short-term, dose-limiting organ toxicity [91, 92]. Therapies with more cytotoxic alpha-emitting radiolabeled

molecules such as meta-211-astatobenzylguanidine ([211]As-MABG) are also being studied [89].

The advent of PET-based iodine-124 ([124]I)-MIBG studies should offer more accurate dosimetric studies than those currently performed using [131]I (difficult quantification) and I-123 [123]I (short physical half-life) [96]. An initial preclinical study has also been performed using meta-bromobenzylguanidine (MBBG) labeled with bromine-76 ([76]Br), a positron emitter [93].

As mentioned before, we know that most NETs of the sympatho-adrenal lineage also express SSTR subtypes. ^{111}In-Octreotide scintigraphy is a very sensitive technique to visualize these tumors and detects more than 90% of known lesions in patients with paragangliomas. Some experts believe that PRRT may have a role in the management of progressive paragangliomas and PCCs. Comparison of PRRT with ^{131}I-MIBG is difficult since no head-to-head trials have ever been done. Essen et al. [97] studied the effects of ^{177}Lu-DOTATATE in patients with paragangliomas, meningiomas, small cell lung carcinoma, and melanoma. They found that regardless of tumor stage and progression, 17% of paragangliomas displayed tumor regression. All other patients showed stable disease or disease progression.

Forrer et al. [98] evaluated the effectiveness and toxicity of radiolabeled DOTATOC in 28 patients with metastatic paragangliomas and PCCs. At restaging, they observed two partial remissions, two mixed responses, and five minor responses with 13 patients showing stable disease and 6 patients showing progressive disease. The treatment was well tolerated with no hematological or renal toxicities occurring. When compared to the therapy of GEP NETs, PRRT seems to be less effective in treating metastatic NETs of the sympatho-adrenal lineage but may still represent a valuable treatment option in these cases since toxicity is very low and long-lasting remissions can still be achieved.

There is also a growing interest in evaluating the hypothesis that PRRT can be used safely and effectively in children and young adults with refractory neuroblastomas that express SSTRs. A phase 1 trial of 90Y-DOTATOC by Menda et al. to determine the dose-toxicity profile in

17 children and young adults with SSTR tumors (including 2 patients with neuroblastoma and 3 patients with paraganglioma) concluded that PRRT is safe, with no dose-limiting toxicities observed. They also showed a 12% partial response and a 29% minor response rate [99].

Summary

NETs are a group of tumors which frequently express SSTRs and represent 1% of all neoplasms that may arise in the body. NETs of the GEP NETs and tumors of the sympatho-adrenal lineage are the most frequent tumors observed in clinical practice. Improved diagnostic techniques, both functional and anatomical, have resulted in an increased incidence of NETs. The variation in biological characteristics of these tumors poses considerable problems when deciding the optimal treatment strategies. PRRT using somatostatin radiolabeled analogues ^{111}In-DTPA-octreotide, ^{90}Y-DOTA-TOC, ^{177}Lu-DOTA-TATE, and ^{90}Y-DOTA-TATE for GEP NETs and radiolabeled ^{131}I-MIBG for NETs of the sympatho-adrenal system have shown promising overall tumor response rates. They appear to be well tolerated by patients with very few side-effects reported. Particular attention to patient selection, pre-therapy preparation, and post-therapy follow-up are essential to ensure optimal treatment efficacy. Various dosimetric calculations are increasingly being employed in PRRT and ^{131}I-MIBG protocols with the aim of personalizing the therapy for the single patient and the radiopharmaceutical used. The use of more specific somatostatin analogues, combination and locoregional therapies in PRRT, and the administration of higher individual doses for ^{131}I-MIBG represent the future for the treatment of NETs.

References

1. Oberg K, Eriksson B. Nuclear medicine in the detection, staging and treatment of gastrointestinal carcinoid tumours. Best Pract Res Clin Endocrinol Metab. 2005;19:265–76.

2. Kaltsas GA, Papadogias D, Makras P, Grossman AB. Treatment of advanced neuroendocrine tumors with radiolabelled somatostatin analogues. Endocr Relat Cancer. 2005;12:683–99.

3. Massironi S, Sciola V, Peracchi M, Ciafardini C, Spampatti MP, Conte D. Neuroendocrine tumors of the gastro-entero-pancreatic system. World J Gastroenterol. 2008;14:5377–84.

4. Kowalsky RJ, Falen SW. Radiopharmaceuticals in nuclear pharmacy and nuclear medicine. 2nd ed. Washington: American Pharmacists Association; 2004.

5. Yao JC, Hassan M, Phan A, et al. One hundred years after "carcinoid": epidemiology of and prognostic factors for neuroendocrine tumors in 35,825 cases in the United States. J Clin Oncol. 2008;26: 3063–72.

6. de Herder WW. Biochemistry of neuroendocrine tumours. Best Pract Res Clin Endocrinol Metab. 2007;21:33–41.

7. O'Toole D, Grossman A, Gross D, et al. Enets consensus guidelines for the standards of care in neuroendocrine tumors: biochemical markers. Neuroendocrinology. 2009;90:194–202.

8. Kloppel G, Couvelard A, Perren A, et al. Enets consensus guidelines for the standards of care in neuroendocrine tumors: Towards a standardized approach to the diagnosis of gastroenteropancreatic neuroendocrine tumors and their prognostic stratification. Neuroendocrinology. 2009;90:162–6.

9. Bosman FT, Carneiro F, Hruban RH, Theise ND. WHO classification of tumours of the digestive system. Lyon: IARC; 2010.

10. Wiedenmann B, Jensen RT, Mignon M, et al. Preoperative diagnosis and surgical management of neuroendocrine gastroenteropancreatic tumors: general recommendations by a consensus workshop. World J Surg. 1998;22:309–18.

11. Sundin A, Vullierme MP, Kaltsas G, Plockinger U. Enets consensus guidelines for the standards of care in neuroendocrine tumors: radiological examinations. Neuroendocrinology. 2009;90:167–83.

12. Kaltsas GA, Besser GM, Grossman AB. The diagnosis and medical management of advanced neuroendocrine tumours. Endocr Rev. 2004;25:458–511.

13. Krenning EP, Kwekkeboom DJ, Bakker WH, et al. Somatostatin receptor scintigraphy with 111In-DTPA-D-Phe1- and 123-Tyr3 octreotide: the Rotterdam experience with more than 1000 patients. Eur J Nucl Med. 1993;20:716–31.

14. Popperl G. Munich interdisciplinary exchange is the key to optimizing diagnosis and therapy. Report on the 3rd Interdisciplinary NET Symposium, Hamburg, Germany, 2008 Apr 18–19.

15. Kwekkeboom D, Krenning E, Scheidhauer K, et al. Enets consensus guidelines for the standards of care in neuroendocrine tumors: somatostatin receptor imaging with ^{111}In-pentetreotide. Neuroendocrinology. 2009;9:184–9.

16. Perri M, Erba P, Volterrani D, et al. Octreo-SPECT/CT imaging for accurate detection and localization of suspected neuroendocrine tumors. Q J Nucl Med Mol Imaging. 2008;52:323–33.
17. Warner RP, O'Dorisio T. Radiolabeled peptides in diagnosis and tumor imaging clinical overview. Semin Nucl Med. 2002;32:79–83.
18. Oksuz MO, Aschoff P, Kemke B, et al. Imaging of somatostatin-receptor expressing neuroendocrine tumours with 68Ga-DOTATOC-PET/CT versus 111-In-DTPA-octreotide SPECT/CT. Eur J Nucl Med Mol Imaging. 2005;32:109S.
19. Haug A, Auernhammer CJ, Wangler B, Tiling R, et al. Intraindividual comparison of ^{68}Ga-DOTA-TATE and ^{18}F-DOPA PET in patients with well-differentiated metastatic neuroendocrine tumours. Eur J Nucl Med Mol Imaging. 2009;36:765–70.
20. Belhocine T, Foidart J, Rigo P, et al. Fluorodeoxyglucose positron emission tomography and somatostatin receptor scintigraphy for diagnosing and staging carcinoid tumors: correlations with the pathological indexes p53 and Ki-67. Nucl Med Commun. 2002;23:727–34.
21. Virgolini I, Andergassen U, Traub-Weidinger T, et al. Therapy of neuroendocrine tumors. In: Bombardieri E, Buscombe J, Lucignani G, editors. Advances in nuclear oncology. London: Informa Healthcare; 2007. p. 315–39.
22. de Herder WW, Hofland LJ, van der Lely AJ, Lamberts SW. Somatostatin receptors in gastroentero-pancreatic neuroendocrine tumours. Endocr Relat Cancer. 2003;10:451–8.
23. Reubi JC, Schar JC, Waser B, et al. Affinity profiles for human somatostatin receptor subtypes SST1-SST5 of somatostatin radiotracers selected for scintigraphic and radiotherapeutic use. Eur J Nucl Med. 2000; 27:273–82.
24. Wild D, Schmitt JS, Ginj M, et al. DOTA-NOC, a high affinity ligand of somatostatin receptor subtypes 2, 3 and 5 for labeling with various radiometals. Eur J Nucl Med Mol Imaging. 2003;30:1338–47.
25. Druce MR, Lewington V, Grossman AB. Targeted radionuclide therapy for neuroendocrine tumours: principles and Application. Neuroendocrinology. 2010;91:1–15.
26. Krenning EP, de Jong M, Kooij PP, et al. Radiolabelled somatostatin analogue(s) for peptide receptor scintigraphy and radionuclide therapy. Ann Oncol. 1999; 10(Suppl):S23–9.
27. de Jong M, Kwekkeboom D, Valkema R, Krenning EP. Radiolabelled peptides for tumour therapy: current status and future directions. Plenary lecture at the EANM 2002. Eur J Nucl Med Mol Imaging. 2003;30:463–9.
28. Slooter GD, Breeman WA, Marquet RL, Krenning EP, van Eijck CH. Anti-proliferative effect of radiolabelled octreotide in a metastases model in rat liver. Int J Cancer. 1999;81:767–71.
29. Valkema R, De Jong M, Bakker WH. Phase I study of peptide receptor radionuclide therapy with [In-DTPA]

octreotide: The Rotterdam experience. Semin Nucl Med. 2002;32:110–22.
30. Anthony LB, Woltering EA, Espenan GD, Cronin MD, Maloney TJ, McCarthy KE. Indium-111-pentetreotide prolongs survival in gastroenteropancreatic malignancies. Semin Nucl Med. 2002;32:123–32.
31. Buscombe JR, Caplin ME, Hilson AJ. Long-term efficacy of high-activity 111 In-pentetreotide therapy in patients with disseminated neuroendocrine tumors. J Nucl Med. 2003;44:1–6.
32. Kong G, Lau S, Ramdave S, Hicks R. High-dose ^{111}In-octreotide therapy in combination with radiosensitizing 5-Fu chemotherapy for treatment of SSR-expressing neuroendocrine tumours. J Nucl Med. 2005;64:437 (abstr).
33. Gancel M, Girault S, Zerdoud S, et al. ^{111}In-pentetreotide therapy in patients with unresectable progressive malignant endocrine and non-endocrine tumours: clinical results in 20 consecutive cases. Eur J Nucl Med Mol Imaging. 2005;32 Suppl 1:378 (abstr).
34. Cremonesi M, Ferrari M, Zoboli S, et al. Biokinetics and dosimetry in patients administered with (111) In-DOTA-Tyr(3)-octreotide: implications for internal radiotherapy with (90)Y-DOTATOC. Eur J Nucl Med. 1999;26:877–86.
35. Jamar F, Barone R, Mathieu I, et al. ^{86}-Y-DOTA0-D-Phe^1-Tyr^3-octreotide (SMT487)-a phase 1 clinical study: pharmacokinetics, bio-distribution and renal protective effect of different regimens of amino acid co-infusion. Eur J Nucl Med Mol Imaging. 2003;30:510–8.
36. Otte A, Mueller-Brand J, Dellas S, Nitzsche EU, Herrmann R, Maecke HR. Yttrium-90-labelled somatostatin analogue for cancer treatment. Lancet. 1998;351(9100):417–8.
37. Waldherr C, Pless M, Maecke HR, Haldemann A, Mueller-Brand J. The clinical value of [90Y-DOTA]-d-phe1-Tyr3-octreotide (90Y-DOTATOC) in the treatment of neuroendocrine tumours: A clinical phase II study. Ann Oncol. 2001;12:941–5.
38. Waldherr C, Pless M, Maecke HR, et al. Tumour response and clinical benefit in neuroendocrine tumours after 7.4 GBq (90)Y-DOTATOC. J Nucl Med. 2002;43:610–6.
39. Bodei L, Cremonesi M, Zoboli S, et al. Receptor mediated radionuclide therapy with 90Y-DOTATOC in association with amino acid infusion: A phase 1 study. Eur J Nucl Med Mol Imaging. 2003;30: 207–16.
40. Bodei L, Cremonesi M, Grana C. Receptor radionuclide therapy with (90)Y-[DOTA](0)-Tyr(3)-octreotide ((90)Y-DOTATOC) in neuroendocrine tumours. Eur J Nucl Med Mol Imaging. 2004;31:1038–46.
41. Valkema R, Pauwels S, Kvols L, et al. Long-term follow up of a phase 1 study of peptide receptor radionuclide therapy (PRRT) with (90Y-DOTA0, Tyr3) octreotide in patients with somatostatin receptor positive tumours. Eur J Nucl Med Mol Imaging. 2003;30 Suppl 2:S232 (abstract).
42. Virgolini I, Britton K, Buscombe J, et al. In- and Y-DOTA-lanreotide: results and implications of the

MAURITIUS trial. Semin Nucl Med. 2002;32: 148–55.

43. de Jong M, Breeman WA, Bakker WH, et al. 1998 Comparison of (111) In labelled somatostatin analogues for tumour scintigraphy and radionuclide therapy. Cancer Res. 1998;58:437–41.

44. de Jong M, Valkema R, Jamar F, et al. Somatostatin receptor targeted radionuclide therapy of tumors: preclinical and clinical findings. Semin Nucl Med. 2002;32:133–40.

45. Kwekkeboom DJ, Bakker WH, Kam BL, et al. Treatment of patients with gastro-entero-pancreatic (GEP) tumours with the novel radiolabelled somatostatin analogue [(177)Lu-DOTA(0), Tyr(3)]octreotate. Eur J Nucl Med Mol Imaging. 2003;30:417–22.

46. Kwekkeboom DJ, Teunissen JJ, Bakker WH, et al. Radiolabelled somatostatin analogue [177Lu-DOTA0, Tyr3]octreotate in patients with endocrine gastroenteropancreatic tumours. J Clin Oncol. 2005;23: 2754–62.

47. Kwekkeboom DJ, de Herder WW, Kam BL, et al. 2008 Treatment with the radiolabeled somatostatin analogue [177Lu-DOTA0, Tyr3]octreotate: toxicity, efficacy, and survival. J Clin Oncol. 2008;26:2124–30.

48. Baum RP, Soldner J, Schmucking M, Niesen A. Intravenous and intra-arterial peptide receptor radionuclide therapy (PRRT) using Y-90-DOTA-Tyr3-octreotate (Y-90-DOTA-TATE) in patients with metastatic neuroendocrine tumours. Eur J Nucl Med Mol. 2004;31 Suppl 2:S238.

49. Kwekkeboom DJ, Krenning EP, Lebtahi R, et al. ENETS Consensus Guidelines for the Standards of Care in Neuroendocrine Tumours: Peptide Receptor Radionuclide Therapy with Radiolabeled Somatostatin Analogs. Neuroendocrinology. 2009;90:220–6.

50. de Keizer B, van Aken MO, Feelders RA, et al. Hormonal crisis following receptor radionuclide therapy with the radiolabeled somatostatin analogue [(177) Lu-DOTA (0), Tyr (3)]. Eur J Nucl Med Mol. 2008;35:749–55.

51. Brans B, Bodei L, Giammarile F, et al. Clinical radionuclide therapy dosimetry: the quest for the "Holy Gray". Eur J Nucl Med Mol. 2007;34:772–86.

52. Stabin MG. MIRDOSE: personal computer software for internal dose assessment in nuclear medicine. J Nucl Med. 1996;37:538–46.

53. Stabin MG, Sparks RB, Crowe E. OLINDA/EXM: the second generation personal computer software for internal dose assessment in nuclear medicine. J Nucl Med. 2005;46:1023–7.

54. Cremonesi M, Botta F, Di Dia A, et al. Dosimetry for treatment with radiolabelled somatostatin analogues — a review. Q J Nucl Med Mol Imaging. 2010;54: 37–51.

55. Cremonesi M, Ferrari M, Di Dia A, et al. Recent issues on dosimetry and radiobiology for peptide receptor radionuclide therapy. Q J Nucl Med Mol Imaging. 2011;55:155–67.

56. Lhommel R, van Elmbt L. Goffette, et al. Feasibility of 90Y TOF PET-based dosimetry in liver metastasis

therapy using SIR-Spheres. Eur J Nucl Med Mol Imaging. 2010;37:1654–62.

57. Warland S, Flux GD, Konijnenberg MW, et al. Dosimetry of yttrium-labelled radiopharmaceuticals for internal therapy: ^{86}Y or ^{90}Y imaging. Eur J Nucl Med Mol Imaging. 2011;38 Suppl 1:S57–68.

58. Pettinato C, Sarnelli A, Di Donna M, et al. 68-Ga-DOTANOC: biodistribution and dosimetry in patients affected by neuroendocrine tumors. Eur J Nucl Med Mol Imaging. 2008;35:72–9.

59. Rolleman EJ, Melis M, Valkema R, et al. Kidney protection during peptide receptor radionuclide therapy with somatostatin analogues. Eur J Nucl Med Mol Imaging. 2010;37:1018–31.

60. Barone R, Borson-Chazot F, Valkema R, et al. Patient-specific dosimetry in predicting renal toxicity with 90Y-DOTATOC: relevance of kidney volume and dose rate in finding a dose-effect relationship. J Nucl Med. 2005;46:99S–106.

61. Valkema R, Pauwels SA, Kvols LK, et al. Long-term follow-up of renal function after peptide receptor radiation therapy with 90Y-DOTA0, Tyr3-octreotide and 177-Lu-DOTA0, Tyr3-octreotide. J Nucl Med. 2005;46:83S–91.

62. Bodei L, Cremonesi M, Ferrari M, et al. Long-term evaluation of renal toxicity after peptide receptor radionuclide therapy with 90-Y-DOTATOC and 177-Lu-DOTATATE: the role of associated risk factors. Eur J Nucl Med Mol Imaging. 2008;35:1847–56.

63. Sgourous G. Dosimetry of internal emitters. J Nucl Med. 2005;46:18S–27.

64. Wild D, Schmitt JS, Ginj M, et al. DOTA-NOC, a high-affinity ligand of somatostatin receptor subtypes 2, 3 and 5 for labeling with various radiometals. Eur J Nucl Med Mol Imaging. 2003;30:1338–47.

65. Seregni E, Maccauro M, Bombardieri E, et al. Treatment with tandem[(90Y)] DOTA-TATE and [(177)]Lu DOTA-TATE of neuroendocrine tumors refractory to conventional therapy: preliminary results. Q J Nucl Med Mol Imaging. 2010;54:84–91.

66. Reubi JC, Waser B. Concomitant expression of several peptide receptors in neuroendocrine tumours: molecular basis for in vivo multi-receptor tumour targeting. Eur J Nucl Med Mol Imaging. 2003;30: 781–93.

67. Tu SM, Millikan RE, Menigistu B, et al. Bone targeted therapy for advanced androgen independent carcinoma of the prostate: a randomized phase II trial. Lancet. 2001;357:336–41.

68. Kwekkeboom DJ, Boen KL, van Essen M, et al. Somatostatin receptor-based imaging and therapy of gastroenteropancreatic tumours. Endocr Relat Cancer. 2010;17:R53–73.

69. Van Eijck CH. Treatment of advanced endocrine gastro-enteropancreatic tumours using radiolabelled somatostatin analogues. Br J Surg. 2005;92:1333–4.

70. Limouris GS, Chatziioannou A, Kontogeorgakos D, et al. Selective hepatic arterial infusion of In-111-DTPA-Phe^1-octreotide in neuroendocrine liver metastases. Eur J Nucl Med Mol Imaging. 2008;35:1827–37.

71. Kim YS, Brechbiel MW. An overview of targeted alpha therapy. Tumour Biol Epub. 2012;33(3):573–90.
72. SNM Advanced Molecular Imaging and Therapy. High impact radiopeptide therapy halts Neuroendocrine Cancer. Accessed 6 June 2011 [cited 28 Dec 2011]. http://www.snm.org/index.cfm?PageID=10766.
73. Lacayo NJ. Paediatric Neuroblastoma [Online]. Accessed 20 Oct 2010 [cited 24 Mar 2011]. http://www.emedicine.com/ped/topic1570.htm.
74. Bénard J, Raguénez G, Kauffmann A, et al. MYCN-non-amplified metastatic neuroblastoma with good prognosis and spontaneous regression: a molecular portrait of stage 4S. Mol Oncol. 2008;2:261–7.
75. Schulte JH, Horn S, Otto T, et al. MYCN regulates oncogenic MicroRNAs in neuroblastoma. Int J Cancer. 2008;122:699–704.
76. Eisenhofer G, Walther MM, Huynh TT, et al. Pheochromocytomas in VHL syndrome and MEN2 display distinct biochemical and clinical phenotypes. J Clin Endocrinol Metabol. 2001;86:1999–2008.
77. Bravo EL, Gifford RW, Manger WM. Adrenal medullary tumours: phaeochromocytoma. In: Mazzaferri L, Samaan NA, editors. Endocrine tumors. Oxford: Blackwell; 1993. p. 426–47.
78. Howman-Giles R, Shaw PJ, Uren RF, Chung DK. Neuroblastoma and other neuroendocrine tumors. Semin Nucl Med. 2007;37:286–302.
79. Rovozky K, Koplewitz B, Krausz Y, et al. Added value of SPECT/CT for correlation of MIBG scintigraphy and diagnostic CT in neuroblastoma and pheochromocytoma. Am J Roentgenol. 2008;190(4):1085–90.
80. Aggarwal G, Obideen K. Wehbi M; Carcinoid tumors: what should increase our suspicion. Cleve Clin J Med. 2008;75(12):849–55.
81. Caplin ME, Buscombe JR, Hilson AJ, et al. Carcinoid tumour. Lancet. 1998;352(9130):799–805.
82. Rufini V, Schulkin B. The evolution in the use of MIBG in more than 25 years of experimental and clinical applications. Q J Nucl Med Mol Imaging. 2008;52:341–50.
83. Giammarile F, Chiti A, Lassmann M, et al. EANM procedure guidelines for ^{131}I-meta-iodobenzylguanidine ([131]-MIBG) therapy. Eur J Nucl Med Mol Imaging. 2008;35:1039–47.
84. Anon. The role of [131I] Metaiodobenzylguanidine in the treatment of neural crest tumors. Proceedings of an international workshop. Rome, Italy 1991. J Nucl Biol Med 1991;35:177–363.
85. Castellani M, Chiti A, Seregni E, Bombardieri E. Role of 131-I Metaiodobenzylguanidine (MIBG) in the treatment of neuroendocrine tumours: experience of the National Cancer Institute of Milan. Q J Nucl Med. 2000;44:77–87.
86. Loh KC, Fitzgerald PA, Matthay KK, et al. The treatment of malignant pheochromocytoma with iodine-131 metaiodobenzylguanidine ([131]-MIBG): a comprehensive review of 116 reported patients. J Endocrinol Invest. 1997;20:648–58.
87. Chrisoulidou A, Kaltsas G, Ilias A, et al. The diagnosis and management of malignant pheochromocytoma and paraganglioma. Endocr Relat Cancer. 2007;14:569–85.
88. Rose B, Matthay KK, Price D, et al. High-dose ^{131}I-metaiodobenzylguanidine therapy for 12 patients with malignant pheochromocytoma. Cancer. 2003;98:239–48.
89. Castellani MR, Chiesa C, Seregni E, Bombardieri E, et al. ^{131}I-MIBG treatment of pheochromocytoma: low versus intermediate activity regimens of therapy. Q J Nucl Med Mol Imaging. 2010;54:100–13.
90. Solanki KK, Bomanji J, Moyes J, et al. A pharmacological guide to medicines which interfere with the bio-distribution of radiolabelled meta-iodobenzylguanidine (MIBG). Nucl Med Commun. 1992;13:513–21.
91. Matthay KK, Panina C, Huberty J, et al. Correlation of tumour and whole-body dosimetry with tumour response and toxicity in refractory neuroblastoma treated with (131)I-MIBG. J Nucl Med. 2001;42:1713–21.
92. Gaze MN, Chang YC, Flux GD, et al. Feasibility of dosimetry based high dose I-131-metaiodobenzylguanidine with topotecan as a radio-sensitizer in children with metastatic neuroblastoma. Cancer Biother Radiopharm. 2005;20:195–9.
93. Flux GD, Chittenden SJ, Saran F, Gaze MN. Clinical applications of dosimetry for MIBG therapy. Q J Nucl Med Mol Imaging. 2011;55:116–25.
94. Mairs RJ, Boyd M. Optimizing MIBG therapy of neuroendocrine tumours: preclinical evidence of dose maximization and synergy. Nucl Med Biol. 2008;35 Suppl 1:S9–20.
95. Bayer M, Kuci Z, Schömig E, et al. Uptake of MIBG and catecholamines in noradrenaline and organic cation transporter-expressing cells: potential use of corticosterone for a preferred uptake in neuroblastoma and pheochromocytoma cells. Nucl Med Biol. 2009;36:287–94.
96. Gregory RA, Hooker CA, Partridge M, Flux GD. Optimization and assessment of quantitative I124 imaging on a Philips Gemini dual GS PET/CT system. Eur J Nucl Med Mol Imaging. 2009;36:1037–48.
97. van Essen M, Krenning EP, Kooij PP, et al. Effects of therapy with [177Lu-DOTA0, Tyr3] octreotate in patients with paraganglioma, meningioma, small cell lung carcinoma, and melanoma. J Nucl Med. 2006;47:1599–606.
98. Forrer F, Riedweg I, Maecke HR, Mueller-Brand J. Radiolabeled DOTATOC in patients with advanced paraganglioma and pheochromocytoma. Q J Nucl Med Mol Imaging. 2008;52:334–40.
99. Menda Y, O'Dorisio MS, Kao S, et al. Phase I trial of 90Y-DOTATOC therapy in children and young adults with refractory solid tumors that express somatostatin receptors. J Nucl Med. 2010;51:1524–31.

Radionuclide Therapy of Bone Metastases

Alain S. Abi-Ghanem and Katherine Zukotynski

Introduction

Bone metastases occur in many patients with solid malignancies. Up to 85% of patients with breast, lung, and prostate cancer at autopsy have bone metastases. Around 80% of patients with prostate carcinoma, 50% of patients with breast carcinoma and 40% of patients with lung carcinoma develop clinically evident osseous metastases. Nearly half of them experience bone pain [1]. Other tumors can also metastasize to bone, including those originating in the kidneys, thyroid gland, endometrium, cervix, bladder, and gastrointestinal tract. However, these tumors account for less than 20% of patients with bone metastases. The clinical implications of bone metastases are serious. When progressive, they often affect the patients' quality of life by contributing to bone pain, use of narcotic analgesics, pathologic fractures, hypercalcemia, nerve entrapment, spinal cord compression, anxiety, depression, and loss of mobility [2, 3].

The recent advances in hormonal treatment and chemotherapy have, paradoxically, improved the longevity of patients with metastatic disease resulting in an increase in the population of patients with osseous metastases seeking pain relief. A comprehensive multidisciplinary approach is usually required not only to elucidate the cause of the pain and its complications but also to treat the patient appropriately. The optimal management of skeletal metastases depends on the underlying biology of the disease, the life expectancy of the patient, the presence and severity of symptoms, and the availability of effective local or systemic therapies. The use of computed tomography (CT) and bone scintigraphy helps to confirm the presence of bone metastases, classify the lesions into osteoblastic, osteolytic or mixed lytic-sclerotic, and determines the lesions that are at risk for pathologic fracture or cord compression.

Currently, the treatment of bone pain remains palliative and may be either systemic (analgesics, hormonal therapy, chemotherapy, steroids, and bisphosphonates) or local (surgery, nerve blocks, and external beam radiotherapy). Many of these treatments have significant side effects and are limited in their efficacy or duration of pain relief. In general, there is no single method that will keep the patient free of pain for an extended period of time. A combination of systemic and local modalities is often required. Narcotic analgesics and external beam radiotherapy are among the most common treatment forms used for palliation of bone pain. External beam radiotherapy is less favorable when the disease has spread globally, because effective radiation delivery can be limited by toxicity in normal adjacent or overlapping critical structures and organs. As an alternative approach, preferential irradiation at multiple

A.S. Abi-Ghanem, M.D. (✉) • K. Zukotynski, M.D.
Department of Radiology, Dana-Farber Cancer
Institute/Brigham and Women's Hospital,
Harvard Medical School, 450 Brookline Avenue,
DL-101, Boston, MA 02115, USA
e-mail: alaina_ghanem@dfci.harvard.edu

metastatic sites can be accomplished internally using bone-seeking radiopharmaceuticals administered orally or intravenously. Radionuclide therapy has shown good efficacy in relieving bone pain secondary to bone metastasis. This form of systemic metabolic radiotherapy is simple to administer and has clear advantages for the treatment of multifocal metastatic bone pain [4–6].

Radionuclide Selection

Bone pain palliation with bone-seeking radiopharmaceuticals selectively delivers ionizing radiation to areas of increased osteoblastic activity, targeting several osseous metastases at the same time, whether symptomatic or asymptomatic [7]. This concept has been successfully used for more than four decades. Phosphorus-32 (^{32}P) sodium orthophosphate, which could be administered intravenously or orally, was the first radiopharmaceutical to be utilized for this purpose [8–10]. Several other radiopharmaceuticals have been developed over the years, including strontium-89 chloride (^{89}SrCl$_2$), samarium-153 ethylenediamine-tetramethylene phosphonate (^{153}Sm-EDTMP), rhenium-186 hydroxyethylidene diphosphonate (^{186}Re-HEDP), ^{188}Re-HEDP, tin-117m diethylenetriamine pentaacetic acid (^{117m}Sn-DTPA), lutetium-177 ethylenediamine-tetramethylene phosphonate (^{177}Lu-EDTMP), and more recently, lutetium-177 methylene diphosphonate (^{177}Lu-MDP) and radium-223 chloride (^{223}RaCl$_2$) (Table 5.1).

The physical properties of these radionuclides vary, and each confers different benefits. Most of them are administered intravenously and target the calcium hydroxyapatite component of the metastatic bone lesion with a high target-to-nontarget ratio and a low concentration in the surrounding tissues such as the healthy bone and bone marrow. Tumor targeting relies on selective uptake in the bone and prolonged retention at sites of increased osteoblastic activity. While some radionuclides (^{89}Sr and ^{223}Ra) have a natural affinity for reactive bone, others (^{153}Sm, ^{186}Re, and ^{188}Re) form stable complexes with bone-seeking cations, such as phosphate and diphosphonate.

The nature of the emissions (β–, conversion electrons, α), the energy of the particles emitted and the range of penetration in the tissues determine the therapeutic suitability of the radionuclide and its treatment-related toxicity. Whereas the energy of short-range electron- or α-particles is largely absorbed within the target cell, longer-range β-particles have the potential to irradiate surrounding normal tissues, contributing to undesirable side effects. The radionuclide should also have a sufficiently long physical half-life that matches the biologic turnover of the radiopharmaceutical in vivo in order to optimally deposit damaging or lethal radiation doses in the target cells [5]. ^{89}Sr is a pure β emitter and has a long physical

Table 5.1 Radionuclides/radiopharmaceuticals used for the therapy of bone metastases

Isotope	Radiopharmaceutical	Half-life (days)	Energy (MeV) (maximum/mean)	γ-Energy (keV) (%)	Soft-tissue range (mm) (maximum/mean)	Usual dose
^{32}P	^{32}P-orthophosphate	14.3	1.7/0.70 (β)	–	8.5/3 (β)	5–10 mCi i.v. 10–12 mCi p.o.
^{89}Sr	^{89}SrCl$_2$	50.5	1.46/0.58 (β)	0.91 (0.01)	7/2.4 (β)	4 mCi i.v. 40–60 μCi/kg i.v.
^{153}Sm	^{153}Sm-EDTMP	1.9	0.81/0.23 (β)	103 (28)	3.4/0.6 (β)	1 mCi/kg i.v.
^{186}Re	^{186}Re-HEDP	3.7	1.07/0.35 (β)	137 (9)	3.7/1.1 (β)	35 mCi i.v.
^{223}Ra	^{223}RaCl$_2$	11.4	5.64 (α) (mean)	154 (5.6) 269 (13.6)	0.05–0.08	1.4 μCi/kg i.v.
^{117m}Sn	^{117m}Sn-DTPA	13.6	0.127, 0.129 and 0.152 (conversion electrons)	159	0.2–0.3 (conversion electrons)	0.05–0.27 mCi/kg i.v.

half-life (50.5 days), while [153]Sm, [186]Re, and [188]Re have much shorter physical half-lives (less than 4 days) and are γ emitters. [223]Ra, with a half-life of 11.4 days, is an α emitter and provides a much more densely ionizing type of radiation that predominantly induces nonrepairable DNA damage [11, 12]. While γ emitters permit dosimetric measurements and posttreatment scintigraphic imaging, there are additional concerns of radiation safety to the public. Bone-seeking radiopharmaceuticals with shorter half-lives could facilitate more rapid bone marrow recovery [13, 14], allowing for safe repeated administration [15].

Regardless the radionuclide utilized, there is persistent concern of cross-irradiation of the adjacent functioning bone marrow contributing to adverse effects and toxicities.

Radiopharmaceuticals for Bone Pain Therapy

Approved Radiopharmaceuticals

The intravenous injection or oral administration of ^{32}P-sodium orthophosphate and the intravenous injection of ^{89}Sr-chloride and [153]Sm-EDTMP (also called [153]Sm-lexidronam) have been approved by the U.S. Food and Drug Administration (FDA) for the treatment of bone pain resulting from osteoblastic metastatic disease, as defined by bone scintigraphy. The administration of these agents falls under the guidelines of the Nuclear Regulatory Commission (NRC), Title 10 CFR Part 35.300 or Agreement State Institutional License. Institutional licenses must specifically list individuals licensed to use Section 35.300 materials.

[32]P-Sodium Orthophosphate

[32]P decays by β-emission to [32]S with maximum energy of 1.71 MeV, mean energy of 0.695 MeV, maximum soft-tissue range of 8.5 mm, average range of 3 mm and no γ emission. However, it may be imaged with moderate success using the low-energy bremsstrahlung emission. [32]P has a physical half-life of 14.3 days. Clearance is mainly renal with 5–10% excreted at 24 h and around 20% at 1 week. The usual administered activity of ^{32}P-sodium phosphate is 5–10 mCi intravenously (often in divided doses) or 10–12 mCi orally, according to the Society of Nuclear Medicine (SNM) Procedure Guidelines [16].

The therapeutic ratio of phosphorus for tumor-to-normal bone is approximately 2:1. Pretreatment with testosterone was shown to increase osteoblastic activity around metastases, enhancing this ratio by up to 20:1. However, testosterone may exacerbate bone pain and cause nausea and vomiting. In addition, the risk of soft-tissue tumor progression in hormone-sensitive tumors increases with testosterone administration [10, 17, 18]. For this reason, some authors have used alternative methods to increase the uptake in the tumor by pretreating with parathormone (PTH). PTH increases bone mineral absorption. It has been postulated that when PTH therapy is withdrawn, a transient rebound effect results in greater deposition of phosphate at metastatic sites associated with increased osteoblastic activity [19].

Total pain relief in patients treated with ^{32}P after androgen stimulation occurs in 20–50% whereas significant pain relief is reported to be around 84% in patients with breast cancer and 77% in patients with prostate cancer. This occurs within 5–14 days after injection, although a flare of pain may occur 2–3 days after injection and lasting for 2–4 days. The mean duration of response is 2–4 months. Dose-dependent pancytopenia is expected after administration of ^{32}P with a nadir at 5–6 weeks [10, 20, 21]. In one study, myelosuppression developed in 8 of 33 patients with metastatic breast carcinoma and in 7 of 15 patients with metastatic prostate carcinoma. Peripheral blood values returned within 8 weeks to 80% of the pretreatment levels in these patients with conservative management. Some patients had transient periods of fever, gastroenteritis, or minor hemorrhagic manifestations at the nadir of the hematological depression [9]. The response in patients who are retreated after recurrence is usually similar to the initial response but may be less intense and shorter in duration.

Currently, intravenous ^{32}P is rarely used for bone pain palliation in the Western world. The significant cost advantage and ease of oral administration compared with licensed alternatives have regenerated interest in this agent as the radiopharmaceutical of choice for bone pain palliation elsewhere in the world. In 1999, a study from India comparing single oral administration of 12 mCi of ^{32}P with intravenous administration of 4 mCi of ^{89}Sr demonstrated equal efficacy and toxicity in 31 patients with painful osseous metastases [22].

[89]Sr-Chloride

[89]Sr emits a β particle with maximum energy of 1.46 MeV, mean energy of 0.58 MeV, maximum soft-tissue range of 7 mm, average range of 2.4 mm and 0.01% abundant nonimageable γ emission with a photopeak of 0.91 MeV. It has a physical half-life of 50.5 days. As a group II metal and similarly to calcium, strontium has a natural affinity for sites within the skeleton that normally metabolize calcium to form new bone. [85]Sr, an isotope of ^{89}Sr, has a physical half-life of 64.8 days and a γ emission at 514 keV that allows imaging for tracer distribution. Biodistribution studies using [85]Sr demonstrated a therapeutic ratio of 10:1 for tumor-to-normal bone [23]. After injection, around 70% of the injected dose is retained in the skeleton while the remaining portion is predominantly excreted in the urine. Renal excretion of strontium is dictated by the skeletal tumor burden: the greater the involvement, the greater the retention. At 90 days, the retention of ^{89}Sr ranges from 11% with minimal metastatic involvement, to 88% with significant involvement [24].

The usual administered activity of [89]SrCl$_2$ is 4 mCi or 40–60 μCi/kg intravenously [16]. There is no dose–response relationship, although some studies suggested a threshold activity of 27 μCi/kg below which ^{89}Sr therapy appeared ineffective and a response plateau above 40 μCi/kg [25].

Total pain relief occurs in about 20% of patients who receive ^{89}Sr, whereas significant pain relief occurs in 70–90% of patients with bone metastases due to breast or prostate cancer. In patients with lung cancer, there is poorer palliation of pain ranging between 20 and 30%. Pain relief usually begins within 2–4 weeks after ^{89}Sr administration. The effects are maintained for 4–15 months, with a mean of 6 months. Pain may flare in 10–20% of patients, 2–3 days after ^{89}Sr is administered. This generally appears subsequent to good responses to the injected [89]Sr. Other side effects include mild hematologic depression, generally occurring after 5 weeks of treatment, with a 15–20% decrease in total platelet and white blood cell count from baseline. Recovery is typically slow over the next 6 weeks, dictated by metastatic extent and bone marrow reserve [25, 26].

Patients with few metastases are more likely to benefit from ^{89}Sr therapy than patients with end-stage disease and an expected survival of less than 3 months. A study by Lee et al. reported unfavorable results in 28 patients with widespread disease who were treated with doses of 2.2–4.4 mCi of ^{89}Sr-chloride (mean of 3 mCi). At 12 weeks, only 29% of patients experienced moderate to dramatic pain relief, 32% had some relief, and 50% had no pain relief. This group of patients had only a 23-week median survival, and 32% required additional palliative external beam radiation. In addition, these patients subsequently had a greater drop in their blood count [27].

Compared with local field and hemibody external beam radiotherapy, [89]SrCl$_2$ was shown to be as effective as both of these approaches in relieving existing bone pain. However, it delayed the development of new pain at preexisting clinically silent sites of disease [28]. This observation was confirmed in the Trans-Canada study in 1993 [29] but later contradicted by a Norwegian study in 2003 [30]. The discrepancy may be reflected by the higher activity used in the Trans-Canada study (10.8 mCi) compared with the licensed 4 mCi activity used in the Norwegian study.

Studies have also examined the role of the combination of ^{89}Sr and chemotherapy in metastatic hormone-refractory prostate cancer. Theoretically, this may add beneficial antitumoral activity to the analgesic effect of ^{89}Sr, and radio-sensitize the tumor cells to the effect of [89]Sr. Whereas preliminary studies of ^{89}Sr with low-dose cisplatin (35 mg/m^2) and doxorubicin (15 and 20 mg/m^2) showed no clear clinical benefit based on pain relief or performance improvement [31, 32], later studies using higher doses of chemotherapy showed not only a benefit in pain relief, but an improvement in overall survival. For instance, Sciuto et al. reported a superior pain response in a prospective randomized controlled trial of 35 patients with hormone-refractory prostate cancer who were treated with ^{89}Sr with low-dose carboplatin (50 mg/m^2 at 0, 10, and 11 days), in comparison with a similar size control group treated with ^{89}Sr alone. In this study, 91% of patients treated with [89]SrCl$_2$ and low-dose cisplatin achieved pain response compared with 63% of patients treated with [89]SrCl$_2$ alone ($P<0.01$). In addition, the combination therapy appeared to slow the rate of skeletal metastatic progression (27% in the first arm vs. 64% in the control arm; $P=0.01$) [33]. There was no increase in myelosuppression by the addition of cisplatin and no significant change in patient survival. However, a randomized phase II study provided provocative data suggesting there was an improvement in overall survival using six weekly administrations of [89]SrCl$_2$ with doxorubicin after induction chemotherapy (consisting of ketoconazole and doxorubicin alternating with estramustine and vinblastine) compared with six weekly administrations of doxorubicin alone. The patients who received [89]SrCl$_2$ and doxorubicin had a median survival time of 27.7 months (4.9–37.7 months), whereas those who received doxorubicin alone had a median survival of 16.8 months (4.4–34.2 months) ($P=0.0014$) [34]. A third nonrandomized study using estramustine phosphate, vinblastine, and [89]SrCl$_2$ provided effective palliation, a ≥50% decline in prostate-specific antigen (PSA) from the pretreatment level in 48% of treated patients, and a probable reduced demand for subsequent palliative radiation therapy [35]. In all these studies, combined chemoradiation was well tolerated with manageable additional hematologic toxicity.

[153]Sm-EDTMP

[153]Sm decays with emissions of both β- and γ-particles. The maximum β-particle energy is 0.81 MeV (mean of 0.23 MeV) with maximum soft-tissue range of 3.4 mm and average range of 0.6 mm. The γ-photon has a 28% abundancy with a photopeak of 103 keV that allows scintigraphic imaging. It has a physical half-life of 1.9 days or 46.3 h. Complexed with the chelator EDTMP, it is supplied as [153]Sm-lexidronam. The usual administered activity of [153]Sm-lexidronam is 1 mCi/kg intravenously [16]. After intravenous administration, [153]Sm-lexidronam is rapidly taken up by the skeleton by bridging the hydroxyapatite bone matrix at sites of increased osteoblastic activity. Clearance from the blood is biexponential with rapid bone uptake (half-life 5.5 min) and plasma renal clearance (half-life 65.4 min) [36] (Fig. 5.1). Skeletal uptake ranges between 55 and 75%, depending on the skeletal tumor burden: the greater the number of metastases, the greater the retention in the bone. The remaining portion is rapidly excreted into the urine by 6–7 h after administration. The tumor-to-normal bone ratio ranges between 4:1 and 7:1 [37–39].

Effective pain relief occurs in 61–80% of patients treated with [153]Sm-lexidronam. The duration of pain relief is typically 8 weeks, ranging between 4 and 35 weeks. Onset of pain palliation is rapid, occurring within 1 week of administration, frequently within 48 h [13, 38, 40]. In a phase I/II trial completed at the University of Washington by Collins et al., symptom benefit was seen in 34 of 46 patients (76%) with hormone-refractory prostate cancer at 4 weeks. Pain relief was observed at each activity level of [153]Sm-lexidronam (0.5–3 mCi/kg with increments of 0.5 mCi/kg) but not in all patients of each cohort. Seventy percent of patients treated at 1 mCi/kg had pain response while 80% of patients treated at 2.5 mCi/kg had a response. Toxicity was limited to dose-related transient myelosuppression, mainly thrombocytopenia with a nadir at 4 weeks recovering at 5 weeks, and leukopenia with a nadir at 2 weeks recovering between 7 and 10 weeks [13]. In all these

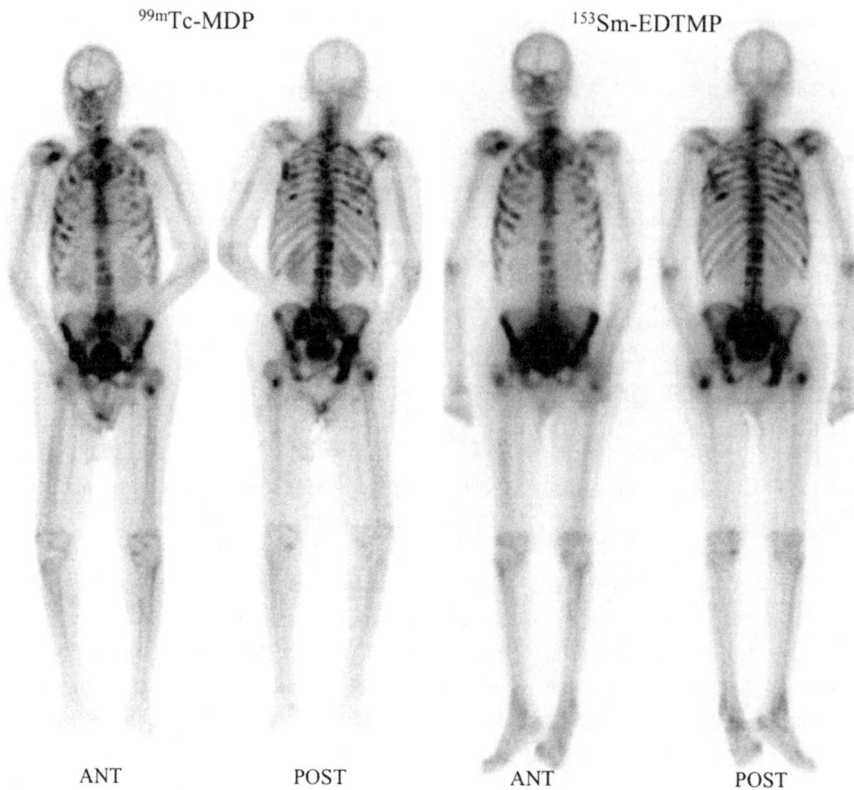

Fig. 5.1 A 77-year-old man with metastatic hormone-resistant prostate cancer and severe bone pain requiring narcotics and causing constipation, somnolence, and inability to function presents for pain palliation with radiopharmaceuticals. A pretherapy bone scan with ^{99m}Tc-methylene diphosphonate (MDP) shows several focal sites of increased radiotracer uptake throughout the axial and proximal appendicular skeleton, confirming the presence of multifocal osteoblastic metastatic disease. He received 49 mCi of samarium-153 ethylenediamine-tetramethylene phosphonate (^{153}Sm-EDTMP) intravenously (1 mCi/kg). A scan obtained 2 h posttherapy using the 103 keV γ-photons shows excellent localization of ^{153}Sm-EDTMP to the sites of metastatic disease demonstrated on the ^{99m}Tc-MDP scan. The excretion of both radiotracers occurs via the kidneys

studies, there was a painful flare response in approximately 10% of patients, noted within 48 h after receiving the treatment.

Based on these studies, larger prospective randomized controlled studies were performed in patients with painful bone metastases secondary to a variety of primary malignancies. These consistently reported high clinical efficacy on the basis of visual analog scores, physician's global assessments and daily opioid analgesic use. They also established the optimal injected activity of ^{153}Sm-lexidronam as 1 mCi/kg. In one study of 118 patients, pain relief was observed in 62–72% of those who received the 1 mCi/kg dose during the first 4 weeks, with marked or complete relief in 31% by 4 weeks. In addition, a significant correlation ($P=0.01$) between reductions in opioid use and pain scores was seen only in those who received the 1 mCi/kg activity [41]. In another study of 114 patients, treatment with ^{153}Sm-lexidronam produced improvement from baseline in all patients. However, the magnitude of improvement was greater in the higher dose group (1 mCi/kg) at each week after initiation of therapy, with statistically significant decreases from baseline at 3 and 4 weeks ($P<0.005$). None of the changes from baseline in the lower dose group (0.5 mCi/kg) were statistically significant. A subset of patients with breast cancer receiving 1 mCi/kg had the most noticeable improvement, with long-term follow-up showing longer survival among those who received the higher dose than among those who received the lower dose [42].

On a different note, there has been a controversy regarding the combined use of bisphosphonates and bone-seeking radiopharmaceuticals such as [153]Sm-EDTMP. Patients with an indication for radionuclide bone palliation usually receive monthly infusions of bisphosphonates to decrease the incidence of skeletal-related events. Based on the hypothesis that both agents have the same binding sites on the hydroxyapatite crystal, there are conflicting data as to whether bisphosphonates inhibit the uptake of radiolabeled phosphonates in bone metastases. While some studies reported a decrease in radiotracer uptake of ^{99m}Tc-labeled phosphonates in patients receiving etidronate intravenously or orally [43–45], other studies reported the possibility of combining both agents [46, 47] as well as an improvement in terms of pain palliation and clinical response using bisphosphonates and [153]Sm-EDTMP [48, 49] and bisphosphonates and [89]SrCl$_2$ [50].

Finally, high activity therapy followed by peripheral blood stem cell transplant has been used to treat locally recurrent or metastatic osteosarcoma and bone metastases that are avid on bone scintigraphy. In a study from Mayo Clinic, 30 patients were treated with activity levels of [153]Sm-EDTMP ranging from 1 to 30 mCi/kg. After peripheral blood progenitor cell (PBPC) or marrow infusion on day 14, recovery of hematopoiesis was problematic in 2 patients treated at the 30 mCi/kg dose level. Reduction or elimination of opioids for pain was seen in all patients suggesting that [153]Sm-EDTMP with PBPC support can provide bone-specific therapeutic irradiation [51]. Furthermore, a case of a 21-year-old woman with nonresectable metastatic pelvic osteosarcoma was reported in the literature. The patient was treated with 4.5 mCi/kg of [153]Sm-EDTMP, peripheral blood progenitor cell support, external beam radiotherapy to the pelvic lesion (total dose of 60 Gy), and multiagent chemotherapy. The treatment led to almost immediate pain relief. She remained alive and without signs of active tumor after 3 years and 4 months following [153]Sm-EDTMP therapy [52].

> **The Principles of Bone Pain Palliation Using Radionuclides**
>
> • Oral or intravenous administration
> • Selective uptake in the bone
> • Prolonged retention at sites of increased osteoblastic activity
> • Therapeutic suitability determined by type of emissions, the energy, path length, and toxicity
> • Improve overall survival with Ra-223

Investigational Radiopharmaceuticals

[186]Re-HEDP

[186]Re-HEDP is supplied as [186]Re-etidronate and approved in some European countries but not in the United States. [186]Re emits a β-particle with maximum energy of 1.07 MeV, mean energy of 0.349 MeV, maximum soft-tissue range of 3.7 mm and average range of 1.1 mm. It also emits a 9% abundant γ-photon of 137 keV that can be used for imaging and dosimetry. The physical half-life is 89 h (3.7 days). Rhenium is chemically similar to ^{99m}Tc and can be easily complexed with diphosphonates such as HEDP with a relatively high radionuclide and radiochemical purity. The biodistribution of [186]Re-HEDP is similar to that of ^{99m}Tc-MDP. Skeletal uptake is maximal 3 h after intravenous injection. Clearance is mainly renal (~70%), with approximately 70% excreted in the first 24 h after injection [53] (Fig. 5.2). The usual administered activity according to the European Association of Nuclear Medicine is 35 mCi intravenously [54]. Using this dose, dosimetric studies found a mean tumor-to-marrow dose ratios of 22:1 [55].

Overall pain relief ranges between 60 and 90% after a single administration of [186]Re-etidronate. Whereas Han et al. showed a 58% response rate in patients with metastatic bone pain in breast cancer [56], Sciuto et al. reported a response of 92% in the same cancer population [57]. In prostate cancer and in a preliminary study on 20 men

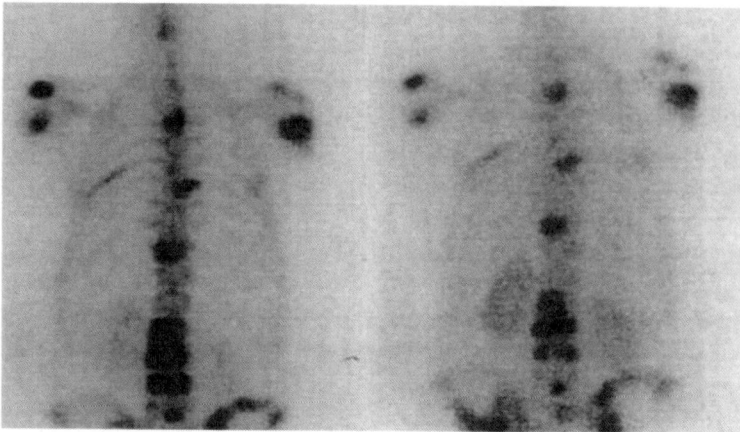

Fig. 5.2 Gamma scintigraphy of ^{99m}Tc-HDP (*left*) and ^{186}Re-HEDP (*right*) in a patient with skeletal metastases. The images were obtained 2 h after the injection of 10.8 mCi ^{99m}Tc-HDP, and 3 h after the injection of 48.3 mCi rhenium-186 hydroxyethylidene diphosphonate (^{186}Re-HEDP). Reprinted by permission of the Society of Nuclear Medicine (SNM) from de Klerk et al. ([53], Fig. 4)

with advanced disease, the authors reported an overall response of 80% (16/20) with partial pain relief in 55% (11/20) and complete pain relief in 25% of patients (5/20). The time to onset was 1–3 weeks after injection of a mean activity of 33.1 mCi ^{186}Re-etidronate, and the duration of response was 7 weeks [58]. The same group later completed a small randomized placebo-controlled study published in 1991 on 13 patients and showed a similar response (~80%) [59]. However, another double-blind placebo-controlled randomized trial published in 2002 showed a lower response rate using more stringent pain assessment criteria and a larger sample size. In this study, the authors evaluated 43 patients in the Rhenium group and 36 patients in the Placebo group. They defined a positive response day as a day on which pain intensity was reduced by ≥25% compared with the baseline values. The total response (%) was then defined as the number of positive response days divided by the number of days of follow-up. With that, they demonstrated a mean response in the treated group of 27% (or 23/84 days) vs. 13% (11/84 days) in the control group ($P < 0.05$) [14].

Pain relief is typically rapid, occurring within 24–48 h of activity administration. The duration of relief ranges from 2 to 8 weeks with a mean of 4 weeks [56]. Toxicity is limited to transient and mild myelosuppression at the recommended dose (35 mCi). In a dose-escalation study of ^{186}Re-HEDP in patients with metastatic prostate cancer, thrombocytopenia proved to be the dose-limiting toxicity, while leukopenia played a minor role. Platelet and neutrophil nadirs were noted at 4 weeks after therapy. Recovery occurred within 4–6 weeks and was complete within 8 weeks [60]. Of note, the maximum tolerated dose (MTD) was found to be 80 mCi vs. 65 mCi in another study of patients with metastatic breast cancer [61]. Other side effects such as pain flare also occur in 7–50% of patients treated with ^{186}Re-HEDP. This has been attributed to intraosseous edema and is usually controlled by temporary analgesic increase and corticosteroids [56, 62]. Because of the early onset of pain relief and the fast time to marrow recovery, ^{186}Re-HEDP seems indicated in patients with unbearable pain and with a low estimated life expectancy.

Finally, the feasibility of high dose therapy followed by peripheral stem cell rescue has been demonstrated in patients with hormone-refractory prostate cancer metastatic to bone in an attempt to maximize the palliative benefit of ^{186}Re-HEDP and deliver ablative doses to each metastasis. PSA reductions of ≥50% lasting at least 4 weeks were seen in some patients (5 of 25 patients) receiving activities greater than 94.6 mCi. However, it remains unclear whether the PSA responses have clinical significance or survival benefit [63].

^{223}RaCl$_2$

The field of radiopharmaceuticals in 2011 was advanced significantly when the results of a well-powered phase III prostate cancer study demonstrated a survival advantage for patients who received the α-emitting radiopharmaceutical ^{223}RaCl$_2$. Overall, they demonstrated efficient pain relief, reduction in tumor marker levels, and improved overall survival in the treatment of skeletal metastases in patients with prostate and breast cancer [12, 64–68].

Investigators have long recognized the potential advantages of α-particle emitters despite the predominant use of β-emitters in radiotherapy trials. α-Particles are positively charged helium nuclei with a higher energy (5–8 MeV) than β-particles and shorter range (50–80 μm) in soft tissue. Compared with electrons and β-particles, α-particles exhibit a high density of ionization events along their track [69], referred to as the linear energy transfer (LET). High-LET radiation also causes more severe chromosomal damage than low-LET radiation, including shattered chromosomes during mitosis and complex chromosomal rearrangements [70]. Thus, the cytotoxicity of α-particles may be extremely effective and less dose-dependent than that of β-particles, and cell death may occur after a single or a few α-particle emissions [71]. In addition, the deposition of energy over a much shorter range than β-emitters is of interest since targeted cells might be destroyed while neighboring cells are spared, making it advantageous in avoiding bone marrow toxicity.

^{223}Ra (half-life 11.4 days) can be obtained from the decay of actinium-227 (^{227}Ac; half-life 21.8 years) using a generator system. Because of its natural affinity for metabolically active bone and similar to calcium, ^{223}Ra, administered intravenously as ^{223}RaCl$_2$, can deliver high-LET radiation to malignant cells. ^{223}Ra decays by the emission of four α-particles and two β-particles via daughter isotopes to stable lead-207 (^{207}Pb). While the mean α-energy released from the decay of ^{223}Ra to radon-219 (^{219}Rn) is 5.64 MeV, the energy associated with the entire decay cascade approximates 28 MeV. ^{223}Ra and bismuth-211 (^{211}Bi) have a characteristic γ-peak at 154 keV (5.6% abundance) and 351 keV (12.8%) respectively. These photons may be used to determine whether daughter radionuclides redistribute in the body. In addition, ^{223}Ra has a 269 keV γ-photon (13.6%) that is difficult to distinguish from that of its ^{219}Rn daughter (271 keV; 9.9%). Preclinical studies in mice show rapid blood clearance after intravenous injection. Peak skeletal uptake occurs within 1 h of injection, with no significant change in the level of uptake after 14 days, indicating excellent skeletal retention. Bone uptake is also high and selective compared with soft-tissue uptake. Unlike calcium, excretion is mainly intestinal with less than 10% renal (Fig. 5.3a, b). It has been postulated that the relatively long half-life of ^{223}Ra allows for incorporation into the bone during remodeling, contributing to better retention of daughter products which could otherwise redistribute in the body and contribute to toxicity [69, 72].

The clinical trials that lead to the conduct of the phase III trial followed a traditional development path. In a phase IA dose-escalation study of 25 patients (15 prostate and 10 breast cancer patients) using single-dose infusion of ^{223}RaCl$_2$ ranging in activity from ~1.2 to 6.8 μCi/kg (46 to 250 kBq/kg), there was no hematologic dose-limiting toxicity. Reversible myelosuppression, mainly neutropenia and leukopenia, occurred with nadirs 2–4 weeks after injection. For platelets, only grade 1 toxicity was observed even at the highest dosage levels. Pain flare occurred in 9 of 25 patients with 7 of the patients during the first week after treatment. Ten of twenty-five patients developed mild and transient diarrhea. Overall, the low-grade toxicities were attributed to the short range of α-particles in soft tissue. Pain relief was observed in more than 50% of the patients after 7 days, 4 and 8 weeks. A decline in total serum alkaline phosphatase (ALP) compared with baseline was observed in greater than 50% of patients with metastatic prostate cancer and elevated pretreatment values [12, 65].

A small phase IB study on 6 patients with prostate cancer was also performed to evaluate the safety profile of repeated injections at two

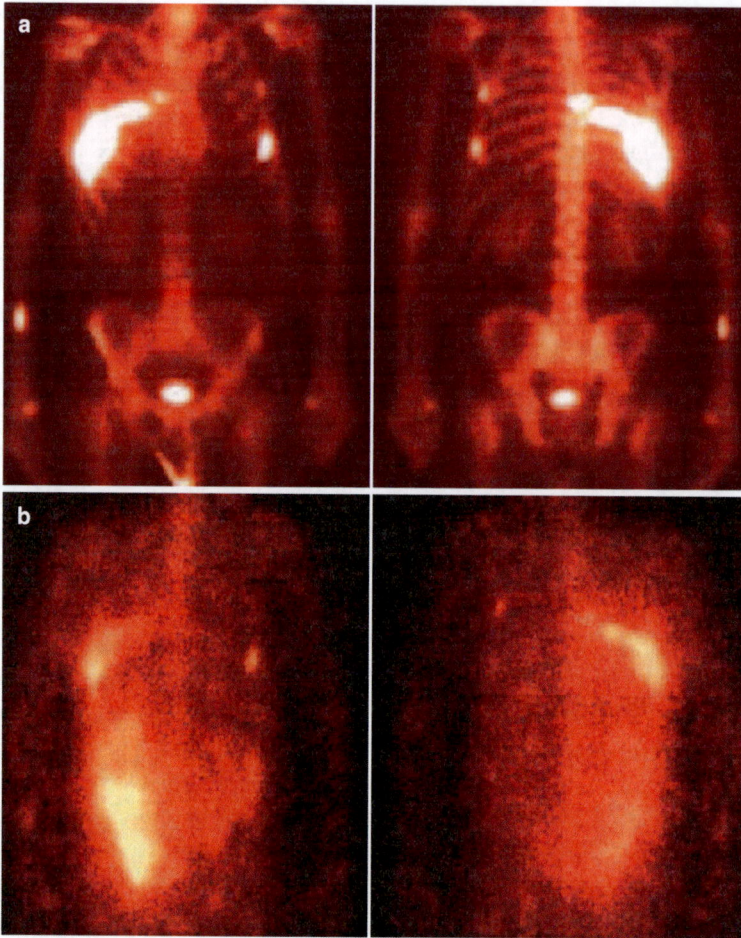

Fig. 5.3 Gamma scintigraphy of ^{99m}Tc-MDP (**a**) and ^{223}RaCl$_2$ (**b**) in a patient with skeletal metastases. ^{223}Ra has γ peaks at 269 and 154 keV, and the ^{219}Rn daughter, which has a very short half-life, has a γ peak at 271 keV. Because of the low levels of injected radioactivity, the number of events is low, necessitating long acquisition times. Clearance of radium-223 chloride (^{223}RaCl$_2$) is predominantly hepatobiliary/intestinal with less than 10% via renal excretion. Reprinted by permission of the American Association for Cancer Research from Nilsson et al. ([12], Fig. 3)

dosage levels: 1.4 μCi/kg (50 kBq/kg) given five times with a 3-week interval (4 patients), or two injections of 3.4 μCi/kg (125 kBq/kg) with a 6-week interval (2 patients). There were no additional toxic effects related to the repeated treatment. The authors suggested that repeated treatment should be scheduled in a way to allow normalization of the blood count before a new injection is given [65, 73].

In a randomized placebo-controlled multicentric phase II trial, 64 patients with hormone-resistant prostate cancer and bone pain needing external beam radiotherapy were randomized to either saline injections given four times with 4-week intervals (31 patients) or 1.4 μCi/kg (50 kBq/kg) ^{223}RaCl$_2$ injections given four times at 4-week intervals (33 patients). Again, ^{223}RaCl$_2$ was well tolerated with minimum myelotoxicity as in the phase I trials. The study showed a significant benefit for ^{223}Ra with respect to all serum bone markers such as bone ALP concentrations (-65.6% at 4 weeks in the ^{223}Ra-treated arm vs. 9.3% in the placebo arm; $P < 0.0001$) and a potential benefit for ^{223}Ra on time to PSA progression (median

26 weeks for ^{223}Ra vs. 8 weeks for placebo; $P=0.048$). The median relative change in PSA from baseline to 4 weeks was −23.8% in the ^{223}Ra group and 44.9% in the placebo group ($P=0.003$). These findings suggested that effective treatment of bone metastases could substantially delay disease progression in hormone-refractory prostate cancer. In addition, median overall survival was improved (65.3 weeks for ^{223}Ra vs. 46.4 weeks for placebo; $P=0.066$) and more patients were alive at 18 months (45% vs. 26%) in the ^{223}Ra-treated arm compared with the placebo arm. However, the survival data were interpreted with caution due to the small sample size [66].

Additional data from the same group from two open-label phase I trials ($N=37$) and three double-blind phase II trials ($N=255$) showed that bone markers and PSA decreased significantly in patients treated with varying doses of ^{223}RaCl$_2$ (0.14–6.8 µCi/kg or 5–250 kBq/kg). More adverse events were seen in the placebo group than in the radium-223 group (174 patients vs. 155 patients), and the median overall survival improved in the radium-223 group compared with the placebo group (65 weeks vs. 46 weeks; $P=0.017$) [68].

In an effort to understand the meaning of ALP normalization (<128 U/L), two other randomized phase II studies were performed. One study showed ALP normalization in 12/26 (46%) patients treated with ^{223}Ra, 1.4 µCi/kg (50 kBq/kg) every 4 weeks for 12 weeks. Median survivals of those with and without ALP normalization were 102 weeks and 42 weeks, respectively ($P<0.001$). The other study, which evaluated ^{223}Ra at different activities (0.7, 1.4, or 2.2 µCi/kg (or 25, 50, or 80 kBq/kg) every 6 weeks for 12 weeks), showed ALP normalization in 25/75 (33%) cases: 5/29 (17%) in the 0.7 µCi/kg group, 10/25 (40%) with 1.4 µCi/kg and 10/21 (48%) with 2.2 µCi/kg, indicating a dose–response relationship. Median survivals for the 25 patients with, and the 50 patients without, ALP normalization were 102 weeks vs. 58 weeks respectively ($P=0.0086$). The authors concluded that, in patients with metastatic castrate-resistant prostate cancer and bone metastases

treated with ^{223}RaCl$_2$, ALP normalization was associated with significantly better overall survival [67].

These encouraging results were supporting the rationale for the larger phase III study that was ongoing around the same time (ALSYMPCA trial). The study design was randomized double-blind placebo-controlled and multicentric, aimed at comparing ^{223}RaCl$_2$ plus best standard of care with placebo plus best standard of care, in patients with prostate cancer. Nine hundred and twenty-two patients were randomly assigned (2:1) either to 1.4 µCi/kg (50 kBq/kg) ^{223}Ra injections given six times at 4-week intervals or to placebo. The majority of patients had received prior chemotherapy with docetaxel. The primary end point of the study was overall survival (OS). In June 2011, press releases from the pharmaceutical company announced that the study was stopped early based on the recommendation of an independent data monitoring committee. The preliminary results from a preplanned interim efficacy analysis showed improved OS in the ^{223}RaCl$_2$ group compared with the placebo group (median 14 months vs. 11.2 months respectively; $P=0.0022$; HR=0.699) [64].

The results of the ALSYMPCA trial represent a major advantage for the future development of ^{223}Ra in the treatment of hormone-refractory prostate cancer with bone metastases. The current standard first-line chemotherapy, docetaxel, has been shown not only to achieve disease responses, but also to improve overall survival. However, the magnitude of the overall survival benefit is modest. In a randomized trial published in the New England Journal of Medicine in 2004, the median duration of survival in the group given docetaxel every 3 weeks was 18.9 months vs. 16.5 months in the group given mitoxantrone ($P=0.009$). Side effects were also more common in the group that received docetaxel. While other chemotherapeutic agents such as estramustine, mitoxantrone, or cyclophosphamide can provide clinical responses including pain palliation, a survival benefit for these drugs has not been demonstrated [74]. In view of the favorable effects and toxicity profile of ^{223}Ra in the treatment of hormone-refractory prostate cancer with bone metastases, combination therapy with docetaxel is considered and could have an additional disease-modifying effect.

For this purpose, a multicentric study is currently underway to explore the safety and efficacy of ^{223}RaCl$_2$ (1.4 μCi/kg or 50 kBq/kg) in combination with docetaxel given every 3 weeks in patients with bone metastases from castrate-resistant prostate cancer. The study has a phase I and a phase IIA components. The phase I part is to establish a recommended dose of ^{223}RaCl$_2$ to be used in combination with docetaxel. The phase IIA part will incorporate a randomized design to investigate the safety and tolerability, and explore efficacy, of ^{223}RaCl$_2$ in combination with docetaxel (with doses defined by the phase I trial) compared with standard dose docetaxel (75 mg/m^2 with prednisone every 3 weeks) [75].

^{117m}Sn-DTPA

Tin-117m (half-life 13.6 days) decays by isomeric transition with emission of a low-abundance γ-photon at 156 keV, and conversion electrons at 127, 129, and 152 keV. It is the conversion electrons that have the therapeutic potential. The conversion electrons have a limited range in soft tissue (0.2–0.3 mm). The γ-photon is useful for imaging. ^{117m}Sn^{4+} is chelated with DTPA and supplied as ^{117m}Sn-pentetate. The chelated compound has bone-seeking properties [76]. After intravenous injection, 22.4% of the administered activity is distributed in the soft tissues with a biologic half-life of 1.45 days while 77.6% is distributed in the bones and shows no biologic clearance. Peak skeletal uptake in normal bone occurs within 24 h whereas uptake in metastatic bone lesions occurs slowly over 3–7 days. Clearance is renal, with a mean of 11.4% of the administered activity excreted within 24 h and 22.4% within 14 days [77]. In a human subject with metastatic prostate cancer who received a therapy dose of 18.6 mCi and who died 47 days later from his primary cancer, there was nonuniform distribution of radioactivity within the same

vertebral body, indicating normal bone between metastatic lesions. While lesion-to-nonlesion ratios ranged from 3 to 5, osteoid-to-marrow cavity deposition ratio was 11:1 on microautoradiography [78].

Preliminary clinical studies have shown that ^{117m}Sn-DTPA is effective in the palliation of bone pain in patients with metastatic breast and prostate cancer. The short range in soft tissue (0.2–0.3 mm) of its conversion electrons may explain the low incidence of myelosuppression and constitute a potential advantage over β-emitters. In a phase I dose-escalation study using activities ranging from 1.8 to 15.5 mCi (66 to 573 MBq) of ^{117m}Sn-DTPA, symptom benefit was observed in 9 of 10 evaluable patients with no significant myelotoxicity [79]. In a later phase I/II study in 47 patients with painful bone metastases from various cancers, pain relief was observed in 75% of the 40 assessable patients. Pain relief was complete in 12 patients (30%). There was no dose–response relationship. The time to onset of pain relief was 19±15 days with doses of ≤0.143 mCi/kg (5.29 MBq/kg) or less and 5±3 days with doses ≥0.179 mCi/kg (6.61 MBq/kg). Toxicity was minimal with only 1 patient experiencing grade 3 reduction in white blood cell count [80]. The potential benefits of this compound are yet to be demonstrated in larger randomized trials.

Criteria for Patient Selection and Guidelines for Treatment

The common indications and contraindications of bone pain palliation using radionuclides are summarized in Table 5.2. In general, the patient should undergo a bone scan using ^{99m}Tc-MDP within 8 weeks prior to therapy in order to document increased osteoblastic activity at the sites of pain. The patient is less likely to have pain relief if he or she has vertebral collapse, pathologic fracture, nerve root entrapment, or visceral pain. In the presence of osteolytic metastases but with a positive bone scan, uptake of radiopharmaceutical is often seen at the tumor sites, but response is less predictable.

Table 5.2 General considerations, indications, and contraindications of bone pain palliation using radionuclides

General considerations	Indications	Contraindications	Precautions
– Bone scan within 8 weeks of treatment – Estimated life expectancy >3 months (especially if ^{89}Sr is being considered) – No chemotherapy or external beam radiation 6 weeks before treatment	– Multifocal painful skeletal metastases, refractory to analgesics – Positive bone scan with uptake correlating to sites of pain	– Pregnancy – Acute spinal cord compression – Impending pathologic fracture – Acute or chronic renal failure – GFR < 30 mL/min – Creatinine > 200 mmol/L – BUN > 12 mmol/L – Hb < 90 g/L – WBC < 3.5 × 10^9/L – Platelets < 60 × 10^9/L	– Urinary incontinence – Bladder outflow obstruction – Vesicoureteric obstruction – Active disseminated intravascular coagulation (DIC)

Contraindications

Contraindications to treatment include acute or chronic renal failure, impending pathologic fracture, and acute spinal cord compression. Cord compression is considered an emergency and should be treated with surgical decompression or external radiotherapy without any delay. Active disseminated intravascular coagulation (DIC) may be a risk factor for severe thrombocytopenia after treatment [81]. Patients should be screened for DIC (D-dimer or fibrin split products) prior to therapy. Urinary incontinence presents a contamination risk and is managed by bladder catheterization before radiopharmaceutical administration.

It is important to be familiar with the physical properties of each radiopharmaceutical and have an estimate of the life expectancy of every patient considered for treatment. It is not clear, however, if these differences provide a basis for the selection of one radiopharmaceutical over the other. In the past, many theories were developed about the potential relationship of half-life (which influences photon flux and therefore dose rate) and β particle energy to therapeutic response but there have been no randomized or controlled studies. Given the many variables involved in assessing the efficacy of these therapies, it is not possible to draw conclusions based on analysis of pain relief variables.

The recent demonstration of improved patient survival following treatment with RaCl$_2$, if confirmed and extended to tumors other than prostate carcinoma, provides a new indication for treatment with this agent and is apt to generate renewed enthusiasm for this approach.

Hospitalization is not required and the patient does not need to fast prior to treatment. A pregnancy test must be negative in women of childbearing age. As in any therapeutic procedure, informed consent is obtained from the patient. The patient is given radiation safety precautions as well as a card documenting the source of radiation in case it is detected by monitoring devices during travel. An intravenous line is inserted. Good blood return and free flow of the saline flush should be verified in order to avoid extravasation of radiotracer in the subcutaneous tissue. The dose is administered by a board-certified nuclear medicine physician listed on the NRC or Agreement State license or specifically designated under a broad license, in the presence of the radiation safety officer. Follow-up is made by the medical oncologist. Blood counts are obtained at least weekly for the first 6 weeks and more frequently if there is evidence of myelotoxicity. Blood counts, mainly platelet and neutrophil counts, should be obtained until the counts are normal. However, this may not always occur. Patients whose blood counts do return to pretreatment values may be retreated, generally not before 12 weeks [16]. In the case of ^{223}RaCl$_2$, dosing is every 6 weeks for up to four doses based on the results of the phase III trial (ALSYMPCA). Long-term follow-up studies are required to document the delayed toxicities such as myelodysplastic syndrome (MDS) which has been seen with repeated administrations of agents like ^{153}Sm-EDTMP [82].

> **Challenges Associated with Bone Pain Palliation Using Radionuclides**
>
> - Cross-irradiation of the adjacent functioning bone marrow
> - Possibility of combination with chemotherapy
> - Unknown long-term toxicities
> - Dose fractionation, repeated treatments, and early treatment of asymptomatic lesions
> - Need for large randomized trials

Conclusion

Bone pain due to osseous metastases represents the most frequent pain among patients with cancer. The treatment approach is multidisciplinary. Pain palliation using bone-seeking radiopharmaceuticals should be considered especially in patients with widespread skeletal metastases. It is particularly efficient and well tolerated, leading to substantial decrease in morbidity and improvement in quality of life. Moreover, the new agent, $^{223}RaCl_2$, has demonstrated a survival benefit. This may provide a new *raison d'être* for radionuclide therapy of bone metastases. Although single therapy has been shown to be effective, retreatment should be carefully administered. Further research is required to examine new radiopharmaceuticals, evaluate the benefits of combination therapy and optimize administration protocols such as dose fractionation and possibly early treatment of asymptomatic lesions if concerns about MDS do not emerge during the expected lifespan of the patients with metastatic disease.

Acknowledgements The authors thank Dr. Christopher J. Sweeney, from the Lank Center for Genitourinary Oncology at the Dana-Farber Cancer Institute—Harvard Medical School, for reviewing the manuscript.

References

1. Campa III JA, Payne R. The management of intractable bone pain: a clinician's perspective. Semin Nucl Med. 1992;22(1):3–10.

2. Nielsen OS, Munro AJ, Tannock IF. Bone metastases: pathophysiology and management policy. J Clin Oncol. 1991;9(3):509–24.

3. Cancer pain relief and palliative care. Report of a WHO Expert Committee. World Health Organ Tech Rep Ser. 1990;804:1–75.

4. Serafini AN. Therapy of metastatic bone pain. J Nucl Med. 2001;42(6):895–906.

5. Lewington VJ. Bone-seeking radionuclides for therapy. J Nucl Med. 2005;46 Suppl 1:38S–47.

6. Silberstein EB. Dosage and response in radiopharmaceutical therapy of painful osseous metastases. J Nucl Med. 1996;37(2):249–52.

7. Silberstein EB. Systemic radiopharmaceutical therapy of painful osteoblastic metastases. Semin Radiat Oncol. 2000;10(3):240–9.

8. Joshi DP, et al. Evaluation of phosphorus 32 for intractable pain secondary to prostatic carcinoma metastases. JAMA. 1965;193:621–3.

9. Cheung A, Driedger AA. Evaluation of radioactive phosphorus in the palliation of metastatic bone lesions from carcinoma of the breast and prostate. Radiology. 1980;134(1):209–12.

10. Silberstein EB. The treatment of painful osseous metastases with phosphorus-32-labeled phosphates. Semin Oncol. 1993;20(3 Suppl 2):10–21.

11. Ritter MA, Cleaver JE, Tobias CA. High-LET radiations induce a large proportion of non-rejoining DNA breaks. Nature. 1977;266(5603):653–5.

12. Nilsson S, et al. First clinical experience with alpha-emitting radium-223 in the treatment of skeletal metastases. Clin Cancer Res. 2005;11(12):4451–9.

13. Collins C, et al. Samarium-153-EDTMP in bone metastases of hormone refractory prostate carcinoma: a phase I/II trial. J Nucl Med. 1993;34(11):1839–44.

14. Han SH, et al. The PLACORHEN study: a double-blind, placebo-controlled, randomized radionuclide study with (186)Re-etidronate in hormone-resistant prostate cancer patients with painful bone metastases. Placebo Controlled Rhenium Study. J Nucl Med. 2002;43(9):1150–6.

15. Palmedo H, et al. Repeated bone-targeted therapy for hormone-refractory prostate carcinoma: randomized phase II trial with the new, high-energy radiopharmaceutical rhenium-188 hydroxyethylidenediphosphonate. J Clin Oncol. 2003;21(15):2869–75.

16. Silberstein EB, et al. Society of Nuclear Medicine procedure guideline for palliative treatment of painful bone metastases 3.0. 25 Jan 2003. http://interactive.snm.org/docs/pg_ch25_0403.pdf. Accessed 25 Jan 2012.

17. Maxfield Jr JR, Maxfield JG, Maxfield WS. The use of radioactive phosphorus and testosterone in metastatic bone lesions from breast and prostate. South Med J. 1958;51(3):320–7.

18. Fowler Jr JE, Whitmore Jr WF. Considerations for the use of testosterone with systemic chemotherapy in prostatic cancer. Cancer. 1982;49(7):1373–7.

19. Tong EC, Rubenfeld S. The treatment of bone metastases with parathormone followed by radiophosphorus. Am J Roentgenol Radium Ther Nucl Med. 1967;99(2):422–34.

20. Silberstein EB, Elgazzar AH, Kapilivsky A. Phosphorus-32 radiopharmaceuticals for the treatment of painful osseous metastases. Semin Nucl Med. 1992;22(1):17–27.

21. Burnet NG, Williams G, Howard N. Phosphorus-32 for intractable bony pain from carcinoma of the prostate. Clin Oncol (R Coll Radiol). 1990;2(4):220–3.

22. Nair N. Relative efficacy of ^{32}P and ^{89}Sr in palliation in skeletal metastases. J Nucl Med. 1999;40(2): 256–61.

23. Blake GM, et al. Strontium-89 therapy: measurement of absorbed dose to skeletal metastases. J Nucl Med. 1988;29(4):549–57.

24. Blake GM, et al. Sr-89 therapy: strontium kinetics in disseminated carcinoma of the prostate. Eur J Nucl Med. 1986;12(9):447–54.

25. Laing AH, et al. Strontium-89 chloride for pain palliation in prostatic skeletal malignancy. Br J Radiol. 1991;64(765):816–22.

26. Robinson RG, et al. Treatment of metastatic bone pain with strontium-89. Int J Rad Appl Instrum B. 1987; 14(3):219–22.

27. Lee CK, et al. Strontium-89 chloride (Metastron) for palliative treatment of bony metastases. The University of Minnesota experience. Am J Clin Oncol. 1996;19(2): 102–7.

28. Quilty PM, et al. A comparison of the palliative effects of strontium-89 and external beam radiotherapy in metastatic prostate cancer. Radiother Oncol. 1994; 31(1):33–40.

29. Porter AT, et al. Results of a randomized phase-III trial to evaluate the efficacy of strontium-89 adjuvant to local field external beam irradiation in the management of endocrine resistant metastatic prostate cancer. Int J Radiat Oncol Biol Phys. 1993;25(5):805–13.

30. Smeland S, et al. Role of strontium-89 as adjuvant to palliative external beam radiotherapy is questionable: results of a double-blind randomized study. Int J Radiat Oncol Biol Phys. 2003;56(5):1397–404.

31. Mertens WC, et al. Strontium-89 and low-dose infusion cisplatin for patients with hormone refractory prostate carcinoma metastatic to bone: a preliminary report. J Nucl Med. 1992;33(8):1437–43.

32. Tu SM, et al. Strontium-89 combined with doxorubicin in the treatment of patients with androgen-independent prostate cancer. Urol Oncol. 1996;2(6):191–7.

33. Sciuto R, et al. Effects of low-dose cisplatin on ^{89}Sr therapy for painful bone metastases from prostate cancer: a randomized clinical trial. J Nucl Med. 2002;43(1):79–86.

34. Tu SM, et al. Bone-targeted therapy for advanced androgen-independent carcinoma of the prostate: a randomised phase II trial. Lancet. 2001;357(9253): 336–41.

35. Akerley W, et al. A multiinstitutional, concurrent chemoradiation trial of strontium-89, estramustine, and vinblastine for hormone refractory prostate carcinoma involving bone. Cancer. 2002;94(6):1654–60.

36. Bayouth JE, et al. Dosimetry and toxicity of samarium-153-EDTMP administered for bone pain due to skeletal metastases. J Nucl Med. 1994;35(1):63–9.

37. Singh A, et al. Human pharmacokinetics of samarium-153 EDTMP in metastatic cancer. J Nucl Med. 1989;30(11):1814–8.

38. Farhanghi M, et al. Samarium-153-EDTMP: pharmacokinetic, toxicity and pain response using an escalating dose schedule in treatment of metastatic bone cancer. J Nucl Med. 1992;33(8):1451–8.

39. Ahonen A, et al. Samarium-153-EDTMP in bone metastases. J Nucl Biol Med. 1994;38(4 Suppl 1):123–7.

40. Turner JH, Claringbold PG. A phase II study of treatment of painful multifocal skeletal metastases with single and repeated dose samarium-153 ethylenediaminetetramethylene phosphonate. Eur J Cancer. 1991;27(9):1084–6.

41. Serafini AN, et al. Palliation of pain associated with metastatic bone cancer using samarium-153 lexidronam: a double-blind placebo-controlled clinical trial. J Clin Oncol. 1998;16(4):1574–81.

42. Resche I, et al. A dose-controlled study of ^{153}Sm-ethylenediaminetetramethylenephosphonate (EDTMP) in the treatment of patients with painful bone metastases. Eur J Cancer. 1997;33(10): 1583–91.

43. Hommeyer SH, Varney DM, Eary JF. Skeletal nonvisualization in a bone scan secondary to intravenous etidronate therapy. J Nucl Med. 1992;33(5):748–50.

44. Krasnow AZ, et al. False-negative bone imaging due to etidronate disodium therapy. Clin Nucl Med. 1988;13(4):264–7.

45. Sandler ED, Parisi MT, Hattner RS. Duration of etidronate effect demonstrated by serial bone scintigraphy. J Nucl Med. 1991;32(9):1782–4.

46. Pecherstorfer M, et al. Effect of clodronate treatment on bone scintigraphy in metastatic breast cancer. J Nucl Med. 1993;34(7):1039–44.

47. Carrasquillo JA, et al. Alendronate does not interfere with ^{99m}Tc-methylene diphosphonate bone scanning. J Nucl Med. 2001;42(9):1359–63.

48. Marcus CS, et al. Lack of effect of a bisphosphonate (pamidronate disodium) infusion on subsequent skeletal uptake of Sm-153 EDTMP. Clin Nucl Med. 2002;27(6):427–30.

49. Lam MG, et al. Combined use of zoledronic acid and ^{153}Sm-EDTMP in hormone-refractory prostate cancer patients with bone metastases. Eur J Nucl Med Mol Imaging. 2008;35(4):756–65.

50. Storto G, et al. Combined therapy of Sr-89 and zoledronic acid in patients with painful bone metastases. Bone. 2006;39(1):35–41.

51. Anderson PM, et al. High-dose samarium-153 ethylene diamine tetramethylene phosphonate: low toxicity of skeletal irradiation in patients with osteosarcoma and bone metastases. J Clin Oncol. 2002;20(1): 189–96.

52. Franzius C, Schuck A, Bielack SS. High-dose samarium-153 ethylene diamine tetramethylene phosphonate: low toxicity of skeletal irradiation in patients with osteosarcoma and bone metastases. J Clin Oncol. 2002;20(7):1953–4.

53. de Klerk JM, et al. Pharmacokinetics of rhenium-186 after administration of rhenium-186-HEDP to patients

with bone metastases. J Nucl Med. 1992;33(5): 646–51.

54. Bodei L, et al. EANM procedure guideline for treatment of refractory metastatic bone pain. Eur J Nucl Med Mol Imaging. 2008;35(10):1934–40.

55. Maxon HR, et al. Re-186(Sn) HEDP for treatment of multiple metastatic foci in bone: human biodistribution and dosimetric studies. Radiology. 1988; 166(2):501–7.

56. Han SH, et al. [186]Re-etidronate in breast cancer patients with metastatic bone pain. J Nucl Med. 1999;40(4):639–42.

57. Sciuto R, et al. Metastatic bone pain palliation with 89-Sr and 186-Re-HEDP in breast cancer patients. Breast Cancer Res Treat. 2001;66(2):101–9.

58. Maxon III HR, et al. Re-186(Sn) HEDP for treatment of painful osseous metastases: initial clinical experience in 20 patients with hormone-resistant prostate cancer. Radiology. 1990;176(1):155–9.

59. Maxon III HR, et al. Rhenium-186(Sn)HEDP for treatment of painful osseous metastases: results of a double-blind crossover comparison with placebo. J Nucl Med. 1991;32(10):1877–81.

60. de Klerk JM, et al. Dose escalation study of rhenium-186 hydroxyethylidene diphosphonate in patients with metastatic prostate cancer. Eur J Nucl Med. 1994;21(10):1114–20.

61. de Klerk JM, et al. Phase 1 study of rhenium-186-HEDP in patients with bone metastases originating from breast cancer. J Nucl Med. 1996;37(2):244–9.

62. Dafermou A, et al. A multicentre observational study of radionuclide therapy in patients with painful bone metastases of prostate cancer. Eur J Nucl Med. 2001;28(7):788–98.

63. O'Sullivan JM, et al. High activity Rhenium-186 HEDP with autologous peripheral blood stem cell rescue: a phase I study in progressive hormone refractory prostate cancer metastatic to bone. Br J Cancer. 2002;86(11):1715–20.

64. Bayer-HealthCare. Bayer's investigational compound radium-223 chloride met its primary endpoint of significantly improving overall survival in a phase III trial in patients with castration-resistant prostate cancer that has spread to the bone. 6 June 2011. http://pharma.bayer.com/html/pdf/news_room115.pdf. Accessed 25 Jan 2012.

65. Nilsson S, et al. Phase I study of Alpharadin™ ([223]Ra), an alpha-emitting bone-seeking agent in cancer patients with skeletal metastases. Oral presentation, annual congress of the EANM, Helsinki, September 8, 2004. Eur J Nucl Med Mol Imaging. 2004; 31(S2):290.

66. Nilsson S, et al. Bone-targeted radium-223 in symptomatic, hormone-refractory prostate cancer: a randomised, multicentre, placebo-controlled phase II study. Lancet Oncol. 2007;8(7):587–94.

67. Nilsson S, et al. Alkaline phosphatase (ALP) normalization and overall survival in patients with bone metastases from castration-resistant prostate cancer

(CRPC) treated with radium-223. ASCO Meet Abstr. 2011;29(15 Suppl):4620.

68. Nilsson S, et al. Radium-223 chloride, a first-in-class alpha-pharmaceutical with a benign safety profile for patients with castration-resistant prostate cancer (CRPC) and bone metastases: combined analysis of phase I and II clinical trials. ASCO Meet Abstr. 2010;28(15 Suppl):4678.

69. Wright HA, et al. Calculations of physical and chemical reactions produced in irradiated water containing DNA. Radiat Prot Dosimetry. 1985;13(1–4):133–6.

70. Kampf G. Induction of DNA double-strand breaks by ionizing radiation of different quality and their relevance for cell inactivation. Radiobiol Radiother (Berl). 1988;29(6):631–58.

71. Raju MR, et al. Radiobiology of alpha particles: III. Cell inactivation by alpha-particle traversals of the cell nucleus. Radiat Res. 1991;128(2):204–9.

72. Henriksen G, et al. Targeting of osseous sites with alpha-emitting [223]Ra: comparison with the beta-emitter ^{89}Sr in mice. J Nucl Med. 2003;44(2):252–9.

73. Bruland OS, et al. High-linear energy transfer irradiation targeted to skeletal metastases by the alpha-emitter [223]Ra: adjuvant or alternative to conventional modalities? Clin Cancer Res. 2006;12(20 Pt 2):6250s–7.

74. Tannock IF, et al. Docetaxel plus prednisone or mitoxantrone plus prednisone for advanced prostate cancer. N Engl J Med. 2004;351(15):1502–12.

75. Algeta ASA and Bayer. A phase I/IIa study of safety and efficacy of Alpharadin® with docetaxel in patients with bone metastasis from castration-resistant prostate cancer. Clinicaltrials.gov NCT01106352.

76. Srivastava SC, et al. The development and in-vivo behavior of tin containing radiopharmaceuticals: I. Chemistry, preparation, and biodistribution in small animals. Int J Nucl Med Biol. 1985;12(3):167–74.

77. Krishnamurthy GT, et al. Tin-117m(4+)DTPA: pharmacokinetics and imaging characteristics in patients with metastatic bone pain. J Nucl Med. 1997; 38(2):230–7.

78. Swailem FM, et al. In-vivo tissue uptake and retention of Sn-117m(4+)DTPA in a human subject with metastatic bone pain and in normal mice. Nucl Med Biol. 1998;25(3):279–87.

79. Atkins HL, et al. Biodistribution of Sn-117m(4+) DTPA for palliative therapy of painful osseous metastases. Radiology. 1993;186(1):279–83.

80. Srivastava SC, et al. Treatment of metastatic bone pain with tin-117m Stannic diethylenetriaminepentaacetic acid: a phase I/II clinical study. Clin Cancer Res. 1998;4(1):61–8.

81. Paszkowski AL, Hewitt DJ, Taylor Jr A. Disseminated intravascular coagulation in a patient treated with strontium-89 for metastatic carcinoma of the prostate. Clin Nucl Med. 1999;24(11):852–4.

82. Sartor O, et al. Safety and efficacy of repeat administration of samarium Sm-153 lexidronam to patients with metastatic bone pain. Cancer. 2007;109(3): 637–43.

Roger F. Uren, Robert Howman-Giles,
and John F. Thompson

Introduction

Melanoma is being diagnosed more often than ever before. This may be due in part to greater vigilance but there is, nevertheless, a steadily increasing incidence of the disease in the western world. Melanoma accounts for less than 5% of skin cancers but is the cause of more than 80% of deaths from skin cancer, and the loss of life years is amplified since some patients die when quite young. If detected early, there is a good prognosis with 10-year survival of around 95% for Stage I melanoma, but if systemic metastases are present, the prognosis is poor with 10-year survival for Stage IV melanoma less than 5%.

These facts have encouraged efforts to decrease the incidence of melanoma through public health campaigns to reduce exposure of the skin to UV radiation and also to improve early diagnosis through education efforts aimed both at medical practitioners and at the general public. They have also prompted efforts to develop therapies to treat distant metastases once they have occurred. One area of this research has involved targeting the melanoma metastases with a radioactive tracer so that the emitted radiation might destroy the tumor cells. Isotopes emitting α and β radiation, high-energy Auger electrons, as well as low-energy γ radiation have all been evaluated.

Clinical Features of Melanoma

- Increasing in incidence
- 80% of deaths from skin cancer
- Large loss of life years
- Stage IV 10-year survival <5%

R.F. Uren, M.D., F.R.A.C.P., D.D.U. (✉)
• R. Howman-Giles, M.D., F.R.A.C.P., D.D.U.
Nuclear Medicine and Diagnostic Ultrasound,
RPAH Medical Centre, Suite 206, 100 Carillon Avenue,
Newtown, NSW 2042, Australia

Sydney Medical School, The University of Sydney,
Sydney, NSW, Australia
e-mail: ruren@usyd.edu.au

J.F. Thompson, M.D., F.R.A.C.S.
Sydney Medical School, The University of Sydney,
Sydney, NSW, Australia

Melanoma Institute Australia, 40 Rocklands Road,
North Sydney, NSW, Australia

Radionuclide Therapy of Systemic Melanoma Metastases

For 30 years, there have been laboratory and animal studies describing new techniques that aimed to effectively treat melanoma metastases using radionuclide therapy. Despite some encouraging results, there have been no human trials of these methods until very recently. This review describes the approaches taken in the past and points to some encouraging signs for future research that offer hope that effective therapies are not far away.

Monoclonal Antibodies

The earliest attempts to target melanoma cells with radionuclides used radiolabeled monoclonal antibodies (mAbs). In the 1980s, DeNardo et al. [1] outlined the requirements for a treatment planning system for radioimmunotherapy and suggested using mAbs for this purpose. At about this time, Larson et al. [2] reported shrinkage of melanoma metastases in a patient treated with ^{131}Iodine (^{131}I)-labeled Fab′ fragments of a mAb against high molecular weight melanoma-associated antigen. Since then, therapy using radiolabeled mAbs has entered clinical practice with the introduction of anti-CD20 mAbs labeled with ^{90}Yttrium (^{90}Y) and ^{131}I to treat B-cell lymphoma, but progress in melanoma has been slower.

Recently, some promising results have been reported in preclinical studies with nude mice harboring human melanoma. Dadachova et al. [3] used a melanin-binding IgM antibody labeled with ^{188}Rhenium (^{188}Re-6D2 mAb) and found tumor growth slowed with only transient effects on white blood cell and platelet counts that resolved within 2 weeks of therapy. A phase I clinical trial in patients with melanoma is underway. A potential problem with this antibody, however, is that melanin lies largely within the melanoma cell and thus necrotic cells are likely to be targeted more effectively than viable tumor cells. Some melanin is also found in the extracellular space and in melanophages [4]. Others have also tried to target the melanin molecule with mAbs [3].

Cetuximab, a chimeric mAb-targeting epidermal growth factor receptor (EGFR), has recently been shown to bind melanoma xenografts in mice [5] with $6.3 \pm 1.1\%$ of the dose/g being found in the tumor at 72 h post injection. This antigenic target offers a potential additional avenue for further investigation.

A mAb against surface antigens that appear on melanoma cells such as the glycoprotein gp57 or the ganglioside GD3 might also have therapeutic benefit [6]. Early studies using mAb against GD3 labeled with the α-emitter ^{213}Bismuth (^{213}Bi) have shown promise [7].

Unwanted irradiation of normal tissues has limited the use of radioimmunotherapy in humans and novel strategies have been suggested to partly overcome these limitations. Siantar et al. [8] have suggested enzymatic linkers to cleave the radioisotope from the mAb in blood and normal tissue after binding to tumor has occurred. This allows excretion of the radionuclide from the blood and normal tissues resulting in reduced radiation exposure to normal tissue while maintaining tumoricidal doses to the tumor. The timing of this intervention would be determined by the pharmacokinetics of the radiopharmaceutical involved. In their modeling, they suggest that therapeutic effectiveness could be increased 1.6–3.2 times that obtained without the intervention.

There is also hope that more precise dosimetry estimates obtained in individual patients using hybrid imaging techniques such as SPECT/CT and PET/CT will lead to more successful radioimmunotherapy with fewer side effects [9]. Using the accurate attenuation correction possible when simultaneous CT data are available alongside the tomographic SPECT or PET data provides precise quantification of radionuclide uptake in the target lesions and the normal tissues. This should allow the maximum killing dose to be delivered to the tumor deposits while remaining below the critical doses to normal tissues.

To avoid unwanted effects on non-melanoma tissue, Allen et al. [10] injected the radiolabeled mAb directly into melanoma metastases. The mAb targeted against melanoma tissue, 9.2.27, was labeled with ^{213}Bi. This is an α emitter and was injected directly into the metastatic melanoma in doses ranging from 5.5 to 50 MBq. There was significant cell death observed without changes in blood proteins or electrolytes. They concluded that such targeted α therapy was a promising therapy for inoperable metastatic melanoma or primary ocular melanoma though this has not yet been tried in human trials.

Radioembolization

Using microspheres labeled with ^{90}Y, Gray et al. [11] showed regression of liver metastases from primary bowel cancer. The microspheres were injected directly into the hepatic artery branches supplying the metastasis, thus embolising the terminal arterioles within the metastatic deposit. The subsequent release of β particles by the ^{90}Y delivered very high dose radiation directly into the metastasis. He called this treatment "selective internal radiation" or SIR and also performed this therapy on some patients with hepatic metastases from melanoma. Using SIR spheres, Cianni et al. [12] treated 110 patients with hepatic metastases, some with melanoma primaries. These patients had all shown no response to chemotherapy. They obtained a complete or partial therapeutic response in 42 patients with acceptable side effects.

Benzamides

Since the first validation in humans by Michelot et al. [13] that radiolabeled benzamides (BZA) target melanoma tissue in humans, there have been many attempts to refine the tracers to increase uptake in the melanoma tissue and increase excretion from normal tissues. A common feature of all BZA derivatives is their avid uptake into melanoma tissue. The precise mechanism of uptake is unknown but several processes are possible including direct binding to the melanin molecule and incorporation into the melanin biosynthesis pathway [14].

One such BZA (MIP-1145) when labeled with ^{131}I [15] was recently shown to bind to melanin in human melanoma tumor xenografts in mice. This significantly reduced tumor growth. Multiple doses caused tumor regression and a durable therapeutic response over 125 days. The compound has a fluoro-benzoate element that has the potential to be labeled with ^{18}F, so that the effectiveness of therapy could be monitored using the uptake of such an agent when imaged by positron emission tomography (PET). MIP-1145 is a small molecule and was found to cross the blood–brain barrier; this bodes well for its use in patients with cerebral metastases from melanoma, traditionally a difficult group to treat effectively because of this barrier.

Chezal et al. [14] synthesized heteroaromatic BZA analogs that incorporated the heteroaromatic structure in place of the benzene ring. These analogs had a stronger affinity for melanin that the original compound showing higher uptake in the melanoma tumor with longer retention, ideal attributes for radionuclide therapy.

The same group of researchers from Clermont-Ferrand in France subsequently described a quinoxaline derivative molecule (ICF01012) that binds melanin with highly specific and long-lasting uptake in melanoma tumors with rapid clearance from normal tissues [16, 17]. In a preclinical study in mice [17], this agent labeled with ^{131}I inhibited tumor growth while the unlabeled compound and ^{131}I-NaI had no effect. The melanoma tumor cells remaining after treatment also showed loss of aggressiveness, thus increasing survival time of the treated mice. Untreated mice developed lung metastases (55%), but lung metastases did not occur in the treated mice. The target to background ratios for this agent was excellent with a tumor to blood ratio of 50:1 at 24 h.

The group also described the addition of a cytotoxic moiety to a heteroaromatic BZA derivative which they termed a DNA intercalating agent [18]. Labeled with ^{125}I that emits Auger electrons delivering localized radiation, they found an acridine derivative to be the most cytotoxic. This would appear to offer excellent potential for radionuclide therapy using ^{125}I. ^{125}I has a half-life of 60 days and decays by electron capture to ^{125}Tellurium (^{125}Te). This decays immediately by releasing a 35 keV γ ray; however, some energy is internally converted to electrons that are ejected at 35 keV or low-energy bremsstrahlung X-rays. Also Auger electrons are produced at low energies ranging from 50 to 500 eV. These low-energy Auger electrons and internally converted electrons deposit their entire energy within the cell that contains the ^{125}I and thus offer effective cell killing ability with no effect on normal cells outside the tumor tissue that have not accumulated the tracer.

Gene Therapy

It is known that the RAS $\rightarrow$ RAF $\rightarrow$ MEK $\rightarrow$ MAP kinase/ERK (MAPK) and the P13K/Akt signaling pathways play an important role in the pathogenesis of melanoma. Genetic mutations can cause over-activation of these pathways such as the BRAF mutation in the MAPK pathway [19] and the PIK3CA amplification and PTEN mutations in the P13K/Akt pathway [20, 21]. By suppressing these pathways in melanoma cells that harbored both these mutations, Hou et al. [22] found potent anti-melanoma cell effects and also expression of genes normally seen in the thyroid such as the sodium/iodide symporter (NIS) and thyroid-stimulating hormone receptor. These affected melanoma cells subsequently had the ability to take up the iodide ion and thus [131]Iodide. The authors concluded that targeting both the MAP kinase and P13K/Akt pathways combined with ^{131}I-NaI therapy could prove to be an effective therapy for melanoma metastases.

In a variation of this approach, Huang et al. [23] infected A375 human melanoma cells with a recombinant adenovirus, Ad-SUR-NIS, that expressed the NIS gene under control of the surviving promoter. Following infection, the cells showed an ability to take up iodide ion 50 times that of control noninfected cells. Ad-SUR-NIS-infected tumors showed significant accumulation of [131]I (13.3±2.85% ID/g at 2 h post injection) and tumor growth was suppressed. At this time, this strategy has not been evaluated in intact animals or clinical trials, but it provides another possible approach for radionuclide therapy of melanoma metastases.

Very recently, Bhang et al. [24] showed that the progression elevated gene-3 (PEG-3) could be used in mouse models of human melanoma to drive imaging reporters selectively to detect melanoma metastases. This also may represent a pathway to deliver therapeutic radionuclides directly to metastatic deposits.

Receptors and Peptides

Melanoma lesions, in general, over-express the melanocortin-1 receptor (MC1R). The peptide, α-melanocyte-stimulating hormone (α-MSH) binds to this receptor. This has led to investigation of analogs of α-MSH that can be labeled with α- or β-emitting radionuclides as a method to deliver therapeutic radiation to melanoma metastases. Initial efforts labeling a native

α-MSH peptide were disappointing with low receptor to background uptake and poor radionuclide stability with the radionuclide leaching off the peptide, resulting in poor target to background ratios [25]. The more recent development of peptide analogs of MSH containing nonnatural amino acids and peptide cyclization have improved receptor affinity and peptide stability in vivo [25] increasing the likelihood of this approach as an effective therapeutic agent.

In 2005, Miao et al. [26] described a melanoma targeting peptide labeled with [188]Re [[188]Re-(Arg(11))Cys(3,4,10), D-Phe(7) α-melanocyte-stimulating hormone(3–13)] or CCMSH that was shown to have a positive therapeutic effect in murine and human melanoma-bearing mouse models. Treatment extended the life of tumor-bearing mice with no toxic effects observed. Later that year, the same group described an analog of this peptide labeled with [212]Pb that was shown to decrease tumor growth and extend survival time in a melanoma-bearing C57 mouse flank tumor model [27]. The peptide, [212]Pb(DOTA)-Re(Arg(11))CCMSH, showed rapid tumor uptake with retention, combined with rapid whole-body clearance. The isotope [212]Pb decays to [212]Bi which then decays via α and β decay releasing high radiation doses to the area of uptake. Survival time increased with increasing dose and 45% of mice receiving the highest dose of 200 mCi survived the study disease free. This is a very promising radionuclide for clinical therapy of melanoma metastases.

One of the potential problems with using such peptides as therapeutic agents is their renal uptake and excretion which can deliver high radiation doses to the kidneys resulting in nephritis and adverse affects on renal function. Froidevaux et al. [28] described a series of melanoma targeting peptides that were DOTA-α-MSH analogs. These analogs retain their affinity for the MC1R which determines their uptake in melanoma tissue but they had significantly less renal uptake making them more desirable as radio-peptide therapeutic agents.

Attempts have been made to use the [177]Lutetium (^{177}Lu)-labeled somatostatin analog

(^{177}Lu-DOTA0, Tyr3) as therapy in melanoma as well as some other tumors [29]. No beneficial therapeutic effect was seen in the melanoma patients who were treated with this agent. All of the patients thus treated died within 5 months showing tumor progression despite treatment.

Liposomes

Almost a decade ago, Asai et al. [30] described the use of liposomes to deliver the potent anticancer agent 2′-C-cyano-2′-deoxy-1-β-D-aribino-pentofuranosylcytosine (CNDAC) to tumor cells in a metastatic pulmonary cancer model. More recently, Fondell et al. [31] harnessed this methodology using a two-stage approach to deliver ^{125}I directly into the cancer cell nucleus. They used PEG-stabilized tumor cell targeting liposomes named "Nuclisome particles." Epidermal growth factor (EGF) was used as a tumor cell specific agent to target the EGFR and the liposomes were loaded with ^{125}I; as described previously, this radionuclide emits Auger electrons and internally converted electrons delivering a high radiation dose directly to the nucleus of the cancer cell. This treatment in the laboratory was 100,000 times more effective than EGFR-targeting liposomes loaded with doxorubicin. The technique may have applicability to treat metastatic cancer cells circulating in the blood stream.

Nanoparticles

A poly(^{198}Au) radioactive gold-dendrimer composite nanodevice with a diameter between 10 and 29 nm was described by Khan et al. [32]. They found a 45% reduction in tumor volume when this was used in a brachytherapy approach and injected directly into melanoma tumors in a mouse model. A single injection of 74 mCi was used. Untreated tumors or those injected with the "cold" nanodevice showed no reduction in tumor volume. There was no clinical toxicity offering the first proof that such nanodevices can safely deliver therapeutic doses of radiation to tumors.

Radionuclide Therapy of Melanoma

- Particle emitters labeled to targeting compounds
- Monoclonal antibodies
- BZA analogs
- Receptors
- Peptides
- Liposomes
- Nanoparticles

Boron Neutron Capture Therapy

Since the first description of this principle in melanoma tissue by Nakanishi et al. [33], there have been many attempts to use this approach in patients with melanoma metastases [34]. The method relies on the uptake of ^{10}Boron-paraboronophenylalanine (^{10}B-BPA) into active melanin producing melanoma tissue. The tissues are subsequently irradiated with thermal neutrons and high-energy α particles are released by the ^{10}B$(n,α)^7$Li reaction. These high-energy α particles deposit 2.33 MeV over a distance of 14 μm, about the size of a melanoma cell, producing a powerful killing effect on the melanoma cells. Only cells that take up the Boron containing compound are targeted by the treatment. Mishima et al. [35] described the first patient with melanoma cured using this technique. Amelanotic melanoma does not accumulate the ^{10}B-BPA, so it is not amenable to this therapeutic approach. Tsuboi et al. [36] induced active melanin biosynthesis by melanogenic gene transfer, which improved the effect of boron neutron capture therapy (BNCT) in amelanotic melanoma tissue. The radiation dose to the skin has been a limiting factor in delivering killing doses to melanoma metastases using BNCT. Recent research has concentrated on increasing the uptake of Boron into the tumor tissue compared to normal tissues such as the skin. Better delivery of Boron to the tumor using carborane derivates loaded into liposomes has achieved cellular concentrations of ^{10}B at least 30 times that seen with ^{10}B-BPA [37]. Uptake into tumor tissue has also found to be superior to ^{10}B-BPA when boronated unnatural cyclic amino acids are used [38]. One of these amino acids, 1-amino-3-boronocyclopentanecarboxylic acid, showed a tumor to blood ratio of 8 and tumor to normal brain ratio of 21 in a melanoma-bearing mouse model. These and other efforts are continuing with the aim of improving the clinical effectiveness of BNCT in humans with melanoma metastases.

Direct Attack on Melanoma Metastases

- Radioembolization
- Gene therapy to make metastases vulnerable
- Delivery via the lymphatics to sentinel node metastases
- Boron neutron capture therapy

Radionuclide Therapy of Primary Melanoma of the Eye

Brachytherapy using radioisotopes is well established and provides very effective treatment for primary ocular melanoma. This therapy is delivered by placing plaques that contain the radionuclide immediately outside the globe, adjacent to the tumor tissue. The most appropriate isotope to use in the plaque varies according to the thickness of the primary tumor and thus the depth of tissue that needs to be penetrated by the emitted radiation. Dosimetry comparisons [39] have shown that for melanoma lesions not greater than 5 mm in thickness, ^{106}Ruthenium (^{106}Ru) plaques are preferred to ^{125}I plaques since an equivalent dose of radiation is delivered to the melanoma with less damage to the normal structures of the eye. This should lead to less loss of vision as a side effect of the treatment.

The long-term outcome of treatment with ^{106}Ru plaques is good, with excellent local control and preservation of the eye. In a series of 425 consecutive patients with choroidal melanoma with a median thickness of 4.2 mm, 5-year over-all and metastasis-free survival rates were 79.6% and 76.5%, respectively [40]. In the survivors, the 5-year enucleation rate was 4.4% and the cosmetic and functional eye preservation rates were 96% and 52%, respectively.

Some researchers have advocated the use of *trans*-pupillary thermotherapy as an adjunct to ^{106}Ru plaque therapy but a retrospective review of 54 patients (24 patients with ^{106}Ru alone and 30 patients combined with transpupillary thermotherapy) showed no additional therapeutic benefit when thermotherapy was added to the plaque radiotherapy [41].

Recently, further efforts have been made to decrease the detrimental effects of radiation to normal eye structures that occur during brachytherapy. Oliver et al. [42] have used liquid vitreous substitutes including silicone oil, heavy oil, and perfluorocarbon liquid to attenuate and absorb the radiation dose from ^{125}I in simulated plaque therapy. They concluded that clinically relevant radiation attenuation could be achieved in humans by endotamponade of the vitreous using silicone oil and that this could significantly reduce radiation injury to critical ocular structures. Similarly, Thomson et al. [43], when treating anterior eye melanomas, found reduced radiation to the normal eye structures using special plaques with a gold alloy backing. These plaques containing ^{125}I or ^{103}Pd showed a reduction in radiation dose to normal eye structures of up to 70% compared to plaques without the gold backing. Of the two radioisotopes, ^{103}Pd showed lower radiation doses to critical structures than ^{125}I.

Lymphoscintigraphy and Sentinel Lymph Node Biopsy

This could be considered as a form of radionuclide therapy since lymphoscintigraphy identifies the lymph node or nodes that have the potential to harbor melanoma metastases [44]. Once a sentinel node has been radiolabeled it can be retrieved by the melanoma surgeon for detailed histological assessment [45]. The application of high-quality lymphoscintigraphy in this fashion has a direct impact on the management of these patients. The use of immunohistochemistry and RT-PCR

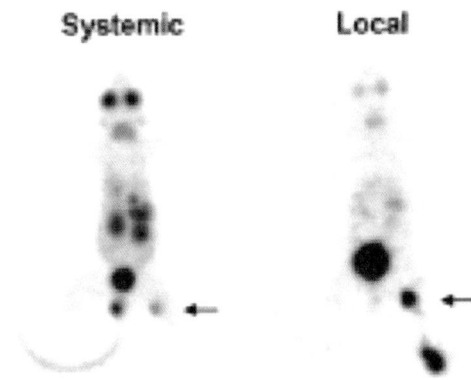

Fig. 6.1 Whole-body ^{18}F-MEL050 PET images of upper-foot-surface B16-BL/6 tumor-bearing mice at 2 h after either intravenous injection of 20 MBq of ^{18}F-MEL050 (systemic administration) or subcutaneous perilesional injection of 1 MBq of ^{18}F-MEL050 at primary tumor site (local administration). *Arrows* indicate left popliteal lymph nodes

analysis has led to unprecedented accuracy in lymph node staging in melanoma and also in a range of other solid tumors that may involve the regional lymph nodes. There is good evidence that this technique will improve survival in some patients with metastatic deposits. In patients with primary cutaneous melanomas of intermediate thickness (1.2–3.5 mm), it has been shown in an interim analysis of a large multicenter randomized trial that identification of a positive sentinel node at initial presentation and an immediate completion lymphadenectomy results in improved disease-free survival and also a substantial benefit in overall survival for node positive patients [46].

Recent work by the group at the Peter MacCallum Cancer Centre in Melbourne [47] has also raised the possibility of using the technology involved in lymphoscintigraphy to deliver cytotoxic doses of radionuclide therapy directly to any metastasis located within a sentinel lymph node. They injected a BZA analog labeled with ^{18}F (^{18}F-MEL050) to image melanoma metastases in the popliteal node of mice. Injections were given intravenously and subcutaneously at the primary tumor site on the dorsum of the mouse foot (Fig. 6.1). Sensitivity for the detection of the metastasis in the popliteal node was 60% for the IV route and 100% for the subcutaneous route. With the subcutaneous injections, 80% of the positive nodes had a node to background ratio

greater than 47 to 1. There was no nonspecific uptake of the tracer in non-metastatic nodes after subcutaneous injection.

These results thus offer the possibility of specifically targeting microscopic melanoma metastases in sentinel lymph nodes. If MEL050 was labeled with a particle emitter and then injected intradermally at the primary site of a cutaneous melanoma before wide excision, a potentially lethal dose of radiation could be delivered to any metastatic cells present in the sentinel node. Screening the sentinel node with targeted ultrasound could be done to exclude the presence of larger metastases [48]. If ultrasound was negative for metastases, this might be a worthwhile treatment option in patients considered unfit for sentinel node biopsy surgery. Wide local excision of the primary melanoma site could be done within a few hours of the injection of the therapeutic radionuclide thus removing the agent remaining at the injection site and preventing any local radiation-induced skin necrosis.

Using this same methodology but without the need for melanin to be effective, antimony sulfide or a similar colloid could be labeled with an α or β emitter and injected intradermally at the primary melanoma excision biopsy site. Since it is known that the radiocolloid particles lodge in the same part of the sub-capsular sinus that contains the metastatic cells, a lethal dose of radiation could be delivered exactly where it is needed to destroy the micrometastasis. The wide local excision performed within a few hours would remove the injection site containing the majority of the injected dose and thus no harmful effects to normal tissues would be expected.

Conclusion

Treatment of melanoma patients with systemic metastases has proved to be challenging, but there are promising therapies now being introduced that aim to induce the metastatic tumor cell to enter the apoptosis cycle, leading to cell death. A major obstacle is the fact that many patients with metastatic melanoma have more than one clone of cancer cells, so that a particular treatment may be only partially (Fig. 6.2) effective or

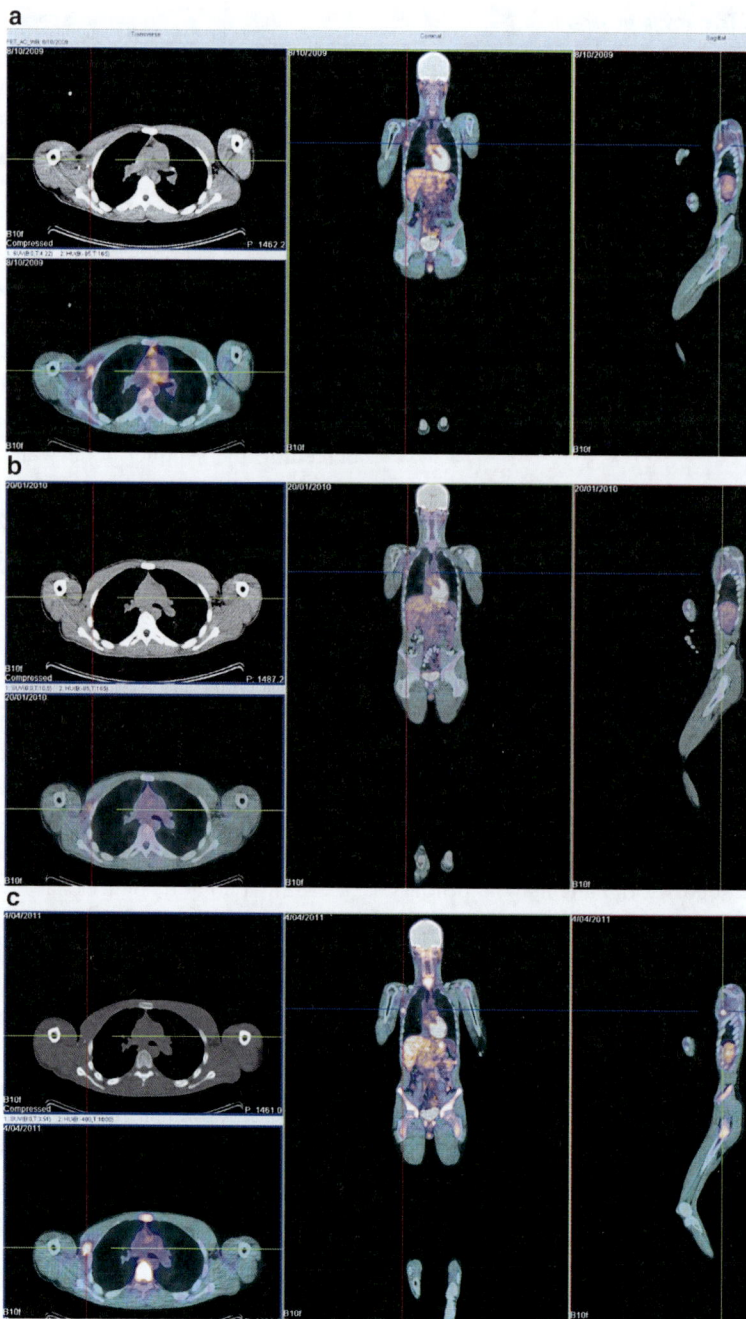

Fig. 6.2 (**a**) Whole-body F18-FDG PET/CT on a 19-year-old male who 2 months previously had undergone a right axillary lymph node dissection for melanoma metastases from an original right forearm primary lesion. Ultrasound had shown recurrent disease in the right axilla against the chest wall that is shown here on the FDG PET/CT scan as being glucose avid. US also showed three abnormal lymph nodes in the right infraclavicular region that were typical of melanoma metastases and had an increased vascular signature. These were also glucose avid on this positron emission tomography (PET) scan (not shown). Fine needle biopsy under ultrasound control confirmed recurrent melanoma. (**b**) Three months later after systemic therapy using a BRAF inhibitor, the chest wall metastasis had become less metabolically active as seen on this F18-FDG PET/CT scan and the lesion had decreased in size on US and had become avascular. This was also seen with the three infraclavicular metastases. (**c**) Eighteen months after the original scan there is now progression of the chest wall disease though the infraclavicular metastases remained dormant. Unfortunately this type of disease recrudescence remains a problem with systemic therapies for melanoma due to the polyclonal nature of the disease in many patients and perhaps a multi-pronged attack including radionuclide therapy at the time of initial therapy could help prevent this pattern of progression in the future

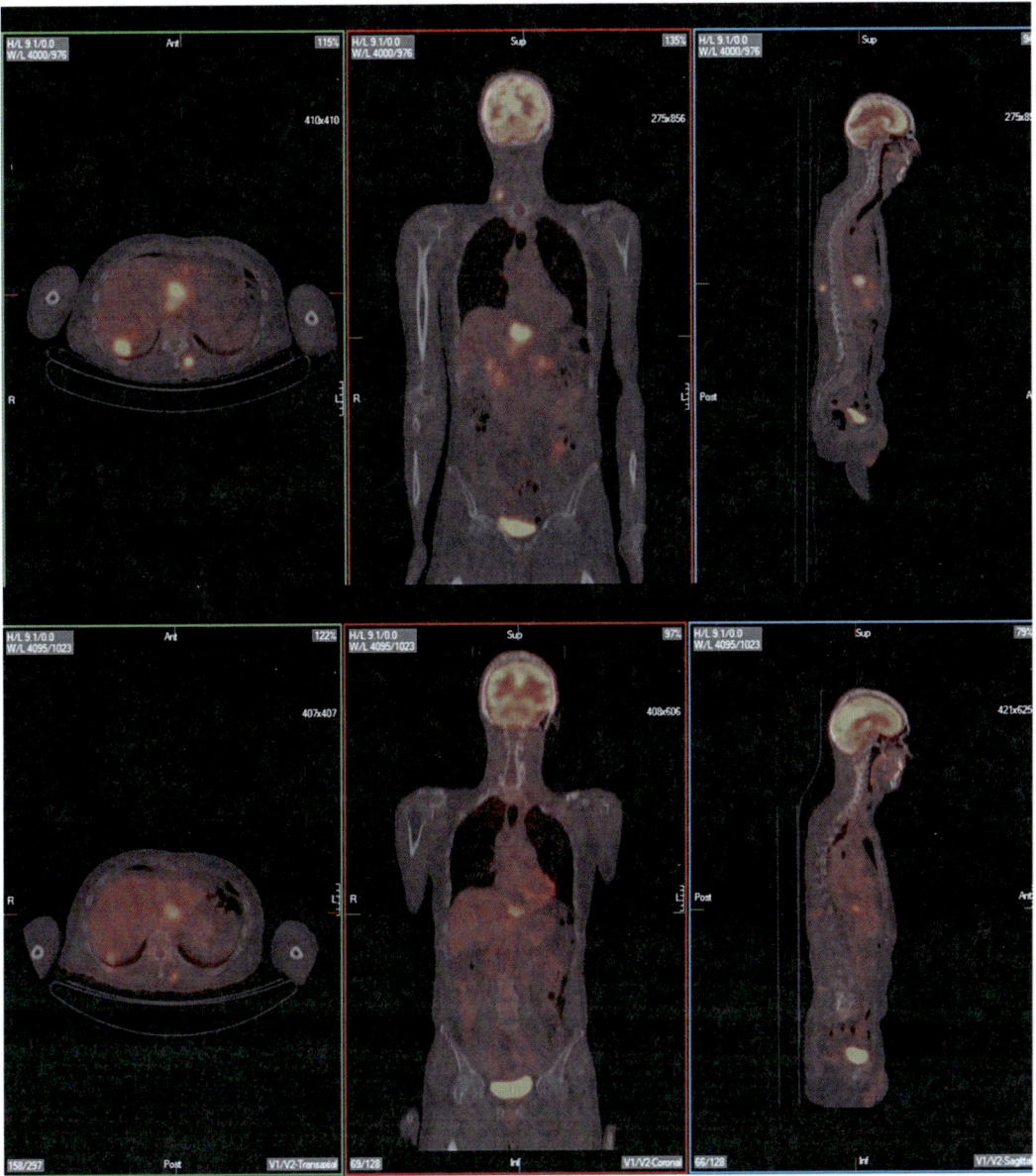

Fig. 6.3 F18-FDG PET images of a patient scanned day 0 (*top row*) and day 15 (*bottom row*) following therapy with an inhibitor of oncogenic mutant BRAF kinase for BRAF mutant metastatic melanoma. Transaxial, coronal and sagittal images are shown. Metastatic melanoma is seen is the liver, paraspinal soft tissues and a right neck node. After 15 days treatment response is almost complete in the right neck node which is barely visible but response to the treatment is less in the liver and para-spinal soft tissue metastases [49]

effective for some metastatic deposits but completely ineffective for others in the same patient (Fig. 6.3) [49]. In the future, the best approach may be to use combination therapy to induce cancer cell death from several different approaches simultaneously.

Radionuclide therapy using one or more of the techniques described above has an opportunity to contribute significantly to this attempt to destroy metastatic cancer cells in patients with melanoma and the future has never looked more promising for this to be successful than it does today.

References

1. DeNardo GL, Raventos A, Hines HH, et al. Requirements for a treatment planning system for radioimmunotherapy. Int J Radiat Oncol Biol Phys. 1985;11:335–48.
2. Larson SM, Brown JP, Wright PW, et al. Imaging of melanoma with I-131-labeled monoclonal antibodies. J Nucl Med. 1983;24:123–9.
3. Dadachova E, Revskaya E, Sesay MA, et al. Preclinical evaluation and efficacy studies of a melanin-binding IgM antibody labeled with [188]Re against experimental human metastatic melanoma in nude mice. Cancer Biol Ther. 2008;7:1116–27.
4. Lazova R, Klump V, Pawelek J. Autophagy in cutaneous malignant melanoma. J Cutan Pathol. 2010;37:256–68.
5. Milenic DE, Wong KJ, Baidoo KE, et al. Cetuximab: preclinical evaluation of a monoclonal antibody targeting EGFR for radioimmunodiagnostic and radioimmunotherapeutic applications. Cancer Biother Radiopharm. 2008;23:619–31.
6. Garin-Chesa P, Beresford HR, Carrato-Mena A, et al. Cell surface molecules of human melanoma. Immunohistochemical analysis of the gp57, GD3 and mel-CSPG antigenic systems. Am J Pathol. 1989;134:295–303.
7. Dadachova E, Casadevall A. Renaissance of targeting molecules for melanoma. Cancer Biother Radiopharm. 2007;21:545–52.
8. Siantar CL, DeNardo GL, Lam K, et al. Selecting an intervention time for intravascular enzymatic cleavage of peptide linkers to clear radioisotope from normal tissues. Cancer Biother Radiopharm. 2007;22:556–63.
9. Williams LE, DeNardo GL, Meredith RF. Targeted radionuclide therapy. Med Phys. 2008;35:3062–8.
10. Allen BJ, Raja C, Rizvi S, et al. Intralesional targeted alpha therapy for metastatic melanoma. Cancer Biol Ther. 2005;4:1318–24.
11. Gray BN, Anderson JE, Burton MA, et al. Regression of liver metastases following treatment with yttrium-90 microspheres. Aust N Z J Surg. 1992;62:105–10.
12. Cianni R, Urigo C, Notarianni E, et al. Radioembolisation using yttrium 90 (Y-90) in patients affected by unresectable hepatic metastases. Radiol Med. 2010;115:619–33.
13. Michelot JM, Moreau MFC, Veyre AJ, et al. Phase II scintigraphic clinical trial of malignant melanoma and metastases with iodine-123-N-(2-diethylaminoethyl 4-iodobenzamide). J Nucl Med. 1993;34:1260–6.
14. Chezal JM, Papon J, Labarre P, et al. Evaluation of radiolabeled (hetero) aromatic analogues of N-(2-diethylaminoethyl)-4-iodobenzamide for imaging and targeted radionuclide therapy in melanoma. J Med Chem. 2008;51:3133–44.
15. Joyal JL, Barrett JA, Marquis JC, et al. Preclinical evaluation of an ^{131}I-labeled benzamide for targeted radiotherapy of metastatic melanoma. Cancer Res. 2010;70:4045–53.
16. Bonnet M, Mishellany F, Papon J, et al. Antimelanoma efficacy of internal radionuclide therapy in relation to melanin target distribution. Pigment Cell Melanoma Res. 2010;23:1–11.
17. Bonnet-Duquennoy M, Papon J, Mishellany F, et al. Targeted radionuclide therapy of melanoma: antitumoral efficacy studies of a new ^{131}I labelled potential agent. Int J Cancer. 2009;125:708–16.
18. Gardette M, Papon J, Bonnet M, et al. Evaluation of new iodinated acridine derivatives for targeted radionuclide therapy of melanoma using (125)I, an Auger electron emitter. Invest New Drugs. 2011;29(6):1253–63.
19. Davies H, Bignell GR, Cox C, et al. Mutations of the BRAF gene in human cancer. Nature. 2002;417:949–54.
20. Curtin JA, Fridlyand J, Kageshita T, et al. Distinct sets of genetic alterations in melanoma. N Engl J Med. 2005;353:2135–47.
21. Marquette A, Bagot M, Bensussan A, Dumas N. Recent discoveries in the genetics of melanoma and their therapeutic implications. Arch Immunol Ther Exp (Warsz). 2007;55:363–72.
22. Hou P, Liu D, Ji M, et al. Induction of thyroid gene expression and radioiodine uptake in melanoma cells: novel therapeutic implications. PLoS One. 2009;4:e6200.
23. Huang R, Zhao Z, Ma X, et al. Targeting of tumor radioiodine therapy by expression of the sodium iodide symporter under control of the survivin promoter. Cancer Gene Ther. 2011;18(2):144–52.
24. Bhang HE, Gabrielson KL, Laterra J, et al. Tumor-specific imaging through progression elevated gene-3 promoter-driven gene expression. Nat Med. 2011;17(1):123–9.
25. Quinn T, Zhang X, Miao Y. Targeted melanoma imaging and therapy with radiolabeled alpha-melanocyte stimulating hormone peptide analogues. G Ital Dermatol Venereol. 2010;145:245–58.
26. Miao Y, Owen NK, Fisher DR, et al. Therapeutic efficacy of a [188]Re-labeled alpha-melanocyte-stimulating hormone peptide analog in murine and human melanoma-bearing mouse models. J Nucl Med. 2005;46:121–9.
27. Miao Y, Hylarides M, Fisher DR, et al. Melanoma therapy via peptide-targeted (alpha)-radiation. Clin Cancer Res. 2005;11:5616–21.
28. Froidevaux S, Calame-Christe M, Tanner H, Eberle AN. Melanoma targeting with DOTA-alpha-melanocyte-stimulating hormone analogs: structural parameters affecting tumor uptake and kidney uptake. J Nucl Med. 2005;46:887–95.
29. van Essen M, Krenning EP, Kooij PP, et al. Effects of therapy with [^{177}Lu-DOTA0, Tyr3] octreotate in patients with paraganglioma, meningioma, small cell lung carcinoma and melanoma. J Nucl Med. 2006;47:1599–606.
30. Asai T, Shuto S, Matsuda A, et al. Targeting and anti-tumor efficacy of liposomal 5'-O- dipalmitoylphosphatidyl 2'-C-cyano-2'-deoxy-1-beta-D-arabino-pentofuranosylcytosine in mice lung bearing B16BL6 melanoma. Cancer Lett. 2001;162:49–56.

31. Fondell A, Edwards K, Ickenstein LM, et al. Nuclisome: a novel concept for radionuclide therapy using targeting liposomes. Eur J Nucl Med Mol Imaging. 2010;37:114–23.
32. Khan MK, Minc LD, Nigavekar SS, et al. Fabrication of (^{198}Au0) radioactive composite nanodevices and their use for nanobrachytherapy. Nanomedicine. 2008;4:57–69.
33. Nakanishi T, Ichihashi M, Mishima Y, Matsuzawa T, Fukuda H. Thermal neutron capture therapy of malignant melanoma: in vitro radiobiological analysis. Int J Radiat Biol Relat Stud Phys Chem Med. 1980; 37:573–80.
34. Allen BJ. Boron neutron capture therapy—a research program for glioblastoma and melanoma. Australas Phys Eng Sci Med. 1983;6:184–6.
35. Mishima Y, Ichihashi M, Tsuji M, et al. Treatment of malignant melanoma by selective thermal neutron capture therapy using melanoma-seeking compound. J Invest Dermatol. 1989;92:321S–5.
36. Tsuboi T, Kondoh H, Hiratsuka J, Mishima Y. Enhanced melanogenesis induced by tyrosinase gene-transfer increases boron-uptake and killing effect of boron neutron capture therapy for amelanotic melanoma. Pigment Cell Res. 1998;11:275–82.
37. Altieri S, Balzi M, Bortolussi S, et al. Carborane derivatives loaded into liposomes as efficient delivery systems for boron neutron capture therapy. J Med Chem. 2009;52:7829–35.
38. Kabalka GW, Yao ML, Marepally SR, Chandra S. Biological evaluation of boronated unnatural amino acids as new boron carriers. Appl Radiat Isot. 2009;67:S374–9.
39. Wilkinson DA, Kolar M, Fleming PA, Singh AD. Dosimetric comparison of ^{106}Ru and ^{125}I plaques for treatment of shallow (< or = 5mm) choroidal melanoma lesions. Br J Radiol. 2008;81:784–9.
40. Verschueren KM, Creutzberg CL, Schalij-Delfos NE, et al. Long-term outcomes of eye-conserving treatment with ruthenium(106) brachytherapy for choroidal melanoma. Radiother Oncol. 2010;95:332–8.
41. Gunduz K, Kurt RA, Akmese HE, et al. Ruthenium-106 plaque radiotherapy alone or in combination with transpupillary thermotherapy in the management of choroidal melanoma. Jpn J Ophthalmol. 2010;54:338–43.
42. Oliver SC, Leu M, DeMarco JJ, Chow PE, Lee SP, McCannel TA. Attenuation of iodine 125 radiation with vitreous substitutes in the treatment of uveal melanoma. Arch Ophthalmol. 2010;128:888–93.
43. Thomson RM, Furutani KM, Pulido JS, et al. Modified COMS plaques for ^{125}I and ^{103}Pd iris melanoma brachytherapy. Int J Radiat Oncol Biol Phys. 2010; 78:1261–9.
44. Uren RF, Howman-Giles RB, Shaw HM, et al. Lymphoscintigraphy in high-risk melanoma of the trunk: predicting draining node groups, defining lymphatic channels and locating the sentinel node. J Nucl Med. 1993;34:1435–40.
45. Morton DL, Wen DR, Wong JH, et al. Technical details of intraoperative lymphatic mapping for early stage melanoma. Arch Surg. 1992;127:392–9.
46. Morton DL, Thompson JF, Cochran AJ, et al. Sentinel-node biopsy or nodal observation in melanoma. N Engl J Med. 2006;355:1307–17.
47. Denoyer D, Potdevin T, Roselt P, et al. Improved detection of regional melanoma metastasis using ^{18}F-6-fluoro-N-[2-(diethylamino)ethyl] pyridine-3-carboxamide, a melanin-specific PET probe, by perilesional administration. J Nucl Med. 2011;52:115–22.
48. Sanki A, Uren RF, Moncrieff M, et al. Targeted high-resolution ultrasound is not an effective substitute for sentinel lymph node biopsy in patients with primary cutaneous melanoma. J Clin Oncol. 2009;27:5614–9.
49. Carlino MS, Saunders CA, Gebski V, Menzies AM, Ma B, Lebowitz PF, et al. Heterogeneity of FDG-PET response to GSK2118436, an inhibitor of oncogenic mutant BRAF-kinase in BRAF-mutant metastatic melanoma. J Clin Oncol. 2011;29 Suppl:Abstract 8539.

Radioimmunotherapy in Brain Tumors

7

Chiara Maria Grana and Giovanni Paganelli

Background

Introduction

Tumors of the central nervous system (CNS) include a number of difficult-to treat neoplasms.

In the United States alone, more than 17,000 new cases of primary malignant brain tumors are diagnosed each year; the incidence of these tumors appears to be increasing.

Studies using data from the Surveillance, Epidemiology, and End Results (SEER) registry report that the incidence of primary tumors of the CNS is between 2 and 19 per 100,000 per year depending on age [1]. From birth to age 4 years, the incidence of primary brain tumors is approximately 3.1 per 100,000 and then slowly declines to a nadir of 1.8 per 100,000 in persons aged 15–24 years. The incidence rises again to a relative plateau around age 65 years with an incidence of approximately 18 cases per 100,000 persons.

The most common and serious malignant neoplasm is glioblastoma multiforme (GBM), which accounts for 23% of cases, and is among the most lethal and difficult-to-treat malignant tumors:

median survival is less than 1 year from the time of diagnosis [2].

The great majority of glioblastoma patients experience local recurrence, and the management of recurrent disease is even less effective, with a median survival of only 16–24 weeks being reported [3].

Pathological Classification

The pathological classification of CNS tumors reflects the many cell types that constitute the CNS, any of which can transform into a neoplastic phenotype. The frequency of individual tumor types roughly parallels the relative frequency of cell types within the CNS and their normal proliferative capacity. Astrocytes are among the most common cell types in the CNS and are mitogenically competent; thus astrocytomas are the most common primary CNS tumor. In contrast, although neurons are also numerous in the CNS, they are postmitotic, and therefore neuronally derived tumors are uncommon.

The recently revised World Health Organization (WHO) Classification of Tumors of the CNS (fourth edition, 2007) follows in the highly successful footsteps of previous editions of this widely used reference [4]. This version is the product of the combined efforts of an international Working Group of 25 pathologists and brain tumor international experts, and is presented as the standard for the definition of brain

C.M. Grana • G. Paganelli (✉)
Division of Nuclear Medicine, European Institute
of Oncology, Via Ripamonti, 435-20141, Milan, Italy
e-mail: chiara.grana@ieo.it;
divisione.medicinanucleare@ieo.it

tumors to the clinical oncology and cancer research communities worldwide.

The WHO scheme for brain tumor classification and grading has been widely adopted worldwide, and it commonly serves as the recommended reference standard for CNS tumor research studies and clinical protocols.

The 2007 WHO Classification includes a number of significant modifications compared with the preceding classification (WHO 2000). Among the modifications are newly introduced tumor entities, variants, patterns, and tumor syndromes, changes in grade for some tumor types, clarification of grading criteria for others, reorganization of some tumor categories, and conceptual shifts for some entities. An illustration of the latter is provided by the evolving view of the most highly infiltrative form of diffuse glioma, gliomatosis cerebri, which has previously been treated by the WHO as an independent tumor entity sui generis but it is now widely viewed as a pattern of widespread brain invasion that, although usually astrocytic in phenotype, can be seen with any diffuse glioma subtype, including oligodendroglioma and oligoastrocytoma.

A complete and proper classification of tumors is important, because tumor subtyping can affect prognosis and treatment recommendations as much as does the general tumor category. Tumor location and patient age are also relevant in tumor classification. For instance, astrocytomas of the spine, brainstem, and cortex may portend very different prognoses. Whether the different natural histories reflect different neuroanatomic constraints or diverse biologic properties of these tumors in various locations, or both, is not known. Finally, patient age may not only influence prognosis but may actually predict a totally different tumor type. For example, tumors in many young adults with glioblastomas (the most aggressive type of astrocytoma) have the genetic and behavioral characteristics of tumors derived from lower-grade gliomas ("secondary glioblastomas"), whereas almost all older patients have *de novo* ("primary") glioblastomas [5].

There has been significant controversy over the pathologic classification of astrocytic tumors. Generally speaking, slower growing and less aggressive tumors have been designated as low grade, and faster growing, more aggressive tumors have been designated as high grade. The first widely used system was devised by Kernohan and coworkers, who proposed a four-tier system with grades 1 and 2 defined as lower-grade tumors and grades 3 (*anaplastic astrocytoma*) and 4 (*GBM*) as high-grade gliomas (HGGs).

Histological grading is a means of predicting the biological behavior of a neoplasm. In the clinical setting, tumor grade is a key factor influencing the choice of therapies, particularly determining the use of adjuvant radiation and specific chemotherapy protocols. The WHO classification of tumors of the nervous system includes a grading scheme that is a "malignancy scale" ranging across a wide variety of neoplasms rather than a strict histological grading system [6, 7]. Grade I applies to lesions with low proliferative potential and the possibility of cure following surgical resection alone. Neoplasms of grade II are generally infiltrative in nature and, despite low proliferative activity, often recur. Some type II tumors tend to progress to higher grades of malignancy, for example, low-grade diffuse astrocytomas can transform to anaplastic astrocytoma and glioblastoma. Similar transformation occurs in oligodendroglioma and oligoastrocytomas. The WHO grade III is generally reserved for lesions with histological evidence of malignancy, including nuclear atypia and high mitotic activity.

The WHO grade IV is assigned to cytological malignant, mitotically active, necrosis-prone neoplasms typically associated with rapid pre- and postoperative disease evolution and a fatal outcome. Examples of grade IV neoplasms include glioblastoma, most embryonal neoplasms, and many sarcomas as well. Widespread infiltration of surrounding tissue and a propensity for craniospinal dissemination characterize some grade IV neoplasms.

Moreover, in recognition of the emerging role of molecular diagnostic approaches to tumor classification, genetic profiles have been emphasized, as in the distinct subtypes of glioblastoma and the already clinically useful 1p and 19q markers for oligodendroglioma and 22q/INI1 for atypical teratoid/rhabdoid tumors.

For histotype characterization, pathologists usually perform immunohistochemical investigations that allow the expression of specific markers of malignancy, which help in the diagnostic definition (standard diagnosis). Through genetic and immunohistochemical investigations it is also possible to study the expression of molecular markers with prognostic/predictive value (individualized diagnosis) and other markers that are associated with different subtypes (experimental diagnosis).

This molecular profile identifies tumoral subtypes with chromosomal, gene, and molecular alterations, which may be indicative of biological behavior, therapeutic response, and thus prognosis. These methods of genetic analysis could be:

- Loss of heterozygosity: PCR after extraction of DNA from tumor tissue (frozen or fixed) and the patient's blood. Alternatively: FISH (Fluorescent in situ hybridization) probes and specific hybridization of histological section prepared from paraffin-embedded.
- Hypermethylation of the MGMT promoter: methylation specific PCR on tumor tissue.
- EGFR gene amplification: PCR or FISH on tumor tissue.
- Mutation of the gene IDH1/IDH2: extraction of DNA from tumor, PCR and subsequent sequence.

Therapeutic Approaches and Procedures

Surgery

An accurate tumor diagnosis requires surgery. With current stereotactic procedures, tissue samples should be obtainable from any location in the brain with few exceptions. In most cases, a surgical resection should be considered and recommended: possible sampling error when only biopsy is performed and the improvement of symptoms related to mass effect of the tumor.

For high grade glioma, the extent of tumor resection and survival are related, favoring any degree of resection beyond biopsy. The major objective of brain tumor surgery is to resect and potentially cure the tumor.

There are several reasons for performing a resection of gliomas in adults whenever it is thought to be safe. First, resection (rather than stereotactic biopsy) provides the best opportunity to obtain an accurate diagnosis. Gliomas are notoriously heterogeneous, and therapy is guided by the most aggressive histological type detected in the specimen. Studies have shown that more complete resections are more likely to provide a high-grade diagnosis [8] and to detect an oligodendroglial component in the tumor [9]. Second, resection relieves symptoms from mass effect in many patients, and more extensive resections are associated with greater chances of neurologic improvement. Third, response to postoperative radiation therapy is more favorable and deterioration during treatment is less probable after resection [10]. Finally, it is likely that resection has a modest survival benefit through cytoreduction. Only one randomized trial of resection of malignant gliomas has been published; survival was approximately twice as long with resection [11]. Many retrospective studies of both low-grade [12] and HGG [13] have shown longer survival with resection, after adjustment for age, performance score, tumor histological type, and other prognostic factors. For deeply situated intrinsic tumors, or for diffuse non-focal tumors, resection is not practical. In these situations, needle stereotactic biopsy is used for diagnosis.

Radiotherapy

Most common brain tumors, such as low-grade and malignant astrocytomas, are infiltrative into surrounding normal brain tissue many centimeters from the primary lesion. Radiation treatment volumes for these tumors generally include the enhancing volume (which contains solid tumor tissue), surrounding oedema (which is comprised of normal brain infiltrated by microscopic tumor), and a margin of normal brain. Thus, even with the use of very conformal techniques, a substantial amount of "normal" brain is included in the full-dose volume. The tolerance of normal brain is a major limiting factor in achieving local control and cure: it depends on the size of the dose per fraction, total dose given, overall treatment time, volume of brain irradiated, host factors, and adjunctive therapies. The probability of injury increases with larger daily doses (2.2 Gy/fraction) and doses in excess of 60 Gy delivered in 30 fractions over approximately 6 weeks.

Approximately 4–9% of patients treated to 50–60 Gy with conventional fractionated radiation for brain tumors develop clinically detectable focal radiation necrosis, but this form of injury may be found in as many as 10–22% of patients at autopsy.

The appropriate volume to encompass within the radiation treatment portal varies with the specific histopathologic tumor type and, with certain histologies, is controversial. Benign tumors typically do not infiltrate beyond the lesional borders seen by MRI. Certain tumors, such as benign meningiomas, pituitary adenomas, craniopharyngiomas, and acoustic neuromas, may be treated with narrow margins of surrounding normal tissue. In contrast, the astrocytic gliomas require larger margins because of their tendency to infiltrate beyond the imaged tumor border.

The across-target volume is defined as a three-dimensional reconstruction of the tumor contour based on operative findings and data from CT and MRI studies. The planning target volume consists of the volume of tissue that must be irradiated to encompass the tumor volume with a margin of surrounding tissue considered to be at risk for microscopic tumor spread and to account for patient movement and daily setup uncertainties. Three-dimensional conformal radiation therapy and the advanced technique of intensity-modulated radiation therapy are new methods of treatment planning and delivery designed to enhance the conformation of the dose to the target volume, while maximally restricting the dose delivered to the normal tissue outside the treatment volume.

Radiosurgery is a method of highly focal, closed-skull external irradiation that uses an imaging-compatible stereotactic device for precise target localization. It is being used to treat other intracranial lesions, including small arteriovenous malformations, pituitary adenomas, acoustic neuromas, meningiomas, gliomas, and brain metastases. The relationship between the stereotactic coordinate system and the radiation

source(s) allows accurate delivery of radiation to the target volume.

Temozolomide (TMZ) is an oral alkylating agent with known activity in patients with malignant gliomas. A pilot phase II trial demonstrated the feasibility of concomitant administration of TMZ with fractionated radiotherapy, followed by up to 6 cycles of adjuvant TMZ, and suggested that this treatment had promising clinical activity (2-year survival rate, 31%) [14].

The European Organization for Research and Treatment of Cancer (EORTC) Brain Tumor and Radiotherapy Groups and the National Cancer Institute of Canada (NCIC) Clinical Trials Group published the long-term findings of the EORT-NCI phase III trial in glioblastoma patients randomized to receive external radiotherapy alone vs. external radiotherapy plus TMZ. Overall survival was 27.2% (95% CI 22.2–32.5) at 2 years. The addition of TMZ to radiotherapy for newly diagnosed glioblastoma resulted so in a clinically meaningful and statistically significant survival benefit with minimal additional toxicity [15].

Brachitherapy has also been suggested to improve the survival and quality of life of patients with recurrent malignant gliomas who meet criteria for implantation [16]. The use of less invasive highly conformal radiation techniques (i.e., radiosurgery) appears to provide results equivalent to those of brachitherapy in patients with recurrent gliomas, and this has become the radiation treatment of choice for patients with small recurrences [17].

Chemotherapy

Chemotherapy offers the theoretical advantage of reaching all tumor cells, regardless of their gross or microanatomic location within the CNS, because all tumor cells must be within the perfusion zone of preexisting or tumor-associated microvasculature. Furthermore, many chemotherapeutic agents have minimum neurotoxic effects, so toxicity concerns are largely confined to systemic toxicity. Finally, because the vast majority of normal cells within the CNS are post-mitotic, chemotherapeutic agents that are preferentially toxic to dividing cells should have a high thera-peutic index within the CNS.

The challenges for successful use of chemo-therapy for CNS tumors, however, are even greater than they are for systemic tumors. Central to this difference is the issue of drug delivery, as the CNS is protected from toxic substances in the blood by the blood brain barrier (BBB).

Physicochemical characteristics largely deter-mine a drug's ability to cross the BBB. Smaller, ionically neutral, lipophilic drugs, are more likely to penetrate the BBB and brain tumor barrier (BTB) [18]. Unfortunately, most drugs lack these characteristics and are excluded by the barrier. For this reason, and because only a tiny portion of any systemically delivered drug finds its way into a relatively small tumor regardless of permeability issues, there are significant problems both in obtaining homogeneous, pharmacologically active concentrations of drugs throughout a brain tumor and in limiting systemic toxicity. This has led to the development of alternate drug administration techniques that either disrupt the BBB and BTB or deliver drugs directly to the region. One way to do this is the surgical placement of biodegradable synthetic polymers impregnated with a drug. The prototype implantable polymer is the Gliadel® wafer, which contains BCNU [19]. After surgical debulking of a malignant glioma the surgeon lines the surgical cavity with Gliadel® wafers that are left in place: over the next several weeks the BCNU diffuses out of the wafers into the sur-rounding brain, providing very high local concen-trations of BCNU with little systemic exposure to the drug. Although theoretically attractive, this approach has pharmacologic constraints: BCNU is highly lipid soluble and crosses the BBB readily in both directions. This carries the drug away from the brain, a phenomenon known as the *sink effect*. Another limitation is that drug penetrates the sur-rounding brain only by passive diffusion, a slow and inefficient process. High concentrations of BCNU are thus found only within a few millime-ters of the wafers, which makes it unlikely that cytotoxic drug concentrations will reach distant infiltrating tumor cells [20].

The agent with the most proven activity against recurrent astrocytomas is TMZ, an orally administered, second-generation imidazotetra-zine prodrug with excellent bioavailability; wide tissue distribution, including the ability to cross the BBB [21].

However alkylating agents, such as TMZ, are highly reactive molecules that cause cell death by forming cross-links between adjacents strands of DNA. However, this cross-linking is inhibited by the cellular DNA-repair protein O6-methylguanine-DNA methyltransferase: the DNA-repair enzyme O6-methylguanine-DNA methyltransferase (MGMT) inhibits the killing of tumor cells by alkylating agents. MGMT activity is controlled by a promoter; methylation of the promoter silences the gene in cancer, and the cells no longer produce MGMT.

Esteller et al. examined gliomas to determine whether methylation of the MGMT promoter is related to the responsiveness of the tumor to alky-lating agents: they found that MGMT promoter was methylated in gliomas from 19 of 47 patients (40%) and this finding was associated with regres-sion of the tumor and prolonged overall and dis-ease-free survival. It was an independent and stronger prognostic factor than age, stage, tumor grade, or performance status. In this paper they concluded that methylation of the MGMT pro-moter in gliomas is a useful predictor of the respon-siveness of the tumors to alkylating agents [22].

New Drugs

Gliomas are highly dependent on vascular endothelial growth factor (VEGF) for angiogene-sis and glioblastoma is one of the most vascular-ised cancers [23]. VEGF is an important regulator of angiogenesis that is highly expressed within brain tumors [24]; the degree of both vasculature density and VEGF expression is correlated with the grade and biologic aggressiveness of tumor, as well as with clinical outcomes [25, 26]. The results from first generation antiangiogenic therapies, as thalidomide, were disappointing showing no addi-tional clinical benefit compared to the standard of care [27, 28]. As a consequence more recent investigations have focused on newer, more potent angiogenic inhibitors such as bevacizumab.

Bevacizumab is the best characterized antiangiogenic therapy and recently received FDA approval as a single agent for the treatment of patients with recurrent GBM following prior upfront, TMZ-based chemoradiotherapy [29, 30]. Overall, treatment with bevacizumab in multiple GBM studies appears to be well tolerated with toxicity similar to that seen with other solid cancers treated with bevacizumab-containing therapies. Because of the extensive clinical experience with bevacizumab, practical issues regarding its administration, safety profile, and response to treatment have been described [31–33]. However, several important questions about the use of bevacizumab in GBM still remain unanswered, for example, the optimal therapeutic dosage, treatment schedule, treatment duration in responding patients, and radiographic response criteria of bevacizumab are all unknown.

Many of these unanswered questions are addressed in on-going clinical trials and results of these trials will likely continue to drive improvements in the treatment of patients with GBM [34].

Radioimmunotherapy

Introduction and Rationale

Despite the modest benefits afforded by radiation therapy and alkylating agent chemotherapy, the new biological drugs, it is clear that more effective treatments are needed.

Monoclonal antibodies against tumor-associated antigens can be used therapeutically as delivery system for chemotherapeutic agents, toxins, and radionuclides. In particular, the utility of MoAbs (MW 150 kDa) for targeting radioactive agents to tumor cells, for diagnostic (radioimmunoscintigraphy and radioimmunoguided surgery) and therapeutic purpose (radioimmunotherapy [RIT]) has been extensively studied [35–38].

Because of its potential for more selectively irradiating tumor cells than conventional radiotherapy, RIT is an attractive strategy for brain tumors: The antitumor effect is primarily due to the associated radioactivity of the radiolabeled

Table 7.1 Radioisotopes characteristics

Isotope	$T_{1/2}$ (days)	E_β (MeV)	R_{max} (mm)	E_γ(KeV)
[131]I	8.0	0.81	3.3	360 (81%)–630 (7%)
[90]Y	2.7	2.27	11.9	–
[177]Lu	6.7	0.50	2.2	113 (6%)–208 (11%)

$T_{1/2}$ half life; $E_\beta max$ (MeV) maximum energy of b particles; R_{max} maximum range; E_g g energy

antibody, which emits continuous slowing-down low-dose-rate irradiation [39, 40]. One of the main therapeutic advantages of radiolabeled MoAbs is their potential to overcome the problem of tumor heterogeneity. Because the radionuclides can penetrate up to several millimeters of tissues, radio-emission can kill those antigen-negative tumor cells, which have no specific radiolabeled antibody localized on their surface (cross fire effect).

The range of radioisotopes available for the production of radiolabeled compounds is ever increasing. Although damaging DNA represents the main mechanism for killing tumor cells, the choice of suitable radioisotopes needs appropriate consideration in order to match their decay properties with the characteristics of the tumor (Table 7.1).

Among the radionuclides used in clinical practice, ^{90}Y has physical and radiobiological features suitable for RIT approach, due to its high-energy β^- particles (maximum energy 2.27 MeV). Moreover, ^{90}Y penetration (maximum particle range in tissue 12 mm, range in tissue after which the 50% of particles are stopped 4 mm) allows high radiation doses to the target area, while sparing surrounding tissues and normal organs and maximizing the tumor to non-tumor dose ratio. In addition, the radiochemistry procedures to conjugate an antibody with a radioisotope vary because of the specific chemistry involved: several isotopes, in particular ^{131}I and ^{125}I, can be directly conjugated to the antibodies. However, radio-metals like ^{90}Y, ^{177}Lu, and [186]Re require more complex reactions, initially involving the binding of a chelator to the antibody and subsequently conjugation with the isotope species [41, 42]. The attractive feature of RIT is the prospect that most normal tissues are spared from high radiation burden. Unfortunately, RIT has thus far failed to fulfill this expectation mainly because only a very small amount of tagged MoAb localizes per gram of tumor (<0.001%) while the remainder stays in the circulation conjugated to the radioisotope with toxic effects on tissues, especially bone marrow [43].

Tumor Pre-targeting

One of the limitations of directly labeled antibodies for targeted radiotherapy is that as a consequence of their macromolecular size they diffuse slowly through tissue, hampering their delivery to tumor cells distant from their site of injection. In an attempt to overcome this problem and the low uptake of radiolabeled MoAbs by the tumor, various studies have examined the concept of tumor pre-targeting consisting in the administration of a modified MoAb (first conjugates) that permits a second component (second conjugates) to bind specifically to it [44]. Conceptually, the modified MoAb is administered first and allowed to distribute throughout the body, to bind to the cells expressing antigen, and to clear substantially from other tissues. Then the radiolabeled second component is administered and, ideally, it localizes at sites where the modified MoAb has accumulated. If the second component has higher permeation, clearance, and diffusion rates than those of MoAb, more rapid radionuclide localization to the tumor and higher tumor selectivity are possible thus achieving higher tumor to non-tumor ratio [45].

The Advantages of Biotin-Avidin Pre-targeting

1. Overcoming the limitations of directly labeled antibodies.
2. Higher tumor to non-tumor ratio, decreased background.
3. Easy biotinylation of antibody.
4. Easy production of other reagents.
5. Possibility of targeting different antigens (cocktail of antibodies).

The Avidin-Biotin System

One of the most clinically used pre-targeting techniques is the Avidin-Biotin system (Fig. 7.1). This pre-targeting approach takes advantage of the extremely high affinity between Avidin and Biotin. Avidin (MW 66 kDa) is a small oligomeric protein made up of four identical sub-units, each bearing a single binding site for biotin (vitamin H, MW 244 Da). They can therefore bind up to four moles of biotin per mole of protein. The affinity of avidin for biotin is extremely high, with a dissociation constant of the avidin-biotin complex in the order of 10^{-15} M. For practical purposes, their binding can be regarded as irreversible [46, 47]. Briefly, this Pre-targeted Antibody-Guided RadioImmunoTherapy (PAGRIT®) is based on intravenous or loco-regional sequential administration of a specific biotinylated antibody, avidin, and radioactive biotin (^{90}Y-Biotin) [48]. The first clinical experience with the avidin-biotin pre-targeting system in cancer therapy was performed more than a decade ago at the European Institute of Oncology in Milan, in patients affected by recurrent HGG [49].

The Steps of Pre-targeting

1. Administration of tumor specific biotinilated monoclonal antibody.
2. Administration of avidin as a chase and as the second step.
3. Chase of biotinilated albumin.
4. Administration of ^{90}Y-biotin.

Clinical Applications

Theoretically, RIT approach could be exploited in all those tumors for which a specific monoclonal antibody is available to target its specific antigen. However, malignant gliomas represent the most favorable model since they are refractory to conventional treatments and a suitable marker, the glycoprotein Tenascin-C, is overexpressed in the extracellular matrix of gliomas, but not in normal cerebral tissues [50]. The level of tenascin

a

b

c

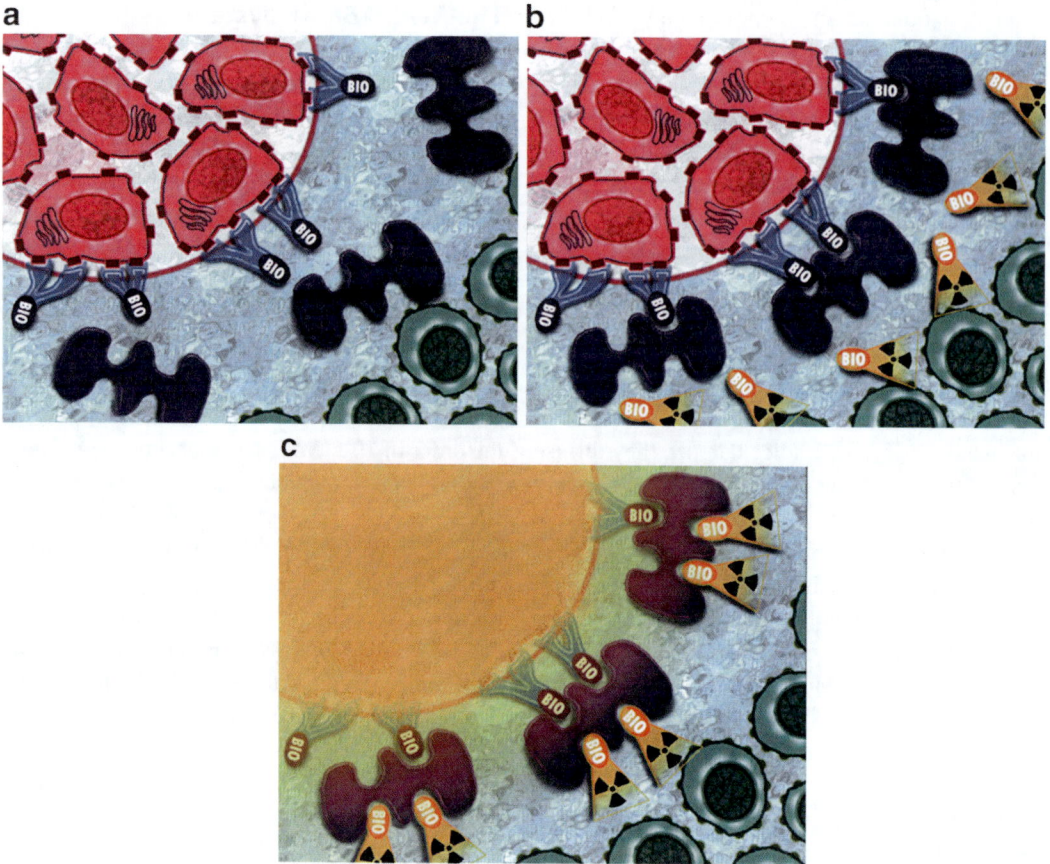

Fig. 7.1 The avidin-biotin model, 3-step radioimmunotherapy. (**a**) First step (binding of biotinylated MoAbs to the antigen tenascin). (**b**) Second step (binding of avidin to biotinylated MoAbs). (**c**) Third step (binding of ^{90}Y-biotin to the biotinylated MoAbs-avidin complex)

expression increases with tumor grade [51]. Important for its role as a target for RIT is the fact that more than 90% of glioblastoma exhibit high levels of tenascin expression [52]. In addition, tenascin is located primarily around tumor blood vessels, with this feature becoming more predominant with advancing tumor grade [53] (Fig. 7.2).

The hope of therapy for brain tumors and, in particular, for HGGs lies in the potential to extend functional life-span with little additional, and possibly reduced, morbidity, as compared with current aggressive treatment modalities. In fact, protocols including aggressive combined therapies, such as surgical debulking, external beam radiotherapy, and chemotherapy, usually provide time-limited results, and local recurrence is a common event occurring in a few months. Surgical resection could potentially represent the

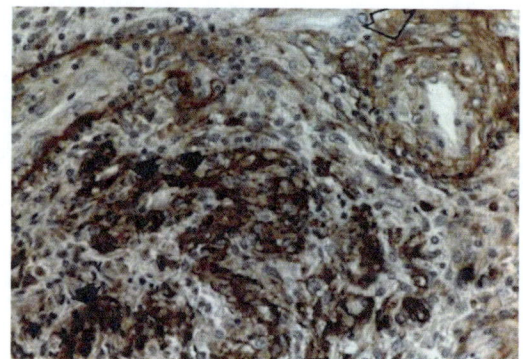

Fig. 7.2 Example of immunoistochemistry, revealing the presence of tenascin in the tumor

only curative option, but, in the clinical practices, it is impossible to remove the microscopic tumor foci, which constantly spread into the Brain

Adjacent Tissue (BAT) giving rise to recurrence. The efficacy of conventional external radiotherapy has been demonstrated, but no more than 60 Gy can be delivered, due to unacceptable risks of neurological toxicity.

RIT, as systemic or loco-regional application has the potential to become a well-tolerated therapeutic option in the management of HGG, complementing traditional regimens.

Systemic Radioimmunotherapy

In a phase I-II study the toxicity and therapeutic efficacy of the Avidin-Biotin pre-targeting approach in a group of 48 eligible patients were evaluated. All patients had histologically confirmed grade III or IV glioma and documented residual disease or recurrence after conventional treatment [49]. The 3-step RIT was performed by intravenous administration of biotinylated anti-tenascin monoclonal antibody (BC2 and BC4 epitopes), followed 36 h later by Avidin and Streptavidin (a non-glycosilated analogue of Avidin) and 18–24 h later by Yttrium-90-labeled Biotin. The injected activity, calculated on the basis of previous studies and dosimetry calculation, ranged from 2.22 to 2.97 GBq/m^2 per cycle. Three major conclusions emerged from this study. First, 3-step radionuclide therapy with high dose ^{90}Y produced acceptable toxicity at the dose of 2.22 GBq/m^2 due to the extremely favorable biodistribution of ^{90}Y-DOTA-Biotin, with the majority of the non-tumor bound activity eliminated in the first 24 h. MTD was determined at the level of 2.96 GBq/m^2. Second, an objective therapeutic response was documented in an encouraging fraction of our patients, who were no longer responsive to conventional treatments: 52% did not progress any further (the majority suspended steroid assumption, had reduction in epileptic seizure rate and improved quality of life), while significant tumor reduction occurred in 25%.

Third, immune response to the murine monoclonal antibody, known to interfere with localization in subsequent administrations, was less frequent than in patients treated with the directly labeled MoAbs used in other studies, possibly because of its shorter residence time in the circulation with our procedure.

The encouraging results obtained in this phase I-II study prompted us to apply the same approach in an adjuvant setting, to evaluate: (a) the time to relapse and (b) the overall survival [54]. We studied 37 HGG patients, 17 with grade III glioma and 20 with glioblastoma, in a controlled open non-randomized study. All patients received surgery and radiotherapy and were disease-free by neuroradiological examinations. Nineteen patients (treated) received adjuvant treatment with RIT. In the treated glioblastoma patients, median disease-free interval was 28 months (range: 9–59); median survival was 33.5 months and one patient is still without evidence of disease. All 12-control glioblastoma patients (non treated) died after a median survival from diagnosis of 8 months. In the treated grade III glioma patients median disease-free interval was 56 months (range: 15–60) and survival cannot be calculated as only two, within this group, died.

A number of points arose from the results of this second study. Firstly, 3-step RIT was confirmed as highly active against malignant glioma, yet did not cause major adverse events, as previously described. Secondly the effect RIT on glioblastoma was interesting: it considerably prolonged disease-free interval and overall survival relative to the untreated group.

A recent evaluation [55] was performed by our group concerning all the patients treated with 3-step RIT in a period of 11 years at our Institute: 3-step RIT was administered 502 recurrent glioblastoma patients, already treated with standard treatment: the results from this retrospective analysis suggest that ^{90}Y-biotin PAGRIT® interferes with the progression of glioblastoma, prolonging survival in a larger number of patients.

Loco-Regional Radioimmunotherapy

RIT, as systemic or loco-regional (LR) application has the potential to become an option in the management of HGG, complementing the above mentioned treatment regimens. One of the main therapeutic advantages of radiolabeled moAbs is their potential to overcome the problem of tumor heterogeneity. Because the radionuclides can penetrate up to several millimeters of tissues, radio-emission can kill those antigen-negative

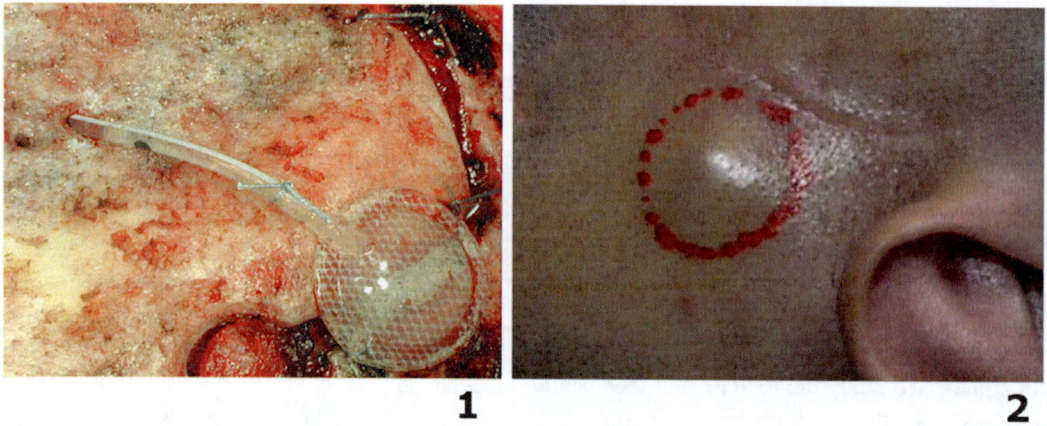

Fig. 7.3 Catheter placed into the surgical cavity (1). In LR RIT, all reagents are injected through the reservoir (2)

tumor cells, which have no specific radiolabeled antibody localized on their surface (cross fire effect).

Many early RIT trials on brain tumor involved the intravenous administration of radiolabeled moAbs. Although some positive responses were described, more encouraging survival benefits have been reported when the radiolabeled moAbs were administered loco-regionally, either into non-resected tumor or into the surgically created resection cavity (SCRC).

High grade glioma recurs at or near the site of origin and are characterized by a high tendency to infiltrate adjacent brain tissue, and only rarely do they metastasize outside the CNS.

Based on these observations, loco-regional therapies are fully justified; in selected cases a second operation to remove recurrence is offered to patients; in the treatment of not operable HGG recurrences, radiosurgery has been confirmed its important role. Brachitherapy (BRT) is defined as an irradiation modality where a radioactive source (seeds or needles) is directly located in a short distance or into the local tumor site. Iodine-125 (^{125}I) can be considered, at present, the preferred agent for intracranial BRT, especially for HGG. Promising results are documented in some retrospective trials from single institutions, though a higher incidence of steroid dependence and re-operation, caused by radiation necrosis, is reported [56].

Since the constant presence of a SCRC after operation for HGG, the injection of drugs directly into the surgical bed might be considered an interesting therapeutic option. In order to facilitate such administrations, a catheter into SCRC connected with a subcutaneous reservoir should have to be permanently implanted during surgical procedures (Fig. 7.3).

The rationale for intracavitary administered therapies for malignant glioma patients is based on two fundamental factors. First, locally administered therapeutics may circumvent the blood–brain barrier and thus potentially achieve higher intratumoral concentrations than the systemic administration. Second, systemic exposures associated with LR therapies are typically minimal, leading to less systemic toxicity.

Clinical experiences using LR techniques to treat malignant gliomas, including intra-tumor injection of interleukin-2, lymphokine-activated killer cells, toxins, and various chemotherapeutic agents, have been reported over the last 30 years.

The principal advantages of a locally delivered compound (chemotherapeutic agent or radiopharmaceutical) consist mainly in bypassing the blood–brain barrier, minimizing systemic toxicity, and in achieving prolonged local drugs concentration.

Several studies demonstrated that the loco-regional infusion of ^{131}I or ^{90}Y-labeled anti-Tenascin MoAbs in glioma patients provided a safety profile and the possibility to control the growth of the tumor in the long-term [57, 58]. Riva et al. [59] evaluated the efficacy of ^{131}I-labeled and ^{90}Y-labeled BC2 and BC4 MoAbs for the loco-regional treatment of malignant gliomas. The phase II study with ^{131}I involved 91 patients including 74 with GBM and 9 with anaplastic astrocytoma (AA). The study population consisted of 47 newly diagnosed and 44 recurrent tumors. Patients received 3–10 cycles of ^{131}I-labeled MoAb, at intervals of either 1 or 3 months, with a cumulative administered activity of up to 20.35 GBq (550 mCi). The median survival was >46 months in AA and 19 months in GBM, with no distinction between newly diagnosed and recurrent patients groups. The response rate was better in those with small volume (56.7%), compared with larger tumors. A subsequent study was performed using ^{90}Y in order to investigate the potential effects of a radionuclide emitting beta particles with greater tissue penetration. Patients received between 3 and 5 cycles of ^{90}Y-labeled MoAbs with a cumulative activity of 3.145 GBq (85 mCi). The median survival for patients with AA and GBM was 90 and 20 months, respectively.

In a more recent study, the therapeutic potential of [131]I- and ^{90}Y-labeled BC4 MoAb were evaluated in 37 patients, consisting of 13 with AA and 24 with GBM [60]. Multiple cycles of labeled MoAbs were administered (mean, three per patients) at various activity levels. The median survival for GBM was 17 months. No attempt was made to stratify analyses according to the radionuclide used or whether the patients had recurrent or newly diagnosed lesions.

Investigators at Duke University Medical Center have assessed the potential therapeutic benefits using the 81C6 MoAb labeled with ^{131}I-labeled in patients with GBM and other malignant brain tumors [61, 62]. Preliminary diagnostic-level studies have demonstrated that delivery of radiolabeled MoAbs by intravenous route would not yield therapeutically relevant tumor doses without unacceptable toxicity for patients. For these reasons, RIT trials with anti-tenascin MoAbs have involved intra-compartmental (loco-regional) administration of the labeled protein,

into either tumor, spontaneous tumor cysts, or, most frequently, surgically created glioma resection cavities.

In the first phase I study, 42 patients with recurrent glioma were included and the maximal tolerable dose (MTD) was assessed in a dose-escalation study after intracavitary administration of ^{131}I-labeled 81C6. This study showed that the MTD was 100 mCi, with neurotoxicity being the dose-limiting factor. The results of this study suggested that there was a potential survival benefit, as compared to patients treated with stereotactic radiotherapy and high-dose brachytherapy (a median survival of 60 weeks in the present study, as compared to 41 and 46 weeks, respectively). In the second study, 42 patients with newly diagnosed glioma were included in order to investigate dosimetry and dose–response relationships. In these patients, the MTD was 120 mCi, with neurotoxicity being the dose-limiting factor. The median survival of these patients was 79 weeks, as compared to 46 weeks of historic controls, when patients were treated with surgery, chemotherapy, and radiotherapy. Based on these encouraging results, a phase II trial was performed in 33 patients with newly diagnosed, previously untreated patients. The median survival after treatment with 120 mCi of ^{131}I-labeled 81C6 in this study was 79–85 weeks, depending on the pathologic type of glioma (patients with astrocytic oligodendroglioma showed a better response than those with GBM). When 100 mCi of radiolabeled antibody was administered to 43 patients with recurrent glioma, survival was still 69 weeks. The results of these trials warranted a phase III trial, which is currently ongoing.

Subsequently, a human/mouse chimeric MoAb, originating from 81C6, was developed, showing better tumor targeting in animal studies. The targeting capabilities of the antibody were subsequently tested in a phase I study that included 47 patients with recurrent disease. This chimeric antibody showed a prolonged retention time within the SCC, as compared to the antibody of murine origin. Based on the enhanced circulatory half-life of the chimeric antibody, a MTD of 80 mCi was found, as compared to 120 mCi found in previous studies with the murine antibody.

Fig. 7.4 PAGRIT®
distribution after
loco-regional injection
of reagents

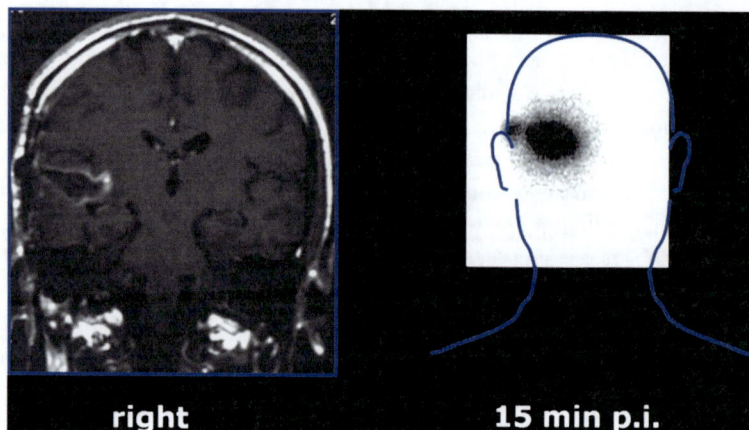

In this phase I dose-escalation study, the median survival was 87 weeks for patients with newly diagnosed glioma and 65 weeks for those patients with recurrent disease.

A more recent clinical experience from the same group was concerning the use of alfa-particles instead of beta-particles in LR-RIT [63]. Eighteen patients were treated with [211]At-labeled chimeric 81C6 ([211]At-ch81C6) administered into a SCRC and then with salvage chemotherapy. Serial gamma-camera imaging and blood sampling over 24 h were performed. A total of $96.7 \pm 3.6\%$ (mean $\pm$ SD) of 211At decays occurred in the SCRC, and the mean blood-pool percentage injected dose was ≤ 0.3. No patient experienced dose-limiting toxicity, and the maximum tolerated dose was not identified. Six patients experienced grade 2 neurotoxicity within 6 weeks of 211At-ch81C6 administration; this neurotoxicity resolved fully in all but one patient. No toxicities of grade 3 or higher were attributable to the treatment. No patient required repeat surgery for radionecrosis. The median survival times for all patients, those with GBM, and those with anaplastic astrocytoma or oligodendroglioma were 54, 52, and 116 weeks, respectively. The authors concluded that the regional administration of [211]At-ch81C6 was feasible, safe, and associated with a promising antitumor benefit in patients with malignant CNS tumors.

The Experience of the European Institute of Oncology, Milan

After the encouraging results from the experiences in gliomas using the intravenous route [49, 54], investigators at the European Institute of Oncology experimented the 3-step pre-targeting method also for loco-regional applications [64]. In this phase I-II study the safety profile and antitumor efficacy of the 3-step method in the loco-regional therapy of recurrent high grade gliomas was assessed. Twenty-four patients with recurrent HGG (8 AA and 16 GBM) underwent second surgical debulking with implantation of an indwelling catheter (connected with a subcutaneous recervoir) into the SCRC, in order to receive the radioimmunotherapeutic agents.

Biotinylated anti-tenascin MoAbs (BC2 or BC4), avidin and, finally, 90Y-Biotin were subsequently injected through the catheter. Each patient received two of these treatments 8–10 weeks apart and the injected activity ranged from 0.5 to 1.1 GBq. Dosage was escalated by 0.2 GBq in four consecutive groups. Bremsstrahlung images were acquired to confirm the correct localization of the 90Y-biotin (Fig. 7.4). The treatment was well tolerated without acute side effects up to 0.7 GBq. The maximum tolerated activity was 1.1 GBq limited by neurologic toxicity. None of the patients developed hematological toxicity. In three patients, catheter infection occurred.

The average absorbed dose to the normal brain was minimal compared with the one received at the surgical resection cavity interface.

This study assessed that with activity ranging from 0.7 to 0.9 GBq per cycle, "3-step" LR RIT was safe and produced an objective response (partial and stable disease in 75% of patients).

Multi-Modal Approach: Loco-Regional RIT in Association with Chemotherapy

The role of chemotherapy in HGG, either in an adjuvant setting or at recurrence, has often been controversial. In 1999, due to the positive results assessed in preclinical and clinical trials a new alkylating drug, TMZ was approved for the treatment of relapsing GBM. Since then, TMZ has been studied in different treatment schedules both in primary and recurrent GBM. In a randomized clinic trial investigators report a median survival of 16 months in 64 GBM patients treated with EBRT in combination with TMZ [15]. The rationale for combining TMZ and radiotherapy is based on preclinical data suggesting additional or, at least, synergistic activity against GBM cell-lines.

Since 1999 at the European Institute of Oncology, TMZ was proposed in association with LR RIT to the new enrolled patients [65]. The rationale for combining LR RIT and TMZ include toxicity independence (the two treatments have different toxicity profiles) and the possibility to eliminate microscopic disease outside the radiation LR RIT field with TMZ. This hypothesis is supported by a retrospective analysis performed in a group of 73 patients with histologically-proven recurrent GBM and immuno-histochemical demonstration of tenascin expression in tumor. All patients had a catheter implanted at second surgery and underwent at least 2 cycles of LR-RIT (range 2–7) with 2 months interval. Thirty-five out of 73 pts were also treated with oral chemotherapy TMZ. Two cycles of TMZ (200 mg/m^2/day, for 5/28 days) were administered in between each course of LR-RIT. Radiological objective response occurred in nine patients (3 PR, 6 MR). In a large number of patients (63%) a stabilization of disease was obtained. In the 38 pts treated with LR-RIT alone, median overall survival and progression-free survival were respectively 17.5 and 5 months, while in the 35 treated with the combined treatment (LR-RIT + TMZ) respective values were 25 months and 10 ($p < 0.01$). The addition of TMZ to LR-RIT did not increase neurological toxicity, and no major hematological toxicity was observed.

This study confirmed the efficacy and safety of LR-RIT in recurrent GBM patients with a significant increase in survival compared to the one obtained with surgery and external radiotherapy alone. In particular, this study showed that this improvement in survival can be further increased by the multi-modal approach of combining LR-RIT with TMZ.

More recently, the same group has assessed another multi-modal therapeutic strategy in co-operation with the Neuro-Oncology Department of the National Neurological Institute "C.Besta" in Milano [66]. Twenty-six recurrent GBM patients sequentially treated at the "C.Besta" Institute were enrolled for a second surgery in order to remove recurrent tumor and to place the indwelling catheter into SCRC in order to allow local delivery of chemotherapy and local pre-targeted RIT. All patients had partial tumor resection and 75% of them had a residual tumor mass after excision larger than 2 cm. After surgery all patients were treated with a second line systemic chemotherapy (PCV). Moreover, the protocol scheduled 2 cycles of loco-regional RIT, according to the "3-step" method, with an activity ranging from 0.2 to 1.0 GBq (depending on the cavity volume), with a 10-week interval. Moreover, Mitoxantrone-based chemotherapy was locally delivered as a single dose of 4 mg every 20 days. Responses to treatment were assessed by monthly neurological examination and by MRI or contrast-enhanced CT scan performed every 2 months. For the whole group of patients the progression-free survival after second surgery, at 6 and 12 months was 61 and 22% respectively and survival after recurrence at 6, 12, and 18 months was 80%, 53%, and 42%, respectively. Neither major side effects occurred systemically nor related on the site of local injections. The percentage of long-tem survivors was very high, being 42% of patients still alive at 18 month.

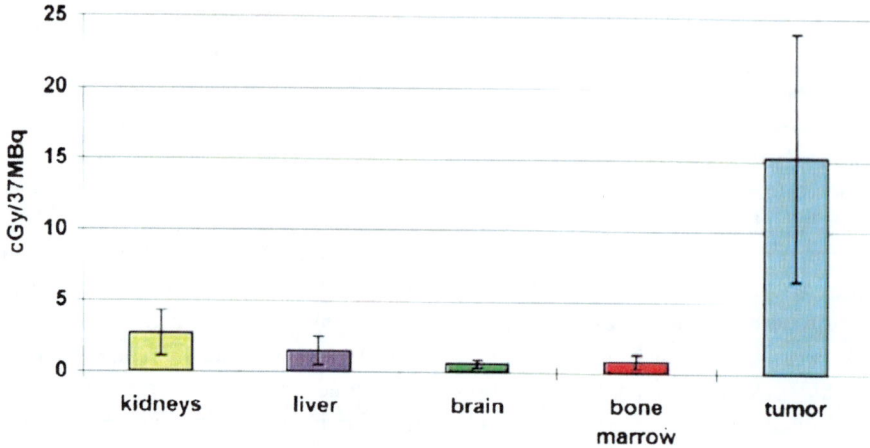

Fig. 7.5 Absorbed doses (cGy/37MBq) in critical organs and in tumor. Mean values are calculated in 12 patients. Note higher uptake in tumor, compared with non-target organs. Reproduced from Paganelli et al. [49]

Radiation Dosimetry

The challenge for internal therapy is to deliver the highest possible dose to the tumor while sparing normal organs from damage. Response and toxicity prediction is essential to rational implementation of cancer therapy.

The appropriate term for the quantity of interest in dosimetry, however, is absorbed dose (D), expressed in units of Gray. This is defined as the energy (E) absorbed in a particular mass of tissue, divided by the tissue mass (M): $D = E / M$

In particular, in radionuclide therapy: E is the number of radionuclide disintegrations in a particular volume × energy emitted per disintegration of the radionuclide × fraction of emitted energy that is absorbed by a particular (target) mass.

The biologic effects of radionuclide therapy are mediated via the absorbed dose.

Thus, accurate dosimetry method that would provide reliable dose estimates to critical organs and to tumors before therapy would allow the clinician to plan a specific therapeutic regimen and also select those patients who would benefit the most from treatment.

In radionuclide treatment, differently from external beam radiotherapy, dosimetry is strongly time and space dependent: radiopharmaceuticals may in fact show different distribution patterns.

The normal brain is the critical organ for external beam radiotherapy, as it is inevitably included in the field of treatment. On the contrary, during RIT, the normal brain received negligible doses. The mean absorbed dose in normal brain resulted 0.16 ± 0.08 and 0.015 ± 0.005 mGy/MBq in the systemic and in the loco-regional treatments, respectively.

Compared to systemic treatment [67], local administration has been demonstrated to be advantageous in the minimization of systemic toxicity. The adsorbed dose to red marrow resulted to be 0.22 mGy/MBq in the systemic treatment compared to 0.03 mGy/MBq in the loco-regional treatment.

In the systemic treatment the biodistribution images showed a rapid clearance of the radio-compound. The normal organs mainly involved in the biodistribution of the ^{90}Y-biotin were liver (1.5 ± 1.0 cGy/37 MBq) and kidneys (2.7 ± 1.6 cGy/37 MBq); $65 \pm 28\%$ of the injected activity was eliminated via the kidneys in the first 24 h after the treatment (Fig. 7.5).

As ^{90}Y is a pure beta-emitter it is difficult to evaluate the exact biodistribution of the radiopharmaceutical by Bremsstrahlung imaging. Therefore, the activity in the SCRC at any time can be assumed equal to the total injected activity minus the activity in the blood at that time and minus the cumulative activity excreted in the urine by that time. Blood samples and urine collection must be taken at regular intervals. The urinary tract can be assumed to be the only elimination route, as is the case when ^{90}Y-DOTA-biotin is administered systemically. In our evaluation [67] the absorbed doses (D) to the tumor and normal organs were evaluated using the MIRD formalism combining the residence time (τ) obtained from the experimental data, and the constant S obtained from Monte Carlo simulations (FLUKA code). As it was not possible to exactly determine the distribution of radioconjugate and the percentage of injected activity in the tumor, without invasive procedures, penetration of activity in adjacent brain tissue was not considered. Tumor dosimetry was obtained considering the SCR radius as the varying parameter and defining the target tissue as a rim of tissue 6 mm thick around the SCRC, which is the distance through which the ^{90}Y particles transfer 95% of their energy in tissue.

Scintigraphic images acquired up to 48 h after RIT showed that the radiolabeled compound remained well localized at the injection site and that the activity in the remainder of the body was minimal. The blood activity curve increased progressively up to 5–6 h to reach a maximum of 4% of the injected activity, after which blood activity decreased slowly. Based on the cumulative activity recovered from urine from 0 to 48 h, approximately 70% of the injected activity was retained in the SRC. The residence time of 90Y within the cavity was 47 h (range: 41–58 h).

For a cavity of radius 1.0 cm (volume, 4 cm^3), the mean absorbed dose to the target tissue (rim of 6 mm) was 230 Gy/GBq, reducing to 15 Gy/GBq for a cavity of radius of 2.5 cm (volume 65 cm^3).

The mean absorbed dose to normal brain tissue was 15 mGy/GBq and the average absorbed dose to the total body was 3 mGy/GBq.

The LR approach, whenever feasible, guarantees a higher irradiation of the tumor resected cavity, while sparing normal brain.

Peptide Receptor Radionuclide Therapy in Menigiomas

Among brain tumors, meningiomas have a relatively favorable course. After traditional treatment consisting of surgery and radiotherapy, most patients remain disease-free for long periods or indefinitely. However, about 10–15% of meningiomas recur. Tumor size, shape and location, as well as infiltrating or multifocal presentation, can render complete surgical eradication impossible, so it is important to have effective systemic treatments. However, no chemotherapy protocols have proven effective, so investigators have focused on defining the molecular profiles of meningioma cells in order to develop targeted therapies that may improve outcomes and spare the patient the morbidity arising from repeated surgery. Most meningiomas express multiple receptors, and various receptor-mediated therapies have been investigated. Close to 100% of meningiomas express somatostatin receptors, especially subtype 2 (SST2) and usually do so at high density. As a result, the approach of specifically targeting receptors on meningioma cells by radiolabeled somatostatin analogues has been developed over the past two decades. Tracer doses of somatostatin analogues, radiolabeled with ^{111}In or ^{68}Ga via linking moieties, have been administered for diagnostic imaging, post-surgical follow up, and differential diagnosis against neurofibromas and neurinomas. Moreover, radiodetection of somatostatin receptors with a handheld gamma probe has been employed to improve the surgical radicalization of somatostatin receptor expressing meningiomas. Based on these diagnostic experiences, the further obvious step was to employ radiolabeled somatostatin analogues for therapeutic purposes.

Investigators at the European Institute of Oncology [68] assessed peptide receptor radionuclide therapy (PRRT) using ^{90}Y-DOTATOC in a group of patients with meningioma recurring after standard treatments in all of whom somatostatin receptors were strongly expressed on cell surfaces. In particular, 29 patients with scintigraphically proven somatostatin subtype 2 receptor-positive meningiomas were enrolled: 14 had benign (grade I), 9 had atypical (grade II), and 6 had malignant (grade III) disease. Patients received intravenous injections of ^{90}Y-DOTATOC, for 2–6 cycles, for a cumulative dose in the range of 5–15 GBq. The treatment was well tolerated in all patients and magnetic resonance controls, performed 3 months after treatment completion, showed disease stabilization in 66% of cases.

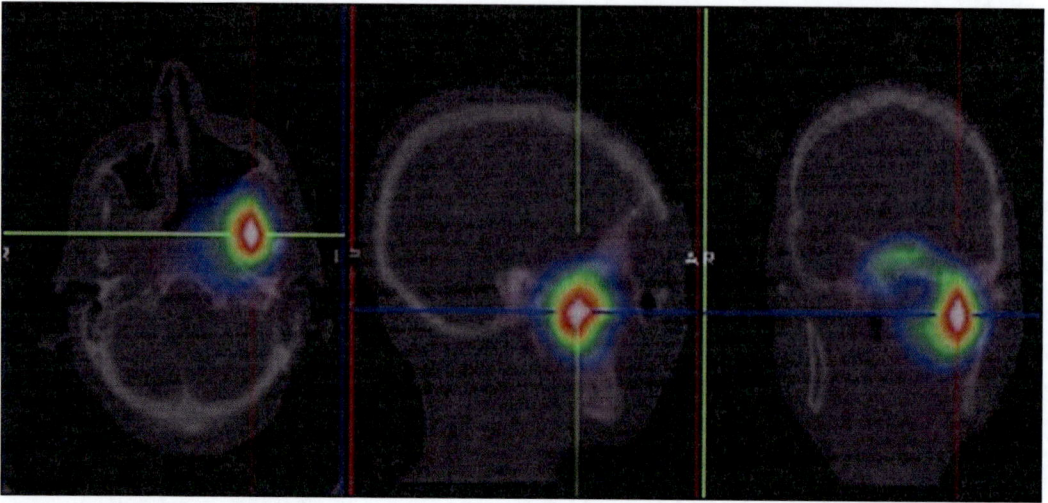

Fig. 7.6 Bremsstrahlung brain SPECT-CT confirms a high tumor uptake of ^{90}Y-DOTATOC intravenously administered in a patient with recurrent meningioma

Despite high tumor uptake of ^{90}Y-DOTATOC (Fig. 7.6) in all cases, no significant reduction in lesion size occurred. Outcomes were better in patients with benign meningiomas, where time to progression was significantly longer than in the group with grade II/III disease, suggesting that the efficacy of PRRT with ^{90}Y-DOTATOC in meningiomas depends more on tumor type than extent of radiopharmaceutical uptake, which did not differ between the two groups. Large tumor size is known to limit the efficacy of radionuclide treatment. In this series, regardless of tumor size a fixed activity per cycle to all patients was administered in order to avoid possible renal toxicity, and this resulted in undertreatment in some cases. For example, dosimetry in one of the patients who received ^{111}In-DOTATOC showed that the absorbed dose to the tumor was approximately 10 Gy, which is well below the therapeutic dose. Despite high uptake (0.6% at 1 h, 0.4% at 24 h, 0.3% at 48 h), the tumor was large (6 cm, 120 g) and intra-tumor activity was correspondingly low, probably representing the main factor limiting efficacy. Intrinsic radioresistance may also have limited efficacy. High-grade meningiomas in particular have large areas of poorly vascularized and hence hypoxic tissue, so radiation-induced oxygen radical formation is reduced. Although no significant reduction of lesions were

obtained after PRRT, the authors conclude that disease stabilization obtained in 66% of patients might be considered as a positive result, particularly in view of the unfavorable prognostic factors affecting the group: high prevalence of atypical and malignant lesions, high recurrence rate (26/29 patients) after surgery and radiotherapy; and high proportion of large size tumors (about 60% with tumors 5–10 cm).

The authors conclude that PRRT with ^{90}Y-DOTATOC can slow meningioma growth, even though the dose to the tumor was well below the therapeutic dose in many patients. Nonetheless, the outcomes of this study are sufficiently encouraging to justify a prospective study in which the activity administered and the timing of cycles is determined in relation to lesion size, lesion uptake, and tumor-kidney dose balance.

Conclusive Considerations and Future Directions

Reported results provide evidence of the efficacy and safety of the radionuclide-based targeted therapies in HGG patients, with a significant increase in survival compared to those series who obtained surgery and external radiotherapy alone. These data represent a basis for further prospective trials to assess timing and schedule of radiopharmaceuticals in the therapeutic algorithm of glioma, and glioblastoma in particular. Probably the best results will be obtained when loco-regional radioisotopes treatments are applied as an adjunct to initial surgery. Moreover, as patients tolerate the catheter very well, it could be inserted already during the first surgical intervention. The 2–4 week gap between surgical intervention and external radiotherapy, should be a very convenient period to start isotope treatments, in order to exploit the greater permeability of the blood–brain barrier at that time. This would be expected to expose more malignant cells to the radionuclide and hence limit the local spread of the cancer.

The multi-modality approach for treating brain tumors was introduced about 30 years ago and remains the most effective approach we have so far: the association of surgery, radiotherapy, chemotherapy, and radioisotope-based techniques may provide, at least, a way of increasing life expectancy and improving quality of life of patients with HGGs.

Concerning meningiomas, PRRT might be applied to patients with smaller lesions, or in an adjuvant setting, particularly as part of a multimodal approach with surgery and radiotherapy, outcomes would be expected to improve, provided kidney toxicity could be avoided. In the event of subtotal resection, with preservation of vascular and neurological integrity (a strategy increasingly favored by neurosurgeons), PRRT could be administered directly after surgery, as a preliminary radiation therapy boost, with a view to conserving quality of life. The utility of a combination of radiopeptides and anti-angiogenic agents in high-grade radioresistant meningiomas should also be investigated.

Acknowledgments We thank Mrs. Deborah Console for editing the manuscript.

References

1. Davis FG, Preston-Martin S. Epidemiology, incidence and survival in central nervous system neoplasia. In: Bigner DD, McLendon RE, Bruner JM, editors. Russell and Rubinstein's pathology of tumors of the nervous system. 6th ed. London: Arnold; 1998. p. 5–145.

2. Stewart LA. Chemotherapy in adult high-grade glioma: a systematic review and meta-analysis of individual patient data from 12 randomised trials. Lancet. 2002;359(9311):1011–8.

3. Wong ET, Hess KR, Gleason MJ, et al. Outcomes and prognostic factors in recurrent glioma patients enrolled onto phase II clinical trials. J Clin Oncol. 1999;17(8):2572–8.

4. Louis DN, Ohgaki H, Wiestler OD, Cavenee WK, Burger PC, Jouvet A, Scheithauer BW, Kleihues P. The 2007 WHO classification of tumours of the central nervous system. Acta Neuropathol. 2007;114(2):97–109.

5. Maher EA, Furnari FB, Bachoo RM, et al. Malignant glioma: genetics and biology of a grave matter. Genes Dev. 2001;15(11):1311–33.

6. Kleihues P, Burger PC, Scheithauer BW. The new WHO classification of brain tumours. Brain Pathol. 1993;3(3):255–68.

7. Zülch KJ, editor. Histological typing of tumours of the central nervous system. Geneva: World Health Organization; 1979.

8. Jackson RJ, Fuller GN, Abi-Said D, et al. Limitations of stereotactic biopsy in the initial management of gliomas. Neuro Oncol. 2001;3(3):193–200.

9. Perry A, Jenkins RB, O'Fallon JR, et al. Clinicopathologic study of 85 similarly treated patients with anaplastic astrocytic tumors. An analysis of DNA content (ploidy), cellular proliferation, and p53 expression. Cancer. 1999;86(4):672–83.

10. Barker 2nd FG, Chang SM, Larson DA, et al. Age and radiation response in glioblastoma multiforme. Neurosurgery. 2001;49(6):1288–98.

11. Vuorinen V, Hinkka S, Färkkilä M, Jääskeläinen J. Debulking or biopsy of malignant glioma in elderly people—a randomised study. Acta Neurochir (Wien). 2003;145(1):5–10.

12. Keles GE, Lamborn KR, Berger MS. Low-grade hemispheric gliomas in adults: a critical review of extent of resection as a factor influencing outcome. J Neurosurg. 2001;95(5):735–45.

13. Hess KR. Extent of resection as a prognostic variable in the treatment of gliomas. J Neurooncol. 1999;42(3):227–31.

14. Stupp R, Dietrich P-Y, Ostermann Kraljevic S, et al. Promising survival for patients with newly diagnosed glioblastoma multiforme treated with concomitant radiation plus temozolomide followed by adjuvant temozolomide. J Clin Oncol. 2002;20(5):1375–82.

15. Stupp R, Hegi ME, Mason WP, et al.; European Organisation for Research and Treatment of Cancer Brain Tumour and Radiation Oncology Groups; National Cancer Institute of Canada Clinical Trials Group. Effects of radiotherapy with concomitant and adjuvant temozolomide versus radiotherapy alone on survival in glioblastoma in a randomised phase III study: 5-year analysis of the EORTC-NCIC trial. Lancet Oncol. 2009;10(5):459–66.

16. Leibel SA, Gutin PH, Wara WM, et al. Survival and quality of life after interstitial implantation of removable high-activity iodine-125 sources for the treatment of patients with recurrent malignant gliomas. Int J Radiat Oncol Biol Phys. 1989;17(6):1129–39.
17. Shrieve DC, Alexander E, Wen PY, et al. Comparison of stereotactic radiosurgery and brachytherapy in the treatment of recurrent glioblastoma multiforme. Neurosurgery. 1995;36(2):275–84.
18. Greig NH, Yu QS, Utsuki T, et al. Optimizing drugs for brain action. In: Koliber D, Lustig S, Shapira S, editors. Blood–brain barrier drug delivery and brain pathology. New York: Kluwer Academic/Plenum; 2001.
19. Brem H, Mahaley Jr MS, Vick NA, Black KL, Schold Jr SC, Burger PC, Friedman AH, Ciric IS, Eller TW, Cozzens JW, et al. Interstitial chemotherapy with drug polymer implants for the treatment of recurrent gliomas. J Neurosurg. 1991;74(3):441–6.
20. Strasser JF, Fung LK, Eller S, Grossman SA, Saltzman WM. Distribution of 1,3-bis(2-chloroethyl)-1-nitrosourea and tracers in the rabbit brain after interstitial delivery by biodegradable polymer implants. J Pharmacol Exp Ther. 1995;275(3):1647–55.
21. Clark AS, Deans B, Stevens MF, et al. Antitumor imidazotetrazines: 32. Synthesis of novel imidazotetrazinones and related dicyclic heterocycles to probe the mode of action on the antitumor drug temozolomide. J Med Chem. 1995;38(9):1493–504.
22. Esteller M, Gargia-Foncillas J, Andion E, et al. Inactivation of the DNA-repair gene MGMT and the clinical response of gliomas to alkylating agents. N Engl J Med. 2000;343(19):1350–4.
23. Brem S, Cotran R, Folkman J. Tumor angiogenesis: a quantitative method for histologic grading. J Natl Cancer Inst. 1972;48(2):347–56.
24. Salmaggi A, Eoli M, Frigerio S, et al. Intracavitary VEGF, bFGF, IL-8, IL-12 levels in primary and recurrent malignant glioma. J Neurooncol. 2003;62(3):297–303.
25. Leon SP, Folkerth RD, Black PM. Microvessel density is a prognostic indicator for patients with astroglial brain tumors. Cancer. 1996;77(2):362–72.
26. Zhou YH, Tan F, Hess KR, Yung WK. The expression of PAX6, PTEN, vascular endothelial growth factor, and epidermal growth factor receptor in gliomas: relationship to tumor grade and survival. Clin Cancer Res. 2003;9(9):3369–75.
27. Fine HA, Figg WD, Jaeckle K, et al. Phase II trial of the antiangiogenic agent thalidomide in patients with recurrent high-grade gliomas. J Clin Oncol. 2000;18(4):708–15.
28. Drappatz J, Wong ET, Schiff D, et al. A pilot safety study of lenalidomide and radiotherapy for patients with newly diagnosed glioblastoma multiforme. Int J Radiat Oncol Biol Phys. 2009;73(1):222–7.
29. National Comprehensive Cancer Network. NCCN practice guidelines in oncology: central nervous system cancers. v.1.2008. Fort Washington: National Comprehensive Cancer Network; 2009. Available from URL: http://www.nccn.org/professionals/physician_gls/PDF/cns.pdf. Accessed 21 May 2009.
30. Cohen M, Shen Y, Keegan P, et al. FDA approval summary: bevacizumab (Avastin) as treatment of recurrent glioblastoma multiforme. Oncologist. 2009;14(11):1131–8.
31. Van Meir EG, Hadjpanayis CG, Norden AD, Shu HK, Wen PY, Olson JJ. Exciting new advances in neuro-oncology: the avenue to a cure for a malignant glioma. CA Cancer J Clin. 2010;60(3):166–93.
32. Norden AD, Drappatz J, Wen PY. Antiangiogenic therapies for high-grade glioma. Nat Rev Neurol. 2009;5(11):610–20.
33. Prados M, Cloughesy T, Samant M, et al. Response as a predictor of survival in patients with recurrent glioblastoma treated with bevacizumab. Neurooncology. 2011;13(1):143–51.
34. Chamberlain MC. Bevacizumab for the treatment of recurrent glioblastoma. Clin Med Insights Oncol. 2011;5:117–29.
35. Epenetos AA, Munro AJ, Stewart S, et al. Antibody-guided irradiation of advanced ovarian cancer with intraperitoneally administered radiolabelled monoclonal antibodies. J Clin Oncol. 1987;5(12):1890–9.
36. Larson SM. Radiolabelled monoclonal anti-tumor antibodies in diagnosis and therapy. J Nucl Med. 1985;26(5):538–45.
37. Buraggi GL, Callegaro L, Mariani G, et al. Imaging with 131I-labeled monoclonal antibodies to a high-molecular-weight melanoma-associated antigen in patients with melanoma: efficacy of whole immunoglobulin and its F(ab')2 fragments. Cancer Res. 1985;45(7):3378–87.
38. Kim JA, Triozzi PL, Martin Jr EW. Radioimmuguided surgery for colorectal cancer. Oncology. 1993;7(2):55–64.
39. Fazio F, Paganelli G. Antibody-guided scintigraphy: targeting of the "magic bullet". Eur J Nucl Med. 1993;20(12):1138–40.
40. Hazra DK, Britton KE, Lahiri VL, Gupta AK, Khanna P, Saran S. Immunotechnological trends in radioimmunotargeting: from 'magic bullet' to 'smart bomb'. Nucl Med Commun. 1995;16(2):66–75.
41. Wessels BW, Rogus RD. Radionuclide selection and model absorbed dose calculations for radiolabeled tumor associated antibodies. Med Phys. 1984;11(5):638–45.
42. Chinol M, Hnatowich DJ. Generator-produced yttrium-90 for radioimmunotherapy. J Nucl Med. 1987;28(9):1465–70.
43. Goldenberg DM, Griffiths GL. Radioimmunotherapy of cancer: arming the missiles. J Nucl Med. 1992;33(6):1110–2.
44. Chetanneau A, Barbet J, Peltier P, et al. Pretargetted imaging of colorectal cancer recurrences using an In-111-labelled bivalent hapten and a biospecific antibody conjugate. Nucl Med Commun. 1994;15(12):972–80.
45. Magnani P, Paganelli G, Modorati G, et al. Quantitative comparison of direct antibody labeling and tumor

pretargeting in uveal melanoma. J Nucl Med. 1996; 37(6): 967–71.

46. Wilchek M, Bayer EA. The avidin biotin complex in bioanalytical applications. Anal Biochem. 1988; 171(1):1–32.

47. Paganelli G, Magnani P, Zito F, et al. Three-step monoclonal antibody tumor targeting in carcinoembryonic antigen-positive patients. Cancer Res. 1991;51(21):5960–6.

48. Paganelli G, Chinol M, Grana C, et al. Optimization of the three-step pretargeting approach for diagnosis and therapy in cancer patients. J Nucl Med. 1995; 36(abs):225P.

49. Paganelli G, Grana C, Chinol M, et al. Antibody-guided three-step therapy for high grade glioma with yttrium-90 biotin. Eur J Nucl Med. 1999;26(4): 348–57.

50. Zagzag D, Friedlander DR, Dosik J, et al. Tenascin-C expression by angiogenic vessels in human astrocytomas and by human brain endothelial cells in vitro. Cancer Res. 1996;56(1):182–9.

51. Leins A, Riva P, Lindstedt R, Davidoff MS, Mehraein P, Weis S. Expression of tenascin-C in various human brain tumors and its relevance for survival in patients with astrocytoma. Cancer. 2003;98(11):2430–9.

52. Wilkstrand CJ, Zalutsky MR, Bigner DD. Therapy of brain tumors with radiolabeled antibodies. In: Liau LM, Becker DP, Cloughsey TF, Bigner DD, editors. Brain tumor immunotherapy. Totwa: Humana Press; 2001. p. 205–29.

53. Herold-Mende C, Mueller MM, Bonsanto MM, Schmitt HP, Kunze S, Steiner HH. Clinical impact and functional aspects of tenascina-C expression during glioma progression. Int J Cancer. 2002;98(3): 362–9.

54. Grana C, Chinol M, Robertson C, et al. Pretargeted adjuvant radioimmunotherapy with yttrium-90-biotin in malignant glioma patients: a pilot study. Br J Cancer. 2002;86(2):207–12.

55. Grana CM, Chinol M, De Cicco C, et al. Eleven-year experience with the Avidin-Biotin pretargeting system in glioblastoma: toxicity, efficacy and survival. The Open Nuclear Medicine Journal. 2012;4:14–20.

56. Liu BL, Cheng JX, Zhang X, Zhang W. Controversies concerning the application of brachitherapy in central nervous system tumours. J Cancer Res Clin Oncol. 2010;136(2):173–85.

57. Riva P, Franceschi G, Frattarelli M, et al. Loco-regional radioimmunotherapy of high-grade malignant gliomas using specific monoclonal antibodies labeled with 90Y: a phase I study. Clin Cancer Res. 1999;5 Suppl 10:3275s–80.

58. Cokgor I, Akabani G, Kuan CT, et al. Phase I trial results of iodine-131–labeled antitenascin monoclonal antibody 81C6 treatment of patients with newly diagnosed malignant gliomas. J Clin Oncol. 2000; 18(22):3862–72.

59. Riva P, Franceschi G, Riva N, Casi M, Santimaria M, Adamo M. Role of nuclear medicine in the treatment of malignant gliomas: the locoregional radioimmunotherapy approach. Eur J Nucl Med. 2000;27(5):601–9.

60. Goetz C, Riva P, Poepperl G, et al. Locoregional radioimmunotherapy in selected patients with malignant gliomas: experiences, side effects and survival times. J Neurooncol. 2003;62(3):321–8.

61. Reardon DA, Rich JN, Friedman HS, Bigner DD. Recent advances in the treatment of malignant astrocytoma. J Clin Oncol. 2006;24(8):1253–65 (review).

62. Zalutsky MR. Current status of therapy of solid tumors: brain tumour therapy. J Nucl Med. 2005; 46(Suppl 1):151S–6S (review).

63. Zalutsky MR, Reardon DA, Akabani G, et al. Clinical experience with alpha-particle emitting 211At: treatment of recurrent brain tumor patients with 211At-labeled chimeric antitenascin monoclonal antibody 81C6. J Nucl Med. 2008;49(1):30–8.

64. Paganelli G, Bartolomei M, Ferrari M, et al. Pre-targeted locoregional radioimmunotherapy with 90Y-biotin in glioma patients: phase I study and preliminary therapeutic results. Cancer Biother Radiopharm. 2001;16(3): 227–35.

65. Bartolomei M, Mazzetta C, Handkiewicz-Junak D, et al. Combined treatment of glioblastoma patients with locoregional pre-targeted 90Y-biotin radioimmunotherapy and temozolomide. Q J Nucl Med Mol Imaging. 2004;48(3):220–8.

66. Boiardi A, Bartolomei M, Silvani A, et al. Intratumoral delivery of mitoxantrone in association with 90-Y radioimmunotherapy (RIT) in recurrent glioblastoma. J Neurooncol. 2005;72(2):125–31.

67. Cremonesi M, Ferrari M, Chinol M, et al. Three-step radioimmunotherapy with yttrium-90 biotin: dosimetry and pharmacokinetics in cancer patients. Eur J Nucl Med. 1999;26(2):110–20.

68. Bartolomei M, Bodei L, De Cicco C, et al. Peptide receptor radionuclide therapy with (90)Y-DOTATOC in recurrent meningioma. Eur J Nucl Med Mol Imaging. 2009;36(9):1407–16.

Radioiodine Therapy of Differentiated Thyroid Cancer

8

Ettore Seregni, Andrew Mallia, Carlo Chiesa,
Gabriele Scaramellini, Maura Massimino,
and Emilio Bombardieri

Introduction

The incidence of thyroid carcinomas is steadily increasing. Primary tumors of the thyroid gland include carcinomas that originate from epithelial cells (carcinomas of thyrocytes and C-cells), and from non-epithelial cells (lymphomas and sarcomas). Thyrocytes are the main functional cells that produce thyroid hormones (T3 and T4), which are vital for human metabolism. The epithelial tumors can be divided into the well-differentiated (papillary and follicular carcinomas), poorly-differentiated, undifferentiated (anaplastic carcinomas) carcinomas, and tumor of the parafollicular or C-cells (medullary carcinoma). Three common histopathological diagnosis of papillary thyroid carcinomas (PTC) include classical PTC, follicular variant PTC and mixed PTC, and follicular thyroid carcinomas (FTC). Mixed medullary and follicular carcinomas are rare neoplasms which show morphologic features of both follicular and C-cell differentiation. These neoplasms must be distinguished from the follicular variant of medullary carcinoma and from medullary carcinoma with entrapped normal follicles. Table 8.1 summarizes the WHO classification of thyroid tumors published in 2004 [1]. According to the American Cancer Society there are 37,000 new cases of thyroid cancer annually in the United States, with approximately 75% occurring in women [2].

The main risk factors for thyroid carcinoma include: age, sex (female > male), radiation exposure, family history, dietary factors, and inherited medical conditions such as Gardner's syndrome, Cowden's disease, and multiple endocrine neoplasia type 2 (MEN2) [3]. Although chronic inflammation, leading to neoplastic transformation, is a well-established clinical phenomenon, the link between Hashimoto's thyroiditis and thyroid cancer remains controversial.

Most cases of differentiated thyroid cancer are sporadic: rearranged forms of the RET proto-oncogene have been identified as the susceptibility genes for the development of sporadic forms of papillary thyroid cancer. The RET proto-oncogene is located on chromosome 10q11.2 and encodes a transmembrane receptor of the tyrosine

E. Seregni • C. Chiesa • E. Bombardieri (✉)
Department of Nuclear Medicine, Fondazione IRCCS
Istituto Nazionale Tumori, Milan, Italy
e-mail: bombardieri@istitutotumori.mi.it

A. Mallia
School of Specialization in Nuclear Medicine,
University of Milano, Milan, Italy

G. Scaramellini
Division of ORL Surgery, Fondazione IRCCS
Istituto Nazionale Tumori, Milan, Italy

M. Massimino
Division of Pediatric Oncology, Fondazione IRCCS
Istituto Nazionale Tumori, Milan, Italy

C. Aktolun and S.J. Goldsmith (eds.), *Nuclear Medicine Therapy: Principles and Clinical Applications*, 133
DOI 10.1007/978-1-4614-4021-5_8, © Springer Science+Business Media New York 2013

Table 8.1 Simplified WHO classification of thyroid tumors [1]

Thyroid carcinomas	Other thyroid tumors	Thyroid adenomas
Papillary	Primary lymphoma	Follicular adenoma
Follicular	Angiosarcoma	Hyalinizing trabecular tumor
Poorly-differentiated	Teratoma	
Undifferentiated (anaplastic)	Ectopic thymoma	
Medullary	Secondary tumors	
Mixed medullary and follicular		

kinase family. Loss of heterozygosity on chromosomes 10q, 3p, and 17p appears to be more common in follicular thyroid cancer.

Familial thyroid cancer which tends to be more often multi-focal, advanced, and aggressive occurs mainly in younger patients: however specific genes responsible for familial thyroid cancer without an associated co-morbidity have not been identified. With increasing acceptance that there are familial cases a careful family history and screening should be taken if two family members are identified with thyroid cancer [3].

Well differentiated thyroid cancer (WDTC) account for approximately 90% of all thyroid cancers [4]. The content of this chapter is limited to the radionuclide therapy of WDTC, and medullary carcinoma of thyroid is addressed in another chapter. Treatment of anaplastic carcinomas is beyond the scope of this book.

WDTC is derived from the follicular epithelium and retains the basic biologic characteristics of healthy thyroid tissue. Its behavior may range from an indolent, clinically insignificant disease found incidentally to an aggressive pattern of locally invasive disease or distant metastases. WDTC is known to have a good long-term prognosis and cure rate, however recurrence is not uncommon, usually affecting 10–30% of patients with the disease [5].

Papillary thyroid cancer (PTC) accounts for 90% of DTC [6]. They are often multi-focal, bilateral, and slow-growing but frequently metastasizes to loco-regional lymph nodes, cervical lymph nodes being the most common site of metastases, followed by the lung [7, 8]. Metastasis to more distant lymph nodes including axillary lymph nodes can also be seen. Several variants of

PTC exist. These range from the most common variants called the follicular variants to the more aggressive rarer poorly-differentiated types known as tall-cell, columnar cell, insular, and diffuse sclerosing variants. Hürthle cell (oncocytic) tumor is a variant of WDTC. There is recently increasing interest in the relation between the prognosis, response to therapy, iodine avidity, and variants of PTC.

FTC are usually unifocal, locally invasive, and tend to metastasize to distant organs including the lung, bones, and brain [7]. It is not uncommon for patients with FTC to present itself with distant metastasis (e.g., a pathologic fracture) as the first and only clinical finding. Although not as frequent as FTCs, follicular variant PTCs can also spread to distant organs and tissues.

The poorly-differentiated forms of both papillary and follicular thyroid cancer cause diagnostic and therapeutic difficulties as they tend to have a low or lack of avidity for radioiodine. Tumors that do not concentrate radioiodine may require chemotherapy, but the results of this are poor and associated with toxicity as discussed below [9].

Thyroid Nodules

Thyroid nodules represent the most common presentation of thyroid cancer. Although the higher risk of scintigraphically hypoactive nodules are well known, normoactive and hyperactive nodules also have the risk of malignancy. They are described as discrete lesions which are radiologically distinct from the surrounding thyroid parenchyma and may be palpable or non-palpable [10].

It is worth to note that either scintigraphic or ultrasonographic findings are not reliable indicators for malignancy, but they provide useful information, which is essential for the management of thyroid nodules.

Thyroid cancer occurs in 5–15% of nodules, scintigraphically hypoactive (cold) nodules have the highest risk [11]. Non-palpable nodules have the same risk of malignancy as palpable nodules of the same size [12]. Generally only nodules >1 cm in size should be evaluated. Suspicious ultrasonographic findings and/or presence of associated risk factors mean that nodules <1 cm warrant further evaluation [13]. This includes fine-needle aspiration (FNA) biopsy under ultrasonographic guidance. FNA has been shown to be the most cost-effective and accurate method for evaluating thyroid nodules even though problems of inadequate sample collection and indeterminate cytology may occur [14]. With the increasing use of ^{18}F-FDG-PET for oncological imaging, FDG positive incidental nodules (incidentalomas) are being discovered. These nodules particularly require further investigations since the risk of malignancy in FDG positive nodules is about 33% [15]. Although a significant portion of patients are asymptomatic and most of the patients present with incidentally detected nodules, the signs and symptoms of thyroid cancer include a lump in the thyroid region, cervical lymphadenopathy, dysphagia, pathologic fracture, hoarseness (due to vocal cord paralysis), neck pain, coughing, and symptoms of hyperthyroidism.

Once a diagnosis of thyroid cancer has been made, most experts now advocate for a total/near-total thyroidectomy as the treatment of choice (with the exception of micro-carcinoma), including cervical lymph node dissection when lymph node disease is suspected or evident, followed by post-operative radioiodine remnant ablation (RRA) and thyroid hormone suppressive therapy [13, 16]. Since 20–50% of patients with PTC have central lymph node involvement at time of initial diagnosis, current evidence suggests that prophylactic central lymph node dissection may decrease recurrence rates and mortality [17]. Care must be taken since some reports have implicated central node dissection as the cause of increased morbidity such as transient hypoparathyroidism and recurrent laryngeal nerve injury.

Radioiodine Therapy

Currently, thyroidectomy followed by radioiodine therapy (RAIT) is the most widely accepted therapeutic methodology in WDTC with size-dependent exception. RAIT was introduced for the treatment of thyroid disease since its first use in 1946 by Siedlin et al. [18]. The radionuclide used for therapy is iodine-131 (^{131}I), a gamma and beta emitter with a physical half-life of 8.02 days. Most of its radiation is delivered by beta particles with a maximum energy of 0.61 MeV and a medium path length in tissue of about 0.4 mm. ^{131}I gamma ray emission, with an energy of 364 KeV, enables post-therapy imaging and plays an important role from a diagnostic point of view and in terms of dosimetric calculations. The disadvantages of gamma radiation include additional unwanted radiation for the patient himself as well as to the medical staff, patient's family, and the public causing a radiation protection challenge.

The mode of uptake and retention of ^{131}I by thyrocytes is similar to that of nutritional iodine. It involves the sodium/iodine symporter (NIS) and is promoted by thyroid peroxidase, under the influence of thyroid stimulation hormone (TSH), before being organified and stored in the colloid of the thyroid follicles. Thyroid cancer cells may differ in two ways: reduced expression of NIS resulting in a decreased uptake of ^{131}I and defects in organification leading to a shortening in the biological half-life and a defect in hormone synthesis [19].

The aim of RAIT includes radioiodine ablation and treatment of loco-regional or metastatic disease. The term "ablation" is used when radioactive iodine is administered to destroy or ablate residual healthy thyroid tissue remaining (remnant) after thyroidectomy. The term "treatment" however refers generally to the administration of radioactive iodine to destroy or ablate the metastatic disease.

Radioiodine Ablation

RRA is a selective irradiation of thyroid remnants (including microscopic foci) and of incompletely resectable WDTCs in order to:

1. To destroy microscopic foci of thyrocytes and thus decrease the long-term risk of recurrent disease.
2. To destroy any remaining normal thyroid tissue and therefore increase the specificity of detectable serum thyroglobulin for follow-up purposes.
3. To allow post-ablative scanning and thus help detect persistent or metastatic carcinoma [7] (Fig. 8.1).

There are still discussions on the role of RAIT based on the lack of prospective controlled randomized trials and due to the use of different "staging" systems in various studies. The main points of discussion involve the use of ^{131}I therapy for cancers smaller than 10 mm and those between 10 and 20 mm. Keeping this in mind, there have been many studies over the years, which showed the advantages of RAIT. It is now recommended as part of the standard protocol for the treatment of WDTC after total thyroidectomy.

In 1994, Mazzaferri and Jhiang showed the beneficial effects of RAIT in all patients except those with Stage 1 disease (defined as unifocal non-metastasized carcinomas <1.5 cm) [20]. In 2000, Mazzaferri also demonstrated that the recurrence rate was significantly lower after RAIT, 38% vs. 16% [21]. According to data from the Ohio State University published in 2001, remnant ablation with ^{131}I is an independent variable that significantly reduces cancer recurrence, distant metastases, and cancer death [22]. Another study by the National Cooperative Thyroid Cancer Treatment Study Group (2006) demonstrated the beneficial effect of RAIT in all patients except those with Stage 1 disease [23]. In 2008, a meta-analysis performed by Sawka et al. [24] resulted in two important conclusions: the first being that RAIT may be effective with regard to tumor-specific survival in low-risk patients but a definite verification could not be given on the basis of the present literature, and secondly

that following RAIT therapy, patients had a significantly reduced number of new distant metastases.

Recently, Shattuk et al. [25] showed that in at least 50% of patients with multifocal disease, the different foci were of independent clonal origin thus suggesting that RAIT treatment would prevent the development of second primaries in any remaining thyroid tissue.

The American Thyroid Association (ATA) Guidelines for Patients with Thyroid Nodules and WDTC (2009) recommend the routine ^{131}I ablation for all patients with T3-T4 or M1 stage diseases. RAIT is recommended for selected patients with T1-T2 disease stage confined to the thyroid with documented lymph node metastases, or higher risk features (age, tumor size, lymph node status, tumor histology). ATA does not recommend ablation for patients with unifocal cancer <1 cm and those with multifocal cancer when all foci are <1 cm, when no other high risk features are present [13].

The European Thyroid Association (ETA) consensus report and guidelines advise RRA ablation for T3-T4, N1, or M1 stages of the disease giving only a relative indication for RRA ablation therapy in young patients (<18 years) and in those with primary tumors between 1 and 2 cm without lymph node or distant metastases. RRA ablation therapy is not indicated in patients with DTCs which are <1 cm with no metastases [26].

The Society of Nuclear Medicine (SNM) Procedure Guideline for The Therapy of Thyroid Disease (2005) states that treatment of WDTC with radioiodine should be considered post-surgically in patients with: tumor size >1.5 cm; tumor size <1.5 cm if there is unfavorable histology; lymph node metastases; multifocal disease, which could represent intra-thyroidal metastases; lymphatic or vascular invasion, capsular invasion or penetration including peri-thyroidal soft tissue involvement; distant metastases. [27].

The Guidelines for RAIT of WDTC published by the European Association of Nuclear Medicine (EANM) in 2008 state that RAIT after total or near-total thyroidectomy is a standard procedure in patients with DTC, with the only exception

Fig. 8.1 Post-operative
successful thyroid remnant
ablation (together with
suspicious para-tracheal
lymph nodes) using 3.7 GBq
^{131}I in a patient with a
follicular variant of papillary
thyroid cancer

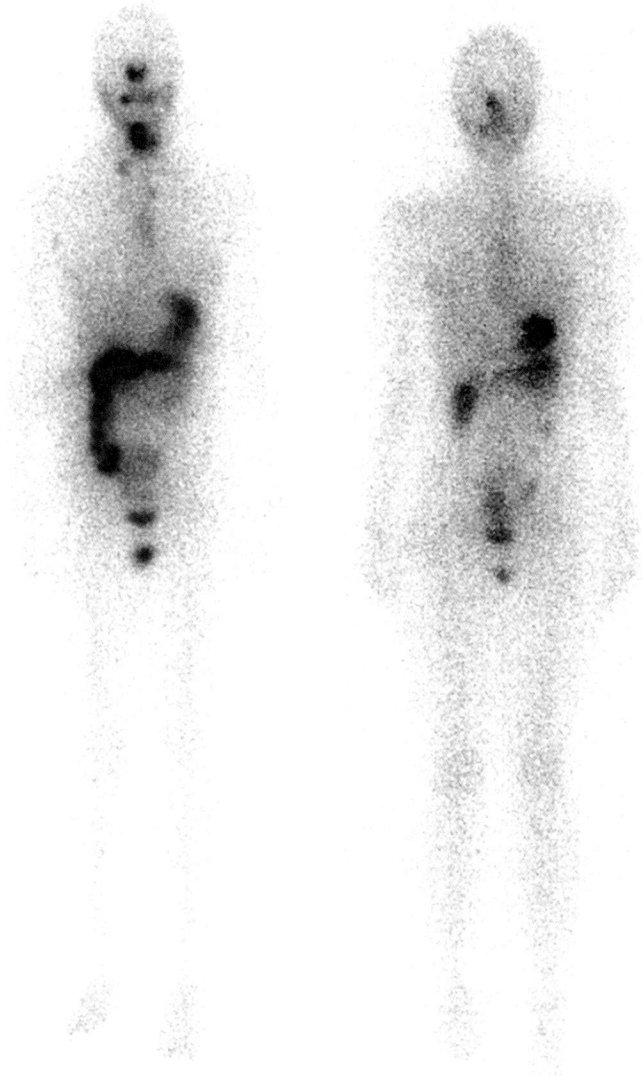

being patients with unifocal thyroid carcinoma
≤1 cm in diameter who lack:

1. Evidence of metastases.
2. Thyroid capsule invasion.
3. History of radiation exposure.
4. Unfavorable histology (tall-cell, columnar
   cell, or diffuse sclerosing subtypes).

They also conclude that radioiodine ablation
should be considered when potential risk factors
for recurrence or mortality, such family history

of WDTC, presence of vascular invasion, and
closeness of the tumor to the thyroid capsule are
present [28].

Radioiodine Treatment of Metastases

The overall 10-year survival rate of patients
with WDTC who have distant metastases is
reduced to 40%. One selected compendium of 13

studies found that among 1,231 patients, 49% of metastases were to the lung, 25% to the bone, 15% to both lung and bone, and 10% to other soft-tissues [29]. A more recent study by Durante et al. [30]. shows that the survival of patients older than 40 years with macro-nodular lung metastases or multiple bone metastases drops to 14%. Levothyroxine therapy is the most fundamental systemic therapy in such patients. RAIT remains the primary therapy for patients with iodine-avid metastatic thyroid carcinoma. Multiple retrospective studies have suggested that use of RAIT confers an overall survival benefit by eradicating cancer cells, controlling disease progression, and providing symptomatic relief [31].

Patients with pulmonary micro-metastases have the best prognosis, with high rates of complete remission with RAIT repeated at 6- to 12-month intervals (whilst the disease is responsive). On the other hand, those with pulmonary metastases which are >than 1 cm in size show prolonged survival but complete remission rates are low [32]. Osseous metastases are rarely cured with RAIT, especially when disease involvement is diffuse, but patients may benefit from symptomatic improvement, partial tumor response or disease stabilization [31]. Bernier et al. [33] showed a significant survival benefit associated with RAIT therapy in patients with osseous metastases that were further improved with higher cumulative doses. A retrospective study by Petrich et al. [34] in 2001 evaluated the therapeutic outcome, total administered activities, and side-effects in 107 patients with initial bone metastases. They concluded that initial bone metastases in selected WDTC patients up to 45 years and those with less than three bone metastases can be treated with curative intent (Figs. 8.2 and 8.3).

Overall, treatment with RAIT improves the disease specific survival rate of those with iodine avid metastases (10-year survival 30–55%) when compared to those with iodine negative metastases, which remains poor (10-year survival, 10–18%) [32].

The major problem encountered when treating patients with extra-cervical thyroid disease who may have to undergo multiple RAIT treatments is the threshold cumulative activity that can be used before stopping the treatment. This is especially true when dealing with young patients. Some authors advocate stopping fractionated ^{131}I therapy after a cumulative activity of 20 GBq because of the small risk of inducing leukemia or developing pulmonary fibrosis. Hindié et al. [35] advocate continuing fractionated RAIT treatment even after a cumulative activity of 18.5 GBq. On the other hand, other groups have reported better results following the administration of a lower cumulative amount of ^{131}I.

Indications and Contraindications of Rait

Indications

The decision to give RAIT has to be considered for each patient and should take different factors into account:

(a) Operability of the tumor
(b) Iodine avidity
(c) Location of disease
(d) Tumor characteristics
(e) Patient age and health status
(f) Potential risks
(g) Contraindications [28]

Radical surgery (total or near-total thyroidectomy), when possible, is the modality of choice that yields the highest potential to improve survival, especially in the presence of loco-regional lesions (thyroid bed or lymph nodes). Surgery is therefore always considered the first choice of treatment, and RAIT has to be adopted as an adjuvant therapy after surgery. The evaluation of the iodine avidity of cancer tissue is the basis of successful RAIT; therefore diagnostic whole-body scintigraphy should be carried out with optimal technical conditions for imaging and in the absence of iodine excess. With regards to the site of tumor deposits, considerable clinical evidence shows that lymph node, soft tissue, and lung metastases can be cured with a high rate of successes by RAIT; on the contrary; this is not observed with brain and skeletal metastases. Some histological subtypes of thyroid cancer (tall-cell, columnar cell) have a particularly high

Fig. 8.2 Fifty-five-year-old female patient with mediastinal lymph nodes and lung metastases from follicular thyroid carcinoma (*left*). Partial reduction of lesions following 1 cycle of RAIT (*right*) (activity administered 7.2 GBq)

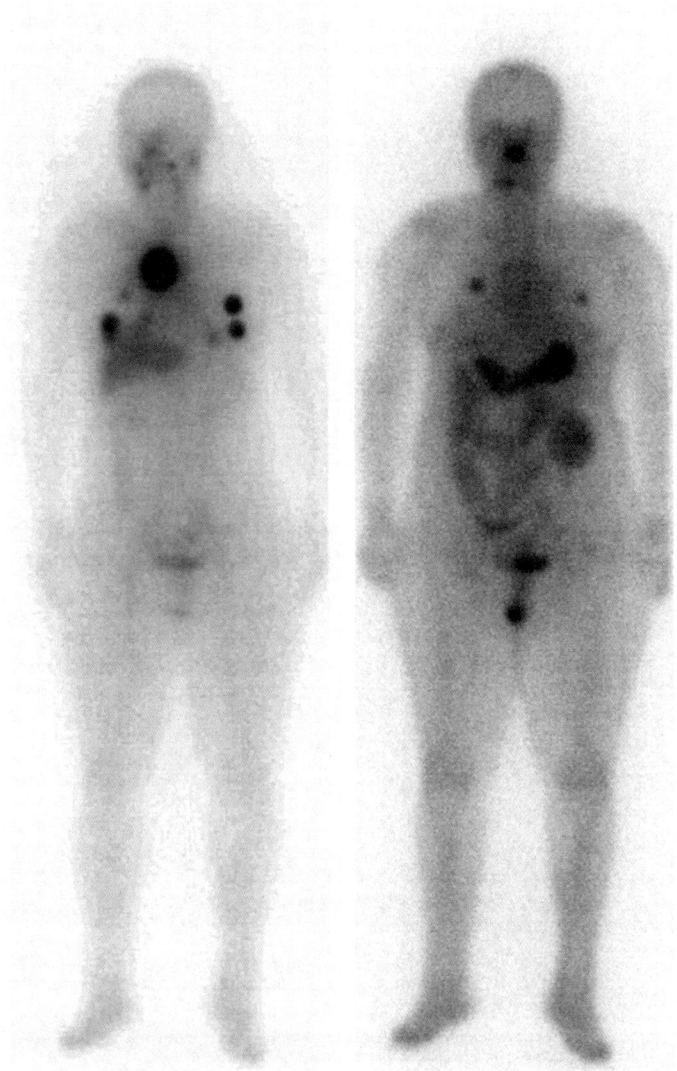

aggressiveness and/or invasive behavior, which in spite of reduced NIS expression may still show a good response to RAIT. On the contrary, some metastatic DTCs progress very slowly and can be considered stable disease. In these cases, RAIT treatment is not effective and the best strategy is to "wait and see." The patient's age at initial diagnosis is usually related to tumor aggressiveness since patients older than 55 years present with more aggressive cancers justifying the use of RAIT if surgery is excluded. Patient's general health status is another factor that affects the therapeutic strategy: a poor health status may exclude surgery or other possible therapies making RAIT the preferred option especially in situations where the use of recombinant human thyroid-stimulating hormone (rhTSH) is economically feasible.

Fig. 8.3 Complete remission after 1 cycle of RAIT (*right*) in a 40-year-old female patient with mediastinal lymph nodes and lung metastases (*left*) from papillary thyroid cancer (activity administered 9.2 GBq)

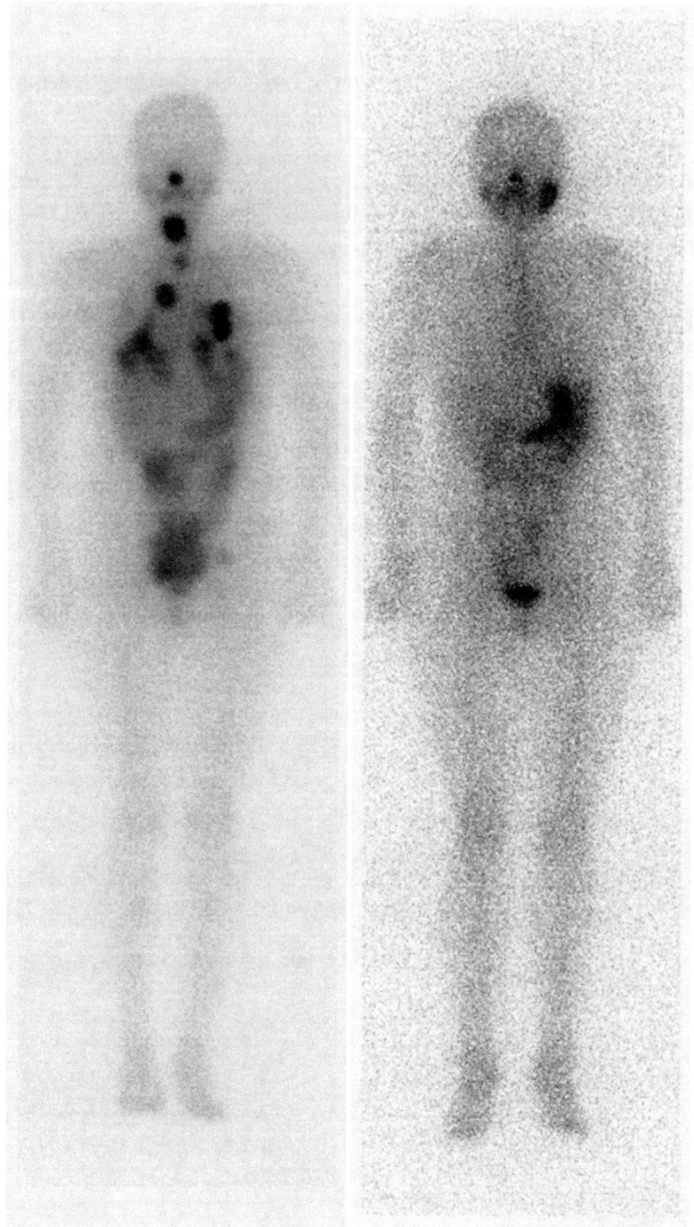

Contraindications

RAIT, like all nuclear medicine modalities, has absolute and relative contraindications.

Pregnancy and breast-feeding are absolute contraindications to RAIT. A careful menstrual history and identification of pregnancy and breast-feeding status is required. Pregnancy is excluded by a beta-HCG test and in some cases by ultrasound. Patients are advised to discontinue breast-feeding 6–8 weeks before radioiodine treatment. If high dose, multiple therapies are planned resulting in high cumulative activities pre-RAIT sperm banking should be offered to young male patients. Relative contraindications to RAIT include: significant bone marrow suppression; presence of pulmonary disease together with multiple lung metastases; relevant salivary gland restriction; presence of neurological symptoms and damage [28].

The Choice of Radioidine Activities: Standard Activity or Dosimetry

Standard Activity

RAIT is usually given as a standard amount. Most centers administer between 3.7 and 7.4 GBq. Doses may be adjusted according to the location of the tumor. In general, the standard dose activities are as following: 3.7 GBq is given for presumed residual thyroid tissue, 5.5–6.4 GBq for lymph node metastases, 6.4–7.4 GBq for lung metastases, and finally 7.4 GBq for bone metastases. Several differences exist, however, among various centers, since the RAIT activities are usually empirically determined according to the tumor characteristics and the patients age. For ablation, the activity ranges from 1 to 5 GBq with many controversies regarding the choice of dose between 1.11 GBq, 1.85 GBq, or 3.7 GBq [36]. It is thought that higher ablative doses may reduce the risk of recurrence since it may have a tumoricidal effect for occult metastases not detected by radioiodine scans. Recent studies however suggest that even though higher doses for ablation purposes are associated with a higher rate of ablation success, this is not necessarily associated with a reduction in disease recurrence. Experts are now recommending the use of lower activities (1.85 GBq) without a preceding radioiodine scan in low-risk patients. We believe that the optimal dose for ablation must be adjusted according to the risk group of individual patients to avoid unnecessary radiation and maximize therapeutic efficacy.

When ablation is not successful, one or more additional RAIT are recommended in order to achieve a successful ablation. For radioiodine ablation in children, some centers adjust the activity according to body weight, surface area, age or 24-h thyroid bed uptake of a radioiodine tracer.

Iodine-avid distant metastases in adolescents and adults are treated with multiple administrations (ranging from 3.7 to 7.4 GBq), given every 6 months during the first 2–3 years and at longer intervals thereafter. When dealing with children, some centers use standard activities (ranging from 1.1 to

7.4 GBq), whilst others use activities ranging from 37 MBq/kg to 92.5 MBq of body weight [37].

RAIT should be carried out until the iodine-avid tumor disappears in the absence of serious side-effects. At the present time, the maximum limit for the cumulative ^{131}I activity given to patients with persistent iodine-avid disease is yet to be defined. Nearly all remissions are obtained with cumulative activities less than 22 GBq. Higher activities should be used only on an individual basis, particularly in patients with metastatic disease since some reports claimed that the risk of secondary tumors is increased when the cumulative activities exceeds 20–30 GBq.

Dosimetry

The activity to be used for RAIT still remains as a topic of discussion. The standard activities described earlier fail to individualize the therapy and thus pose a risk of either under and/or over treating the patient. Within this context, we expect the role of dosimetry to expand and lead us to deliver what we consider as the "optimal" activity to the patient, that is, the lowest possible amount of individualized activity of radioiodine that delivers a lethal dose of radiation to the entire lesion/metastases while minimizing side-effects.

Dosimetric Methods

Currently there are two dosimetric methods used for the treatment of thyroid cancer using [131]I: *bone marrow (blood) dosimetry* and *lesion-based dosimetry*.

The bone marrow (blood) approach was originally described by Benua et al. [38] in 1962: assuming that the bone marrow is the critical organ, it deals mainly with avoiding myelotoxicity by ensuring a blood absorbed dose of not more than 2 Gy. The method involves the measurements of radiation counts of serial blood samples and serial uptake probe measurements of the patient's whole-body activity over the course of 4 or more days after administration of a tracer activity of [131]I (usually 10–15 MBq). Recently the EANM Dosimetry Committee published a standard operating procedure guideline in order to calculate the activity for the systemic treatment of DTC with the goal of not exceeding 2 Gy for the blood absorbed dose [39]. The equation for the mean absorbed dose $[\bar{D}_{blood}]$ to the blood per unit administered activity is:

$$\frac{\bar{D}_{blood}}{A_0}\left[\frac{Gy}{GBq}\right] = 108 \cdot \tau_{mL\,of\,blood}[h] + \frac{0.0188}{(wt[kg])^{2/3}} \cdot \tau_{total\,body}[h]$$

where τ_{source} stands for the residence time in a source organ representing the integral of the activity-time curve in the source organ (cumulated activity) divided by the administered activity.

Lesion-based dosimetry aims to deliver the recommended absorbed dose of radiation in order to ablate thyroid remnant (≥300 Gy) or to treat metastatic disease (≥80 Gy) whilst minimizing the risk to the patient [40]. In order to perform these calculations, one must measure the uptake and clearance of ^{131}I in each lesion. Selected regions of interest (ROIs) on images (planar, SPECT, or [124]I PET) are required to determine the ^{131}I activity in lesions, which are usually acquired at different time-points, up to 96 h after administration. In certain situations, later images may be required, for example to reach a complete ^{131}I fecal excretion.

Attenuation and scatter correction is advised, obtained through transmission ([57]Co flood in planar, CT in SPECT, or PET imaging) or scatter images (triple energy window). Another important parameter required for the calculation is the mass of the lesion which is being treated. Currently the best way to do this is using higher spatial resolution images such as those obtained with computed tomography (CT). The final calculation is often based on adaptations of the generic MIRD equation for the mean absorbed dose:

$$\bar{D} = \frac{\tilde{A} \times S \times m_r}{m_t}$$

Where $\bar{D}$ is the lesion mean absorbed dose, $\tilde{A}$ is the cumulative activity, m_r is the reference mass of the thyroid (20.7 g) and m_t is the remnant/lesion mass, and S is the MIRD defined S value for thyroid self irradiation.

Some centers combine the lesion and blood based dosimetric approaches, aiming for an individualized optimized therapy. Nevertheless, additional studies are needed to support this approach, since so far only three reports are available in the literature. The calculation of lesion volume with sufficient accuracy remains one of the main problems since this is difficult to determine for metastases and almost impossible for remnants.

The shortcomings of planar and SPECT diagnostic procedures are reduced by I-124 PET/CT which also allows precise dosimetry to be performed. An accurate estimation of the maximum tolerated dose to the lesions is possible. Original I-124 PET dosimetry protocols used five PET measurements at 4, 24, 48, 72, and 96 h after [124]I administration. However, recent protocols rely on fewer measurements reducing the inconvenience to both patients and staff. In general, the protocol involves estimating the lesion absorbed dose per administered ^{131}I activity (LDpA) for each positive lesion. The LDpA allows calculation of a putative minimum effective therapeutic activity [41].

Patient Preparation and Treatment

Intact thyrocytes are more avid for radioiodine than malignant thyroid carcinoma cells, particularly metastatic cells. Radical removal of intact thyroid tissue together with the primary tumor is thus of vital importance for providing the metastatic cells with sufficient amount of radioiodine to obtain a satisfactory tumoricidal effect. For malignant diseases of the thyroid, the percentage storage in residual thyroid tissue and metastases is considerably lower than that in the intact thyroid (<1–20% of the radioactivity administered orally).

Of the radioactivity not taken up, considerably more than 90% is excreted within 2 days of oral administration. For this reason, depending upon local regulations, the patient may need to be hospitalized in an approved ward with personnel qualified in radiation protection for at least 48 h after the radioiodine treatment has been given. In recent years, this requirement has been relaxed in the United States. Appropriate pre-therapy counseling should be offered to the patient regardless of whether or not they are hospitalized for isolation purposes or released to supervise themselves.

The use of low sensitivity pre-therapy imaging after surgery remains controversial. In some centers, 4–5 weeks after surgery, a diagnostic study using low dose [131]I (activity upto 100 MBq) is performed to assess the amount of residual thyroid tissue. Large remnants with 24 h radioiodine uptake above 10% should preferably be re-operated upon.

Whole-body scanning (WBS) also allows detection of unknown metastases so that the administered activity can be adjusted according to neck uptake and extent of metastases. Nevertheless, the pre-therapy scan after surgery has been abandoned in many Institutions. Both European and American guidelines only recommend the pre-ablation scan in cases of uncertainty concerning extent of thyroidectomy or when the result would alter either the decision to treat or the dose to be administered to the patient. The SNM guidelines state that *one must recognize the low but finite details such scanning can uncover*. All agree that low activities of ^{131}I should be used for pre-ablative imaging scanning at least 72 h before the therapeutic activity is given [13, 26, 28, 42].

Some believe that pre-therapy scanning may cause a phenomenon known as "stunning," which was first described by Rawson et al. [43]. "Stunning" is defined as diminution of radioiodine uptake and efficacy due to suboptimal therapeutic effects, biological effects, or both of prior diagnostic radioiodine administration. Such an observation is still being debated. Some authors do not recognize the stunning effect, especially if the diagnostic activity administered is low. Recently Dam et al. [44] demonstrated that ^{131}I therapeutic efficacy is not influenced by stunning after a diagnostic 185 MBq WBS. An alternative to the ^{131}I diagnostic scan is the use of ^{123}I or Tc-99 m pertechnetate, which are pure γ emitters with a shorter half-life, thus avoiding stunning. However, the lower imaging sensitivity of ^{123}I has hindered its use, but use of Tc-99 m pertechnetate as a "remnant scan" is not uncommon in Europe.

The effectiveness of the treatment depends on the patient having an elevated serum TSH level. Usually a TSH level of ≥30 mU/L is believed to increase the NIS expression and therefore optimize radioiodine uptake [45]. In order to achieve the required TSH stimulation of thyroid tissue, it is necessary to wait at least 3–4 weeks after thyroidectomy, without hormone replacement therapy. Alternatively, adequate levels of TSH can be reached 4–5 weeks after discontinuing therapy with Levothyroxine (LT4) in patients who had been receiving hormone therapy. As a second option, triiodothyronine (LT3) can be used instead of LT4 until 2 weeks prior to RAIT.

Thyroid hormone replacement should be resumed 2 days after radioiodine administration. The third option to obtain high levels of TSH is the use of recombinant human TSH (rhTSH). The biggest advantage of this technique is that the TSH levels may be increased without inducing hypothyroidism with its associated physical and psychological morbidities. This is especially useful when dealing with patients who have concomitant medical conditions with risk of clinical deterioration (unstable coronary artery disease, psychiatric disease etc.). It is difficult to achieve high levels of TSH in patients with significant metastatic tumor burden. rTSH is clinically useful in this subgroup of patients to maintain the highest radioiodine uptake in malignant cells. Also, rTSH is of help in some patients, in whom satisfactorily high level of TSH cannot be achieved weeks after surgery despite low-iodine diet and lack of T3 or T4 therapy, most probably due to considerable amount of remnant thyroid tissue.

Approval to use rhTSH in the United States was granted by the Food and Drug Administration in 1998, and approval to use it in Europe was granted by the European Agency for the Evaluation of Medicinal Products in 2001. It is usually given in two consecutive daily intra-muscular injections of 0.9 mg with ^{131}I given one day after the second injection. Side-effects are not common but include nausea, headaches, and generalized weakness. Many studies have been published confirming the safety and efficacy of rhTSH.

Overall, these studies have also shown that a euthyroid state at the time of treatment is better from a dosimetric point of view, in that the renal clearance is increased, and that the stimulation of thyroid cells is less prolonged than after thyroid hormone withdrawal. The EANM Guidelines state that unless it is not economically feasible, the use of rhTSH is generally the preferred TSH stimulation method before radioiodine ablation with medium-high activities of radioiodine. For ablation with smaller activities, either preparation method may be used [28].

The importance of a low-iodine diet by avoiding intake of iodinated multivitamins, seafood, and iodized salt must be explained to the patient. A low-iodine diet with <50 μg of iodine per day is recommended for 2–3 weeks before radioiodine treatment [46]. Iodine containing drugs such as amioderone, disinfectants, and eye-drops should also be discontinued (following medical advice). Radiologic contrast agents should be avoided and any CT scan including PET/CT, if required, should be performed without the use of iodinated contrast agents. One must wait for at least 3 months before undergoing radioiodine treatment following the administration of iodinated contrast agents or amioderone. These considerations aim to avoid iodine excess which could result in a decreased efficacy of RAIT (Table 8.2)

Patients should be fasting at least 8–12 h before radioiodine administration. Some physicians advise patients to keep fasting for at least 2 h after ingestion of ^{131}I to avoid any interference with the absorption of iodine. Adequate oral hydration is required for the duration of the treatment. Diluted lemon juice is given for 2–4 days starting 24 h after the radioiodine treatment to stimulate saliva flow since this is believed to reduce salivary gland radiation exposure and thus minimize eventual side-effects. Other alternatives include chewing gum and sucking on hard candy. This line of thought has been questioned recently by Jentzen et al. [47] who studied salivary gland dosimetry using [124]I PET/CT and indicated that lemon juice stimulation shortly after RAIT increases the absorbed doses to the salivary glands.

Two to three days after RAIT, the use of an oral laxative reduces colonic radiation exposure and allows better interpretation of the post-treatment

Table 8.2 Basic instructions given to the patient pre-RAIT to ensure a low total body iodine pool

Diet
The following foods should be avoided for 2–3 weeks before RAIT
Iodized salt, sea salt
Seafood and any sea products
Dairy products (including milk, cheese, yogurt, ice-cream)
Eggs (and any food containing eggs, including chocolate)
Soybeans and soybean products
Bakery products made with iodate dough conditioners
Sulfured molasses
Rhubarb and potato skins
Radiologic contrast agents
Contrast enhanced CT scan (including Ce PET/CT) should be performed at least 3 months before RAIT
Medications
Iodine containing drugs (amioderone), vitamins, food supplements, and any red-colored medications may have to be discontinued (following medical advice)

whole-body scan. The presence of large thyroid remnants or diffuse pulmonary disease may warrant treatment with glucocorticoids to reduce symptoms.

Post-therapy Whole-body Scan

The high dose of administered therapeutic ^{131}I activity makes possible a highly sensitive post-therapy whole-body scan (WBS). This detects the residual thyroid remnant and may detect previously unidentified metastasis upstaging the patient. Approximately 20% of patients are upstaged (due to lung and bone metastases) when compared to the pre-ablation WBS with either ^{131}I or [123]I [48]. Better specificity is now achieved by fusing the functional SPECT images with the anatomical tomographic images, SPECT/CT.

Discharge

In 1997, the U.S. Nuclear Regulatory Commission (USNRC) revised Title 10 of the Code of Federal Regulations (10CFR 35.75), allowing the release

Table 8.3 Some discharge instructions for both patient and family

Diet and nutrition	Contact with other people	Personal hygiene
Keep fasting for 2 h after ingestion of [131]I	Avoid prolonged contact with other people for 7 days (especially infants, children, and pregnant women)	Use separate towels; flush toilet twice after use; men are advised to sit down whilst urinating (for 4–7 days)
Drink plenty of fluids for the first 48 h	Avoid long automobile trips with others, air, and railway travel for 4–7 days	Have a daily shower and wash hands each time you go to the toilet (for 4–7 days)
Drink diluted lemon juice for 2–4 days starting 24 h after treatment (alternatively chew gum or suck hard candy)	Avoid kissing and sexual intercourse for 4–7 days; use contraception for at least 6 months after RAIT	Wash all clothed items separately after 7 days
Do not share cooking utensils and wash them separately for 4–7 days. Preferably use disposable utensils		Should you vomit outside a toilet after receiving the therapy, use paper towels to collect the material and flush them down the toilet

The amount of days may vary according to the dose of radioiodine which has been administered

of patients immediately after ^{131}I therapy if the total effective dose equivalent from the patient to an individual does not exceed 5 mSv in any 1 year (a dose rate of 0.05 μSv per hour at 1 m from the patient). Theoretically, patients requiring doses as high as 9.25 GBq could be discharged from the hospital immediately after receiving the radioiodine dose. This method has been shown to be safe and cost-effective. Previously, patients treated with doses greater than 1.1 GBq had to be hospitalized and isolated [49].

Two important requirements for discharging patients include:

1. Patient assessment and selection: patients should be mentally alert and physically able to take care of themselves without much assistance from family members or friends and be able to use the toilet as necessary without urine contamination outside the toilet.
2. Written and oral instructions for radiation protection should be given both to the patient and to his/her family members or close friends who would be responsible for ensuring that the patient follows all of the instructions [50].

Family planning issues should be discussed with young patients and contraception use for at least 6 months after RAIT is advised. Incontinent patients require special measures and professional supervision, and it is recommended to hospitalize this subgroup of patients for RAIT.

Out-Patient Therapy

Table 8.3 shows a list of the most important instructions that need to be followed after administration of radioiodine. Panzegrau et al. [49] analyzed 48 patients who were treated as out-patients and found that no levels of contamination above regulatory levels were observed and the cost of the treatment was favorable. Since this method represents a dramatic change from past practice, some physicians feel uneasy about not hospitalizing patients undergoing RAIT.

Controversies Associated with RAIT

- [131]I therapy in patients with primary tumors smaller than 10 mm
- [131]I therapy in patients with primary tumors between 10 and 20 mm
- High dose ablation to reduce recurrence rates
- Whole-body I-131 imaging prior to RAIT

Side-Effects

The side-effects of RAIT are not serious, especially when considering the potential benefits of this therapy. The most common early side-effects include radiation thyroiditis if there is a significant remnant, neck pain, swelling, larynx edema, which may cause compressive symptoms, sialadenitis, xerostomia, xerophthalmia, and gastritis. Bone-marrow toxicity, which is usually transient, occurs more frequently in patients receiving large cumulative activities and in those with multiple bone metastases. Chronic sialadenitis associated with xerostomia and abnormalities of taste and smell are the most frequent long-term side-effects. Keratoconjunctivitis sicca, chronic bone-marrow depression, early onset of menopause, chronic hypospermia are rare long-term side-effects. Amongst these, radiation pulmonary fibrosis affects patients with diffuse iodine-avid pulmonary metastases, receiving multiple cycles of RAIT [28].

Secondary primary malignancies (leukemia and solid tumors) following RAIT for DTCs is a risk that has been recognized over the last decade. The incidence of WDTCs has increased steadily over the years with the majority of patients (80–85%) being considered as low-risk patients. The current situation has created open questions regarding the use of radioiodine remnant ablation, with some experts in the field claiming that there is no evidence that RRA is beneficial in low-risk patients and therefore should rarely be used. They believe that this approach would avoid putting patients at risk of developing secondary tumors, especially when we know that they have

a less than 1% chance of dying from their disease. A review of 6,841 patients who had undergone RAIT at several European centers showed that, compared with the general population, these patients were at an increased risk (27%) for solid tumors and leukemia [51]. On the other hand, we know that the absolute risk of death due to recurrent thyroid carcinoma exceeds the risk of death from leukemia by 4- to 40-fold, depending on the age at which the patient is treated. In addition, soon later, Iyher et al. performed a re-analysis to determine the pattern of increase in the use of RAIT and the pattern of increase of secondary primary malignancies in low-risk patients with DTC. They showed that the rises in secondary primary malignancies and the use of RAIT are not similar and suggest that other factors may be involved in the development of these malignancies. Such factors include specific gene alterations, genetic predisposition, and/or common risk factors for the development of these malignancies [52] (Table 8.4).

Common Side-effects of RAIT

- Radiation thyroiditis,
- Sialadenitis, xerostomia
- Gastritis
- Bone-marrow toxicity
- Radiation pulmonary fibrosis

Treatment Failure

Good patient compliance (hormone withdrawal, low-iodine diet, etc.) resulting in high TSH levels

Table 8.4 Common early/short-term and late/long-term side effects follow

Early/short-term side-effects	Late/long-term side-effects
Sialadenitis (30%)	Chronic sialadenitis with xerostomia (10–20%) (especially following multiple treatments)
Gastritis (30%)	Radiation pulmonary fibrosis (<1% of patients with lung metastases)
Radiation thyroiditis (10–20%)	Chronic bone marrow depression (rare)
Bone-marrow depression (depending on the administered activity)	Chronic dry eye (rare)
Xerostomia (rare)	Second primary malignancy (rare)
Nausea and vomiting (transient)	Chronic hypospermia or azoospermia (rare)

together with iodine depleted cells before RAIT increases the chances of successfully ablating any remaining thyroid tissue. Failure to do so may hinder the therapeutic efficacy. Surgical removal of submaximal amount of thyroid tissue may also contribute to a poor success rate in radioiodine ablation. Another important cause of treatment failure occurs when the tumor has low-iodine avidity and, as already mentioned, this may occur with the less differentiated histological subtypes or in patients with rapidly de-differentiating tumors. In such cases alternative treatment strategies need to be sought.

Demonstration of abnormal foci of radioiodine on the post-ablative scan or during follow-up radioiodine scans may require re-treatment with radioiodine using higher therapeutic doses. In patients with bulky disease such as palpable masses or lymph nodes, repeat surgery may be necessary prior to RAIT. In patients with disseminated metastatic disease, a higher cumulative dose should be divided and administered least 3–6 months apart.

Evaluation Response and Follow-Up

The exact time course for complete thyroid remnant ablation after radioiodine administration is not well known. Biochemical response is seen as early as 2 months, recent reports suggest that complete thyroid remnant ablation could take at least 18 months [48]. The time period needed for therapeutic response in patients with metastasis depends on the size, number, and location of metastasis.

Follow-up After RAIT

- Measurement of thyroglobulin & anti-thyroglobulin antibody
- Ultrasonography
- CT/MRI,
- ^{131}I-Whole-body imaging
- ^{18}F-FDG PET/CT
- ^{124}I-PET/CT (future studies)

The evaluation of response is based on the measurement of thyroglobulin (Tg) and anti-thyroglubulin antibody levels and use of imaging modalities

The ablation success after the RAIT procedure is indicated by:

(a) Undetectable level of Tg in the absence of interference by anti-Tg antibodies.
(b) Negative radioiodine uptake in the thyroid bed or a very faint uptake under an arbitrary threshold (less than 0.1%).
(c) Absence of thyroid tissue on neck ultrasonography.

Follow-Up

The patients should be seen at the end of first month following RAIT in order to assess the possible local and systemic effects of radiotoxicity. The nuclear medicine physician should be involved in the first visits. There is no consensus on the frequency and the duration of follow-up visits. As a general rule, the time interval between follow-up visits should not exceed 3 months in the first year, and 6 months thereafter in patients with moderate risk while in patients with high risk parameters and metastatic disease, the frequency of visits and the diagnostic procedures should be tailored to each patient's needs and requirements.

Following successful ablation an accurate life-long follow-up is recommended since WDTC can recur at any time, with two-thirds of recurrences occurring in the first 10 years [53]. The follow-up plan is influenced by the overall risk of the patient, which in turn is determined by patient and tumor characteristics (Table 8.5). In low-risk patients radioiodine WBS can be performed 1 year after ablative therapy. On the other hand, when dealing with high-risk patients, a radioiodine scan 6 months after therapy is usually recommended. Following a first negative radioiodine scan, repeat scans can be done yearly for the next 2 years. Recently, the role of radioiodine scans in the follow-up of patients with WDTC has been becoming controversial since the combination of

Table 8.5 Factors which influence prognosis and follow-up

	High risk for recurrence and death	Moderate-low risk for recurrence and death
Age	<15 or >45 years	Age between 15 and 45 years
Sex	Male	Female
Family history	Family history of thyroid cancer	No family history of thyroid cancer
Tumor		
Primary tumor >3.9 cm	Yes	No
Tumor subtypes	Hürthle, tall, columnar, diffuse sclerosing, insular	Papillary, encapsulated, micro-carcinoma
Vascular invasion	Yes	No
Low radioiodine avidity	Yes	No
Loco-regional metastases	Yes	No
Distant metastases	Yes	No

stimulated thyroglobulin and neck ultrasonography is known to have a high if not equivalent diagnostic accuracy for detection of disease recurrence [54]. This is in addition to the inconvenience and associated health risk the patient experiences due to the 4–5 weeks of thyroxin withdrawal. Currently, the combination of a reliable measurement of serum thyroglobulin and high resolution neck ultrasonography is accepted the most preferable method for the follow-up by endocrinologists, and ATA encourages its members to be involved in learning and performing thyroid ultrasonography.

Stimulated thyroglobulin may be obtained following two successive intra-muscular injections (each 0.9 mg at days 0 and 1) of recombinant human TSH (rhTSH) achieving a TSH peak at days 2 and 3. Stimulated levels of thyroglobulin greater than 2 ng/mL should trigger diagnostic assessment, usually in the form of rhTSH stimulated ^{131}I WBS. In patients with a negative stimulated thyroglobulin 1 year after treatment, the chance of a subsequent positive result during follow-up is low. Detectable thyroglobulin levels on suppressive therapy reliably indicate ongoing disease whereas a negative result does not always exclude the presence of recurrence or metastasis. An increased level of thyroglobulin in the presence of anti-thyroglobulin antibodies is also a strong indicator of ongoing disease or recurrence/metastasis. Recent reports indicate that the development and use of ultrasensitive thyroglobulin assays may render TSH stimulation unnecessary for identification of patients with persistent tumor.

Apart from radioiodine scans and stimulated thyroglobulin levels patients should also undergo periodical physical examinations, chest X-rays and appropriate blood tests.

Hybrid Imaging: SPECT/CT and PET/CT

Radioiodine WBS is highly specific but is limited by lack of anatomical detail. A number of false positive results are seen in non-thyroid conditions such as physiological uptake in the salivary glands, stomach and liver, gastrointestinal and urinary excretion, and non-thyroidal neoplasms. In such cases, SPECT images should complement the planar images obtained. Precise anatomical localization of ^{131}I can be achieved by co-registration with CT images, which is possible with the hybrid SPECT/CT imaging systems currently available. Studies have shown that SPECT/CT has a management impact on 25–41% of patients with thyroid cancer [55].

The impact of ^{124}I-PET/CT in the treatment of WDTC deserves special mention: from a clinical imaging point of view, ^{124}I-PET/CT has been shown to have a high rate of lesion detectability, and therefore improves detection of local recurrences or metastases. Regarding the treatment of WDTC, ^{124}I-PET/CT can have a significant impact on lesion-based pre-therapy dosimetry, which, as discussed previously allows safer and more effective radioiodine activities to be administered. This is because PET images have a higher sensitivity and higher spatial resolution when compared to planar/SPECT gamma-camera images using ^{131}I or ^{123}I-124 PET/CT can be used more frequently in future, but its exact role in this setting is yet to be defined, and I-124 is not commonly available.

Diagnostic and Therapeutic Approach for Patients with Positive Thyroglobulin and Negative Iodine Uptake

Physicians are increasingly being faced with patients presenting with positive thyroglobulin levels and a negative iodine scan. Dealing with these patients is a real challenge. It is important to exclude artifactual suppression of ^{131}I uptake, false positive thyroglobulin levels and the presence of normal thyroid tissue that decreases the sensitivity for imaging of metastatic disease. The most common cause is tumor cell de-differentiation. Many of these patients also have normal conventional imaging studies (CT, MRI, neck ultrasonography). In these cases ^{18}F-FDG/PET has become a valuable diagnostic tool with an 85% increase in sensitivity. ^{18}F-FDG-PET/CT also has a prognostic value (Fig. 8.4). Robbins et al. [56] showed a significant inverse relationship between patient survival and lesion number and intensity of uptake on FDG-PET/CT scans. Other imaging agents that may be used to detect the presence of recurrent/metastatic disease include 111-In-octreotide, 99mTc-sestamibi/tetrofosamin, and 201-Thallium. If diagnostic workup fails to confirm tumor cell de-differentiation and artifactual causes therapeutic doses of radioiodine can be given inspite of negative diagnostic radioiodine imaging, and a significant proportion (about 60%) of patients benefited from this administration.

Alternative or Additional Treatments

Besides surgery, hormone suppression and RAIT other treatment modalities are available for some clinical situations such as tumor cell de-differentiation and poorly-differentiated histological

subtypes with poor iodine avidity (Hürthle, tall, and columnar cell). These include chemotherapy, external beam radiotherapy (EBRT), localized interventions, and molecular targeted therapies. These are not *options* or *alternatives* but *solutions* which can be used when I-131 cannot be used or it is ineffective in special clinical situations. Currently, they are usually employed in the setting of symptomatic progressive WDTCs not amenable to surgery and failing to respond to RAIT (Table 8.6).

Generally, in well-differentiated carcinomas, chemotherapy is not as effective as in undifferentiated carcinomas. Clinical studies studying the effect of chemotherapy in WDTC are limited in number and include only small number of patients. Doxorubicin is an anthracycline and, in the case of thyroid cancer, is the most widely studied chemotherapeutic agent by oncologists. Common side-effects include myelosuppression, gastrointestinal toxicity, and cardiotoxicity. It has also been used under TSH stimulation and in combination with other chemotherapeutic agents such as cisplatin and bleomycin, but so far only partial response rates of 10–20% have been achieved [57].

EBRT plays a role in the management of unresectable, partially resectable, and locally invasive WDTCs. In addition, EBRT should be used when treating non-operable bone metastases from WDTC that may cause pathological fractures and associated neurological symptoms.

Systemic therapy with bisphosphonates can be used to reduce skeletal morbidity and achieve pain control in patients with bone metastases. Localized interventions include chemoembolisation, radiofrequency ablation, or cement injection.

Over the last decade, a great amount of attention has been given for the development of molecular target therapies. These include cell signaling or angiogenesis inhibitors, in particular those targeting vascular endothelial growth factor receptors (VEGF), RET tyrosine kinase (Sunitinib, Vandetanib, Motesanib), and BRAF kinase (Sorafenib). These molecules were studied in limited number of patients (most of them having anaplastic carcinomas and medullary

Fig. 8.4 Negative radioiodine total body scan (*left*) and
^{18}F-FDG PET/CT scan
showing pathological right
sided latero-cervical
lymphadenopathy (*right*) in a
patient who had previously
undergone RAIT for thyroid
remnant ablation and who
presented with raised levels
of thyroglobulin

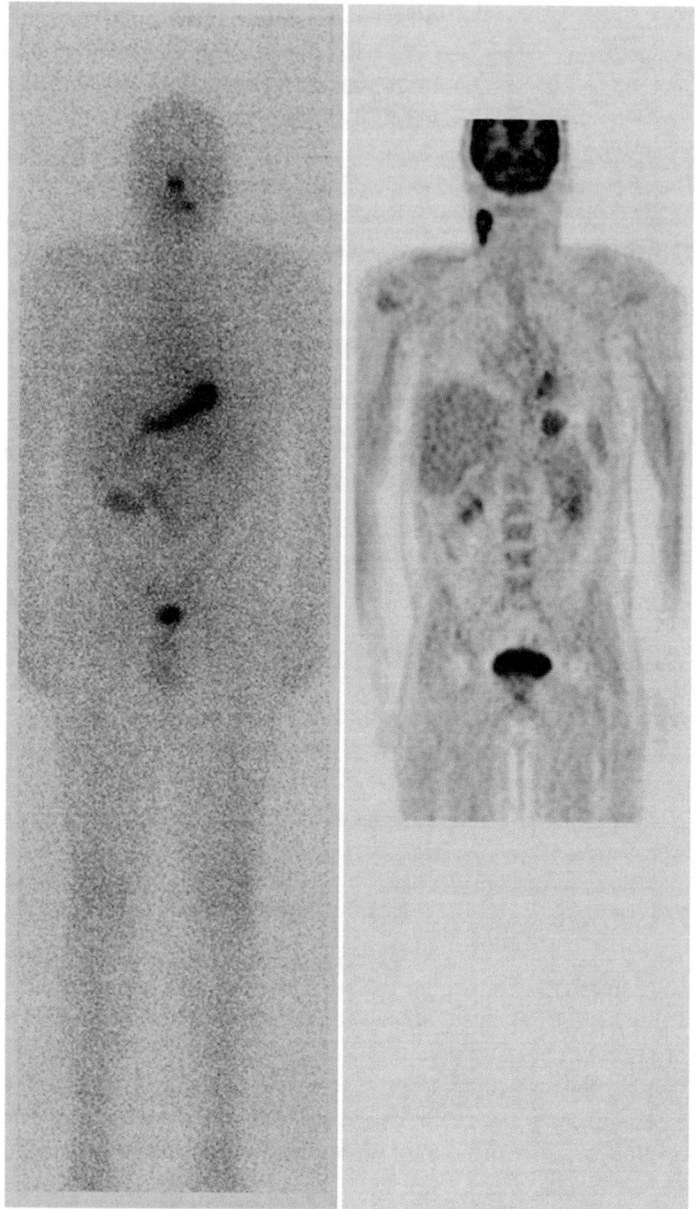

Table 8.6 Overview of the treatment modalities used in the management of DTC after surgery

Therapy	Advantages	Disadvantages
Radioiodine	Targeted therapy, safe	Non-iodine avid tumors Associated side effects
Hormone suppression therapy with Levothyroxine (post-RAIT)	Increased overall survival Decreased recurrence rates	Bone loss Atrial dysrhtmias
Chemotherapy (doxorubicin)	Wide experience in clinical oncology	Poor response rate (PR:10–20%)
Molecular target therapies	Low toxicity; oral preparations	Only clinical trials so far
Bisphosphonates	Pain control; reduce skeletal morbidity	Osteonecrosis; renal failure
Radiotherapy	Loco-regional control; no systemic effects	Long duration of treatment; associated localized side-effects

carcinoma) without reliable comparison to RAIT, but can be tried in iodine negative metastatic disease while there are no convincing studies and cumulative experience in WDTC.

Vitamin A analogs (Isotretinoin), also known as retinoids are capable of re-differentiating cells by increasing thyroid cell NIS expression and subsequent radioiodine uptake. However, relatively low response rates have been achieved to date; the most likely reason being that there are other defects, other than impaired NIS expression, that explain poor radioiodine uptake by de-differentiated cells [58]. Further research is required in this field before a reliable conclusion can be made.

The expression of somatostatin receptors in thyroid tissue, both benign and malignant, has been observed. From a diagnostic point of view this may allow the use of somatostatin receptor scintigraphy (which has been used predominantly for imaging of medullary thyroid cancer), to be used for WDTCs. This may also represent a promising avenue for therapy of advanced thyroid cancer with high activities of β-emitting radioisotopes labeled with somatostatin analogs, which has already been shown to be effective when treating neuroendocrine tumors over-expressing somatostatin receptors [59].

Summary

Differentiated thyroid cancer (papillary and follicular) accounts for approximately 90% of all thyroid cancers and is associated with a wide range of behavior patterns. Disease recurrence occurs in approximately 10–30% of patients. Surgery represents the first form of treatment once a diagnosis of thyroid cancer has been made. With the incidence of well-differentiated thyroid cancers steadily increasing number of patients is being referred for radioiodine therapy. RAIT still remains the mainstay of the treatment strategy in thyroid cancer. It is used for ablation of thyroid remnants following surgery and for treatment of loco-regional or distant metastases. Most of the radiation is delivered by the beta particles of ^{131}I whereas its gamma emission allows WBS to be performed. The effectiveness of RAIT depends on optimal patient selection and preparation with all patients required to have an elevated serum TSH level. The aim of dosimetric calculations (lesion and blood based) is to achieve individualized optimized therapies. When considering the potential benefits of RAIT, the side-effects are not serious. Therapy response is based on tumor detection imaging modalities and measurement of thyroglobulin (Tg) levels. Fused functional and anatomical imaging (SPECT/CT, ^{18}F-FDG-PET/CT, and ^{124}I-PET/CT) are expected to improve RAIT efficacy by increasing diagnostic specificity and sensitivity and by improving dosimetric protocols.

Besides surgery, hormone suppression and RAIT, other treatment options are available when dealing with thyroid cancer. These include chemotherapy, external beam radiotherapy (XRT), localized interventions, and molecular targeted therapies

There are still many areas to improve in this respect. The lack of randomized controlled trials has left vital questions unanswered in RAIT; these include the comparison of treatment and on-treatment, high dose vs. low dose, role of follow-up radioiodine scans, treatment in iodine negative metastatic disease. Well designed clinical researches are needed to improve the efficacy of RAIT as alternative therapies have not been effective so far.

References

1. DeLellis R, Lloyd R, Heitz P, Eng C. World Health Organization classification of tumors: pathology and genetics of tumours of endocrine organs. Lyon: IARC Press; 2004.
2. Enewold L, Zhu K, Ron E, et al. Rising thyroid cancer incidence in the United States by demographic and tumor characteristics, 1980–2005. Cancer Epidemiol Biomarkers Prev. 2009;18:784–91.
3. IAEA. Nuclear medicine in thyroid cancer management: a practical approach [online]. 2009 [cited 2011 Mar 4]; Available from URL: http://nucleus.iaea.org/HHW/NuclearMedicine/Endocrinology/IAEA_Publications/Thyroid_Cancer_Management/index.html.
4. Sherman SI. Thyroid caricinoma. Lancet. 2003;361: 501–11.

5. Eustatia-Rutten CF, Corssmit EP, Biermasz NR, Pereira AM, Romijn JA, Smit JW. Survival and death causes in differentiated thyroid cancer. J Clin Endocrinol Metab. 2006;91(1):313–9.

6. Tuttle RM, Leboeuf R, Martorella AJ. Papillary thyroid cancer: monitoring and therapy. Endocrinol Metab Clin North Am. 2007;36:753–8; vii.

7. Schlumberger MJ. Papillary and follicular thyroid carcinoma. N Engl J Med. 1998;338:297–306.

8. Mazzaferri EL, Kloos RT. Clinical review 128: current approaches to primary therapy for papillary and follicular thyroid cancer. J Clin Endocrinol Metab. 2001;86:1447–63.

9. Montone KT, Baloch ZW, LiVolsi VA. The thyroid Hürthle (oncocytic) cell and its associated pathologic conditions: a surgical and pathology and cytopathology review. Arch Pathol Lab Med. 2008;132:1241–50.

10. Marqusee E, Benson CB, Frates MC, et al. Usefulness of ultrasonography in the management of nodular thyroid disease. Ann Intern Med. 2000;1339:696–700.

11. Hegedus L. Clinical practice. The thyroid nodule. N Engl J Med. 2004;351:1764–71.

12. Hagag P, Strauss S, Weiss M. Role of ultrasounded-guided fine-needle aspiration biopsy in the evaluation of non-palpable thyroid nodules. Thyroid. 1998;8:989–95.

13. American Thyroid Association (ATA) Guidelines Taskforce on Thyroid Nodules and Differentiated Thyroid Cancer, Cooper DS, Doherty GM, et al. Revised American Thyroid Association management guidelines for patients with thyroid nodules and differentiated thyroid cancer. Thyroid. 2009;19(11): 1167–214.

14. Danese D, Sciacchitano S, Farsetti A, Andreoli M, Pontecorvi A. Diagnostic accuracy of conventional versus sonography-guided fine-needle aspiration biospy of thyroid masses. Thyroid. 1998;8:283–9.

15. Are C, Hsu JF, Ghossein RA, Schoder H, Shah JP, Shaha AR. Histological aggressiveness of flurodeoxyglucose positron-emission tomogram (FDG-PET)-detected incidental thyroid carcinomas. Ann Surg Oncol. 2007;14:3210–5.

16. Pacini F, Castagna MG, Brilli L, Pentheroudakis G. Thyroid cancer: ESMO Clinical Practice Guidelines for diagnosis, treatment and follow-up. Ann Oncol. 2010;21:v214–9.

17. Carter WB, Tourtelot JB, Savell JG, Lilienfeld H. New treatments and shifting paradigms in differentiated thyroid cancer management. Cancer Control. 2011;18(2):96–103.

18. Siedlin SM, Marinelli LD, Oshry E. Radioactive iodine-therapy: effect on functioning metastases of adenocarcinoma of thyroid. JAMA. 1946;132: 838–47.

19. Klain M, Ricard M, Leboulleux S, et al. Radioiodine therapy for papillary and follicular thyroid carcinoma. Eur J Nucl Med. 2002;29:S479–85.

20. Mazzaferri EL, Jhiang SM. Long-term impact of initial surgical and medical therapy on papillary and follicular thyroid cancer. Am J Med. 1994;97:418–28.

21. Lind P, Igerc I, Kohlfürst S. Radioiodine therapy: malignant thyroid disease. In: Biersack HJ, Freeman LM, editors. Clinical nuclear medicine. Berlin: Springer; 2007. p. 418–32.

22. Reiners C. Radioiodine therapy in patients with pulmonary metastases of thyroid cancer: when to treat, when not to treat? Eur J Nucl Med Mol Imaging. 2003;30(7):939–42.

23. Jonklaas J, Sarlis NJ, Litofsky D, et al. Outcomes of patients with differentiated thyroid carcinoma following initial therapy. Thyroid. 2006;16:1229–42.

24. Sawka AM, Brierley JD, Tsang RW, et al. An updated systematic review and commentary examining the effectiveness of radioactive iodine remnant ablation in well-differentiated thyroid cancer. Endocrinol Metab Clin North Am. 2008;37:457–80.

25. Shattuk TM, Westra WH, Ladenson PW, Arnold A. Independent clonal origins of distinct tumor foci in multifocal papillary thyroid carcinoma. N Engl J Med. 2005;352:2406–12.

26. Pacini F, Schlumberger M, Dralle H, et al. European consensus for the management of patients with differentiated thyroid carcinoma of the follicular epithelium. Eur J Endocrinol. 2006;154:787–803.

27. Society of Nuclear Medicine. Procedure guideline for therapy of thyroid disease with iodine-131 (sodium iodide): version 2.0. 2005. http://interactive.snm.org.

28. Luster M, Clarke SE, Dietlein M, et al. Guidelines for radioiodine therapy of differentiated thyroid cancer. Eur J Nucl Med Mol Imaging. 2008;35(10):1941–59.

29. Muresan MM, Olivier P, Leclère J, et al. Bone metastases from differentiated thyroid carcinoma. Endocr Relat Cancer. 2008;15(1):37–49.

30. Durante C, Haddy N, Baudin E, et al. Long-term outcome of 444 patients with distant metastases from papillary and follicular thyroid carcinoma; benefits and limits of radioiodine therapy. J Clin Endocrinol Metab. 2006;91:2892–9.

31. Haugen BR, Kane MA. Approach to the thyroid cancer patient with extracervical metastases. J Clin Endocrinol Metab. 2010;95(3):987–93.

32. O'Neill CJ, Oucharek J, Learoyd D, Sidhu SB. Standard and emerging therapies for metastatic differentiated thyroid cancer. Oncologist. 2010;15(2): 146–56.

33. Bernier MO, Leehardt L, Hoang C, et al. Survival and therapeutic modalities in patients with bone metastases of differentiated thyroid carcinomas. J Clin Endocrinol Metab. 2001;86:1568–73.

34. Petrich T, Widjaja A, Musholt TJ, et al. Outcome after radioiodine therapy in 107 patients with differentiated thyroid carcinoma and initial bone metastases: side-effects and influence of age. Eur J Nucl Med. 2001;28: 203–8.

35. Hindié E, Mellière D, Lange F, et al. Functioning pulmonary metastases of thyroid cancer: does radioiodine influence the prognosis? Eur J Nucl Med. 2003;30(7):974–81.

36. Hachshaw A, Harmer C, Mallick U, Haq M, Franklyn JA. 131I activity for remnant ablation in patients with

differentiated thyroid cancer: a systematic review. J Clin Endocrinol Metab. 2007;92:28–38.

37. Jarzab B, Handkiewicz-Junak D, Wloch J. Juvenile differentiated thyroid carcinoma and the role of radio-iodine in its treatment: a qualitative review. Endocr Relat Cancer. 2005;12:773–803.

38. Benua RS, Cicale NR, Sonenberg M, Rawson RW. The relation of radioiodine dosimetry to results and complications in the treatment of metastatic thyroid cancer. Am J Roentgenol Radium Ther Nucl Med. 1962;87:171–82.

39. Lassman M, Hänscheid H, Chiesa C, Hindorf C, Flux G, Luster M. EANM Dosimetry Committee series on standard operational procedures for pre-therapeutic dosimetry I: blood and bone marrow dosimetry in differentiated thyroid cancer therapy. Eur J Nucl Med Mol Imaging. 2008;35(7):1405–12.

40. Maxon 3rd HR, Smith HS. Radioiodine-131 in the diagnosis and treatment of metastatic well differentiated thyroid cancer. Endocrinol Metab Clin North Am. 1990;19(3):685–718.

41. Freudenberg LS, Jentzen W, Stahl A, Bockisch A, Rosenbaum-Krumme SJ. Clinical applications of ^{124}I-PET/CT in patients with differentiated thyroid cancer. Eur J Nucl Med Mol Imaging. 2011;38 Suppl 1:S48–56.

42. Society of Nuclear Medicine: Procedure Guideline For Scintigraphy For Differentiated Papillary and Follicular Thyroid Cancer. 2006. http://interactive.snm.org.

43. Rawson RW, Rall JE, Peacock W. Limitations and indications in the treatment of cancer of the thyroid with radioactive iodine. J Clin Endocrinol Metab. 1951;11:1128–31.

44. Dam HQ, Kim SM, Lin HC, Intenzo CM. ^{131}I therapeutic efficacy is not influenced by stunning after diagnostic whole-body scanning. Radiology. 2004;232:527–33.

45. Cooper DS, Doherty GM, Haugen BR, et al. Management guidelines for patients with thyroid nodules and differentiated thyroid cancer. Thyroid. 2006;16(2):109–42.

46. Pluijmen MJ, Eustatia-Rutten C, Goslings BM, et al. Effects of low-iodide diet on postsurgical radioiodide ablation therapy in patients with differentiated thyroid carcinoma. Clin Endocrinol (Oxf). 2003;58(4):428–35.

47. Jentzen W, Balschuweit D, Schmitz J, et al. The influence of saliva flow stimulation on the absorbed radiation dose to the salivary glands during radioiodine therapy of thyroid cancer using ^{124}I PET(/CT)

imaging. Eur J Nucl Med Mol Imaging. 2010;37(12):2298–306.

48. Abrosetti MC, Colato C, Dardano A, Monzani F, Ferdeghini M. Radioiodine ablation: when and how. Q J Nucl Med Mol Imaging. 2009;53:473–81.

49. Panzegrau B, Gordon L, Goudy GH. Outpatient therapeutic ^{131}I for thyroid cancer. J Nucl Med Technol. 2005;33:28–30.

50. Parthasarathy KL, Crawford ES. Treatment of thyroid carcinoma: emphasis on high-dose ^{131}I outpatient therapy. J Nucl Med Technol. 2002;30:165–71.

51. Rubino C, de Vathaire F, Dottorini ME, et al. Second primary malignancies in thyroid cancer patients. Br J Cancer. 2003;89(9):1638–44.

52. Iyer NG, Morris LG, Tuttle RM, Shaha AR, Ganly I. Rising incidence of second cancers in patients with low-risk (T1N0) thyroid cancer who receive radioactive iodine therapy. Cancer. 2011;117(19):4439–46.

53. McLeod DS. Current concepts and future directions in differentiated thyroid cancer. Clin Biochem Rev. 2010;31(1):9–19.

54. Pacini F, Molinaro E, Castagna MG, et al. Recombinant human thyrotropin-stimulated serum thyroglobulin combined with neck ultrasonography has the highest sensitivity in monitoring differentiated thyroid carcinoma. J Clin Endocrinol Metab. 2003;88(8):3668–773.

55. Wong KT, Choi FP, Lee YY, Ahuja AT. Current role of radionuclide imaging in differentiated thyroid cancer. Cancer Imaging. 2008;8:159–62.

56. Robbins RJ, Wan Q, Grewal RK, et al. Real-time prognosis for metastatic thyroid carcinoma based on 2-[^{18}F]fluoro-2-deoxy-$_D$-glucose-positron emission tomography scanning. J Clin Endocrinol Metab. 2006;91:498–505.

57. Shimaoka K, Schoenfeld DA, DeWys WD, Creech RH, DeConti R. A randomized trial of doxorubicin versus doxorubicin plus cisplatin in patients with advanced thyroid carcinoma. Cancer. 1985;56(9):2155–60.

58. Baudin E, Schlumberger M. New therapeutic approaches for metastatic thyroid carcinoma. Lancet Oncol. 2007;8:148–56.

59. Klagge A, Krause K, Schierle K, Steinert F, Dralle H, Fuhrer D. Somatostatin receptor subtype expression in human thyroid tumours. Horm Metab Res. 2010;42(4):237–40. Epub 2010 Jan 21.

60. Carlisle MR, McDougall IR. Familial differentiated carcinoma of the thryoid. In: Biersack HJ, Grünwald F, editors. Thyroid cancer. Berlin: Springer; 2005. p. 57–70.

Medullary Thyroid Carcinoma

9

Jean François Chatal, Jacques Barbet,
Francoise Kraeber-Bodéré,
and David M. Goldenberg

Introduction

Medullary thyroid carcinoma (MTC) originates from parafollicular cells (C-cells) of the thyroid gland. Calcitonin is a hormone secreted by

J.F. Chatal (✉)
GIP ARRONAX, 1, rue Aronnax,
BP 10112, Nantes 44817, Saint-Herblain,
Cedex, France
e-mail: chatal@arronax-nantes.fr

J. Barbet
GIP ARRONAX, 1, rue Aronnax,
BP 10112, Nantes, 44817 Saint-Herblain,
Cedex, France

Oncology Research Center,
Nantes University, Inserm UMR 892,
Nantes, France
e-mail: Jacques.Barbet@univ-nantes.fr

F. Kraeber-Bodéré, M.D., Ph.D.
Oncology Research Center,
Nantes University, Inserm UMR 892,
Nantes, France

Nuclear Medicine Department, University Hospital and
ICO Gauducheau Cancer Institute, Nantes, France
e-mail: francoise.bodere@chu-nantes.fr

D.M. Goldenberg, Sc.D., M.D.
IBC Pharmaceuticals, Inc. and Immunomedics, Inc,
Morris Plains, NJ, USA

Garden State Cancer Center, Center for Molecular
Medicine and Immunology, 300 The American Road,
Morris Plains, NJ, USA
e-mail: dmg.gscancer@att.net

parafollicular cells. The exact role of calcitonin is not understood, but it modulates bone mineral turnover. Medullary carcinoma accounts for less than 5% of all thyroid cancers and is a clinically heterogeneous disease with quite variable growth rates and survival extending from months to years, sometimes decades, even when the disease is metastatic [1]. The primary treatment for this neuroendocrine tumor is surgical consisting of total thyroidectomy, with dissection of ipsilateral and central lymph nodes, which may be extended to contralateral nodes. Following surgery, patients, without lymph node involvement who have an undetectable calcitonin serum level, can be considered to be cured. For patients with persistent abnormal calcitonin serum levels, indicating residual disease or relapse, imaging generally becomes positive when calcitonin levels exceed 200 ng/L [2]. When the relapse is localized in the neck or mediastinum, single or repeated surgical resection(s) is (are) performed but are rarely followed by a normalization of calcitonin serum level. This situation is compatible, nevertheless, with long survival extending to some years and even decades without additional therapy [3]. It is important to take into consideration reliable prognostic indicators before planning systemic treatment (targeted radionuclide therapy and/or chemotherapy). Indeed, systemic treatment can be highly toxic with only a modest survival benefit. Thus, it is necessary to carefully balance the potential toxicity and benefit.

C. Aktolun and S.J. Goldsmith (eds.), *Nuclear Medicine Therapy: Principles and Clinical Applications*,
DOI 10.1007/978-1-4614-4021-5_9, © Springer Science+Business Media New York 2013

Selection of Patients for Systemic Treatment

Several prognostic factors have been identified in the past, including age at initial diagnosis, gender, TNM stage, RET protooncogene mutation, Cdc25b phosphatase or Ki67 expression level [1, 4–9]. These are considered good predictors of probability of cure after primary surgery but they do not predict life expectancy for patients with persistently elevated calcitonin serum level after single or repeated surgery. Serum calcitonin and/or carcinoembryonic antigen (CEA) doubling time (DT) have been identified as the most reliable predictors of survival [10]. More recently, the results of a structured meta-analysis initially utilizing 60 publications and finally comprising 6 studies which included 73 patients, confirmed that calcitonin-DT and CEA-DT are strong indicators for disease-related survival and recurrence-free survival, indicating an aggressive disease and, consequently, the need for systemic treatment [11]. Two points still need additional studies for clarification. The most appropriate cutoff value for calcitonin-DT and CEA-DT, allowing a clear stratification between high-risk and low-risk patients, is currently 2 years. Moreover, there is a debate concerning whether CEA-DT or calcitonin-DT has a higher predictive value. It is generally agreed, however, that for patients with rapidly progressing metastatic MTC, the simultaneous determination of calcitonin-DT and CEA-DT allows proper risk stratification between those who need "watchful waiting" and those who might benefit from systemic treatment.

Role of Imaging

For a long time, imaging techniques in MTC included computed tomography and bone scintigraphy. Recently, we have shown that bone/bone marrow MRI detected a high rate of previously unknown metastatic involvement (75% bone marrow involvement) [12]. This detection had an impact on the effectiveness of pretargeted radioimmunotherapy (pRAIT) with an overall

survival (OS) significantly longer in patients with positive post-pRAIT bone-marrow immunoscintigraphy than in those without bone/bone-marrow uptake of radioactivity. Thus, it was speculated that pRAIT efficacy in MTC could be related in part to bone marrow tumor response because of findings in animal and clinical studies that the best indication for pRAIT is in disseminated microscopic disease, in which a much higher uptake and consequently higher tumoricidal dose of the radiotherapeutic agent are achieved [13]. Positron emission tomography/computed tomography imaging with ^{18}F-2-fluoro-2-deoxyglucose (F18-FDG PET/CT) proved to be sensitive for visualization of tumors in the neck and mediastinum in patients with progressive metastatic disease, with possible prognostication by SUV (standardized uptake value) quantification, whereas computed tomography was the most sensitive technique for detection of liver and lung metastases [14] ^{18}F-DOPA-PET/CT is another functional whole-body imaging procedure that appears to provide useful results in neuroendocrine tumors including MTC [15].

Before deciding on a systemic treatment such as radioimmunotherapy (RAIT) in a patient with rapidly progressing metastatic MTC, as documented by a short calcitonin-DT, it is useful to identify tumors in the neck and mediastinum because, in the situation of bulky tumors, it is appropriate to perform a surgical resection first, if technically possible, to enhance the potential therapeutic effect of RAIT. Surgery to clear the neck of gross lymph nodes should be considered also before systemic-targeted therapy using multikinase inhibitors because of a possible better tissue-specific response of well perfused parenchymal relative to nonparenchymal target lesions [16].

Systemic Treatment Modalities

Chemotherapy

Currently, there is a general consensus that chemotherapy using different drugs as monotherapy or in combination is not effective enough to compensate for the serious toxicity observed.

Moreover, it is difficult to conduct a useful meta-analysis, because the results of only a few clinical studies using different regimens in a limited number of patients have been reported.

Chemoembolization is an alternative modality for patients with metastases involving only the liver. Some transient partial remissions or stabilizations have been reported in 70% of cases with liver involvement when disease is limited to less than 30% of the liver parenchyma, which is a relatively rare situation [17, 18].

Radionuclide Therapy

Radioimmunotherapy

For a long time, RAIT clinical studies have been performed using an anti-CEA MAb labeled with iodine-131. The rationale for targeting this antigen is the high expression of CEA by tumor cells and the generally good vascularization of tumors, providing easy access of radioimmunoconjugate to its antigenic target. In 2 successive phase I clinical trials, with a total of 27 patients, efficacy was documented by objective responses in a small number of patients and, interestingly, by long-term radiological stabilization in a substantial number of patients [19, 20]. With the aim of increasing the therapeutic index in relatively radioresistant tumors, we have developed a novel approach to RAIT, termed pRAIT. It consists of decoupling the injection of an unlabeled bispecific anti-CEA/anti-hapten antibody and that of a small, rapidly diffusible, radiolabeled bivalent hapten which is injected 4–6 days after the first injection of the bispecific antibody [21]. This two-step approach allows the decrease of radioactive concentration in blood and normal organs while maintaining a tumoricidal effect. Consequently, the therapeutic index is increased by a factor between 2 and 5.

The first pRAIT clinical study was performed to evaluate whether it could deliver radiation absorbed doses to tumors comparable to those delivered by iodine-131 in patients with differentiated thyroid cancer since efficacy of this approach has been documented for 50 years. The results showed that estimates of absorbed doses

delivered to small tumors after pRAIT were in the same range as those delivered after conventional iodine-131 therapy to thyroid cancer metastases [22] supporting the conclusion that efficacy of pRAIT could be expected in the clinical setting of small disseminated tumors.

Since 1996, three successive phase I and II clinical trials have been conducted in a total of 77 patients with rapidly progressing metastatic MTC. The first study was performed using a murine unlabeled bispecific antibody given 4 days before injection of 1.5–3.7 GBq of di-DTPA-^{131}I-hapten. In the second phase I/II and the subsequent phase II study, murine antibody was replaced by a human–mouse chimeric antibody using the same methodology and allowing repeated injections to be given while achieving a decrease in the immune response rate (development of human anti-murine antibodies [HAMA]).

In all clinical studies, dose-limiting toxicity was hematological and was always manageable using blood-product transfusions and/or hematopoietic growth factors. Myelodysplastic syndrome (MDS) was observed in three patients, two of whom were heavily pretreated with external beam radiotherapy. One case of MDS could be related to pRAIT. Cytogenetic testing before RAIT may identify existing chromosomal abnormalities in previously-treated patients who would be at higher risk for MDS.

Due to the large variability of growth rates, it is necessary to refer to an untreated control group to evaluate clinical effectiveness of systemic treatment in metastatic MTC. In published studies, it appears that patients with calcitonin-DT or CEA-DT longer than 2 years have a long life expectancy extending over some years and decades. Thus 'watchful waiting' is advisable in these patients. On the other hand, patients with short calcitonin-DT or CEA-DT, below 2 years, have a poor prognosis and are candidates for systemic treatment.

In a retrospective study, the overall survival of 29 MTC patients included in 2 phase I/II trials was compared with that of 39 untreated patients in a control group [13]. In the treated group, responders were arbitrarily defined as showing at least a 100% increase in calcitonin-DT in the

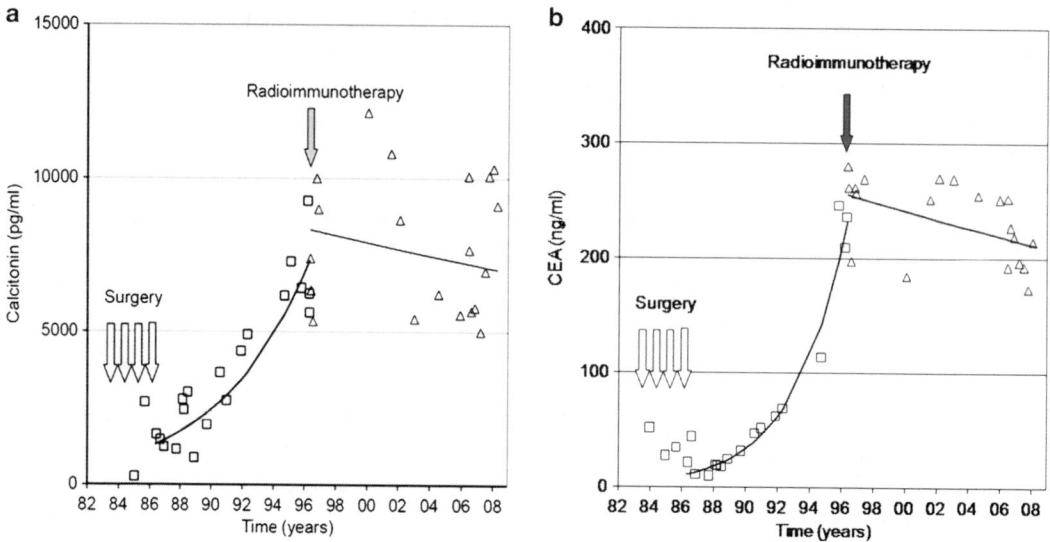

Fig. 9.1 Serum biomarkers kinetics in a patient with several bone metastases and showing fast progression (*squares*) after four surgeries (*arrows*) and before pRAIT. (**a**) Serum calcitonin kinetics and (**b**) serum carcinoem- bryonic antigen (CEA) kinetics. Following pRAIT, long- term (12 years) decrease of serum calcitonin (common large fluctuation to be noted) and CEA levels (*triangles*) and stabilization of bone metastases

most frequent situation of still continuing increase of serum calcitonin and/or CEA, after pRAIT but at a slower rate or showing a decrease of these biomarkers. In the treated group of high-risk patients, OS was significantly longer than in the high-risk untreated patients (median OS: 110 vs. 61 months; $P<0.03$). OS was also longer in bio- logical responders than in nonresponders (median OS: 159 vs. 109 months; $P<0.035$). This indi- cates that 100% increase of calcitonin-DT or decrease of serum calcitonin is a good surrogate marker for overall survival. In a limited number of patients, biological response was defined as showing a post-pRAIT decrease in calcitonin and/or CEA serum levels (Fig. 9.1a, b).

A recently completed phase II prospective clinical trial included 42 patients with calcitonin- DT less than 2 years (Fig. 9.2). Overall survival after pRAIT was significantly longer in combined responders (as defined by RECIST, PET and bio- logical criteria) than in nonresponders (median OS 67 vs. 25 months $P<0.04$) (Fig. 9.3).

Thus, it appears that pRAIT is a promising systemic treatment modality resulting in a significant survival gain in high-risk, metastatic patients.

Radiopeptide Therapy

[^{90}Y-DOTA]-TOC, a somatostatin analog, has been used for systemic treatment of metastatic MTC patients. In a clinical study enrolling 21 patients who progressed after conventional treat- ment, a clinical benefit (objective responses plus stable disease) was observed in 67% of patients with the duration of response ranging from 3 to 40 months [23]. In a more recent phase II clinical study with 31 patients, using the same definition of biological response as in the pRAIT study, namely prolongation of calcitonin-DT of at least 100%, a biological response was observed in 58% of patients, with a significantly longer sur- vival in responders than in nonresponders [24]. However, from these two studies, it is not possi- ble to draw any valid conclusion with regard to a potential survival benefit because of a lack of pre-therapeutic selection based on a validated prognostic factor, such as calcitonin-DT. In both studies, patients were progressing before

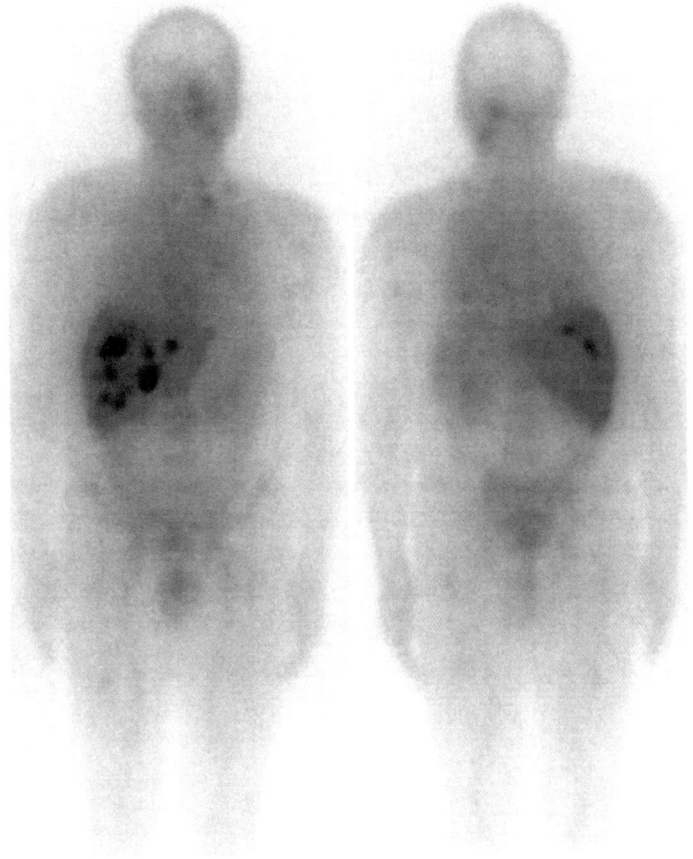

treatment but the rate of progression was not
evaluated.

^{131}I-MIBG Therapy

In a recent review reporting cumulative results of
^{131}I-MIBG in a total of 50 patients, an objective
response rate (CR + PR + SD) was observed in
64% of patients but without precise information
on PFS or OS [25]. As with the ^{90}Y-DOTA-TOC
studies, it is quite difficult to draw any valid conclusion without data on the progression prior to
^{131}I-MIBG therapy. If patients included in that
report had predominantly slowly-progressing
disease, long-term survival might have been
observed irrespective of ^{131}I-MIBG therapy
efficacy.

Targeted Biotherapy Using Multikinase Inhibitors

In MTC, several transduction pathways lead
to neoplastic transformation. Among signaling
components, receptors for vascular endothelial
growth factor (VEGF), epidermal growth factor
(EGFR), platelet-derived growth factor (PDGFR),
and RET protein have been targeted with multikinase inhibitors. Two of these inhibitors have been
clinically evaluated in a substantial number of
MTC patients. Motesanib diphosphate (AMG
706; from AMGEN, Inc; Thousand Oaks CA,
USA), which inhibits VEGFR 1–3, PDGFR, and
stem-cell factor receptor (c-kit), was evaluated in

2005

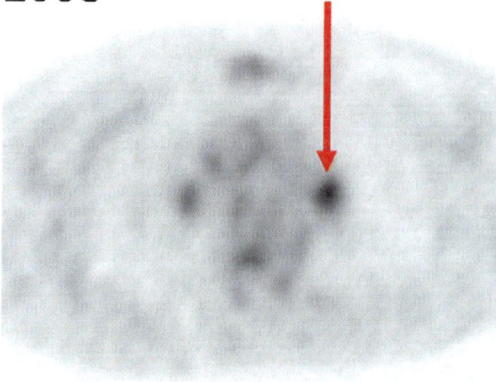

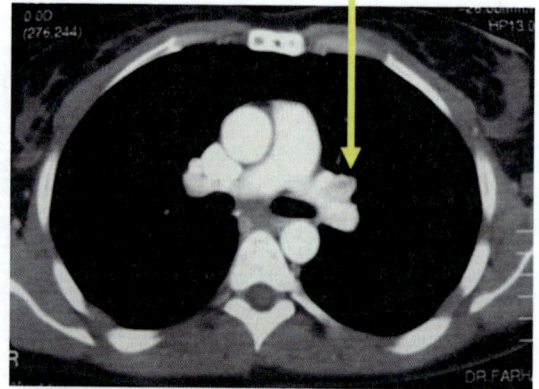

2007

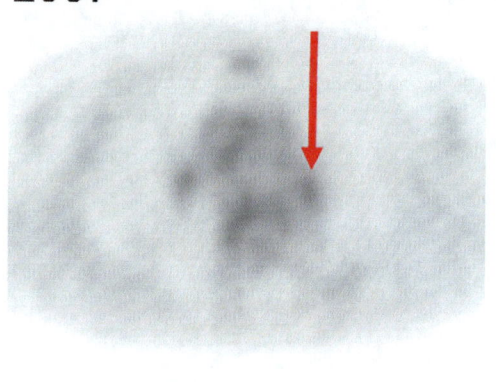

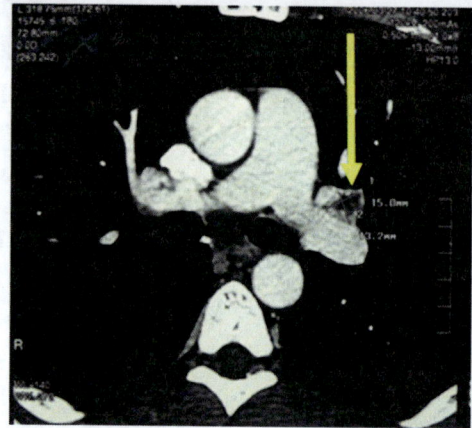

Fig. 9.3 Patient with high-risk medullary thyroid carcinoma (calcitonin doubling time of 1.5 years). After pRAIT in 2005, treatment efficacy was documented 2 years later (2007) with PET-FDG showing a decrease in lymph node uptake (*red arrows*) and with CT showing a lymp node necrosis (*yellow arrows*)

a phase II clinical study of 91 patients with locally advanced or metastatic disease [26]. Some clinical efficacy was documented including two objective responses with a duration of 21 and 32 weeks. There were 81 cases of stable disease with 48% of the patients clinically stable for more than 24 weeks. A clinical benefit rate, defined as confirmed objective response or durable stabilization (SD) of 51% was obtained in the overall population, but only 21% SD in the 42 patients with proven progression before inclusion. The median progression-free survival was 48 weeks. Treatment with motesanib was tolerable but 41% of patients experienced treatment-related grade 3 and 4 adverse events including 3 patients with grade 3 acute cholecystitis.

Vandetanib (Caprelsa®), ASTRAZENECA (London, United Kingdom) which inhibits VEGFR, EGFR and RET, was evaluated in a phase II clinical trial of 30 patients with locally-advanced or metastatic disease with at least one measurable lesion. Some clinical efficacy was documented by a confirmed partial response in 20% of patients; disease stabilization longer than 6 months was observed in 53% of patients [27]. Vandetanib dosing had to be reduced or interrupted in 24 patients, due to adverse events. The most common grade 3 adverse events were QTc prolongation, diarrhea, nausea, and hypertension. A phase III, randomized, double-blind, multicenter study enrolled 331 patients with inclusion criteria including the presence of measurable tumor but without reference to the progression kinetics before treatment [28]. Interestingly, median progression-free survival was longer in the vandetanib arm (22.6 months) than in the placebo arm (16.4 months). However, some serious adverse effects were observed, such as cardiac risks, which could lead to death (unpublished data). Based on these results vandetanib was approved by FDA on April 6, 2011, with a Risk Evaluation and Mitigation Strategy (REMS) to inform health care professionals about the serious heart-related risks.

tyrosine kinase [30]. Consequently, a new multikinase inhibitor, cabozantinib (XL184), EXELIXIS San Francisco CA, USA has been developed and inhibits MET in addition to VEGFR2 and RET. It was evaluated in a phase I study of 37 patients with MTC. A confirmed partial response was observed in 29% of patients, and stabilization of more than 6 months in 41%. The clinical significance of such stabilization is uncertain due to lack of evidence of disease progression before trial inclusion [31].

Conclusions

For decades, no efficient systemic treatment was available for patients with rapidly progressive metastatic MTC. Recently, several types of targeted therapy have shown some effectiveness, including pRAIT, radiolabeled peptide therapy, ^{131}I-MIBG and multikinase inhibitors, in addition to chemotherapy (Table 9.1). In the two types of targeted therapy, some efficacy was documented in patients with metastases but without any clearly defined disease progression kinetics, which can vary from months to decades. pRAIT was the only treatment modality used in patients with a bad prognosis based on documented biomarker doubling time. pRAIT clearly showed a survival benefit with manageable hematologic toxicity.

> **Systemic Therapy Options for Medullary Carcinoma of Thyroid**
>
> - Pretargeted radioimmunotherapy (pRAIT)
> - 90Y-DOTA-TOC
> - 131I-MIBG
> - Multikinase Inhibitors
> - Chemotherapy

It has been reported recently that VEGF inhibitors can promote tumor aggressiveness with metastatic extension to distant sites [29]. This adverse effect has been reported based on the upregulation of MET, a proinvasive receptor

Table 9.1 Compared survival between three therapeutic modalities

	PFS (months)	OS (months)	References	Comments
Chemotherapy	4–29 median: 10	8.5–33 months median: 17.5	[13]	87 pts in 4 studies
Vandetanib	Median: 22.6	ND	[26]	Phase III 331 pts median control PFS arm: 16.4
pRAIT	Median: 13.6	Median: 43.9	[13]	Phase II 42 pts

Comparison of progression-free survival (PFS) and overall survival (OS) in three therapeutic modalities: chemotherapy, a multikinase inhibitor, and pretargeted radioimmunotherapy [13, 26]. These results are not from a randomized comparison but rather represent simply an amalgam of results from separate studies. Thus, they should be considered with due caution (Wu LT et al., Cancer 73;432–436, 1994, Schlumberger M et al., Br J Cancer 71; 363–365, 1995, Petursson SR et al., Cancer 62; 1899–1902, 1988, Shimaoka K, Cancer 56; 2155–2160, 1985, [13, 28]). Nevertheless, it appears that a much longer OS is observed after pRAIT than after chemotherapy. On the other hand, median PFS is longer after vandetanib than after pRAIT, but patients treated after pRAIT were rapidly progressing, whereas progression rate in patients treated after vandetanib was unknown, which could explain the longer PFS if a majority of patients were slowly progressing. In this comparison, vandetanib and pRAIT are more effective than chemotherapy

References

1. Kebebew E, Ituarte PH, Siperstein AE, et al. Medullary thyroid carcinoma: characteristics, treatment, prognostic factors, and a comparison of staging systems. Cancer. 2000;88:1139–48.

2. Giraudet AL, Vanel D, Leboulleux S, et al. Imaging medullary thyroid carcinoma with persistent elevated calcitonin levels. J Clin Endocrinol Metab. 2007;92:4185–90.

3. Bergholm U, Bergstrom R, Ekbom A. Long-term follow-up of patients with medullary carcinoma of the thyroid. Cancer. 1997;79:132–8.

4. Modigliani E, Cohen R, Campos JM, et al. Prognostic factors for survival and for biochemical cure in medullary thyroid carcinoma: results in 899 patients. The GETC Study Group. Clin Endocrinol. 1998;48:265–73.

5. Miccoli P, Minuto MNMN, Ugolini C, et al. Clinically unpredictable prognostic factors in the outcome of medullary thyroid cancer. Endocr Relat Cancer. 2007;14:1099–105.

6. Byar DP, Green SB, Dor P, et al. A prognostic index for thyroid carcinoma. A study of the EORTC Thyroid Cancer Cooperative Group. Eur J Cancer. 1979;15:1033–41.

7. Elisei R, Cosci B, Romei C, et al. Prognostic significance of somatic ret oncogene mutations in sporadic medullary thyroid cancer: a 10-year follow-up study. J Clin Endocrinol Metab. 2008;93:682–7.

8. Ito Y, Yoshida H, Tomoda C, et al. Expression of Cdc25b expression level predicts a poor prognosis. Cancer Lett. 2005;229:291–7.

9. Tisell LE, Oden A, Muth A, et al. The Ki67 index a prognostic marker in medullary thyroid carcinoma. Br J Cancer. 2003;89:2093–7.

10. Barbet J, Campion L, Kraeber-Bodéré F, Chatal JF, The GTE study group. Prognostic impact of serum calcitonin and carcinoembryonic antigen doubling-times in patients with medullary thyroid carcinoma. J Clin Endocrinol Metab. 2005;90:6077–84.

11. Meijer JAA, le Cessie S, van den Hout WB, et al. Calcitonin and carcinoembryonic antigen doubling times as prognostic factors in medullary thyroid carcinoma: a structured meta-analysis. Clin Endocrinol. 2010;72:534–42.

12. Mirallie E, Vuillez JP, Bardet S, et al. High frequency of bone/bone marrow involvement in advanced medullary thyroid cancer. J Clin Endocrinol Metab. 2005;90:779–88.

13. Chatal JF, Campion L, Kraeber-Bodéré F, et al. Survival improvement in patients with medullary thyroid carcinoma who undergo pretargeted anti-carcinoembryonic antigen radioimmunotherapy: a collaborative study with the French Endocrine Tumor Group. J Clin Oncol. 2006;24:1705–11.

14. Oudoux A, Salaun PY, Bournaud C, et al. Sensitivity and prognostic value of Positron Emission Tomography with F-18-Fluorodeoxyglucose and sensitivity of immunoscintigraphy in patients with medullary thyroid carcinoma treated with anticarcinoembryonic antigen-targeted radioimmunotherapy. J Clin Endocrinol Metab. 2007;92:4590–7.

15. Beheshti M, Pöcher S, Vali R, et al. The value of 18F-DOPA PET-CT in patients with medullary thyroid carcinoma: comparison with 18F-FDG PET-CT. Eur Radiol. 2009;19:1425–34.

16. Machens A, Dralle H. Parenchymal versus nonparenchymal target lesion response in clinical trials for metastatic medullary thyroid cancer. J Clin Oncol. 2010;28:e534: author reply e535–6.

17. Lorenz K, Brauckhoff M, Behrmann C, et al. Selective arterial chemoembolization for hepatic metastases from medullary thyroid carcinoma. Surgery. 2005;138:986–93.

18. Fromigue J, De Baere T, Baudin E, et al. Chemoembolization for liver metastases from medullary thyroid carcinoma. J Clin Endocrinol Metab. 2006;91:2496–9.

19. Juweid ME, Hajjar G, Stein R, et al. Initial experience with high-dose radioimmunotherapy of metastatic medullary thyroid cancer using ^{131}I-MN-14F(b)$_2$ anticarcinoembryonic antigen MAb and AHSCR. J Nucl Med. 2000;41:93–103.

20. Juweid ME, Hajjar G, Swayne LC. Phase I/II trial of (131)I-MN-14F(ab)2 anti-carcinoembryonic antigen monoclonal antibody in the treatment of patients with metastatic medullary thyroid carcinoma. Cancer. 1999;85:1828–42.

21. Barbet J, Kraeber-Bodéré F, Vuillez JP, et al. Pretargeting with the affinity enhancement system for radioimmunotherapy. Cancer Biother Radiopharm. 1999;14:153–66.

22. Bardies M, Bardet S, Faivre-Chauvet A, et al. Bispecific antibody and iodine-131-labeled bivalent hapten dosimetry in patients with medullary thyroid or small-cell lung cancer. J Nucl Med. 1996;37:1853–9.

23. Bodei L, Handkiewicz-Junak D, Grana C, et al. Receptor radionuclide therapy with ^{90}Y-DOTATOC in patients with medullary thyroid carcinomas. Cancer Biother Radiopharm. 2004;19:65–71.

24. Iten F, Müller B, Schindler C, et al. Response to [^{90}Y-DOTA]-TOC treatment is associated with long-term survival benefit in metastasized medullary thyroid cancer: a phase II clinical trial. Clin Cancer Res. 2007;13:6696–702.

25. Castellani MR, Seregni E, Maccauro M, et al. MIBG for diagnosis and therapy of medullary thyroid carcinoma: is there still a role? Q J Nucl Med Mol Imaging. 2008;52:430–40.

26. Schlumberger MJ, Elisei R, Bastholt L, et al. Phase II study of safety and efficacy of motesanib in patients with progressive or symptomatic, advanced or metastatic medullary thyroid cancer. J Clin Oncol. 2009;27:3794–801.

27. Wells SA, Gosnell JE, Gagel RF, et al. Vandetanib for the treatment of patients with locally advanced or metastatic hereditary medullary thyroid cancer. J Clin Oncol. 2010;28:767–72.

28. Wells SA, Robinson BG, Gagel RF, et al. Vandetanib (VAN) in locally advanced or metastatic medullary thyroid cancer (MTC): a randomized, double-blind phase III trial (ZETA). J Clin Oncol. 2010;28:15s (suppl; abstr 5503).
29. Loges S, Mazzone M, Hohensinner P, et al. Silencing or fueling metastasis with VEGF inhibitors. Cancer Cell. 2009;15:167–70.
30. Stellrecht CM, Gandhi V. MET receptor tyrosine kinase as a therapeutic anticancer target. Cancer Lett. 2009;280:1–14.
31. Kurzrock R, ShermanSI BDW, et al. Activity of XL184 (Cabozantinib), an oral tyrosine kinase inhibitor, in patients with medullary thyroid cancer. J Clin Oncol. 2011;29:2660–6.

Local Accelerated Radionuclide Breast Irradiation: Avidin-Biotin Targeting System

10

Concetta De Cicco and Giovanni Paganelli

Introduction

Breast cancer remains the most common cancer in women in the developed world and the most frequent cause of cancer-related death among women worldwide [1]. In 2010 in the United States, the estimated number of new cases of breast cancer was 207,090 (28% of all cancer in women), with 39,840 expected deaths (second cause of death after lung and bronchus carcinoma) [2]. Fortunately, thanks to the screening campaigns carried out in the Western countries, breast cancer can be treated in its early phase. The conventional surgical treatment for early breast cancer consists of either a mastectomy or breast conserving surgery (BCS), often accompanied by axillary dissection or sentinel node biopsy. If BCS is performed, whole breast external beam radiotherapy (EBRT) with doses around 50–60 Gy remains the gold standard for local control. The benefit of postoperative radiotherapy is well known since the completion of few prospective randomized trials conducted in the years 1976–1990, which compared conservative surgery and radiation with conservative surgery alone. Several clinical trials compared also breast conservative surgery (BCS) alone vs. BCS

C. De Cicco • G. Paganelli (✉)
Division of Nuclear Medicine,
European Institute of Oncology, Via Ripamonti,
435-20141 Milan, Italy
e-mail: divisione.medicinanucleare@ieo.it

followed by whole breast (WB) EBRT: 10–35% of women receiving BCS alone showed locoregional recurrence, whilst it occurred only in 0.3–8% of women after BCS plus WB-EBRT (follow-up range: 39–102 months), although both treatments produced the same 10-year overall survival rates [3]. However, there is some recent evidence that lack of radiotherapy is associated with an increased hazard ratio for death [4]. Current accepted treatment protocol takes advantage of the above experiences and consists of BCS, usually accompanied by axillary node dissection or sentinel node biopsy. If BCS is performed, it is almost always accompanied by postoperative regional radiotherapy; 2 Gy per day delivered five times a week for 6–8 weeks, for a total dose of 50–60 Gy to eliminate microscopic cancer foci remaining after surgery [5]. A substantial benefit of an additional boost with 16 Gy to the tumor bed was then confirmed by the EORTC [6] particularly in premenopausal women.

The standard EBRT protocol requires more than a month and a half to perform a whole breast conventional 60 Gy EBRT cycle (50 Gy in 25 fractions over 5 weeks + postoperative sequential boost, 2 Gy/day over 5 days). This has a negative impact on the quality of life (QoL) of the patients (absence from the family and from work, heavy financial commitment) and often many are not able to complete their radiation treatment.

A substantial benefit of an additional boost with 16 Gy to the tumor bed was recently confirmed by the EORCT [7] especially in premenopausal women. However, irradiation of normal organs (lung, heart) and long-lasting EBRT are major drawbacks. Alternative modalities have been proposed with the aim of reducing the EBRT treatment. The so-called IORT (Intra Operative RadioTherapy) is a new procedure for intraoperative electron radiotherapy (also known as ELIOT) that employs a linear accelerator (LA) placed into the operation room. This technique has been applied at the European Institute of Oncology (Milan, Italy) in several trials as full dose for partial breast irradiation (PBI) or as a boost followed by whole breast irradiation (WBI). Recently, several examples of intraoperative radiotherapy followed by accelerated EBRT reported encouraging results and excellent local tumor control rate [8–10]. An update of the IEO study [8] shows no recurrences out of 171 patients with a median follow-up of 55 months. Toxicity evaluated in 204 patients was observed at the end of EBRT and was 28% grade 3 and 67% grade 2.

However, the ELIOT approach is limited to hospitals with a dedicated linear accelerator. In terms of target volume, the field of irradiation is limited to 4–6 cm diameter; in patients with multifocal multicentric tumors, this is a serious limitation.

In an effort to develop a versatile and easy procedure to deliver radiation (electron) therapy combined with reduced EBRT post quadrantectomy, investigators at the European Institute of Oncology designed the so-called IART® method: a radionuclide targeted therapy based on the high affinity between avidin and biotin based on the experience with the ROLL [11] and the avidin-biotin pretargeting technique [12–14].

Avidin is injected into the tumor bed intraoperatively and remains in the breast parenchyma for several days, acting as "new receptor" for ^{90}Y radio-labeled biotin which is administered intravenously to the patients 16–24 h after surgery.

Clinical studies conducted at the European Institute of Oncology have involved 10 patients in a Phase I dosimetric study and 35 patients in a Phase II protocol [15, 16]. Detailed dosimetry data from both studies show that intravenous administration of a fixed activity of 3.7 GBq ^{90}Y-ST2210 after 100 mg of avidin provides a boost of 20 Gy absorbed dose, corresponding to a Biological Effective Dose (BED) of 21 Gy, in the tumor bed (mean BED ± standard deviation 21.2 ± 4.3 Gy).

Based on the positive results of the above studies, we may today affirm that IART® is able to provide, in a reproducible manner, a boost of 20 ± 4.0 Gy to the operated tumor bed as for IORT, without the need of a linear accelerator.

The advantage of the IART® boost is mainly logistical. In fact, IORT + EBRT require special facilities equipped with linear accelerators. The avidin injected intraoperatively by the surgeon into the tumor bed is retained at the site of injection for several days acting as "new receptor" for ^{90}Y radio-labeled biotin which is administered intravenously to patient 16–24 h after surgery by the nuclear medicine physician. Two studies have been published so far on IART®:

– Phase I (biodistribution) study ($n = 11$ patients). Local as well as systemic distribution data have underlined the very specific uptake of radiation to the operated tumor area, with a limited amount of radiation in the rest of the mammary gland, as well as the sparing of surrounding/distant organs [17].

– Phase II (efficacy/safety) study ($n = 35$ patients). Detailed dosimetry data showed that patients receiving an intramammary injection of 100 mg avidin in the tumor bed, when systemically injected with a fixed activity of 3.7 GBq ^{90}Y biotin-DOTA, received a radiation boost of 20 Gy (BED equal to 21.2 ± 4.3 Gy). This was equivalent to the dose achieved with an intraoperative injection of 150 mg of avidin (BED = 19.7 ± 3.9 Gy). These data clearly indicate the performance of IART® in delivering the required radiation locally [16].

The IART® method is a radionuclide targeted therapy based on the high affinity between avidin and biotin. Avidin is a 66-kDa highly glycosylated and positively charged (isoelectric point, $pI \cong 10$) tetrameric protein derived from eggs. It shows extremely high affinity for the 244 Da vitamin H, biotin ($K_d = 10$–15 M) [18].

The avidin, intraoperatively injected to the tumor bed, is retained at the sites of injections for several hours, thus acting as "a new receptor" for radio-labeled biotin [15].

The IART® procedure consists of two steps:
1. Intraoperative injection of native avidin immediately after quadrantectomy (pre-targeting);
2. Targeting of the tumor by intravenous injection of ^{90}Yttrium-Biotin-DOTA (ST2210) 24 ± 12 h after surgery.

^{90}Yttrium (^{90}Y) is a high-energy pure β^- emitter, with a relatively short physical half-life ($T_{1/2}$ = 64.1 h) and a mean penetration range in tissue of 2.5 mm (R_{max} = 11.3 mm). Thus, ^{90}Y-ST2210 is particularly suitable for radionuclide therapy and the probability of killing the majority of neoplastic cells is related to the so-called cross-fire effect [19]. In addition, it is known that early administration of radiotherapy shows a positive effect in tumor control [20–22].

Two clinical studies were conducted on IART® at IEO: a phase I dosimetric study [15, 17] and a phase II dose-range study enrolling 35 patients [16].

Two-Step IART® Procedure

Step 1: Avidination of the tumor bed with native avidin by surgeon.
Step 2: Intravenous injection 90Y-labeled biotin.

Pharmacokinetics Biodistribution and Dosimetry

In the IEO S208/204 study [17], ten patients received ^{111}In-ST2210 infusion (108 ± 9 MBq) the day after the surgical intervention. Indium-111 (^{111}-In) is a gamma emitting radionuclide used to provide pharmacokinetics of the ^{90}Y labeled ST2210. Thus, it is possible to predict the dosimetry with ^{90}Y-biotin. On average, the ^{111}In-ST2210 was administered 21 ± 3h after the avidin injection. Patients showed no clinical adverse reactions. The injection of avidin during the surgical intervention was well tolerated and no side effects after the i.v. injection of ^{111}In-ST2210 were observed.

ST2210 cleared rapidly from the blood stream, decreasing to less than 1% of the injected activity within 12 h after injection and the mean activity in blood at 12 h post injection was $0.15 \pm 0.11\%$ of the injected activity.

The cumulative activity excreted in the urine 24 h after injection was $81.4 \pm 12.2\%$ of the injected activity.

The mean uptake of the breast region was equal to $6 \pm 2.5\%$ of the injected activity (IA). The radioactivity — labeled to avidin — was localized to the breast region only, without diffusion to the organs surrounding the operated breast (lung, ribs, heart). The radiation dose released to the tumor bed was more than 5 Gy/GBq, consistent with a boost of 20 Gy in the tumor bed for a standard activity of 3.7 GBq ^{90}Y-ST2210. The absorbed doses to the normal organs (urinary bladder, kidneys) were far from the threshold doses of tissue side effects reported in the literature [23, 24]. In particular, for an injection of 3.7 GBq, the absorbed dose to the kidney resulted to be 4.4 ± 1.5 Gy, corresponding to a kidney BED of 4.8 ± 1.8 Gy, clearly lower than the threshold dose for kidney toxicity [25].

The above results provided the rationale for a further phase I/II clinical trial conducted at IEO which included 35 patients. The main objective was to determine the optimal dose of avidin with a fixed activity of ^{90}Y-DOTA BIOTIN ST2210 able to provide a boost of 20 Gy (BED 21 Gy). This early boost was followed, 3–4 weeks after quadrantectomy (as soon as the conditions of the surgical wound as well as of the breast and/or of the lymph nodes allow the administration of the radiotherapy on the radiotherapist's judgment), by an accelerated EBRT of an additional 40 Gy in 20 fractions of 2 Gy each [16].

Thirty-eight subjects were included: 3 screening failures and 35 treated patients grouped in three consecutive cohorts according to different doses of avidin administered into the tumor bed immediately after surgical resection: 15 patients received 100 mg native avidin (group 1), 10 patients 50 mg avidin (group 2), and 10 patients received 150 mg avidin (group 3). The day after surgery all patients received a slow intravenous infusion of 3.7 GBq ^{90}Y-ST2210 spiked with ^{111}In (185 MBq) in order to obtain dosimetric data for each patient. All patients underwent partial breast

a

b

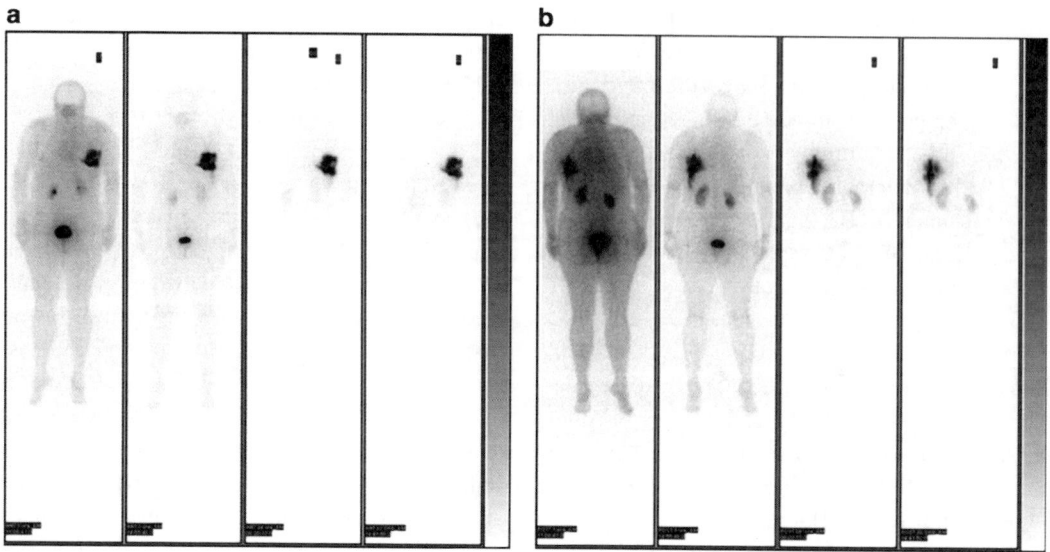

Fig. 10.1 Whole body scans in anterior (**a**) and posterior (**b**) projection acquired at 1, 3, 24 and 32 h post injection of ^{90}Y-biotin and ^{111}In-biotin in a patient operated in the left breast

resection (quadrantectomy). Sentinel node biopsy alone was carried out in 28 patients; 7 patients had sentinel node positive and axillary dissection followed. Pathological examination demonstrated an infiltrating ductal carcinoma in 24 cases, 2 mucinous carcinoma, 3 infiltrating lobular carcinoma, an infiltrating tubular carcinoma in 1 case, 2 infiltrating mixed carcinoma, 1 infiltrating papillary carcinoma; in 2 patients an intraepithelial neoplasia was diagnosed as DIN1 c, DIN G2, respectively.

After completion of IART® procedure, the WBS images (Fig. 10.1) showed a fast and intense uptake of the radio-labeled biotin in the breast area of all patients. Dosimetric data and estimated masses of the irradiated breast, obtained from the three cohorts of patients, showed that a considerable mass of breast parenchyma (mean value of 250 g) was irradiated (Fig. 10.2). Data from the 15 women given 100 mg avidin showed a mean absorbed dose to the breast of 19.5 ± 4.0 Gy in the area of highest uptake, with a corresponding BED of 21.2 ± 4.3 Gy. The dose of 100 mg of avidin resulted to be the most appropriate (and the minimum needed) in terms of dose delivery into the index quadrant. The gap between surgery and biotin injection did not influence the percentage uptake in the operated breast, which was up to ~12% with a mean value of ~8% (Table 10.1).

The absorbed dose to the red marrow was 0.2 ± 0.1 Gy, never exceeding 0.4 Gy, giving no concern for hematological toxicity.

The results obtained supported the conclusions of the phase I study: the injection of 3.7 GBq ^{90}Y-ST2210 provides a boost of 20 Gy in the tumor bed. One hundred milligrams has been identified as the minimum quantity of avidin that reliably provides the required BED, since 50 mg provides a slightly lower dose, while 150 mg does not appreciably increase it. The dose of 100 mg of avidin acts as an "interstitial molecular device" that specifically binds ^{90}Y-labeled-DOTA-biotin in a considerable mass of breast tissue without any significant side effects.

A tolerability issue can be raised as avidin is known to induce an immune response in the majority of human subjects [26, 27]. Despite the human anti-avidin antibody (HAVA) response, the clinical use of avidin, in hundreds of patients treated with either Pre-targeted Antibody Guided RadioImmunoTherapy (PAGRIT®), where avidin is injected intravenously, or IART®, where avidin is injected in the breast, has not been associated to any adverse event [5, 15, 18, 28, 29].

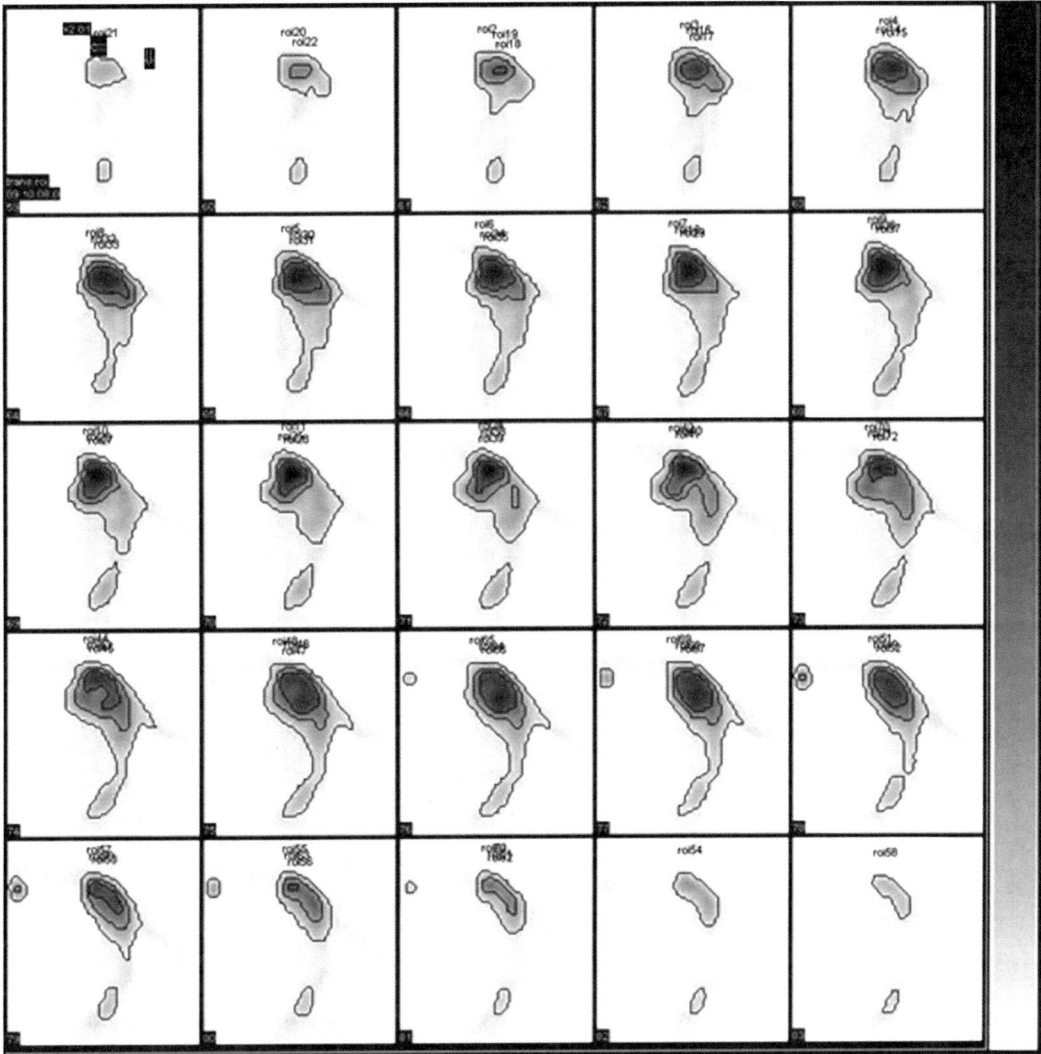

Fig. 10.2 Isorois referred to different grades of uptake in the tumor bed drawn on transassial SPECT images

Table 10.1 Dosimetric data (mean values ± SD) of the high uptake areas of the irradiated breast

Cohort	Avidin (mg)	Number of patients enrolled	%IA of ^{90}Y-biotin in the breast area	Uptake region	Absorbed doses (Gy)	Involved masses (g)	BED (Gy)
I	100	15	8.0 ± 3.3	high	19.5 ± 4.0	250 ± 100	21.2 ± 4.3
II	50	10	4.6 ± 1.2	high	13.0 ± 5.1	190 ± 50	13.8 ± 5.8
III	150	10	8.6 ± 3.5	high	18.4 ± 3.5	230 ± 130	19.7 ± 3.9

The scintigraphic images demonstrated rapid and stable uptake of labeled ^{90}Y-DOTA-biotin at the operated breast site. Moreover, in 20 out of 35 patients, the axillary lymph nodes or the internal mammary chain nodes were visualized. This observation indicates that avidin, as albumin colloids for the sentinel node biopsy, is drained into the blood stream through the lymphatic system, and so lymph node irradiation with IART® would also be possible.

Table 10.2 Local toxicity in 35 patients at different time points (after IART®, at the EBRT completion, 1 and 6 months after EBRT) evaluated by RTOG Scale

Local toxicity over the time	Number of patients				
	G0	G1	G2	G3	G4
Post IART®	12	23	0	0	0
Post EBRT (40 Gy)	0	4	25	3	0
4 weeks after EBRT	20	10	2	0	0
6 months after EBRT	27	5	0	0	0

Radionuclide therapy with IART® allows to:

1. Targeting only in the region of "interest"
2. Sparing the vital organs (lung, heart)
3. Reducing Less local damage and external burning
4. Reducing hospital visits by up to a third

Toxicity and Quality of Life

No side effects were observed after avidin administration and biotinylated HSA chase, nor after radio-labeled biotin, both ^{111}In or ^{90}Y labeled. Systemic toxicity, assessed by evaluating hematological, liver, and renal functions, was not found. The overall cosmetic result was good.

Table 10.2 reports local toxicity results in the patients who received EBRT after IART®. The majority of patients experienced low-grade toxicity during EBRT, starting from the second week. At the end of EBRT in 25 patients local toxicity was classified as G2, in 4 patients as G1. Grade 3 skin toxicity was observed in 3 patients. Four weeks after the completion of WB-EBRT, no local toxicity (G0) was observed in 20 cases, while 10 patients had residual G1 and 2 patients G2 toxicity. All patients completed the 6-month follow-up and showed an excellent tolerance to the whole treatment schedule. Figure 10.3 is an example of mild local toxicity through the time, with a complete recovery of 6 months after EBRT treatment. No local relapse has occurred to date in any patient with a median follow-up of 41 months (range 32–51).

Moreover, IART® plus short 4-week EBRT treatment was very well accepted by the patients. The quality of life, evaluated by EORTC QoL questionnaire, demonstrated no significant changes in patients' quality of life.

The rapid renal elimination of labeled DOTA-biotin is important for the radiation protection point of view, allowing a short period of hospitalization (ideally 1 day).

IART® could be an interesting nuclear medicine procedure for breast irradiation similar to the other techniques of PBI, offering many practical advantages over other methods.

One of the main advantages is its potential applicability to every kind of breast cancer patient scheduled for conservative surgery, without limitations of tumor location and size or multifocality. Importantly, with IART®, the irradiation field is identified with precision by the surgeon, who knows exactly where the tumor was located and therefore injects avidin under visual control directly into the tumor bed, thus preparing the remaining mammary gland to receive ^{90}Y-biotin. With a surgeon of average experience, avidin injection around the tumor bed should be simple and uniform throughout the target area of the breast. Another IART® advantage is that neither dedicated linear accelerator nor other sophisticated devices are needed. IART® is a procedure that may be applied worldwide in all hospitals where breast surgery is performed and a nuclear medicine unit is present. Moreover, the possibility to inject ^{90}Y-radio-labeled biotin 16–24 h after avidin administration makes the procedure suitable even if the nuclear medicine department is not close to the surgical unit. A future possible clinical scenario could be the production of ^{90}Y-radio-labeled biotin in a GMP central radio pharmacy and delivered within few hours to the surrounding hospitals. This should facilitate worldwide use of BCS and accelerated radiotherapy especially when logistical barriers to traveling are present, with consequent rebound on both the patient's quality of life and socioeconomic aspects.

Several studies support the rationale of intraoperative radiation therapy (RT) as an adjuvant therapy after surgery, including systematic

Fig. 10.3 Patient who received IART® plus EBRT: mild local toxicity (classified as G1) after delivery of 10 Gy (**a**), 40 Gy (**b**) by EBRT; partial recovery after 1 month after completion of EBRT (**c**); No residual signs of local toxicity 6 months after EBRT. Cosmetic outcome was judged good (**d**)

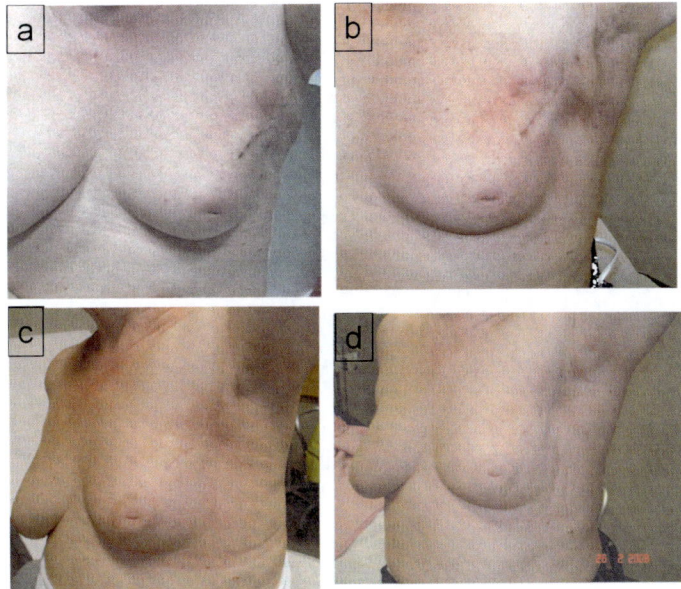

reviews [22]. Specifically, a short time interval between surgery and RT should increase the probability of local tumor control [30]. An analysis of the surviving fraction (SF) and the tumor control probability (TCP), evaluated after different schemes of radiation delivery to breast cancer cells, shows a decrease of the SF and an increase of the TCP when intraoperative radiation techniques are used, as compared to standard EBRT alone.

IART® can be considered as an "anticipated boost" 3–4 weeks before whole breast irradiation with EBRT. This will turn out in a new approach for accelerated whole breast irradiation after BCS, with considerable economical and social impact. As for sentinel node lympho-scintigraphy and biopsy [26, 31], we hope that this Nuclear Medicine technique will contribute to a better management of breast cancer patients.

The results of these pilot studies suggest that the IART® is a safe Nuclear Medicine Therapy procedure which delivers, 1 day after surgery, a 20 Gy dose in women who undergo BCS for breast cancer.

This approach is a useful, economical treatment in patients of nations with limited healthcare resources, as notoriously BCS and radiation therapy requires more economic resources than mastectomy. IART® could also improve breast cancer outcomes in such cases.

Accelerated Breast Irradiation: The Use of IART® + EBRT in Early Breast Cancer. The IEO Protocol

IART® Procedure

Step I: intraoperative phase

After the tumor has been removed, the surgeon injects native avidin, 100 mg, directly into and around the tumor bed, by several injections using an ad hoc syringe and a dedicated multi-hole needle device (Fig. 10.4). Avidin is diluted in 20 ml and each injection deposits 2 ml. Ten injections are perfomed in a Clock map to homogeneously cover the index quadrant (h 12-6-9-3-1-7-10-4 plus two more injections along the margins between 12 and 6).

Step II: postoperative phase

From 24 ± 12 h after the surgical intervention, and 10 min before the i.v. injection of radioactive biotin, 10 mg of HSA-biotin are administered intravenously in 1–2 min, in order to reduce the

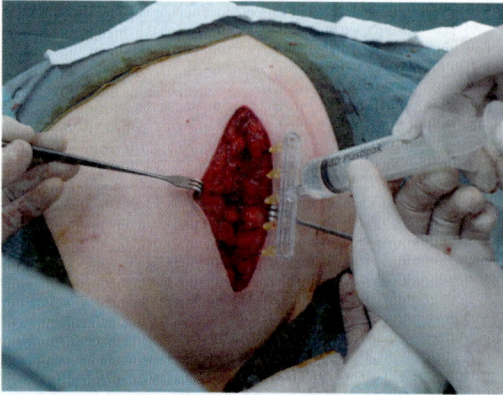

Fig. 10.4 A multihole needle conceived in order to deliver avidin at different depths into the breast parenchyma at each injection site

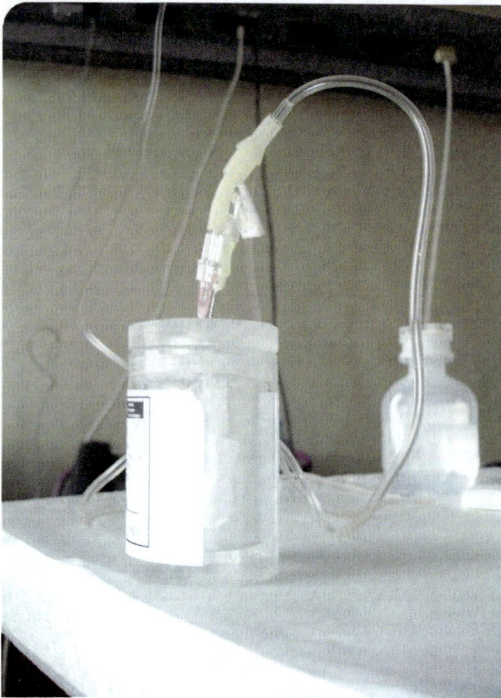

Fig. 10.5 Dedicated disposable system to intravenous injection of radiopharmaceuticals by slow infusion. The system allows to minimize the radiation exposure to the personnel

circulating levels of avidin and consequently the liver uptake of ^{90}Y-ST2210.

Thereafter, a dose of 100 mCi (3.7 GBq) of ^{90}Y-ST2210 (SA about 4 GBq/1 mg ST2210) + 185 (±10%) MBq of ^{111}In-ST2210 at the same SA are

injected intravenously in 30 minutes (slow infusion) using a dedicated disposable system (Fig. 10.5) [32].

Dosimetry

To evaluate the biodistribution (site of surgery, lymph nodes, and other tissues) and the percentage of the administered activity into the tumor bed, the following scans have to be performed:

- Whole body scintigraphic images within 30 min after the infusion of radiolabeled Biotin as well as 4±1, 16–20, 24–30, and 40–48 h after the radio-labeled drug administration, using a double-head γ-camera equipped with a medium-energy general-purpose collimator;
- Whole body transmission scan prior to ^{90}Y/^{111}In-ST2210 infusion;
- Hybrid SPECT/CT, 17–21 h after the radiolabeled drug administration, in order to provide maps of activity distribution of the index quadrant;
- Whole body low dose CT, concomitantly to SPECT in order to evaluate the patient-specific organ masses, especially the kidneys.

Before SPECT, three radioactive and radio-opaque markers are positioned on the skin of the patient to allow appropriate image matching. SPECT/CT fused images are used to assess the correct tracer localization in the breast (Fig. 10.2). Time activity curves are obtained for the normal organs from whole body images and the breast gland (SPECT and whole body images). The breast region is divided into three different areas:
1. High uptake area (uptake higher than 50% of the maximum—isorois 50%);
2. Medium uptake area (between 50 and 30% isorois);
3. Low uptake area (between 30 and 10% isorois).

For each patient, dose calculations have to be performed entering the number of decays (ND) estimated for normal organs (kidneys, heart, lungs, red marrow, urinary bladder contents, and remainder of the body) and irradiated breast in the OLINDA/EXM software [23], applying the correction for the individual patient weight and organ masses. In particular, the self-dose in the three breast areas are calculated considering the ND values derived for the three areas identified (high, medium, low uptake), with the approximation of uniform activity distribution in lesions (OLINDA/EXM, sphere model).

The linear quadratic model enables the comparison of doses released through EBRT to those from IART® for the analysis of possible effects on the operated breast and non-target organs. In particular, we adoptes the BED expression defined by [33].

$$\mathrm{BED} = D + \frac{1}{\alpha/\beta} \left(\frac{T_{1/2\,\mathrm{rep}}}{T_{1/2\,\mathrm{rep}} + T_{1/2\,\mathrm{eff}}} \right) \times D^2,$$

where D is the dose delivered; $T_{1/2\mathrm{rep}}$ is the repair half-time of sub-lethal damage; $T_{1/2\mathrm{eff}}$ is the effective half-life of the radiopharmaceutical in the specific tissue. The α/β ratio relates the intrinsic radio-sensitivity (α) and the potential sparing capacity (β) for a specified tissue or effect. For the breast region, we used a $T_{1/2\mathrm{rep}}$ equal to 1.5 h, α/β 10 Gy; for the kidneys, we used a $T_{1/2\mathrm{rep}}$ equal to 2.8 h, α/β 2.6 Gy [25, 33, 34].

Radiation Therapy (RT)

All patients receive accelerated postoperative EBRT to the entire breast with tangent fields: 2.85 Gy × 13 fractions equal to 37 Gy BED. EBRT should start at least 3 weeks after the quadrantectomy, as soon as the conditions of the surgical wound as well as of the breast and/or of the lymph nodes allow the administration of the radiotherapy on the radiotherapist's judgment.

Patients undergo virtual simulation including a treatment-planning CT scan. At the time of CT scanning, the patient is placed on a breast board to ensure setup reproducibility, in the supine position with both arms raised above the head. Radio-opaque markers are placed beyond the superior, inferior, lateral, and medial border of the palpated ipsilateral breast tissue. Contiguous 5-mm CT axial images are obtained extending from the pulmonary apex to the upper abdomen including the entire breast and lungs. Dataset are then transferred to a 3D treatment planning workstation for treatment planning. The residual breast, the contra lateral breast, the heart, and lungs are outlined (manually or automatically) on each of the acquired CT slices.

Conclusion

BCS followed by postoperative EBRT is the treatment of choice in patients with early breast cancer (stage I–II). There are over 700,000 new cases of breast cancer patients/year in EU and US, 88% are stage I–II and 70% of them (around 450,000) need radiotherapy. Irradiating the mammary gland using a nuclear medicine technique (IART®) is possible. IART® is a simple technique that consists of two steps:

1. Intraoperative "avidination" of the anatomical area of the tumor after its removal by the surgeon, who injects with a syringe a solution of avidin into the mammary gland;
2. Postoperative (16–24 h after surgery) delivery of a radiation dose by targeting the "avidinated" area of the mammary gland with ^{90}Y-labeled biotin, via a slow intravenous injection. The two steps are based on the incredible high affinity between avidin and biotin, the highest affinity known in nature.

Phase I and II studies conducted at the European Institute of Oncology in Milan, Italy, showed that IART® can safely deliver a dose of radiation (23–25 Gy), targeting the mammary region of interest, sparing the surrounding organs (lungs and heart), with minimal skin damage.

IART® peri-operative timing allows starting adjuvant treatment after conservative surgery immediately, thus minimizing the negative outcomes associated with delayed radiotherapy. This, in turn, permits abbreviated EBRT, that can reduce the burden for patients from the usual 5–7 weeks of daily sessions to just 2 weeks. In low risk patients such as postmenopausal women, IART® has the potential to replace EBRT after BCS. From the technical and logistic point of view, IART® offers several advantages over other irradiation methods. It is applicable to the majority of breast cancers, without limitation to location, size, or multifocality; it can be carried out in any hospital, independently of the availability of radiotherapy, thus facilitating a wider adoption of conservative breast surgery. This standard of care is not practiced in many areas of the world because radiotherapy centers are unable to cope with the current demand (which is expected to further increase in the next 10 years), or are too distant from patients' homes.

Future Considerations

IART® is a "molecular brachytherapy" approach for delivering an appropriate amount of radiation in a very selected anatomical area. As such, it can be used in a variety of solid tumors, such as those of bladder, prostate, peritoneum, pleura, and brain, both in an adjuvant and in a palliative setting. For superficial bladder cancer and stage I–II prostate cancer, IART® might represent an alternative option to BCC therapy and 125I seeds, respectively. In malignant brain tumors such as glioblastoma, ^{90}Y biotin associated to Moabs biotinylated and avidin has been reported in phase I-II studies. However, in these very aggressive diseases, IART® as anticipated boost to conventional EBRT might improve PFS and OS. Only phase III dedicated randomized trials will give us the answer. The real problem remains the lack of financial support for such randomized trials.

References

1. Anderson BO, Shyyan R, Eniu A, Smith RA, Yip CH, Bese NS, et al. Breast cancer in limited-resource countries: an overview of the Breast Health Global Initiative 2005 guidelines. Breast J. 2006;12 Suppl 1:S3–15.
2. Jemal A, Siegel R, Xu J, Ward E. Cancer statistics, 2010. CA Cancer J Clin. 2010;60(5):277–300.
3. Veronesi U, Luini A, Galimberti V, Zurridda S. Conservation approaches for the management of stage I/II carcinoma of the breast: Milan Cancer Institute trials. World J Surg. 1994;18:70–5.
4. Dragun AE, Huang B, Tucker TC, Spanos WJ. Disparities in the application of adjuvant radiotherapy after breast-conserving surgery for early stage breast cancer: impact on overall survival. Cancer. 2011; 117(12):2590–8.
5. NHI Consensus Conference. Treatment of early breast cancer. JAMA. 1991;265:391–5.
6. Bartelink H, Horiot JC, Poortmans P, et al. European Organization for Research and Treatment of Cancer Radiotherapy and Breast Cancer Groups. Recurrence rates after treatment of breast cancer with standard radiotherapy with or without additional radiation. N Engl J Med. 2001;345:1378–87.
7. Jones HA, Antonini N, Hart AAM, et al. Impact of pathological characteristics on local relapse after breast-conserving therapy: a subgroup analysis of the EORTC boost versus no boost trial. J Clin Oncol. 2009;27:4939–47.
8. Ivaldi GB, et al. Preliminary results of electron intraoperative therapy boost and hypofractionated external beam radiotherapy after breast conserving surgery in premenopausal women. Int J Radiat Oncol Biol Phys. 2008;72(2):485–93.
9. Reitsamer R, Peintinger F, Sedlmayer F, Kopp M, Menzel C, Cimpoca W, et al. Intraoperative radiotherapy given as a boost after breast-conserving surgery in breast cancer patients. Eur J Cancer. 2002;38(12): 1607–10.
10. Lemanski C, Azria D, Thezenas S, Gutowski M, Saint-Aubert B, Rouanet P, et al. Intraoperative radiotherapy given as a boost for early breast cancer: long-term clinical and cosmetic results. Int J Radiat Oncol Biol Phys. 2006;64(5):1410–5.
11. De Cicco C, Pizzamiglio M, Trifirò G, Luini A, Ferrari M, Prisco G, et al. Radioguided occult lesion localisation (ROLL) and surgical biopsy in breast cancer: technical aspects. Q J Nucl Med. 2002;46:145–51.
12. Goldenberg DM, Sharkey RM, Paganelli G, Barbet J, Chatal JF. Antibody pretargeting advances cancer radioimmunodetection and radioimmunotherapy. J Clin Oncol. 2006;24:823–34.
13. Grana C, Chinol M, Robertson C, Mazzetta C, Bartolomei M, De Cicco C, et al. Pretargeted adjuvant radioimmunotherapy with Yttrium-90-biotin in malignant glioma patients: a pilot study. B J Cancer. 2002; 86:207–12.
14. Paganelli G, Grana C, Chinol M, Cremonesi M, De Cicco C, De Braud F, et al. Antibody-guided three-step therapy for high grade glioma with yttrium-90 biotin. Eur J Nucl Med. 1999;26(4):348–57.
15. Paganelli G, Ferrari M, Cremonesi M, De Cicco C, Galimberti V, Luini A, et al. IART®: intraoperative avidination for radionuclide treatment. A new way of partial breast irradiation. Breast. 2007;16:17–26.
16. Paganelli G, De Cicco C, Ferrari M, Carbone G, Pagani G, Leonardi MC, et al. Intraoperative avidination for radionuclide treatment as a radiotherapy boost in breast cancer: results of a phase II study with ^{90}Y-labeled biotin. Eur J Nucl Med Mol Imaging. 2010;37:203–11.
17. Paganelli G, Ferrari M, Ravasi L, Cremonesi M, De Cicco C, Galimberti V, et al. Intraoperative avidination for radionuclide therapy: a prospective new development to accelerate radiotherapy in breast cancer. Clin Cancer Res. 2007;13 Suppl 18:5646s–51.

18. Wilchek M, Bayer EA. The avidin-biotin complex in immunology. Immunol Today. 1984;5:39–43.
19. Schubiger PA, Alberto R, Smith A. Vehicles, chelators, and radionuclides: choosing the "Building Block" of an effective therapeutic radioimmunoconjugate. Bioconjug Chem. 1996;7:165–79.
20. Wyatt RM, Beddoe AH, Dale RG. The effects of delays in radiotherapy treatment on tumour control. Phys Med Biol. 2003;48:139–55.
21. Mackillop WJ, et al. The effect of delay in treatment on local control by radiotherapy. Int J Radiat Oncol Biol Phys. 1996;34(1):243–50.
22. Mackillop WJ, et al. Does delay in starting treatment affect the outcomes of radiotherapy? A systematic review. J Clin Oncol. 2003;21(3):555–63.
23. Cassady JR. Clinical radiation nephropathy. Int J Radiat Oncol Biol Phys. 1995;31:1249–56.
24. Emami B, Lyman J, Brown A, et al. Tolerance of normal tissue to therapeutic irradiation. Int J Radiat Oncol Biol Phys. 1991;21:109–22.
25. Wessels BW, Konijnenberg MB, Dale RG, Breitz HB, Cremonesi M, Meredith RF, et al. MIRD Pamphlet No. 20: the effect of model assumptions on kidney dosimetry and response: implications for radionuclide therapy. J Nucl Med. 2008;49:1884–99.
26. Poortmans PM, et al. The addition of a boost dose on the primary tumour bed after lumpectomy in breast conserving treatment for breast cancer. A summary of the results of EORTC 22881-10882 "boost versus no boost" trial. Cancer Radiother. 2008;2(6–7):565–70.
27. Reitsamer R, et al. The Salzburg concept of intraoperative radiotherapy for cancer: results and considerations for breast. Int J Cancer. 2006;118:2882–7.
28. Veronesi U, Salvadori B, Luini A, et al. Breast conservation is a safe method in patients with small cancer of the breast. Long term results of three randomized trials on 1973 patients. Eur J Cancer. 1995;31:1574–9.
29. Fisher B, Anderson S, Bryant J, et al. Twenty-year follow-up of a randomized trail comparing total mastectomy, lumpectomy plus irradiation for the treatment of invasive breast cancer. N Engl J Med. 2002;347:1233–41.
30. The START Trialists' Group. The UK Standardisation of Breast Radiotherapy (START) Trial A of radiotherapy hypofractionation for treatment of early breast cancer: a randomised trial. Lancet Oncol. 2008;9:331–41.
31. The START Trialists' Group. The UK Standardisation of Breast Radiotherapy (START) Trial B of radiotherapy hypofractionation for treatment of early breast cancer: a randomised trial. Lancet. 2008;371:1098–107.
32. Paganelli G, Ferrari M, De Cicco C, et al. Intraoperative avidination for radionuclide treatment (IART®) post quadrantectomy in breast cancer: predicted dosimetry with ^{90}Y-biotin. JNM. 2006;47:488P.
33. Dale R, Carabe-Fernandez A. The radiobiology of conventional radiotherapy and its application to radionuclide therapy. Cancer Biother Radiopharm. 2005;20(1):47.
34. Rosenstein BS, Lymberis SC, Formenti SC. Biologic comparison of partial breast irradiation protocols. Int J Radiat Oncol Biol Phys. 2004;60:1393–404.

Radiomicrosphere Therapy of Liver Tumors

11

Seza A. Gulec, Rekha Suthar, and Tushar Barot

Introduction

Radiomicrosphere therapy (RMT) using Yttrium-90 (Y-90) microspheres has entered the contemporary management paradigm of a number of primary and metastatic liver neoplasms. There has been a remarkable improvement in clinical techniques of the modality since its first entry to the United States in 2000 and clinical applications of Y-90 microspheres are steadily expanding. The growing experience brings more responsibility onto the nuclear medicine community, as some of the most critical questions and controversies in the practical daily clinical use of RMT are related to nuclear medicine techniques.

RMT refers to intra-arterial administration of microspheres of *any chemical composition* labeled with *any radioisotope*. The first clinical applications of the technique date back early 1960s [1]. The beta particle-emitting Y-90 is currently the radioisotope of choice for the commercially available resin and glass microspheres. Y-90 has a high energy beta particle. It is incorporated into

S.A. Gulec, M.D., F.A.C.S. (✉) • R. Suthar, M.D.
Department of Radiology/Nuclear Medicine,
Florida International University College of Medicine,
11200 SW 8th Street, Miami 33199 FL, USA
e-mail: sgulec@fiu.com

T. Barot, M.D.
Departments of Surgical Oncology and Radiology/
Nuclear Medicine, Florida International University
College of Medicine, 11200 SW 8th Street,
Miami 33199 FL, USA

biocompatible microspheres measuring 30–40 μm. These preparations are approved for use in the treatment of primary and metastatic liver tumors. Other uses are currently under investigation.

The intellectual basis for Y-90 microsphere treatment is the preferential distribution of microspheres into the tumor compartment as opposed to normal hepatocellular parenchyma. Tumor blood supply is mostly derived from the hepatic artery since the neovasculature resulting from tumor angiogenesis is based on hepatic arterial branches. Therapeutic materials infused into the hepatic artery preferentially target tumor in proportion to the tumor blood flow. Y-90 microspheres infused into the hepatic artery are entrapped in the microvasculature with a high tumor-to-liver concentration ratio. The result is delivery of a tumoricidal dose of radiation with limited radiation injury to the normal hepatocellular parenchyma (Fig. 11.1).

RMT differs from nonradioactive transarterial particle therapies directed at tumor in one important aspect: namely that the goal is non-occlusive delivery of particles. In bland embolization or chemoembolization, the goal is to achieve occlusion of the tumor vasculature in order to produce tumor killing by hypoxia. In RMT, the therapeutic effectiveness requires continued blood flow to enhance free radical-dependent cell death [2]. Radiation combined with embolization-induced hypoxia is undesirable because the radio-biologic response is optimized by preservation of blood flow, and hence oxygenation, to the target area.

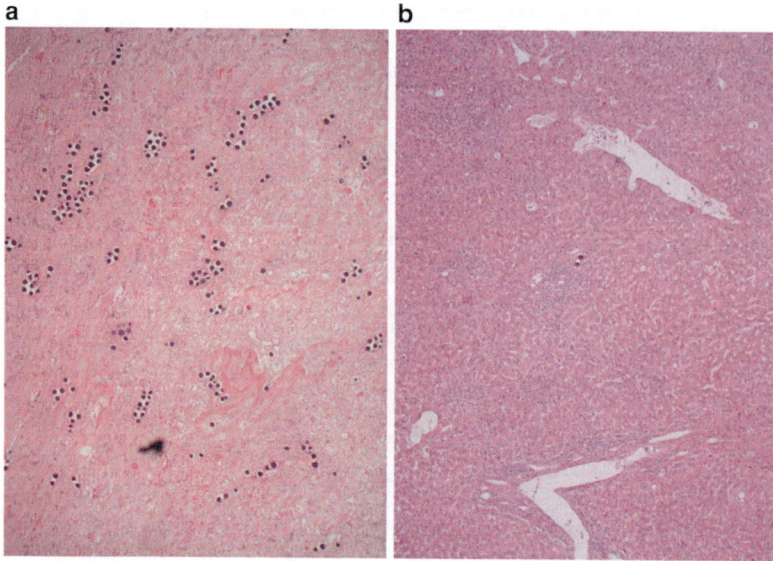

Fig. 11.1 Distribution of microspheres infused by transarterial route into the liver. Note the arterial position of the microspheres within the tumor (*left panel*). The *right* *panel* shows the rare deposit of microsphere within the normal liver parenchyma

Y-90 Microsphere Products

Two commercial products are available in the United States at the present time. SIR-Spheres® (Sirtex Medical, Wilmington, MA) resin microspheres are polymer beads designed to be 20–40 μm in diameter and bound with Y-90 with a specific activity of 40–70 Bq/sphere. Thera Sphere® (MDS Nordion, Kanata, Canada) are glass microspheres, 20–30 μm in diameter, with a Y-90 specific activity of 2,400–2,700 Bq/sphere. Typical treatment doses are in the range of 2–6 GBq; the maximum administered activity for resin microspheres has generally been limited to 3 GBq while it may be as high as 9 GBq for glass microspheres [3, 4].

The incorporation of Y-90 in resin and glass microspheres is essentially different. The Y-90 resin microspheres are constructed with chemical labeling of Y-90 to the surface of the resin matrix whereas the Y-90 glass microspheres are produced by the neutron bombardment of a Y-90 yttrium-oxide bearing substrate that is integrally bound within the glass matrix of the microsphere in a high flux reactor. There are two main methods for producing Y-90 for the radiolabeling of resin microspheres: (1) nuclear-reactor produc-

tion (neutron activation); and (2) Sr-90/Y-90 generator production. The generator produces "carrier-free" (no carrier added) Y-90 ($T_{1/2}$=64.1 h); the only significant potential radionuclide impurity is Sr-90 ($T_{1/2}$=29.1 year). Reactor-produced Y-90 contains several parts per million of radioactive impurities, the most significant being Y-88, which decays by electron capture or positron emission with a physical half-life of 106.6 days. By virtue of its generation process, long-lived radiocontaminants such as Eu-152 may be present in Y-90 glass microspheres. The radiocontaminant profiles of resin and glass microspheres show differences related to their production mechanisms. Resin microspheres were shown to contain detectable amounts of Y-88, and glass microspheres may have Y-88, Eu-154 ($T_{1/2}$=8.8 year), Eu-152 ($T_{1/2}$=13.3 year), Co-57 ($T_{1/2}$=270.9 day), and Co-60 ($T_{1/2}$=5.27 year). Dose calculations indicated that the radiocontaminant dose contribution did not exceed the medical event limit, but licensees may need to be concerned with disposal of the microspheres due to the long-lived contaminants that may be present and detectable long after all the Y-90 has decayed. Glass microspheres are not known to have free Y-90 in the treatment vial, nor is there any significant amount of Y-90 that leaches from the glass matrix. Resin microspheres, on the other hand, may have trace amounts of free Y-90 in solution, perhaps as high as 0.4% of the Y-90 administered activity, which can be excreted in the urine during the first 24 h. Trace amounts (25–50 kBq/L/GBq) of urinary excretion are a possibility in the first 24 h after administration [5].

Y-90 Microsphere Products

- SIR-Spheres® (Sirtex Medical, Wilmington, MA)
- Resin microspheres (polymer beads) 20–40 μm in diameter
- Y-90 label—specific activity: 40–70 Bq/microsphere
- Typical treatment activity: 2–6 GBq; generally limited to 3 GBq
  - Thera Sphere® (MDS Nordion, Kanata, Canada)
- Glass microspheres, 20–30 μm in diameter
- Y-90 label—specific activity: 2,400–2,700 Bq/sphere
- Typical treatment activity: as high as 9 GBq

Clinical Applications

Hepatic Colorectal Metastases

There have been numerous studies testing the use of RMT using Y-90 microspheres as treatment for unresectable metastatic colorectal cancer including retrospective studies from New Zealand and the United States. More recently, encouraging data from phase I and II trials have led to two phase III trials [6–10].

Retrospective data from New Zealand: The RMT technique adapted by Stubbs et al. involved administration of 2–3 GBq Y-90 microspheres into the hepatic artery via a subcutaneous port followed at 4 weeks intervals by regional chemotherapy with 5-fluorouracil. An early report on 50

patients with advanced, unresectable colorectal liver metastases who were treated with RMT between February 1997 and June 1999 demonstrated that RMT was well tolerated with no treatment-related mortality. Morbidity including duodenal ulceration, however, was noted in 12 of 50 patients (24%). Median carcinoembryonic antigen (CEA) values 1 and 2 months after RMT (expressed as percentage of initial CEA) were 19% and 13%, respectively. Median survival for patients who developed extrahepatic disease within 6 months of RMT ($n = 26$) was 6.9 months (range 1.3–18.8 months). In those who did not develop extrahepatic disease ($n = 24$), the median survival was 17.5 months (range 1.0–30.3 months) [11].

Retrospective data from the United States in the salvage setting: Cumulative data analyzed by Kennedy et al. on 208 patients who were treated from April 2002 to April 2005 at seven institutions with a median follow-up of 13 months (1–42 months) indicated a median survival of 10.5 months for responders, and 4.5 months in nonresponders. No treatment-related procedure deaths or radiation-related liver failure was encountered. Response rates as defined by CT, CEA, and FDG PET were 35%, 70%, and 91%, respectively [12].

Phase I/II dose escalation study in combination with oxaliplatin: Twenty patients were studied in a phase I/II dose escalation trial of systemic chemotherapy using FOLFOX 4 plus RMT. The study population consisted of patients with nonresectable liver-dominant metastatic colorectal adenocarcinoma, who had not previously been treated with chemotherapy. The investigators were successful at achieving safe delivery of standard doses of oxaliplatin (85 mg/m²). The toxicity profile of combined FOLFOX and RMT was very similar to that observed in other phase III trials of FOLFOX 4 alone. The only difference was the presence of abdominal pain, which was reported at grade 1–3 levels in 50% of patients within 48 h of RMT administration. These episodes of abdominal pain were self-limiting. The overall response as measured by RECIST was 90% (CR + PR), with the remaining patients (10%) having stable disease. Of note, two of the

20 patients in this study had their disease sufficiently down-staged to allow subsequently surgically resection [8].

Phase I/II dose escalation study in combination with irinotecan: A phase I/II dose escalation trial of systemic chemotherapy using irinotecan plus RMT was also performed. Twenty-five patients who had failed previous chemotherapy, but were naive to irinotecan, were entered into the study. Irinotecan was given, starting the day before RMT, for a maximum of nine cycles. The irinotecan dose was escalated from 50 to 100 mg/m^2. Early stage acute and self-limiting nausea, vomiting, and liver pain were experienced by most patients. Mild lethargy and anorexia were also common. Grade 3/4 toxic events were seen in four out of six patients at 50 mg/m^2, four out of 13 patients at 75 mg/m^2, and two out of six patients at 100 mg/m^2. Of evaluable patients, partial responses were seen in nine out of 17 patients. Median time to liver progression was 7.5 months and median survival was 12 months [9].

Randomized phase II comparison of chemotherapy vs. chemotherapy plus SIRT as first-line treatment (Chemo-SIRT Trial): A phase II clinical trial using resin microspheres concomitantly with modern chemotherapy regimens as a frontline application was completed at the Center for Cancer Care in Goshen, IN [10]. Patients with disease limited predominantly to the liver were eligible for the study. SIRT was administered to either one lobe or to the whole liver on day 2 of the first chemotherapy course. Chemotherapy (FOLFOX or FOLFIRI) was repeated on a biweekly schedule. CEA levels, response evaluation criteria in solid tumors (RECIST), and metabolic response by PET/CT were used to determine tumor response at 4, 8, and 12 weeks after therapy. Fifteen patients were enrolled. Mean tumor absorbed dose was 137 Gy (range 50–285 Gy). Mean liver absorbed dose was 39 Gy (range 6–93 Gy). All tumors in chemo-RMT treated lobes showed a response by PET criteria (V_F) (Fig. 11.2). Mean percent decreases in V_F for

chemo-RMT and chemo-alone treated fields were 86% and 35%, respectively. Mean percent decreases in VA for chemo-RMT and chemo-alone treated fields were 59% and 22%, respectively. A V_F decrease of >90% (complete metabolic response) was observed in 73% of chemo-RMT and 40% of chemo-alone treatment fields. No disease progression was observed in the chemo-RMT treated fields, whereas 27% of the chemo-alone treated fields showed disease progression during the course of therapy. Changes in V_F preceded the changes in cross-sectional scanning and were documented as early as 4 weeks (Fig. 11.3).

Randomized phase III regional chemotherapy vs. RMT plus regional chemotherapy: A randomized phase III trial was performed comparing hepatic arterial chemotherapy (FUDR 0.3 mg/kg/day for 12 days and repeated every 4 weeks for 18 months) alone vs. combined RMT (2–3 GBq of Y-90 activity) plus HAC with FUDR. The outcome documented in this 74 patient trial showed significant improvement resulting from the addition of RMT to systemic chemotherapy. Toxicity data showed no difference in grade 3 or 4 toxicity between the two treatment arms. There was a significant increase in the complete and partial response rate (CR + PR = 17.6–44%, $p = 0.01$) and prolongation of time-to-disease progression in the liver (9.7–15.9 months, $p = 0.001$) for patients receiving the combination treatment. Although the trial design was not of sufficient statistical power to detect a survival difference, there was a trend observed towards improved survival for the combination treatment arm (Fig. 11.4). Exploratory subset regression analysis suggested improved survival for those patients who survived at least 15 months ($p = 0.06$) [6]. Despite the high response rate from regional treatment of the liver metastases, failure to control the disease at extrahepatic sites was problematic among the patients in this phase III trial. This is consistent with findings from the meta-analysis of HAC and indicates the need to add systemic treatment to this management strategy.

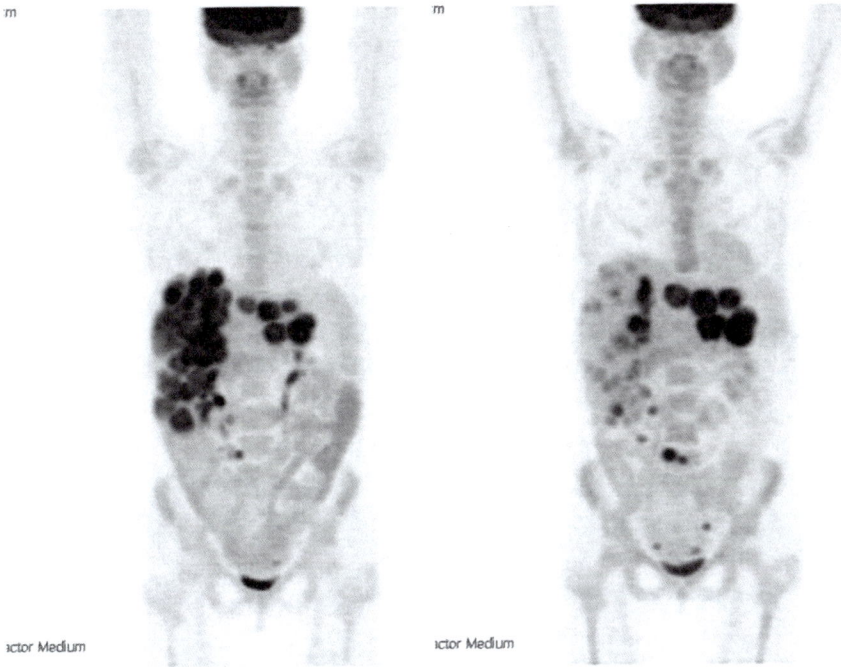

Fig. 11.2 Positron emission tomography demonstrating response of tumor in the right lobe of liver to combined RMT and chemotherapy

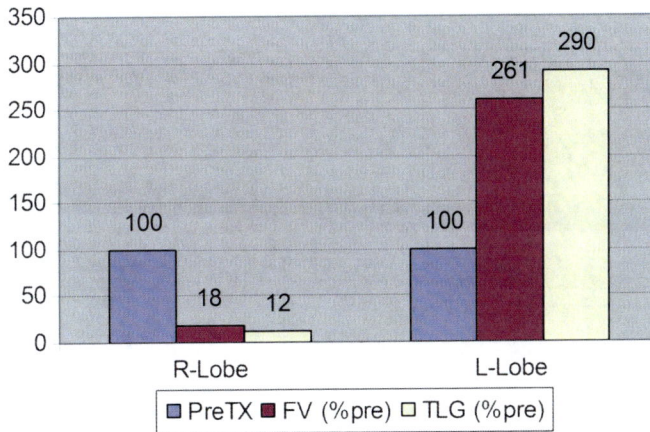

Fig. 11.3 Fluorodeoxyglucose uptake before (PreTX) and after combined RMT (delivered to right lobe) and chemotherapy. Results are shown for right (R-lobe) and left lobe (L-Lobe) of liver

Randomized trial of systemic chemotherapy vs. RMT plus chemotherapy: A study combining RMT with systemic chemotherapy (5-FU/LV) was designed as a randomized phase II/III trial. RMT was used in combination with systemic chemotherapy and was compared to chemotherapy alone. The hypothesis tested in this study was that systemic chemotherapy potentiates RMT and results in better response rates in the liver. In addition, a beneficial effect of systemic chemotherapy

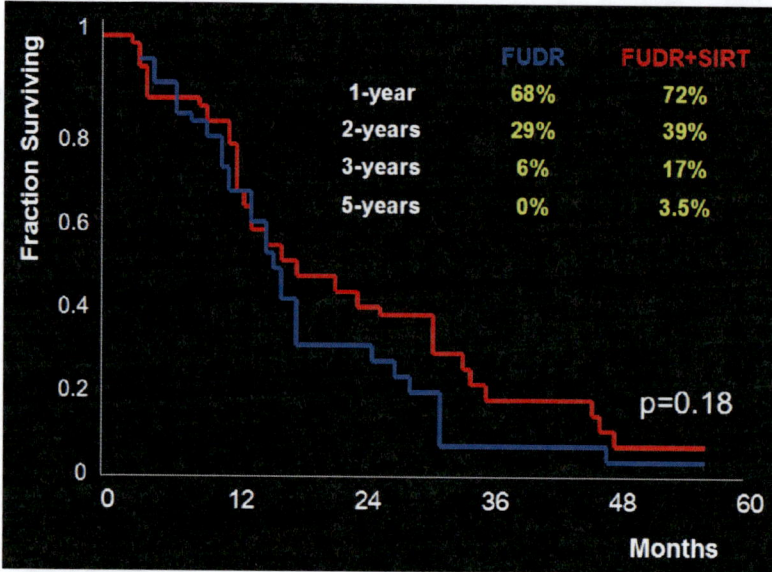

Fig. 11.4 Overall survival of patients subjected to regional chemotherapy alone (*blue curve*) vs. those subjected to combined RMT and chemotherapy (*red curve*)

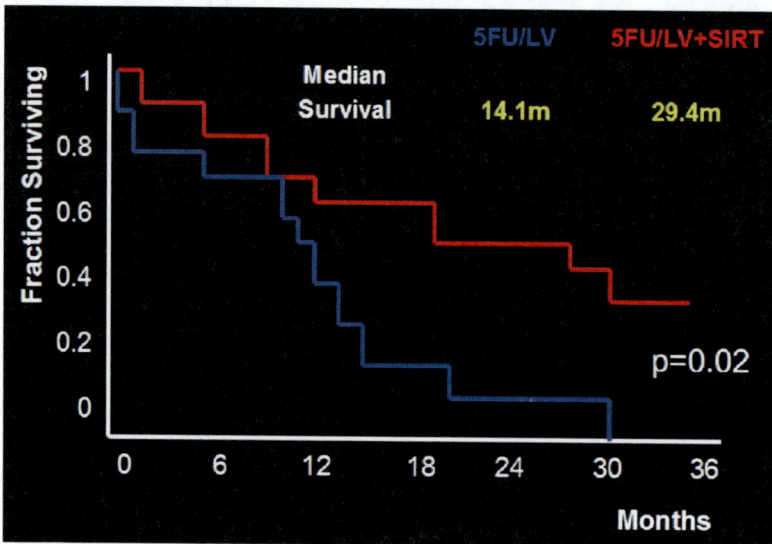

Fig. 11.5 Overall survival of patients subjected to systemic chemotherapy alone (5-FU/LV) (*blue curve*) vs. those subjected to RMT and systemic chemotherapy (*red curve*)

on extrahepatic metastases was sought. This trial accrued only 21 patients because of the impressive response to combined therapy (Fig. 11.5). The toxicity profile was higher in patients receiv- ing the combination treatment, although a dose modification of RMT decreased the toxicity profile to an acceptable level. Progression-free survival in the combination therapy arm was 18.6

months compared to 3.4 months in the chemotherapy alone arm ($p < 0.0005$). Overall median survival was 29.4 months in the combination therapy arm, compared to 12.8 months in the chemotherapy alone arm ($p = 0.02$). There was no difference in quality-of-life over a 3-month period between the two treatments when rated by patients ($p = 0.96$) or physicians ($p = 0.98$) [7].

Hepatocellular Carcinoma

There have been no randomized clinical trials with Y-90 microsphere treatment in hepatocellular carcinoma (HCC). However, an extensive world-wide clinical experience in this patient population has been reported.

Data from Hong Kong: Given the high prevalence of HCC in the region, Hong Kong has been a pivotal site for early (and ongoing) experience with Y-90 microsphere safety and efficacy studies. Early Y-90 microsphere trials by Hong Kong investigators concentrated on issues of safety and efficacy. In 1998, Lau et al. reported that the objective response with respect to changes in alpha-fetoprotein level was 89% (PR 67%, CR 22%). Of additional importance, this study reported that non-tumorous liver appears more tolerant to internal radiation than external beam radiation [13]. These investigators also correlated treatment efficacy with yttrium dose [14]. In a series of 18 patients treated with Y-90 microspheres for inoperable HCC, tumor regression was found to be dose-related with statistically improved survival for those patients treated with tumor dose exceeding 120 Gy. In 2001, Lau et al. reported, in a series of 82 patients, variables which may predict a more favorable outcome (improved survival) following Y-90 microsphere therapy: lower pretreatment level of alpha-fetoprotein and higher tumor-to-normal Y-90 microsphere uptake ratio. This study was also important in suggesting Y-90 microsphere treatment is effective for large tumors as well as tumor recurrence following surgical resection [15].

Data from the United States: Most early clinical work in the United States has focused on patient selection criteria. In a series of 121 patients, Goin et al. reported poor prognostic indicators: infiltrative or bulky disease, increase in liver enzyme levels, tumor volume at least 50% in combination with decreased serum albumin, elevated bilirubin, or predicted lung dose of greater than 30 Gy [16]. Patients with any of these risk factors were at greater risk for early death (<3 months) and were at increased risk of adverse events related to therapy. In the absence of these risk factors, patients demonstrated improved survival (median, 466 days) relative to patients in the high-risk group (median, 108 days). Salem et al., who has published extensively on Y-90 microsphere therapy, has further stressed the importance of patient selection in order to optimize treatment outcomes and avoid unnecessary morbidity and mortality. One study with 43 patients reported a median survival of 24.4 months for early stage disease and 12.5 months for later stage disease [17]. Factors found to be associated with decreased survival included those reported by Goin et al., presence of ascites, Eastern Cooperative Oncology Group (ECOG) performance status >0, presence of extrahepatic disease, >25% tumor burden, infiltrative disease, main portal vein thrombosis, and alpha fetoprotein >400 ng/mL. Salem et al. has also shown that, using appropriate selection and technique, Y-90 microsphere therapy can be administered to patients with compromised portal venous flow in the presence of portal vein thrombosis [18]. This report helped expand the patient population that can be safely treated with Y-90 microspheres.

Clinical Application of Intrahepatic Arterial-Radiolabeled Microspheres

- Colorectal hepatic metastases
- HCC
- Neuroendocrine hepatic metastases
- Cholangiocarcinoma
- Breast cancer
- Pancreatic cancer
- Other

Neuroendocrine Metastases to the Liver

To date there have been no randomized clinical trials with Y-90 microsphere SIRT in carcinoid or other neuroendocrine tumors (NET). In a retrospective analysis by Kennedy et al., both glass and resin Y-90 microspheres were evaluated in the treatment of 40 patients with NET. Radiographic responses were demonstrated (CR, PR) in 93% ($n=34$). There was low toxicity, and a subset of patients were able to discontinue palliative somatostatin therapy [19]. A recent report by Rhee et al. evaluated 42 patients treated with ceramic and resin microspheres. Greater radiotherapeutic activity was administered with ceramic microspheres without a significant difference in radiographic response (92% in the case of ceramic microspheres, and 94% in the case of resin microspheres) with overall medial survival of 25 months [20]. Kennedy et al. has reported median survival of 70 months in a 148 patient cohort undergoing resin microsphere therapy for metastatic NET [21]. Therapy was well tolerated with only 13% of patients reporting toxicities of three or higher (nausea, fatigue, pain, or ascites). Radiographic response reported as complete in 3% ($n=5$), partial in 60.5% ($n=112$), stable in 22.7% ($n=42$), and progressive in 4.9% ($n=9$).

An earlier retrospective study of 20 patients by Gulec et al. providing dosimetric data demonstrated that Y-90 microsphere therapy produced a significant objective response rate with no significant toxicity [22]. This study reviewed liver and tumor radiation doses using the medical internal radiation dosimetry (MIRD) technique. Liver toxicity was assessed clinically and by liver function tests, and the response to treatment was evaluated by *Octreoscan®*, Computed Tomography, and tumor markers. All patients had unresectable liver disease. Fifteen of the 20 patients (75%) were symptomatic despite maximal medical treatment and 2 of 20 patients had extrahepatic disease. The average administered activity was 1.6 GBq (0.6–3.2 GBq). Liver absorbed doses ranged from 0.3 to 99.5 Gy (mean: 28.9 Gy). Tumor absorbed doses ranged from 19.2 to 262.7 Gy (mean: 128.5 Gy). No treatment-related mortality, clinical radiation hepatitis, or veno-occlusive liver failure was seen. An objective response by CT and/or Octreoscan was observed in 18/20 (90%) and symptom control was achieved in 11 of 15 (73%) patients.

Other Primary and Metastatic Cancers

Much of the Y-90 microsphere research to date has concentrated on primary HCC and CRC liver metastases. Many other tumors also demonstrate liver metastases, and those patients with liver-dominant disease have been considered potential candidates for Y-90 microsphere therapy. Successful RMT in small series has been reported in a number of other primary and metastatic liver cancers. These include cholangiocarcinoma [23], breast cancer [24], pancreatic cancer [25], and other [26]. All series have demonstrated a therapeutic profile similar to more definitively studied liver cancers.

Clinical Practice of RMT

Pretreatment Evaluation/ Patient Selection

Evaluation of Liver Function: Liver reserve is affected by neoplastic replacement and prior hepatotoxic treatments. ALT/AST, and alkaline phosphatase/GGT are the markers for acute and subacute hepatocellular and bilio-canalicular injury, respectively. More difficult to evaluate is the real "functional volume" in the anatomically intact appearing liver regions. Bilirubin is a composite marker of liver reserve and has been widely used in many classification systems as a predictive measure. In practical terms, a bilirubin level above 2 mg/dL in the absence of correctable obstructive etiology precludes RMT.

CT and PET/CT
Standard imaging for detection and characterization of liver lesions is a multi-phase liver scan.

The initial examination is a non-contrast acquisition. This is followed by three additional acquisitions obtained at various times during the different phases of contrast medium distribution: (1) arterial phase acquisition, (2) portal phase acquisition, and (3) delayed phase acquisition (also termed an "equilibrium phase" study). Portal phase imaging has the highest yield for lesion detection in colorectal cancer liver metastases (CRCLM) as it shows the liver during highest parenchymal enhancement and consequently allows depiction of most lesions with greater lesion-to-liver contrast when compared to other phases. Arterial phase imaging best depicts tumors with a greater degree of neovascularity such as HCC and carcinoid/neuroendocrine tumors (NET). Arterial phase imaging also offers a fairly detailed overview of the arterial anatomy to the liver and dominant arteries contributing to tumor vascularity.

Tissue characterization by cross-sectional imaging to assess for tumor viability is based mainly on flow dynamics of the contrast medium and on changes in tumor size. FDG PET/CT technology adds a new phase to liver imaging through utilization of a metabolic tracer. F-18 Fluorodeoxy glucose (FDG) PET/CT clearly improves the diagnostic yield in patients based on CRCLM with superior detection of extrahepatic metastases. It is also very useful in the evaluation of response in Y-90 microsphere treatment [27–32]. The sensitivity of FDG PET/CT is low for HCC and NET lesions. There may still be a role for FDG PET imaging, however, for prognostication and for detection of extrahepatic lesions with aggressive clinical course. A practical imaging protocol for Y-90 microsphere workup includes FDG PET/CT, immediately followed by multi-phase contrast CT acquisition. The digital interface of PET/CT with radiation treatment planning software allows image quantitation with tumor and liver volume determinations.

Angiography

Angiography has a paramount importance in the planning and administration of RMT. Angiography depicts the vascular anatomy, identifies variant blood vessels, and allows exclusion of gastrointestinal branches with coil embolization. A methodical interrogation of the hepatic and visceral vasculature should be performed in all patients using digital subtraction imaging and power-injection technique to define tumor vascularity and discover variant anatomy. Major complications of RMT are a result of nontarget Y-90 microsphere localization.

It is critical to identify and investigate any and all potentially extra-hepatic branches. These extrahepatic branches may contribute to the tumor volume in question or supply visceral structures at risk for nontargeted embolization. These branches typically include the GDA, right and left gastric, phrenic, supraduodenal, and retroduodenal arteries. It is typically standard practice to identify and coil embolize any enteric branches that may be a source for nontarget embolization. Aside from the GDA, the right gastric is the extra-hepatic artery which is most commonly encountered. An active search for this vessel should be routine as this is a potential source of morbidity. The right gastric artery most commonly originates from the left hepatic artery, but may also arise from the common hepatic artery, the right hepatic artery, or the gastroduodenal artery. Liu et al. have published a comprehensive review detailing angiographic technique and visceral anatomy pertinent to delivery of Y-90 microspheres [33]. These authors have reported a gastrointestinal toxicity rate below 1%. This angiographic diligence is crucial as the deposition of Y-90 microspheres into gastroenteropancreatic vessels can result in significant morbidity (gastrointestinal inflammation/ulceration, pancreatitis, dermal pain/ulceration) if proper angiographic technique is not followed.

Detailed understanding of patient specific vascular anatomy also allows for accurate lobar volume calculations in order to prescribe the optimal Y-90 microsphere dose. In order to maximize tumor response and conserve normal liver function, it is extremely important that dosimetry calculations be based on the liver volume supplied by the arterial distribution that is to be catheterized at the time of treatment.

Table 11.1 Comparison of physical characteristics of resin microspheres, glass microspheres, and MAA particles

Characteristic	Resin	Glass	MAA
# Spheres (particles) per injected activity	60 million/3 GBq	1.2 million/3 GBq	0.8 million/0.3 GBq
Density (g/cc)	1.6	3.7	1.3

Hepatic Arterial Macroaggregated Albumin Imaging

^{99m}Tc-labeled macroaggregated albumin (MAA) is used clinically as a surrogate for the distribution of therapeutic microspheres. MAA is a biodegradable protein that is fragmented with sizes ranging between 10 and 100 μm. The majority of particles range from 20 to 60 μm in size. The density of MAA particles is less than that of the available microsphere products (Table 11.1).

Biologic degradation of MAA is size-dependent, ranging from 1 to 18 h. There are differences in the biologic half lives of commercially available MAA products. In general, a 6 h $T_{1/2}$ is accepted as the average. Approximately $4-6 \times 10^5$ fragments are injected (the standard for pulmonary perfusion imaging). Given the physical differences in quality, size, and particle number, MAA may not be an optimal surrogate for therapeutic microspheres. Despite these concerns, ^{99m}Tc-MAA is the current standard for evaluation of hepatic arterial flow. There are three objectives of Tc-99MAA study.

1. *Detection and quantitation of pulmonary shunting.* Intrahepatic shunting is thought to be related to abnormal tumor vasculature. Underlying cirrhotic changes may also lead to shunting. If significant, pulmonary shunting could result in radiation pneumonitis. A 30 Gy limit has been reported to be restrictive.
2. *Identification of extrahepatic GI uptake.* Extrahepatic activity may be caused by an unrecognized hepatofugal vascular run off. A scintigraphically detectable extrahepatic uptake is very likely to associate with symptomatic GI complications such as ulceration. This finding, depending on its size, might preclude further treatment with Y-90 microspheres unless a safe interventional plan for prevention of extrahepatic flux can be made.
3. *Determination of the blood flow ratio between the tumor and normal liver compartments.* The tumor-to-liver perfusion ratio, a major index of the effectiveness of tumor targeting, is associated with higher therapeutic profile.

Lung shunt fraction (LSF) is determined by ROI analysis on Tc-99m MAA planar images. Tumor-to-liver uptake ratio is best determined using SPECT images. The absolute activity quantification in SPECT depends on reconstruction methods, collimator-detector response compensation, attenuation correction, scatter correction, partial volume effects, dead time, and the activity calibration. Software programs have been specifically developed to assist in quantitative SPECT activity. Utilization of specific acquisition and processing protocols improves accuracy of quantitation, which is a prerequisite for reliable dosimetry. SPECT/CT is particularly useful for precise localization of extrahepatic uptake and accurate registration of tumor perfusion.

A Tc-99m MAA unit dose is injected via the hepatic arterial catheter at the completion of the visceral angiography. Typical injection activity/concentration/volume is 4 mCi/400,000 particles/4 cc. These quantities can be doubled if preferred. The injection site along the hepatic artery could be the anticipated treatment injection point or the proper hepatic artery. It is important to start imaging as early as safely possible to avoid MAA degradation-related artifacts. Activity has been observed in the stomach, salivary glands, thyroid, kidneys, and bladder due to these degradation artifacts.

Planar images are obtained in anterior and posterior projections over chest and abdomen regions. SPECT images are obtained using 128 × 128 matrix, 64 Azimuth at 10-s/stop duration. The LSF is calculated using geometric mean technique on planar images (Fig. 11.1 and (11.1)), and the tumor-to-liver perfusion ratio (TLR) is calculated using a ROI technique on SPECT images (Fig. 11.6b and (11.2)).

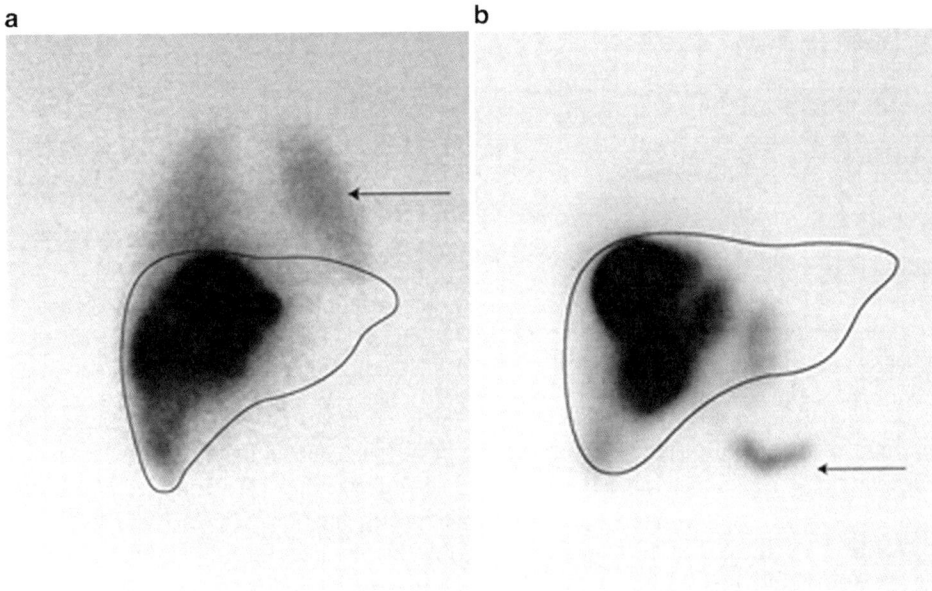

Fig. 11.6 Technitium-99m macroaggregated albumin scanning demonstrating extrahepatic perfusion. Radioactive particles in the lungs on *left panel*, duodenal perfusion on the *right panel*

$$LSF = \sqrt{\frac{Counts_{Lung\langle Anterior\rangle} \times Counts_{Lung\langle Posterior\rangle}}{Counts_{Lung+Liver\langle Anterior\rangle} \times Counts_{Lung+Liver\langle Posterior\rangle}}} \qquad (11.1)$$

$$TLR = \frac{Counts/Pixel_{tumor}}{Counts/Pixel_{liver}} \qquad (11.2)$$

Dosimetry and Treatment Planning

The strict definition of dosimetry is the calculation of radiation absorbed dose in the target lesions and organs. The term, however, is being used rather loosely in the clinical practice of Y-90 microsphere treatment. A decision regarding a reasonably safe or acceptable amount of administered activity is being referred as dosimetry. In actuality, this is merely an activity prescription or written directive.

There are three recommended methods for a written directive for Y-90 microsphere therapy:

1. Body surface area (BSA) method
2. MIRD, non-compartmental macrodosimetry method
3. MIRD, compartmental macrodosimetry method (partition method)

Written Directive/Activity Prescription Based on Body Surface Area Method

The BSA Method is used for resin microsphere activity prescription. The BSA method is based on the presumed correlation between the size of the liver and the patient's size and is meant to protect smaller patients with less tumor burden. The user manual for the resin Y-90 microspheres recommends (11.3) for the determination of the activity to be administered.

Table 11.2 Dose modifiers for lung shunting and lobular treatment

Lung shunt (%)	Dose modifier	Part of liver	Dose modifier
10–15	0.8	Right lobe	0.7
15–20	0.6	Left lobe	0.3
>20	No treatment		

$$\text{Activity(GBq)} = \frac{(\text{BSA} - 2) + \text{Tumor volume}}{\text{Liver volume}} \tag{11.3}$$

The recommended activity is reduced further for percent lung shunting and for lobular or sequential liver treatments as given in Table 11.2.

Written Directive/Activity Prescription Based on Medical Internal Radiation Dosimetry, Non-compartmental Macrodosimetry Method

This method, essentially, is the calculation of the absorbed dose to the liver from an administered activity. This methodology has been recommended in the dose calculations for glass microsphere treatment. The adopted methodology uses a simplistic method and does not consider tumor and liver compartments separately. The method assumes that distribution of the microspheres is even in the tumor and the liver compartments, which leads to an overestimation of the absorbed dose in the liver. The use of this approach requires an understanding of important limitation of this application. The activity required to achieve the "intended" dose in this approach is calculated using (11.4).

$$\text{Activity(GBq)} = \frac{\text{Desired dose(Gy)} \times \text{Target liver mass(g)}}{50 \times (1 - \text{LSF})} \tag{11.4}$$

Written Directive/Activity Prescription Based on Medical Internal Radiation Dosimetry, Compartmental-Macrodosimetry Method (Partition Model)

The administered Y-90 microsphere activity is distributed in tumor and normal liver compartments. The distribution profile is determined by the relative vascularity and volume of these two compartments and is expressed as the TLR. When lung shunting occurs due to intrahepatic peritumoral arteriovenous communications, a third compartment (lung) is encountered and is expressed as the LSF. The TLR and LSF can be determined using Tc-99m MAA scans. Region of interest (ROI) analysis of tumor and normal liver compartments on SPECT images are used to determine the TLR. The LSF is calculated on planar images using the formula given in the MAA imaging section. It is assumed that the administered activity is distributed evenly within the normal liver and tumor compartments. The tumor compartment, as expected, receives a higher concentration proportional to the TLR.

Fractional liver uptake (The fraction of the administered activity accumulated in the normal liver) is:

$$\text{Fractional uptake}_{\text{liver}} = (1 - \text{LSF}) \left[\frac{\text{Mass}_{\text{liver}}(g)}{[\text{Mass}_{\text{tumor}}(g) \times \text{TLR}] + \text{Mass}_{\text{liver}}(g)} \right] \tag{11.5}$$

Activity to be administered for a desired liver dose can be calculated from:

$$Activity_{admin}(GBq) = \frac{Dose_{liver}(Gy) \times Mass_{liver}(g)}{50 \times Fractional\ uptake_{liver}}$$ (11.6)

The dose to the liver delivered from a given administered activity is:

$$Dose_{liver}(Gy) = \frac{Activity_{admin}(GBq) \times 50 \times Fractional\ uptake_{liver}}{Mass_{liver}(g)}$$ (11.7)

Fractional tumor uptake (The fraction of the administered activity accumulated in the tumor) is:

$$Fractional\ uptake_{tumor} = (1 - LSF)\left[\frac{TLR \times Mass_{tumor}(g)}{(TLR \times mass_{tumor}(g)) + mass_{liver}(g)}\right]$$ (11.8)

The dose to the tumor can be determined using the following equation:

$$Dose_{tumor}(Gy) = \frac{Activity_{admin}(GBq) \times 50 \times Fractional\ uptake_{tumor}}{Mass_{tumor}(g)}$$ (11.9)

The dose to the lungs can be determined using the following equation:

$$Dose_{lung}(Gy) = \frac{Activity_{admin}(GBq) \times 50 \times LSF}{Mass_{lung}(g)}$$ (11.10)

Mass is assumed to be equal to volume for tumor and liver tissues, based on their densities being close to that of soft tissue (1.04 g/cm³). Therefore, "mass" can be replaced with "volume" in equations for liver and tumor dose determination for simplicity. The density of lung, however, is approximately 0.30 g/cm³. Therefore, measured lung volumes on CT images need to be multiplied by this factor to obtain the mass. A lung mass of 1,000 g can be used based on

anthropomorphic phantom design used in MIRD modeling if CT calculation is not available.

Use of this method requires three measurements: (1) volume of tumor and normal liver generally obtained from CT scans; (2) proportion of the total administered activity that lodges in tumor and normal liver as determined from a Tc-99m MAA SPECT scan; and (3) fraction of the total administered activity lodged in the lungs, LSF, as determined from a Tc-99m MAA planar scan. Thus, the TLR and the LSF are measured. The partition model can best be used when tumor mass is localized in a discrete area within the liver and tumor regions-of-interest (ROIs) can be identified and reliably drawn. This is usually relatively easy to perform in patients with primary HCC where there is often a large single tumor mass. The technique would be more demanding for routine application in the presence of metastatic disease with multiple tumors. Despite the technical challenges, the compartmental model has been successfully adapted for clinical use in both primary and metastatic settings [34, 35].

Written Directive

For regulatory purposes, "prescribed dose" means the total activity documented in the written directive. *The written directive should include*:
1. Activity determined for administration
2. The type of radiomicrosphere (the radionuclide, and the chemical of the microsphere [resin or glass])
3. The treatment site (whole liver, lobe, or segment)

The written directive should also include a statement that "the administration of the microspheres could be terminated if a stasis is reached" (This provision is only relevant to SIR-Spheres®)

Treatment and Follow-Up Procedures

The administration of Y-90 microspheres is performed in an angiography suite, by an interventional radiologist and the authorized user. The catheter is usually positioned at a location determined by the desired treatment mode (whole liver, lobar, or segmental). Both Y-90 microsphere products have their own dedicated delivery device designed to facilitate the administration. Because the resin microspheres have a much higher number of microspheres per unit dose, there is an embolic tendency especially towards the last stages of administration which is performed in a manually controlled manner with fluoroscopic monitoring. Observation of increasing reflux is a sign of increased embolic effect and risk for hepatofugal flux and therefore might be an indication to discontinue the administration. Strict adherence to radiation safety guidelines is critically important in patient and personnel safety.

Y-90 microsphere treatment is usually an outpatient treatment. Patients who experience moderate embolic syndrome can be admitted for less than 24 h. Symptomatic treatment might be indicated for pain or nausea. Prophylactic use of antibiotics, proton pump inhibitors, or steroids should be considered individually. Patients are provided with radiation safety instructions upon discharge.

Bremsstrahlung Imaging

Y-90 being a pure beta emitter, Bremsstrahlung imaging is the only method of obtaining a posttreatment localization study. Bremsstrahlung imaging is rather challenging due to its continuous broad energy spectrum. Bremsstrahlung imaging is suggested as a quality assurance procedure, to document absence of pulmonary or extrahepatic GI uptake, and hence it became a routine imaging procedure. However, due to its inherent poor imaging quality, the technique is far from being an accurate or reliable document of safe delivery of microspheres. A negative scan does not assure nontarget delivery of microspheres.

Bremsstrahlung imaging is started any time between immediate posttreatment period and before the patient is discharged. Anterior and posterior planar images and SPECT of the abdomen/liver were obtained using a medium or high energy collimator and with camera settings at 78 keV photopeak and 57% window. These collimators are effective since while there is a broad peak in the low energy range, 10–20% of the counts come from γ photons in the 270–540 keV range. The SPECT protocol typically uses a 128×128 matrix, 120 images (60/head), 20–30 s/image, and a total time of 20–30 min

Follow-Up Functional Imaging

Quantitative PET/CT provides highly sensitive information regarding objective tumor responses.

Responses can be documented as early as 4 weeks posttreatment. Routine use of FDG PET/CT is recommended for evaluation of patients with metastatic disease originating from CRC, breast cancer, lung cancer, esophageal cancer, melanoma, head and neck cancers, and cervical cancer, all of which are CMS-approved clinical indications. Tumor SUV is used as a standard clinical tool for determining disease prognosis, as a marker for tumor biology, and also as an evaluation of treatment response. SUV provides a snapshot of the biological function and activity of the tumor. A more comprehensive approach involving the determination of functional tumor volume (FTV), total lesion glycolysis (TLG), and Larson-Ginsberg Index was first described by Larson et al. [36]. The clinical validity and reproducibility of these measures were demonstrated in a more recent study on 20 patients with CRCLM [37]. The median survival in the study group was 14.8 months (range 2.0–27.7 months). The median survival for patients with pretreatment FTV values of above and below 200 cc was 11.2 and 26.9 months, respectively ($p < 0.05$), while the median survival for patients with 4-week posttreatment FTV values of above and below 30 cc was 10.9 and 26.9 months, respectively ($p < 0.05$). The median survival for patients with pretreatment TLG values of above and below 600 g was 11.2 and 26.9 months, respectively ($p < 0.05$), while the median survival for patients with 4-week posttreatment TLG values of above and below 100 g was 10.9 and 26.9 months, respectively ($p < 0.05$).

Complications of Y-90 Microsphere Therapy

Commonly Observed After-Effects

Post-Y-90 microsphere therapy lethargy and mild nausea are common symptoms lasting up to 10 days and may require medication. Most patients develop mild fever for several days following Y-90 microsphere therapy that does not require treatment.

Post-embolization Syndrome

Post-embolization syndrome (PES) refers to a clinical picture of acute abdominal pain, nausea, vomiting, and fever resulting from acute ischemic insult to the liver. PES in its most severe form is seen after chemoembolization. RMT is not (and should not be) a devascularization treatment. Nevertheless, in approximately one-third of patients, administration of Y-90 microsphere therapy causes early, short-term abdominal pain requiring narcotic analgesia. This side effect is more common with increasing number of microspheres administered. This can be avoided with slow, well-controlled administration of microspheres and has been uncommon in experienced hands. PES typically does not occur with glass microsphere treatment given the difference in embolic load [38].

Hepatic Injury

The pathogenesis of radiation damage to the liver from conventional external beam radiation is dominated by vascular injury in the central vein region. Early alterations in the central vein caused by external beam radiation include intimal damage which leads to eccentric wall thickening. This process, when diffuse and progressive, results in clinical "veno-occlusive disease" characterized by the development of post-sinusoidal portal hypertension, ascites, and deterioration of liver function tests [39].

Y-90 microsphere therapy-associated radiation injury has a different pattern. Radiation from microspheres is deposited primarily in the region of the portal triad away from the central vein and thus is distinct from the damage pattern seen in radiation hepatitis from external beam sources. Radiation-induced liver disease secondary to radioembolization is not common, but has been reported and may be more common in patients also treated with systemic chemotherapy [40]. Chemo-SIRT patients' post-resection specimens commonly demonstrate steatosis or steatohepatitis, which are not typically seen in SIRT-alone specimens. It is important to note that sinusoidal obstruction, perisinusoidal fibrosis, and veno-occlusive disease are not uncommon with chemotherapy-associated hepatic toxicity.

Particularly in patients with CRC liver metasta-ses who have received prior or concomitant che-motherapy, the hepatic toxicity picture may be a combination pattern [41].

A review by Atassi et al. involving 569 Y-90 microsphere treatments in 327 patients reported a 10% incidence of grade 3 bilirubin toxicity [42]. Portal hypertension, as a sequela of Y-90 micro-sphere therapy, has been described in early stud-ies and case reports [43]. Subclinical portal hypertension may manifest by splenomegaly.

Radiation Pneumonitis

A fraction of microspheres may shunt through the liver and into the lungs. Radiation pneumoni-tis has been reported to occur at estimated lung dose levels of 30 Gy [44]. Proper lung shunting studies and incorporation of this information in dosimetry models should be practiced univer-sally. The risk of radiation pneumonitis is miti-gated if the cumulative lung dose is limited to 50 Gy [44].

GI Complications

The most commonly affected site in the GI tract is the gastroduodenal segment due to rich hepatof-ugal collaterals. Collateral vessels posing height-ened risk for nontarget embolization should be coiled. The Y-90 microsphere therapy-induced GI ulceration rate is under 5% and is close to minimal in experienced hands. However, when these ulcers occur, RMT-induced ulcers are more challenging than accustomed peptic ulcerations and might be refractory to standard treatment regimens. Y-90 microsphere therapy may cause radiation cholecystitis. Although clinically rele-vant radiation cholecystitis requiring cholecys-tectomy is rare, imaging findings of gallbladder injury (i.e., enhancing wall, mural rent) are quite common. Other possible biliary complications reported include biliary necrosis, biloma, and stricture [42].

Conclusion

Y-90 radiomicrosphere treatment for primary and metastatic liver cancer is no longer purely experimental or investigational. This treatment modality has been shown to be safe and efficacious and is approved for the treatment of metastatic colorectal cancer and HCC. Treatment paradigms have significantly evolved and con-tinue to be refined. Based on the literature to date, this therapy is increasingly being utilized to treat primary and metastatic liver cancer. Y-90 RMT is increasingly considered earlier in the course of treatment as opposed to the salvage set-ting and ongoing trials are currently accruing patients to support this role. There is, however, a need for development of a clinically practical dosimetry technique and more unified patient selection criteria for treatment planning and execution.

Appendix 1: Radiation Safety Procedures and Guidelines

Pre- and Intra-procedural Safety Considerations and Standard Procedures in the Interventional Radiology Suite

Shielding is accomplished with plastic and acrylic materials during dose preparation and adminis-tration; lead should be avoided due to the external exposure risk due to bremsstrahlung production. Routine radiation surveys, as with any other ther-apeutic radionuclide administration, must be per-formed at the end of each day in all areas where the ^{90}Y-microsphere treatment was prepared or administered.

Microspheres can cause significant problems if spilled. Unlike liquid isotope spills, which can be mopped up, the tiny microspheres can become lodged in crevices from which they are difficult to remove, or they can disperse in the air and be inhaled.

- Pregnant staff and/or pregnant family mem-bers should be excluded from procedural care of Y-90 microsphere patients.
- Infusion personnel must remain behind deliv-ery apparatus containing the dose. Anyone assisting should remain clear of the tubing connected to the catheters.
- The angiographic suite area immediately underneath personnel involved in dose

administration should be draped and plastic covers placed over pedals as a precautionary measure in case of spillage.

- Double gloves, double shoe covering, and protective eyewear are advised for administering staff.
- The delivery catheter should be considered radioactive and disposed of, observing radiation precautions. All other potentially contaminated material (i.e., exit tubing from the dose vial, three-way valve, tube to catheter, needles, gloves, gauzes, hemostat, and drapes) should be considered radioactive and disposed of, observing radiation precautions, after catheter removal.
- Tubing and syringes to deliver and flush and the catheter sheath are not considered "hot" and therefore do not need special radiation precautions for disposal. However, they should be surveyed for radioactivity before routine disposal.
- All personnel within the angiography suite must have their shoe covers checked for radiation at the end of the procedure and before leaving the suite. The suite must be checked at the end of the procedure after all contaminated waste and the patient have been removed from the room to detect any radiation contamination.

All contaminated materials (disposable or recoverable) must be available to stock-take throughout the procedure, and particularly for final reconciliation at the end. Once stock-take is complete, containers can be sealed for removal to the storage or disposal area as appropriate. All gowns and other surgical equipment should be monitored using the radiation monitoring equipment for contamination at the conclusion of the procedure, and if contaminated, bagged and sent to the storage area to wait laundering. Surgical instruments should be cleaned in Decon to decontaminate them. Once decontaminated, they can be handled in the normal manner. Once all materials and staff are removed from the room, a final check with the radiation monitor should verify that the room is not contaminated and is ready for re-use. All staff should be checked, including soles of shoes, hands, and body before leaving the area.

Handling of a Contamination

All contamination with Y-90 Microspheres should be treated seriously. Being a solid suspended in liquid, contamination with microspheres is likely to be on surfaces or people, rather than airborne. In the absence of an obvious event, routine cleaning and monitoring of surfaces, work areas, floors, and equipment should be conducted. Decontamination procedures are the same, regardless of resulting from an occult or obvious event. Contamination may be transferred from one surface to another, such as bench to hand to bench or surface to person via direct contact. In the event of a contamination:

1. The first task is to prevent access to the contaminated area. This protects staff and limits spread of contamination.
2. As Y-90 Microspheres contamination consists of a liquid spill of nonvolatile materials, respiration equipment is generally unnecessary. An appropriate protective wear is necessary for the radiation safety officer or his designee who is involved in decontamination process. A gown should be worn over surgical scrubs. Plastic disposable overshoes and a plastic disposable apron should be considered in light of a liquid spill. Double gloves are considered standard. Generally the hair is covered in a cap and protective eyewear is worn as radiation protection and splash protection.
3. A radiation monitor is required and should be placed in a fixed position on a non-contaminated surface. All measurements should be taken by holding the item in front of the monitor. This provides stable background readings and allows interpretation of the measurements. In the absence of a non-contaminated surface, a second person, also in protective clothing should hold the monitor in a fixed position. The officer performing the decontamination should avoid holding or touching the monitor after decontamination begins.
4. All personnel in the area of the contamination should be monitored and non-contaminated personnel should leave the area.
5. Contaminated personnel should be decontaminated before addressing contamination in the facility.

- Remove all contaminated clothing and place it directly into an appropriate receptacle without placing it on any surface, contaminated or not.
- If there is contamination on the skin, the officer should wipe the area using a disposable paper towel moistened with water or soapy water. Wiping should be from the periphery of the contamination towards the center to avoid spreading the isotope.
- Care needs to be taken not to spread or drip water into the eyes, nose, mouth, or ears.
- After each wipe is used, it should be monitored and then placed directly into the appropriate waste receptacle.
- Wiping should continue until monitored wipes demonstrate that no more contamination can be removed.
- Due to the normal dress standards in an isotope measuring or SIR-spheres facility, the only skin likely to be exposed to the risk of contamination is the face and neck. As such, washing with water and soap is best avoided due to the risk of rinsing spheres into the eyes or nose, etc., and the risk of spreading contamination via splashing.
- Soap is not generally required to remove contamination, as the microspheres and water in which they are suspended are not sticky or tenacious on skin or other surfaces.
- The radiation officer should always perform the personnel decontamination in a controlled manner. Self-removal of contamination generally increases the risk of spreading contamination.
- The first step is to mark out the area of contamination. At no stage should anyone cross through this area, as it will spread contamination.
- As a beta emitter, shielding of the area is not generally required, however this should be at the discretion of the radiation officer.
- Decontamination should begin from the periphery and work towards the center. Forward progress should only occur after objective measurements on the materials used to wipe surfaces or instruments demonstrate that the immediate area is clean.

6. Once all staff have been decontaminated and removed from the area, the facility can be decontaminated.
7. The radiation officer uses reports from the staff involved, direct observation, and objective measurements to determine the extent of contamination.
8. At completion of the decontamination process, the radiation officer should be monitored for contamination and all disposables and protective clothing should be bagged appropriately.
9. All bags should be sealed and tagged (isotope and date) before removal to the disposal area.

Post-procedural Safety Considerations and Standard Procedures in an in Patient/Observation Unit

Although Y-90 is a pure beta emitter, and a gamma exposure is absent, the bremsstrahlung component of the ^{90}Y is not negligible. Bremsstrahlung radiation could be notable for several days. While special shielding requirements are not necessary for post-procedure nursing care, it is advisable that pregnant staff and/or pregnant family members be excluded from post-procedural care of Y-90 microsphere patients.

Yttrium-90 resin microspheres may have trace amounts of free Y-90 on their surface, which can be excreted in the urine during the first 24 h. Patients are advised to wash their hands after voiding. Men should sit to urinate, and the urinal should be double-flushed after voiding. These precautions should be in place for the first 24 h after treatment. In contrast, Y90 glass microspheres are not known to have free Y-90 in trace amounts in the treatment vial; therefore, no special precautions are necessary for the handling of patient urine.

Patient Release

A licensee may release patients, regardless of administered activity, if it can be demonstrated that the total effective dose equivalent (TEDE) to another individual from exposure to a released patient is not likely to exceed 5 mSv (0.5 rem). In addition, licensees must provide a released patient with written instructions on actions recommended to maintain doses to others as low as reasonably achievable (ALARA) if the dose to any other individual is likely to exceed 1 mSv. The patient release dose calculations performed indicated that, consistent with regulatory requirements, patients receiving ^{90}Y-microsphere therapy can be immediately released without the need for radiation safety instructions on actions aimed at maintaining doses to others ALARA, as these doses are all minimal and well below regulatory limits.

Post-discharge Instructions Appropriate for Released Patient

Standard universal precautions to avoid contact with body fluids are all that is required to ensure minimal doses to individuals exposed to patients receiving ^{90}Y-microsphere treatment. Body fluid radioactivity is not problematic for ^{90}Y-microspheres. Therefore, patient release instructions involving hand-washing and clean-up of any contaminated materials are not necessary at all for glass microsphere patients and for longer than 24 h in the case of resin microsphere treatments. For the latter group, it may be prudent to instruct the patients to wash their hands after voiding, and to have men sit to urinate, and to dispose any body fluid-contaminated material (e.g., flush down toilet or place in household trash) during the first day. There is no legitimate radiation protection reason to advise patients to abstain from sex after radiomicrosphere treatment. No release instructions are required for glass microsphere patients (unless activities higher than 9 GBq are administered), while patients receiving resin microspheres may be given simple precaution instructions for the first 24 h only.

Appendix 2: Procedure Coding

Besides reporting the imaging studies, nuclear medicine physicians could/should generate clinical reports directly related to patient care.

Initial Consultation Report

The following two codes can be used for an initial consultation.

99205: Comprehensive evaluation and management of a new patient, which requires these three key components: A comprehensive history; A comprehensive examination; Medical decision making of high complexity. Counseling and/or coordination of care with other providers or agencies are provided consistent with the nature of the problem(s) and the patient's and/or family's needs. Usually, the presenting problem(s) are of moderate-to-high severity. Physicians typically spend 60 min face-to-face with the patient and/or family.

99201: Problem Focused evaluation and management of a new patient, which requires these three key components: A problem focused history; A problem focused examination; Straightforward medical decision making. Counseling and/or coordination of care with other providers or agencies are provided consistent with the nature of the problem(s) and the patient's and/or family's needs. Usually, the presenting problem(s) are self-limited or minor. Physicians typically spend 10 min face-to-face with the patient and/or family.

Treatment Planning and Dosimetry Report

Treatment planning encompasses decisions regarding treatment field (whole liver, lobar, or segmental), hepatic arterial branch of administration, and determination of administered activity. Most of the above decisions are made in a multidisciplinary manner. The following codes are appropriate if the required elements are present in the report.

77263: Therapeutic radiology treatment planning; complex: This code is appropriate when the report contains the elements of treatment field, and treatment venue. Determination of administered activity using SIR-Spheres' BSA method would be part of this code.

77300: Basic radiation dosimetry calculation, calculation of nonionizing radiation surface and depth dose, as required during course of treatment: This code is appropriate when any MIRD methodology is used for dosimetric purposes. Determination of administered activity using TheraSphere's formula would be part of this code.

76377: 3D rendering with interpretation and reporting of computed tomography, magnetic resonance imaging, PET/CT or SPECT; requiring image postprocessing on an independent workstation. This code is appropriate when a comprehensive Dosimetry involving determination of tumor and liver volumes, and differential activity concentrations.

Procedure Report

This report is generated for the actual administration procedure by the authorized user. Although technically the procedure fits to the CPT code 79445; Radiopharmaceutical therapy by intra-arterial particulate administration, currently the reimbursement under this code is substantially low. The recognized code is a brachytherapy code. The following codes are used when/if the procedure report contains the appropriate descriptions.

77778: Interstitial radiation source application; complex

77790: Supervision, handling, loading of radiation source

References

1. Ariel IM, Pack GT (1967) Treatment of inoperable cancer of the liver by intra-arterial radioactive isotopes and chemotherapy. Cancer 20(5):793–804
2. Huang P, Feng L, Oldham EA, Keating MJ, Plunkett W (2000) Superoxide dismutase as a target for the selective killing of cancer cells. Nature 407(6802): 390–5
3. Sirtex Medical. Package Insert for SIR-Spheres® microspheres (Yttrium-90 microspheres). http://www. sirtex.com; http://sirtex.com/files/US20Package20 Insert1.pdf.
4. MDS Nordion. Package Insert for TheraSphere Yttrium-90 glass microspheres. www. nordion.com; http://www.nordion.com/therasphere/physicians-package-insert/package-insert-us.pdf.
5. Gulec SA, Siegel JA (2007) Posttherapy radiation safety considerations in radiomicrosphere treatment with 90Y-microspheres. J Nucl Med 48(12):2080–6
6. Gray B, Van Hazel G, Hope M et al (2001) Randomised trial of SIR-Spheres plus chemotherapy vs. chemotherapy alone for treating patients with liver metastases from primary large bowel cancer. Ann Oncol 12(12):1711–20
7. Van Hazel G, Blackwell A, Anderson J et al (2004) Randomised phase 2 trial of SIR-Spheres plus fluorouracil/leucovorin chemotherapy versus fluorouracil/leucovorin chemotherapy alone in advanced colorectal cancer. J Surg Oncol 88(2):78–85
8. Sharma RA, Van Hazel GA, Morgan B et al (2007) Radioembolization of liver metastases from colorectal cancer using yttrium-90 microspheres with concomitant systemic oxaliplatin, fluorouracil, and leucovorin chemotherapy. J Clin Oncol 25(9):1099–106
9. van Hazel GA, Pavlakis N, Goldstein D et al (2009) Treatment of fluorouracil-refractory patients with liver metastases from colorectal cancer by using yttrium-90 resin microspheres plus concomitant systemic irinotecan chemotherapy. J Clin Oncol 27(25): 4089–95
10. Gulec S, Hall M, Atkinson H, Mesoloras G, Pennington K. Efficacy of 90Y radiomicrosphere and chemotherapy combination treatment in patients with colorectal cancer liver metastases. J Nucl Med. Meeting Abstracts. 2008; 49 (MeetingAbstracts_1): 103P.
11. Stubbs RS, Cannan RJ, Mitchell AW (2001) Selective internal radiation therapy with 90yttrium microspheres for extensive colorectal liver metastases. J Gastrointest Surg 5(3):294–302
12. Kennedy AS, Coldwell D, Nutting C et al (2006) Resin 90Y-microsphere brachytherapy for unresectable colorectal liver metastases: modern USA experience. Int J Radiat Oncol Biol Phys 65(2):412–25
13. Lau WY, Ho S, Leung TW et al (1998) Selective internal radiation therapy for nonresectable hepatocellular carcinoma with intraarterial infusion of 90yttrium microspheres. Int J Radiat Oncol Biol Phys 40(3): 583–92
14. Lau WY, Leung WT, Ho S et al (1994) Treatment of inoperable hepatocellular carcinoma with intrahepatic arterial yttrium-90 microspheres: a phase I and II study. Br J Cancer 70(5):994–9
15. Lau WY, Ho S, Leung WT, Chan M, Lee WY, Johnson PJ (2001) What determines survival duration in hepatocellular carcinoma treated with intraarterial Yttrium-90 microspheres? Hepatogastroenterology 48(38):338–40
16. Goin JE, Salem R, Carr BI et al (2005) Treatment of unresectable hepatocellular carcinoma with intrahepatic

yttrium 90 microspheres: a risk-stratification analysis. J Vasc Interv Radiol 16(2 Pt 1):195–203

17. Salem R, Lewandowski RJ, Atassi B et al (2005) Treatment of unresectable hepatocellular carcinoma with use of 90Y microspheres (TheraSphere): safety, tumor response, and survival. J Vasc Interv Radiol 16(12):1627–39

18. Salem R, Lewandowski R, Roberts C et al (2004) Use of Yttrium-90 glass microspheres (TheraSphere) for the treatment of unresectable hepatocellular carcinoma in patients with portal vein thrombosis. J Vasc Interv Radiol 15(4):335–45

19. Kennedy A, Coldwell D, Nutting C, et al. Hepatic brachytherapy for GI neuroendocrine tumors with 90y-microspheres: long term USA experience (abstract 285). In: Presented at 16th international conference on anti-cancer treatment, Paris, France; 1–4 Feb 2005.

20. Rhee TK, Lewandowski RJ, Liu DM et al (2008) 90Y Radioembolization for metastatic neuroendocrine liver tumors: preliminary results from a multi-institutional experience. Ann Surg 247(6):1029–35

21. Kennedy A, Liu DM, Dezarn WA, et al. Resin 90y-microsphere brachytherapy for unresectable neuroendocrine hepatic metastases. In: Presented at liver directed radiotherapy with microspheres: second annual clinical symposium, Scottsdale, AZ; 27–28 April 2006.

22. Gulec SA, Hostetter R, Schwartzentruber D et al (2007) Treatment of neuroendocrine tumor liver metastases with Y-90 microspheres: an effective cytoreduction for disease consolidation and symptom control. Ann Surg Oncol 14:93

23. Ibrahim SM, Mulcahy MF, Lewandowski RJ et al (2008) Treatment of unresectable cholangiocarcinoma using yttrium-90 microspheres: results from a pilot study. Cancer 113(8):2119–28

24. Bangash AK, Atassi B, Kaklamani V et al (2007) 90Y radioembolization of metastatic breast cancer to the liver: toxicity, imaging response, survival. J Vasc Interv Radiol 18(5):621–8

25. Gulec SA, Hall MJ, Wheller J, et al. A Phase II study of selective internal radiation treatment (SIRT) and selective external radiation treatment (SERT) with chemotherapy in patients with recurrent/metastatic pancreatic cancer: preliminary results. In: Presented at world conference on interventional oncology, Los Angeles, CA; 2008.

26. Lewandowski RJ, Atassi BA, Wong CO, et al. Use of yttrium-90 microspheres for the treatment of liver neoplasia: long-term follow-up. In: Presented at the annual meeting of the cardiovascular and interventional society of Europe, Rome; 2006.

27. Gulec SA, Fong Y (2007) Yttrium 90 microsphere selective internal radiation treatment of hepatic colorectal metastases. Arch Surg 142(7):675–82

28. Fong Y, Saldinger PF, Akhurst T et al (1999) Utility of 18F-FDG positron emission tomography scanning on selection of patients for resection of hepatic colorectal metastases. Am J Surg 178(4):282–7

29. Arulampalam TH, Francis DL, Visvikis D, Taylor I, Ell PJ (2004) FDG-PET for the pre-operative evaluation of colorectal liver metastases. Eur J Surg Oncol 30(3):286–91

30. Bipat S, van Leeuwen MS, Comans EF et al (2005) Colorectal liver metastases: CT, MR imaging, and PET for diagnosis–meta-analysis. Radiology 237(1):123–31

31. Bienert M, McCook B, Carr BI et al (2005) 90Y microsphere treatment of unresectable liver metastases: changes in 18F-FDG uptake and tumour size on PET/CT. Eur J Nucl Med Mol Imaging 32(7):778–87

32. Wong CY, Salem R, Qing F et al (2004) Metabolic response after intraarterial 90Y-glass microsphere treatment for colorectal liver metastases: comparison of quantitative and visual analyses by 18F-FDG PET. J Nucl Med 45(11):1892–7

33. Liu DM, Salem R, Bui JT et al (2005) Angiographic considerations in patients undergoing liver-directed therapy. J Vasc Interv Radiol 16(7):911–35

34. Gulec SA, Mesoloras G, Dezarn WA, McNeillie P, Kennedy AS (2007) Safety and efficacy of Y-90 microsphere treatment in patients with primary and metastatic liver cancer: the tumor selectivity of the treatment as a function of tumor to liver flow ratio. J Transl Med 5:15

35. Gulec SA, Mesoloras G, Stabin M (2006) Dosimetric techniques in 90Y-microsphere therapy of liver cancer: the MIRD equations for dose calculations. J Nucl Med 47(7):1209–11

36. Larson SM, Erdi Y, Akhurst T et al (1999) Tumor treatment response based on visual and quantitative changes in global tumor glycolysis using PET-FDG imaging. The Visual Response Score and the change in total lesion glycolysis. Clin Positron Imaging 2(3):159–71

37. Gulec SA, Suthar RR, Barot TC, Pennington K (2011) The prognostic value of functional tumor volume and total lesion glycolysis in patients with colorectal cancer liver metastases undergoing (90)Y selective internal radiation therapy plus chemotherapy. Eur J Nucl Med Mol Imaging 38(7):1289–95

38. Sato K, Lewandowski RJ, Bui JT et al (2006) Treatment of unresectable primary and metastatic liver cancer with yttrium-90 microspheres (TheraSphere): assessment of hepatic arterial embolization. Cardiovasc Intervent Radiol 29(4):522–9

39. Cheng JC, Wu JK, Huang CM et al (2002) Radiation-induced liver disease after radiotherapy for hepatocellular carcinoma: clinical manifestation and dosimetric description. Radiother Oncol 63(1):41–5

40. Sangro B, Gil-Alzugaray B, Rodriguez J et al (2008) Liver disease induced by radioembolization of liver tumors: description and possible risk factors. Cancer 112(7):1538–46

41. Schouten van der Velden AP, Punt CJ, Van Krieken JH, Derleyn VA, Ruers TJ (2008) Hepatic veno-occlusive disease after neoadjuvant treatment of colorectal liver metastases with oxaliplatin: a lesson of the month. Eur J Surg Oncol 34(3):353–5

42. Atassi B, Bangash AK, Lewandowski RJ et al (2008) Biliary sequelae following radioembolization with Yttrium-90 microspheres. J Vasc Interv Radiol 19(5):691–7

43. Jakobs TF, Saleem S, Atassi B et al (2008) Fibrosis, portal hypertension, and hepatic volume changes induced by intra-arterial radiotherapy with 90yttrium microspheres. Dig Dis Sci 53(9): 2556–63

44. Ho S, Lau WY, Leung TW, Chan M, Johnson PJ, Li AK (1997) Clinical evaluation of the partition model for estimating radiation doses from yttrium-90 microspheres in the treatment of hepatic cancer. Eur J Nucl Med 24(3):293–8

Trans-Arterial I-131 Lipiodol Therapy of Liver Tumors

David K. Leung and Chaitanya Divgi

Introduction

Trans-arterial radiotherapy for liver malignancies began with iodine-131 labeled lipiodol for hepatocellular carcinoma (HCC). This agent continues to be used, labeled with ^{131}I as well as with other radionuclides that emit β-particles, notably rhenium-188. Particulates such as glass and albumin microspheres labeled with yttrium-90 have also been utilized, and their physical characteristics have enabled evaluation of their utility in metastatic liver cancers as well, with considerable success.

While the initial therapies with ^{131}I-lipiodol utilized a standard treatment schema based on amount of administered radioactivity, subsequent trial designs have utilized image-based treatments of varying complexity, in an attempt to account for extent of hepatic/pulmonary shunting as well as extent of dose deposition in normal liver. Imaging of distribution of radioactivity following intra-arterial administration is achieved by use of a surrogate of nontherapeutic radioactivity, usually technetium-99 m labeled macroaggregated albumin (MAA), administered through the intra-arterial catheter situated in a location comparable to that for the actual therapy. Calculation of the amount of radioactivity that may be safely administered relies on shunt quantitation calculated by this method. If fractional flow through the shunt is deemed acceptable, the amount of therapeutic radioactivity that may be safely administered is then calculated by estimating radiation burden to normal liver.

The aim of trans-arterial delivery of therapeutic radionuclides depends on "internal" irradiation of hepatic tumors without significant systemic toxicity. Hepatic trans-arterial radionuclide therapy, commonly known as trans-arterial radioembolization (TARE), although embolization is not the primary therapeutic goal, has been shown to alleviate symptoms in patients with neuroendocrine tumors and HCC. TARE may also have a survival benefit in these diseases. Moreover, it is relatively less toxic compared to trans-arterial chemoembolization (TACE), which has significant embolic effect and also needs to be carried out much more frequently. Direct comparative data are however necessary and may spur more frequent use of this currently underutilized therapy.

Radiopharmaceutical administration in an Interventional Radiology suite needs a coordinated multidisciplinary approach, which is critical to the successful utilization of this therapy. Radiation safety and radioactivity disposal are additional important considerations. Successful multidisciplinary integration results in a safe, effective outpatient therapy for the vast majority of patients.

D.K. Leung, M.D., Ph.D. • C. Divgi, M.D. (✉)
Department of Radiology, PET/Nuclear Medicine
Division, Columbia University, 722 West 168 Street,
New York, NY, USA
e-mail: dkl2@columbia.edu; crdivgi@columbia.edu

C. Aktolun and S.J. Goldsmith (eds.), *Nuclear Medicine Therapy: Principles and Clinical Applications*,
DOI 10.1007/978-1-4614-4021-5_12, © Springer Science+Business Media New York 2013

This chapter traces the development of radio-labeled lipiodol and then discusses the salient features of ^{90}Y-labeled microspheres, highlighting differences between the available agents where relevant. While TARE has been employed in primary as well as metastatic hepatic malignancies, the focus in this chapter is on HCC.

Radiolabeled Lipiodol Therapy

^{131}-I Lipiodol Therapy

Hepatic arterial hyper-vascularization is a feature of most HCC and some neuroendocrine and colorectal metastases [1, 2]. Most patients with HCC (>70%) are inoperable at initial presentation, and trans-arterial techniques have therefore been the mainstay of therapies in this disease with a dismal overall prognosis [3].

Trans-arterial chemotherapy has been utilized with varying success in the therapy of HCC [4]. The first TARE therapies were carried out with ^{131}I-lipiodol. Lipiodol is an iodinated oil that, after selective trans-arterial injection, is retained by the tumor for a very long time, and more than 75% of ^{131}I-lipiodol in HCC remains in the liver after hepatic arterial injection [5]. A dose of 2,400 MBq was determined in a Phase 1 study to provide a meaningful therapeutic dose with an acceptable hospital stay [5]. This dose has been used subsequently in therapeutic studies. TARE with ^{131}I-lipiodol has been used with success rates of up to 40% in Phase 2 studies [6], and subsequently been found to be useful in patients with portal vein thrombosis, for whom chemotherapy was not a viable option [7]. A prospective randomized trial that compared TARE with TACE found comparable efficacy with a far more favorable toxicity profile for TARE [8, 9]. Moreover, monotherapy with ^{131}I-Lipiodol in patients with potentially curable lesions who were not candidates for surgery also had comparable survival to historical surgically resected controls who did undergo surgery [10].

These encouraging results led to the exploration of ^{131}I-lipiodol as adjuvant therapy following surgical resection of HCC. A small randomized trial of 43 patients revealed improved recurrence-free and overall survival in patients who received ^{131}I-lipiodol 6 weeks after curative surgery [11]. Neo-adjuvant therapy with ^{131}I-lipiodol has also been found to be promising [12], and worthy of future evaluation.

In summary [13], ^{131}I-lipiodol has an excellent safety profile, has efficacy at least comparable to TACE and perhaps surgical resection, and can be administered repeatedly without cumulative toxicity. A possible limitation of its use is the need for radiation safety precautions, including hospitalization, associated with the gamma emissions of iodine-131. These precautions, along with their cost as well as the cost of the agent, made it prohibitive for use in developing countries, where HCC is more prevalent, and hence a lower-cost alternative was sought. The development of rhenium-188 labeled lipiodol made that possible.

188-Re-Lipiodol

^{188}Re-lipiodol was successfully synthesized and demonstrated to have physicochemical properties comparable to ^{131}I-lipiodol [14]. The ability to produce ^{188}Re from a tungsten-188 generator is a significant advantage that limits the cost of isotope production and also permits distribution of the generator to developing countries [15]. With its favorable half-life (17 h), and gamma emission of 155 KeV enabling imaging by most gamma cameras, ^{188}Re has the potential to be a therapeutic radionuclide with promise in HCC, since its beta-minus emission is of relatively high energy (maximum energy = 1.12 MeV, average soft-tissue penetration 3 mm). The International Atomic Energy Agency sponsored a dosimetry-based therapy trial in several developing countries, using a simple dosimetric model to calculate radiation-absorbed dose to liver, lung, and tumor. The trial [16] was impressive for several reasons: (1) it demonstrated the feasibility of a standardized approach to therapy using TARE in developing countries like Mongolia and

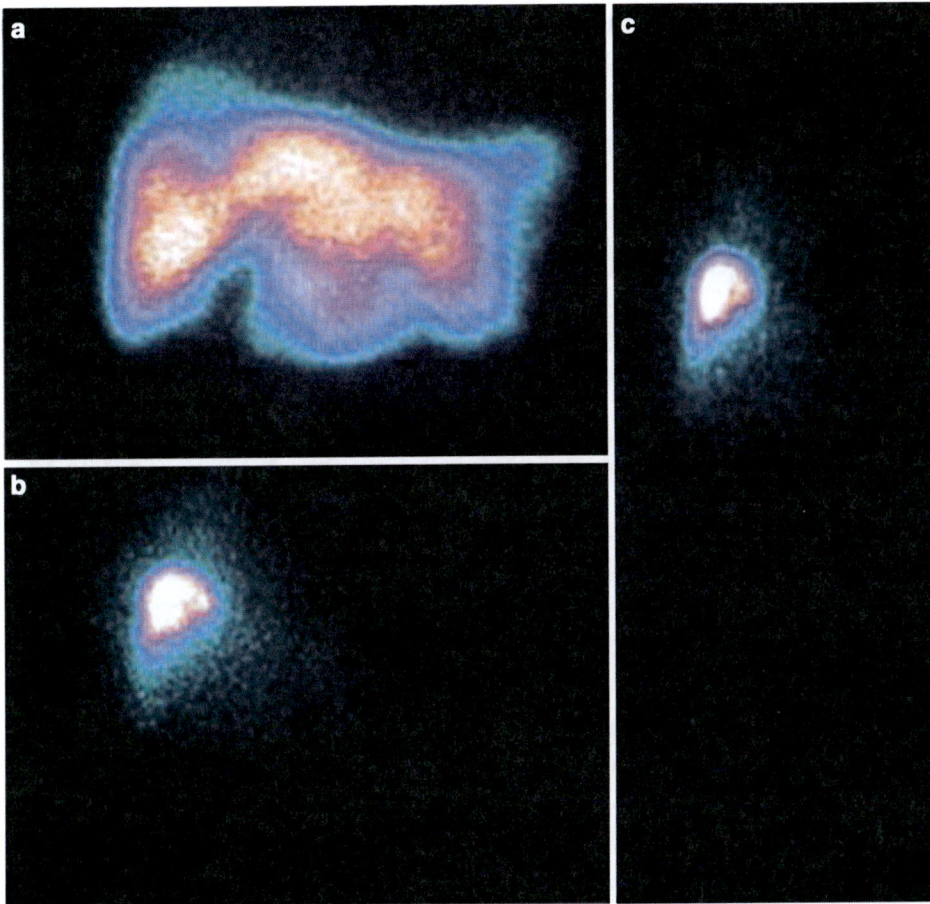

Fig. 12.1 A low dose (185 KBq) of [188]Re-lipiodol was first injected after optimal intra-arterial catheter placement in a patient with hepatocellular cancer. The focal defect caused by the mass is visualized in the anterior sulfur colloid scan (**a**). Accumulation of the low dose of [188]Re-lipiodol is evident in the liver (**b**), with no evidence of significant pulmonary shunting or extrahepatic accumulation in the anterior whole body scan (**c**)

Colombia, as well as more developed nations like Singapore [17]. (2) It provided the validation for a simple dosimetry model that utilized images obtained after a subtherapeutic dose of [188]Re-lipiodol [18]. (3) It demonstrated the utility of this approach, with overall response rates comparable to those with TACE and TARE in developed countries [19]. These results strongly point toward further exploration of this easy-to-use, low-cost therapy, particularly in developing countries; the lack of commercial exploitation may be a factor impeding its development.

The methodology universally employed to calculate radiation absorbed dose to the tumor and normal liver with [188]Re-lipiodol TARE is illustrated in the Figures. A low dose (200 KBq) of [188]Re-lipiodol is first injected after optimal intra-arterial catheter placement (Fig. 12.1). Radiation absorbed dose to tumor and normal liver are estimated assuming only physical decay, using whole body images combined with CT estimates of liver and tumor mass. The therapeutic amount of radioactivity is calculated to deliver no more than 30 Gy to normal liver OR 12 Gy to lung OR

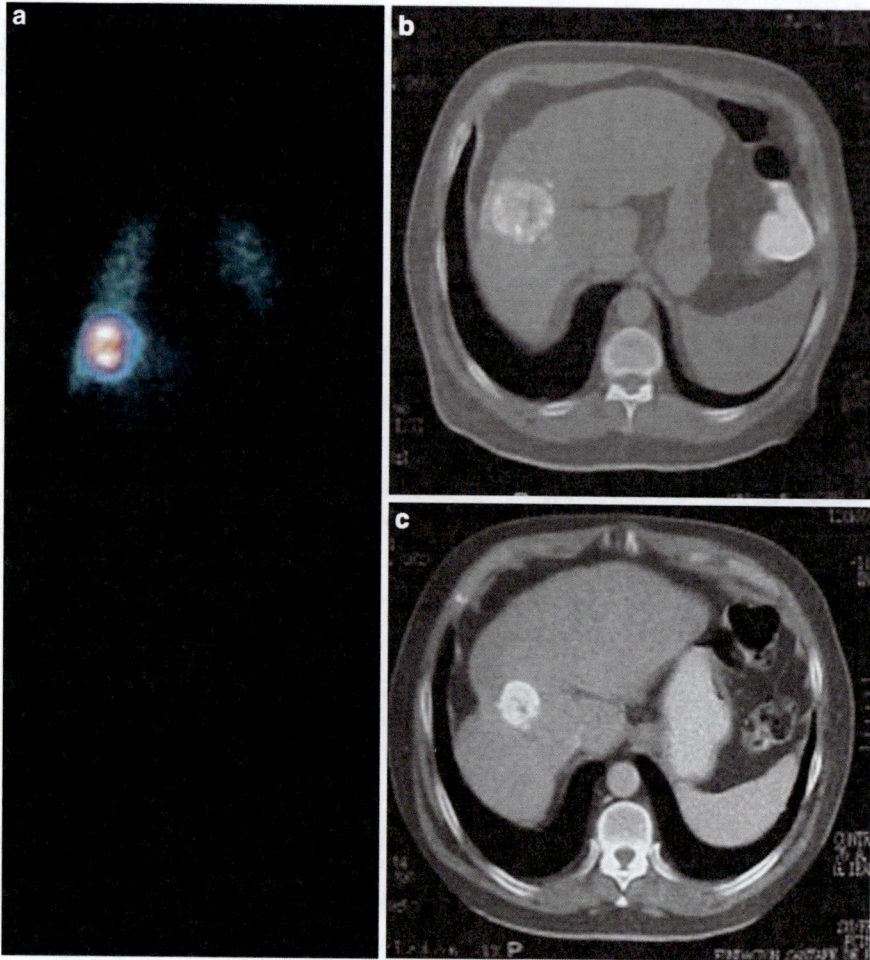

Fig. 12.2 There is continuing hepatic retention of therapeutic radioactivity (**a**) in the patient depicted in Fig. 12.1. Accumulation of lipiodol is visualized in the CT scan immediately after this therapy (**b**) as well as 6 months later (**c**)

1.5 Gy to bone marrow. Median radioactivity has been about 6 MBq of ^{188}Re-lipiodol (Fig. 12.2).

Comparison to Yttrium-90 Microsphere Tare

Commercial development of TARE has focused on yttrium-90, a pure beta emitter with a half-life of 64 h and a maximum beta-minus energy of 2.3 MeV (with an average soft-tissue penetration of about 5 mm). Both the currently used agents— Theraspheres (Theraspheres; MDS Nordion, Ottawa, Ontario, Canada) and SIR-Spheres (SIR-spheres; Sirtex Medical, Lake Forest, IL)—have been approved for use as devices. Theraspheres [20] are glass microspheres while SIR-spheres are resin microspheres [21]. Both contain ^{90}Y as the active carrier; both have an average particle size of around 25 μm; the resin microspheres generally have lower specific activity per sphere than do the glass microspheres. Another important

Table 12.1 Comparison of radionuclides used for hepatic trans-arterial radiotherapy

Nuclide	Half-life	Beta-minus energy (average) (KeV)	Gamma energy
Iodine-131	8 days	182	364 KeV
Rhenium-188	17 h	520	155 KeV
Yttrium-90	64 h	934	None (Bremsstrahlung)

difference is in the method of calculation of dose to be administered, with the calculated activity being more empiric for the resin than for the glass microspheres.

In both instances, however, volume of involved liver is an important criterion for calculation of administered radioactivity, and, as with all TARE, the extent of pulmonary shunting is important and needs to be assessed with planar/SPECT images obtained after trans-arterial injection of ^{99m}Tc-MAA.

Yttrium-90 is a pure beta-minus emitter, and thus therapy can usually be carried out in the outpatient setting. While not required, imaging following therapy—utilizing ^{90}Y Bremsstrahlung—is very feasible [22]. PET has also been attempted, both on time-of-flight [23] as well as other PET/CT devices [24].

The efficacy of ^{90}Y-microsphere TARE has, in large part, been comparable to that of the lipiodol-based therapies discussed above. They have been used widely in both HCC as well as in metastatic liver malignancies [4, 25–32]. Table 12.1 summarizes the major features of the three most commonly utilized radionuclides for TARE.

Multimodality Therapy Including Tare

The potential for combination therapy that includes TARE is compelling. Chemotherapy can potentially reduce tumor size and act as a radiosensitizer, enhancing the effects of TARE. Combination therapy with cisplatinum and ^{131}I-lipiodol resulted in a response rate of 47% with a 2-year survival of 48%, suggesting the additive if not synergistic effects of these therapies [33].

Principles of I-131 Lipiodol Therapy

- Selective trans-arterial delivery of radiation [5].
- Accumulation of lipiodol in HCC [5, 6].
- Dose-limiting toxicity to normal liver [8, 9].
- Radionuclide: Iodine-131, Rhenium-188 [5, 14].
- Improved response rate, survival [6, 16].
- Less toxic than TACE [8, 9].

Radiation Safety Issues

Trans-arterial radioembolization is a multimodality therapy. Nuclear Medicine physicians, physicists and staff are involved in image interpretation, calculation of pulmonary shunt, assessment of extrahepatic perfusion, and calculation of radiation absorbed dose to tumor, normal liver and lungs, where applicable. Nuclear Medicine physicians are also most likely to be the authorized users permitted to administer the therapeutic radioactivity. Interventional radiologists are involved in catheterization and management of the patient during and immediately after both the diagnostic catheterization and the embolization. Radiation safety personnel are closely involved, too, in ensuring that patient and staff radiation safety precautions are adhered to and within reasonable limits, and that the radioactive catheter components are safely disposed of. In many instances, radiation oncologists are also frequently involved in multiple aspects of patient care. Radiation safety precautions need to be observed according to governing laws by these diverse specialties in order for the therapy to be carried out successfully.

There are few radiation safety precautions other than proper disposal of radioactive materials, particularly radioactive syringes and catheters, and appropriate handling of gowns and other items that may be in the radioactive contamination field, when yttrium-90 is the therapeutic nuclide. However, local and national laws governing radiation exposure are particularly relevant for therapy with those radionuclides (^{131}I, ^{188}Re) that emit gamma radiation in addition to the therapeutic beta-minus emission. Most patients need to be admitted after radioactive lipiodol therapy, the duration of stay being dependent on amount of radioactivity administered and clearance characteristics. Such clearance is typically measured using a survey meter, with patient discharge being contingent upon adequate reduction in patient radiation emissions; these regulations vary particularly between the United States and other countries. It is critical to ensure that staff and patients and their families are familiar with relevant aspects of radiation safety and universal precautions.

Conclusion

TARE has the potential to be the therapy of choice in inoperable HCC, and has a role in the control and symptom alleviation of hepatic metastases, particularly from neuroendocrine tumors. Beta-minus emitters labeled to agents that are trapped in the hepatic arterial circulation are agents of choice, and are usually administered after assessment of pulmonary shunting and radiation dose to normal organs and contiguous hepatic tissue. This multidisciplinary effort requires careful coordination and radiation safety planning.

References

1. Gyves JW, Ziessman HA, Ensminger WD, et al. Definition of hepatic tumor microcirculation by single photon emission computerized tomography (SPECT). J Nucl Med. 1984;25:972–7.

2. Bierman HR, Byron Jr RL, Kelley KH, Grady A. Studies on the blood supply of tumors in man. III. Vascular patterns of the liver by hepatic arteriography in vivo. J Natl Cancer Inst. 1951;12:107–31.

3. El-Serag HB. Hepatocellular carcinoma. N Engl J Med. 2011;365(12):1118–27.

4. Liapi E, Geschwind JF. Intra-arterial therapies for hepatocellular carcinoma: where do we stand? Ann Surg Oncol. 2010;17(5):1234–46.

5. Raoul JL, Bourguet P, Bretagne JF, et al. Hepatic artery injection of I-131-labeled lipiodol. Part I. Biodistribution study results in patients with hepatocellular carcinoma and liver metastases. Radiology. 1988;168(2):541–5.

6. Raoul JI, Bretagne JF, Caucanas JP, et al. Internal radiation therapy for hepatocellular carcinoma. Results of a French multicenter phase II trial of transarterial injection of iodine 131-labeled Lipiodol. Cancer. 1992;69(2):346–520.

7. Raoul JL, Guyader D, Bretagne JF, et al. Randomized controlled trial for hepatocellular carcinoma with portal vein thrombosis: intra-arterial iodine-131-iodized oil versus medical support. J Nucl Med. 1994;35(11):1782–7.

8. Bhattacharya S, Novell JR, Dusheiko GM, Hilson AJ, Dick R, Hobbs KE. Epirubicin-Lipiodol chemotherapy versus 131iodine-Lipiodol radiotherapy in the treatment of unresectable hepatocellular carcinoma. Cancer. 1995;76(11):2202–10.

9. Raoul JL, Guyader D, Bretagne JF, et al. Prospective randomized trial of chemoembolization versus intra-arterial injection of 131I-labeled-iodized oil in the treatment of hepatocellular carcinoma. Hepatology. 1997;26(5):1156–61.

10. Boucher E, Garin E, Guylligomarch A, Olivié D, Boudjema K, Raoul JL. Intra-arterial injection of iodine-131-labeled lipiodol for treatment of hepatocellular carcinoma. Radiother Oncol. 2007;82(1):76–82.

11. Lau WY, Leung TW, Ho SK, et al. Adjuvant intra-arterial iodine-131-labelled lipiodol for resectable hepatocellular carcinoma: a prospective randomised trial. Lancet. 1999;353(9155):797–801.

12. Raoul JL, Messner M, Boucher E, Bretagne JF, Campion JP, Boudjema K. Preoperative treatment of hepatocellular carcinoma with intra-arterial injection of 131I-labelled lipiodol. Br J Surg. 2003;90(11):1379–830.

13. Raoul JL, Boucher E, Roland V, Garin E. 131-iodine Lipiodol therapy in hepatocellular carcinoma. Q J Nucl Med Mol Imaging. 2009;53(3):348–55.

14. Garin E, Noiret N, Malbert C, et al. Development and biodistribution of 188Re-SSS lipiodol following injection into the hepatic artery of healthy pigs. Eur J Nucl Med Mol Imaging. 2004;31(4):542–6.

15. Jeong JM, Knapp Jr FF. Use of the Oak Ridge National Laboratory tungsten-188/rhenium-188 generator for preparation of the rhenium-188 HDD/lipiodol complex for trans-arterial liver cancer therapy. Semin Nucl Med. 2008;38(2):S19–29.

16. Bernal P, Raoul JL, Vidmar G, et al. Intra-arterial rhenium-188 lipiodol in the treatment of inoperable hepatocellular carcinoma: results of an IAEA-sponsored multination study. Int J Radiat Oncol Biol Phys. 2007;69(5):1448–55.

17. Sundram F, Chau TC, Onkhuudai P, Bernal P, Padhy AK. Preliminary results of transarterial rhenium-188 HDD lipiodol in the treatment of inoperable primary hepatocellular carcinoma. Eur J Nucl Med Mol Imaging. 2004;31(2):250–7.

18. Zanzonico PB, Divgi C. Patient-specific radiation dosimetry for radionuclide therapy of liver tumors with intrahepatic artery rhenium-188 lipiodol. Semin Nucl Med. 2008;38(2):S30–9.

19. Bernal P, Raoul JL, Stare J, et al. International Atomic Energy Agency-sponsored multination study of intra-arterial rhenium-188-labeled lipiodol in the treatment of inoperable hepatocellular carcinoma: results with special emphasis on prognostic value of dosimetric study. Semin Nucl Med. 2008;38(2):S40–5.

20. Accessed from: http://www.nordion.com/therasphere/physicians_intl/package_insert.asp.

21. Sirtex Medical Training Program manual, downloaded from http://www.sirtex.com.

22. Prompers L, Bucerius J, Brans B, Temur Y, Berger L, Mottaghy FM. Selective internal radiation therapy (SIRT) in primary or secondary liver cancer. Methods. 2011;55(3):253–7.

23. Lhommel R, Goffette P, Van den Eynde M, et al. Yttrium-90 TOF PET scan demonstrates high-resolution biodistribution after liver SIRT. Eur J Nucl Med Mol Imaging. 2009;36(10):1696.

24. Gates VL, Esmail AA, Marshall K, Spies S, Salem R. Internal pair production of 90Y permits hepatic localization of microspheres using routine PET: proof of concept. J Nucl Med. 2011;52(1):72–6.

25. Lewandowski RJ, Geschwind JF, Liapi E, Salem R. Transcatheter intraarterial therapies: rationale and overview. Radiology. 2011;259(3):641–57. Review. PubMed PMID: 21602502.

26. Coldwell D, Sangro B, Salem R, Wasan H, Kennedy A. Radioembolization in the treatment of unresectable liver tumors: experience across a range of primary cancers. Am J Clin Oncol. 2012;35(2):167–77. PMID: 21127414.

27. Kennedy A, Coldwell D, Sangro B, Wasan H, Salem R. Integrating radioembolization (90Y microspheres) into current treatment options for liver tumors: introduction to the International Working Group Report. Am J Clin Oncol. 2012;35(1):81–90.

28. Kennedy AS, Dezarn WA, McNeillie P, et al. Radioembolization for unresectable neuroendocrine hepatic metastases using resin 90Y-microspheres: early results in 148 patients. Am J Clin Oncol. 2008;31(3):271–9.

29. Hendlisz A, Van den Eynde M, Peeters M, et al. Phase III trial comparing protracted intravenous fluorouracil infusion alone or with yttrium-90 resin microspheres radioembolization for liver-limited metastatic colorectal cancer refractory to standard chemotherapy. J Clin Oncol. 2010;28(23):3687–94.

30. Bester L, Meteling B, Pocock N, et al. Radioembolization versus standard care of hepatic metastases: comparative retrospective cohort study of survival outcomes and adverse events in salvage patients. J Vasc Interv Radiol. 2012;23(1):96–105.

31. Lewandowski RJ, Geschwind JF, Liapi E, Salem R. Transcatheter intraarterial therapies: rationale and overview. Radiology. 2011;259(3):641–57.

32. Raoul JL, Boucher E, Rolland Y, Garin E. Treatment of hepatocellular carcinoma with intra-arterial injection of radionuclides. Nat Rev Gastroenterol Hepatol. 2010;7(1):41–9.

33. Raoul JL, Boucher E, Olivie D, Guillygomarc'h A, Boudjema K, Garin E. Association of cisplatin and intra-arterial injection of 131I-lipiodol in treatment of hepatocellular carcinoma: results of phase II trial. Int J Radiat Oncol Biol Phys. 2006;64(3):745–50.

Antibody-Targeted Therapeutic Radionuclides in the Management of Colorectal Cancer

13

Robert M. Sharkey and David M. Goldenberg

Introduction

Colon cancer is the third most common cancer diagnosed in men and women in the USA, with ~103,000 new cases in 2010, but it ranks second among all cancer-related deaths in men and women, with nearly 51,000 deaths (lung cancer is the highest with an estimated 157,000 deaths and breast is third with 40,000 deaths) [1]. Globally, colorectal cancer (CRC) again ranks as the second most common cause of cancer-related deaths [2]. However, the rate of CRC deaths in both men and women is decreasing in the USA, largely because of screening. As with all cancers, the prognosis is largely dependent on the stage of disease when first diagnosed, with the 5-year survival rate decreasing from an average of 90% for stage I to just about 12% for stage IV [3].

Stages I and II colon cancer are treated primarily by surgery, but the use of postsurgical adjuvant chemotherapy for stage II cancer is controversial [4–8]. Stages III and IV colon cancer are primarily

treated with surgery, followed by chemotherapy (5-fluorouracil, leucovorin, oxaliplatin, and irinotecan combinations, such as FOLFOX, FOLFIRI) with or without an antibody-based therapeutic, such as bevacizumab (anti-vascular endothelial growth factor) and cetuximab or panitumumab (anti-epithelial growth factor receptor antibodies), mainly in patients with wild-type *KRAS* expression. In the case of rectal cancer, external beam therapy also is employed [9–20]. Patients with surgically resectable hepatic metastases, occurring at the time of diagnosis or developed later, may benefit from hepatic resection, with or without neoadjuvant chemotherapy [5, 8, 21–29]. There are also indications that postsurgical adjuvant therapy improves survival, but with the changing landscape in available chemotherapeutic regimens, this remains an area of active investigation [30–36]. Studies have supported the use of cetuximab and bevacizumab combinations with chemotherapy for treating patients with stage IV disease [37–43]. However, results from a large randomized study examining resected stage III patients with wild-type or mutant *KRAS* reported that cetuximab added to a FOLFOX6 regimen did not improve the 3-year disease-free survival or overall survival, with evidence that the addition of cetuximab to FOLFOX in mutant *KRAS* patients actually resulted in a poorer outcome than FOLFOX alone [44, 45]. Interestingly, Huang et al. reported the addition of cetuximab to a FOLFIRI regimen appeared to be beneficial, with a trend toward improved disease-free survival ($P=0.09$), regardless of their *KRAS* status. The addition of bevacizumab to

R.M. Sharkey, Ph.D.
Center of Molecular Medicine and Immunology
and the Garden State Cancer Center, 300 The American
Road, Morris Plains, NJ, 07950, USA
e-mail: rmsharkey@gscancer.org; dmg.gscancer@att.net

D.M. Goldenberg, Sc.D., M.D. (✉)
IBC Pharmaceuticals, Inc. and Immunomedics, Inc.,
Morris Plains, NJ, USA

Garden State Cancer Center, Center for Molecular
Medicine and Immunology, 300 The American Road,
Morris Plains, NJ, USA

C. Aktolun and S.J. Goldsmith (eds.), *Nuclear Medicine Therapy: Principles and Clinical Applications*,   207
DOI 10.1007/978-1-4614-4021-5_13, © Springer Science+Business Media New York 2013

mFOLFOX6 for adjuvant treatment of stage II and III patients similarly did not improve disease-free survival [15].

Nonantibody-Based Therapeutics

There are no standard therapies for primary colon cancer that involve radionuclide treatments. Radioembolization, using ^{90}Y-microspheres (selective internal radiation therapy, SIRT), is used for treating primary and secondary tumors (such as CRC) in the liver when patients have unresectable hepatic lesions (without extrahepatic involvement), and where surgery or tumor ablation is not a practical treatment option [46–56]. This procedure received FDA approval initially in 2002 for the treatment of CRC metastases when used in combination with hepatic arterial chemotherapy [54]. Other clinical trials followed, with one randomized trial using the ^{90}Y-microspheres and systemic fluorouracil/leucovorin showing more favorable response rates, time to progression and survival [54], while other trials have shown encouraging results with other chemotherapeutic agent [49, 55, 57]. Another agent, lipiodol, typically used as a contrast agent, also was examined as a possible therapeutic when radiolabeled with ^{131}I or ^{188}Re [58–65]. It was considered as a possible therapeutic for localized disease in the liver, since when injected intra-arterially, this ethiodized oil has high uptake in the liver [66]. This agent was more commonly examined in primary hepatocellular carcinomas, and while there was some evidence it was effective when used as part of an embolism treatment protocol, it is not widely used at this time [65, 67]. The European Association of Nuclear Medicine recently published guidelines for the use of ^{90}Y-microspheres and ^{131}I-lipiodol [68].

Neuroendocrine tumors originating in the colon and rectum (also known as hindgut carcinoids) are relatively rare (e.g., <1% to 3.9% of all CRCs [69, 70]), but these can have a poor prognosis, with a median survival determined from one institution to be 10.4 months [70]. These tumors are being treated with some success using a radio-labeled somatostatin-receptor peptide [71–73],

and there also have been some investigations with ^{131}I-MIBG therapy [74, 75], which is discussed elsewhere (Chap. 20).

Antibody-Targeted Radionuclides Radioimmunotherapy

Radioimmunotherapy (RAIT) is one of the most studied therapeutic procedures in nuclear medicine, having the approval of two therapeutic agents for the treatment of follicular lymphomas [76–78]. However, there also have been considerable preclinical and clinical experiences in RAIT of CRC [79–81]. Goldenberg et al. were the first to demonstrate that a radiolabeled antibody against a human tumor-associated antigen could by itself arrest tumor progression [82]. In this study, an^{131}I-labeled, affinity-purified, polyclonal goat antibody to carcinoembryonic antigen (CEA) successfully inhibited the growth of 4-day-old human colon cancer xenografts (signet-ring-cell histology) implanted in the cheek pouch of hamsters. At 0.5 mCi of the ^{131}I-anti-CEA IgG, no significant antitumor effect was observed, with untreated and treated tumors progressing nearly fourfold 15 days from the baseline measurement. A single 1.0-mCi dose of the specific antibody inhibited tumor growth significantly over the same dose of an^{131}I-labeled goat IgG, with tumors treated with ^{131}I-labeled irrelevant IgG progressing ~2.5 fold in size from baseline, while tumors in animals given the ^{131}I-anti-CEA IgG progressed ~1.5-fold. At 2.0 mCi, both the specific and irrelevant radiolabeled IgG prevented tumor progression equally. This was the first evidence that high doses of an irrelevant radiolabeled IgG could be therapeutic. However, radiation dosimetry estimates predicted the tumors in the animals given 1.0 mCi of the specific antibody received 1,325 cGy, while the irrelevant antibody delivered 411 cGy. No toxicity, as measured by changes in weight, was reported at any of the dose levels.

This study was significant from several perspectives. First, therapy trials with radiolabeled antibodies in patients had only started to begin, but the treatment regimens combined ^{131}I-labeled anti-ferritin and anti-CEA antibodies with chemotherapy and external beam radiation, and therefore the contribution of RAIT to the antitumor effects was unclear [83–88]. The animal studies proved a directly radiolabeled antibody alone can affect tumor progression, with a specific antibody providing a significant benefit over a nonbinding antibody. The efficacy of even a nonspecific antibody was not surprising, since earlier biodistribution studies had indicated that a nonbinding IgG localized in tumors at higher levels than most normal tissues [89, 90]. This occurs because tumors have a unique, albeit dysfunctional, vascular physiology that allows macromolecules, such as an IgG, to localize at higher levels than in normal tissues [91–93]. However, agents that bind to the tumor will accrue at higher levels and be retained longer than nonbinding agents. Indeed, enriching the immunoreactive fraction by affinity-purifying polyclonal antibodies increased the percent uptake in the tumor [94]. Finally, it was interesting to find a therapeutic effect occurred even though the radiation dose delivered to the tumors was estimated to be substantially lower than that typically given as external beam therapy. This stimulated a wide range of studies to understand therapeutic differences between continuous, low-dose-rate radiation delivered with a radiolabeled antibody and fractionated, high-dose-rate radiation delivered by external beam therapy, as well as other issues related to the therapeutic potential of antibody-targeted radionuclides [95–114].

Preclinical and clinical studies continued with radiolabeled polyclonal anti-CEA antibodies, but thanks to the development of the hybridoma technology and the use of murine monoclonal antibody (mMAb), more widespread interest in antibody-based targeting of radionuclides ensued. MAbs had a tremendous production advantage, so adaptation of mMAbs occurred quickly. However, MAbs created a new set of concerns. For example, would an antibody that binds to just one well-defined epitope target tumors as well as a polyclonal antibody that contained multiple clones to diverse epitopes (supposedly on the same molecule)? A few preclinical studies soon dispelled this concern by showing mMAbs localized tumors as well or better than polyclonal antibodies (e.g., [115]). Another issue arose, particularly for CEA MAbs, which was related to their exquisite ability to discern subtle structural differences in molecules (i.e., well-defined epitopes). Even with polyclonal antibodies to CEA, investigators had known that "CEA" was a family of multiple antigens having shared epitopes. For example, Primus et al. developed 4 mMAbs to CEA purified from a hepatic metastasis of human colon cancer, designated NP-1 through NP-4, each having unique specificities that were grouped into three classes based on their binding to purified CEA, NCA (nonspecific cross-reactive antigen) and MA (meconium antigen) [116–118]. In hamsters bearing the GW-39 human colonic cancer cell line, the NP-2 MAb was judged to have the best tumor localization properties, followed by NP-4 [115]. NP-2's binding to CEA also was ion-sensitive, and therefore did not bind to CEA in the blood, but it did bind to CEA affixed to a solid support (i.e., tumor cells) [119–121]. At the onset, NP-1 was known to bind to an epitope shared with NCA, an antigen present on granulocytes, and therefore the likelihood that bone marrow targeting would make unambiguous identification of tumors difficult, it was not considered suitable for targeting of colon cancer in patients. However, the other 3 mMAbs were purified and given to patients, starting with NP-2 [120]. Initial targeting with ^{131}I-NP-2 IgG in patients with diverse CEA-producing cancers (mostly GI) was promising (similar sensitivity as the affinity-purified goat antibody). However, as purification procedures improved the immunoreactive fraction, a previously unknown binding to human granulocytes was revealed, and images then showed strong uptake in the bone marrow (Fig. 13.1a, b). NP-3 very avidly bound to CEA in the blood and, like earlier findings with polyclonal antibodies, where interaction with CEA in the serum did not prevent tumor localization [122], ^{131}I-labeled NP-3 also targeted cancers well. However, the images revealed an enhanced uptake in the colon (Fig. 13.1c). Over time, the activity moved through the intestinal tract, and further analysis revealed the uptake was due to immune complexes in the stool rather than fixed antibody

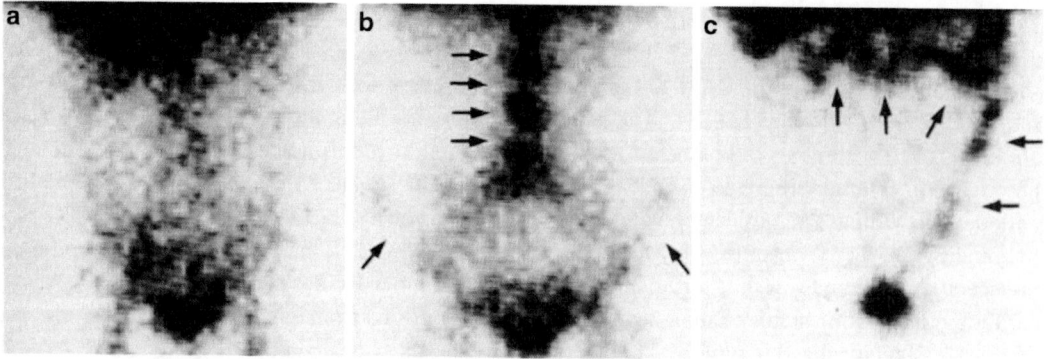

Fig. 13.1 Gamma scintillation (anterior views) images illustrating unfavorable localization patterns for ^{131}I-labeled murine anti-CEA antibodies that recognize different CEA-related antigen. (**a**) ^{131}I-NP-2 (immunoreactive fraction 30–50%) is compared to ^{131}I-NP-2 having an immunoreactive fraction of 70–90% (**b**), where bone marrow targeting in the spine is seen (*arrows*). (**c**) ^{131}I-NP-3 (immunoreactive fraction 90%) shows uptake in the transverse and in portions of the descending colon (*arrows*). Figures reprinted from reference [120] with permission

binding to the intestine. Apparently, the NP-3/CEA complexes formed in the serum were removed in the liver, traveling through the bile duct into the intestines. ^{131}I-NP-4 also targeted known sites of cancer with high sensitivity, but it did not show any uptake in the bone marrow or colon. It did not complex with CEA as readily as NP-3, but NP-4 also had the lowest affinity of the original 4 mMAbs for binding CEA [118]. An international workshop examining anti-CEA MAbs developed a classification system for what eventually became known as carcinoembryonic antigen-related cell adhesion molecules (CEACAMs) [123, 124]. NP-4 was classified in a group of antibodies that only bound to CEA, now called CEACAM5, not including any of the other cross-reactive antigens [5].

A Fab' fragment of the NP-4 mMAb labeled with ^{99m}Tc was developed by Immunomedics, Inc. (Morris Plains, NJ) and approved for imaging metastatic CRC (IMMU-4, CEAScan®) [125, 126], but preclinical and clinical therapy studies with NP-4 continued as well. Behr et al. [127] summarized patient studies where ^{131}I-NP-4 IgG was used to treat diverse, advanced, CEA-producing cancers, including 29 CRC patients. The administered activity for ^{131}I-NP-4 IgG therapy was based on the radiation dose to their red marrow (using blood clearance data and assuming blood/marrow ratio

of 1.0), which was derived from a pretherapy imaging study. Escalating in 100-cGy increments from a starting level of 150 cGy, the MTD was determined to be 450 cGy (no more than 1/6 patients experienced Grade 4 hematologic toxicity for any duration). The average red marrow dose in CRC patients was 2.2 ± 1.1 cGy/mCi. Antitumor responses were found in 12 of 35 assessable patients, with one partial response (PR), four mixed/minor responses, with seven showing marked stabilization of previously rapidly progressing disease. The single PR occurred in a patient with multiple small hepatic lesions from a pancreatic primary. Responses occurred mainly in patients who received >400 cGy to the red marrow, prompting investigators to speculate that more clinically relevant responses would require higher doses, which would need hematopoietic support; alternatively, the treatment would need to focus on patients with less disease burden. It also should be noted that the immunogenicity of the murine antibody prevented any real attempt at fractionating or repeating treatments in these early RAIT studies. The development of chimeric and humanized antibodies would soon mitigate, but not eliminate this problem.

Tumor dosimetry from these clinical studies indicated that smaller tumors received substantially higher radiation doses, mimicking earlier preclinical studies that had emphasized that RAIT would have maximum benefit only when treating minimal disease burden [127–131]. Indeed, other studies showed a large tumor reduces antibody uptake in smaller tumors in the same animals [132], which suggested that clinically, RAIT's therapeutic prospects against small tumors would be masked in a patient with bulky disease. These findings provided further credence for debulking surgery before treating with RAIT.

Another interesting finding from some of these earlier animal studies was related to the effect of antibody protein dose on therapeutic responses. Fujimori et al. [133] reported that in addition to physiological issues that impeded fluidic movement of macromolecules into tumors, substances such as antibodies that specifically bind to tumor cells would not move very far away from the blood vessels where they emerge, due to a "binding-site barrier." Logically, antibodies with higher affinity would be affected more than those with low affinity. Administering additional antibody protein was shown to encourage a more homogeneous distribution, but unless carefully adjusted, competition for antigen between the radiolabeled and nonradioactive antibody could decrease the amount of radioactivity in the tumor, thereby reducing the efficacy potentially elicited by the radiolabeled antibody treatment [134, 135].

While clinical trials were reporting disappointing therapeutic results with ^{131}I-mMAb IgG in patients with advanced disease, preclinical studies were actively exploring ways to improve RAIT, with some suggesting that accelerating the clearance of the radiolabeled IgG from the blood, using a clearing agent (second antibody) [136–140] or with antibody fragments [141–145] might improve responses. Both of these methods reduced red marrow exposure, allowing more activity to be administered, but antibody fragments allowed tumor uptake to reach a maximum level more quickly than an IgG, yielding a higher dose rate that might further enhance therapeutic prospects. Juweid et al. reported a small clinical study included 13 patients (eight were colorectal, one pancreatic, the others were lung and medullary thyroid cancers) who had minimal disease (i.e., no single lesion >3.0 cm) and were treated with ^{131}I-labeled NP-4 anti-CEA F(ab')$_2$ fragments [146]. Three of the CRC patients had disease in the liver, and the others had lung, bone, or lymph node involvement. A pretherapy imaging study using ~10 mCi of the labeled antibody was used initially to gauge the therapeutic dose, which was given based on 450 cGy to the red marrow. However, the trial was modified to increase the pretherapy "imaging" dose to 40 mCi/m^2, followed ≥4 weeks later by a higher therapeutic dose. The total red-marrow dose was not to exceed 450 cGy for treatments given within 8 weeks. Two of the CRC patients received more than one dose exceeding the 40 mCi/m^2 level. There were no objective responses, but four of the eight CRC patients had stable disease for 1–11 months. Ychou et al. [147] reported a clinical trial that included ten CRC patients with unresectable hepatic metastases; five were given 87–300 mCi of ^{131}I-F6 anti-CEA F(ab')$_2$, with the next five patients receiving a fixed dose of 300 mCi. Bone marrow harvested prior to the treatment was used in five of six patients given 300 mCi of ^{131}I-F6 because of severe hematologic toxicity. One patient had a partial response in a 2-cm hepatic tumor, with stable disease in the remaining lesions, while two had stable disease and six progressed. Thus, despite having a shorter residence time in the blood and the ability to administer higher levels of radioactivity, clinically significant responses were not more forthcoming with the ^{131}I-F(ab')$_2$ than with the ^{131}I-IgG. This same group also investigated the prospects for direct intra-arterial injection of the radiolabeled antibody for patients with hepatic metastases as well as combining RAIT with external beam radiation, but these studies never proceeded beyond feasibility testing in a limited number of patients [148–150].

Although targeting with NP-4 appeared adequate, this antibody's affinity to CEA was rather low. Thus, an effort to develop second-generation anti-CEA mMAbs was undertaken [119], ultimately yielding another anti-CEACAM5 specific mMAb, MN-14, that had tenfold higher affinity than NP-4, which animal studies found increased tumor uptake. The ^{131}I-mMN-14 IgG and its F(ab)$_2$ fragment (papain-derived) were used primarily in

Antibodies Evaluated as Colo-Rectal Ca Recognition Reagents

Anti-CEA	Carcinoembryonic antigen
Anti-CA19-9	Tumor marker for pancreatic ca
Anti-EpCam	Epithelial cell adhesion molecule, otherwise known as epithelial glycoprotein-2
TAG-72	Tumor-associated glycoprotein-72
CC49	Colon cancer-49 (second generation anti-TAG-72)
Mu-9	Mucin-9 (anti-colon-specific antigen-p, CSAp)
A33	An antibody to the antigen GPA33, a 43 kDa type I transmembrane cell surface glycoprotein that is a member of the immunoglobulin superfamily, with homology to cell adhesion and tight-junction-associated proteins
F19	Does not bind to tumor cells, directed against surface glycoprotein (fibroblast activation protein)

patients for the therapy of ovarian [151, 152] and medullary thyroid cancers [146, 153, 154]. One ovarian cancer patient with malignant ascites who was refractory to paclitaxel achieved a partial response within 1 month of receiving ~75 mCi of ^{131}I-mMN-14 IgG, which converted to a complete response after receiving a second course of ^{131}I-mMN-14 IgG [151]. However, in an expanded Phase I trial of advanced ovarian cancer, no other significant responses were observed. In medullary thyroid cancer, patients were enrolled in two trials, one using nonmyeloablative doses and the other myeloablative doses of ^{131}I-mMN-14 F(ab)$_2$. In the nonmyeloablative dose trial, administered activity was based on the radiation dose to the red marrow, with patients first having a 8.0 mCi pretherapy imaging study followed 1 week later with a treatment of activities ranging from 100 to 267 mCi of ^{131}I-mMN-14 F(ab)$_2$. There were no partial or complete response in this trial, but there were radiological and biochemical responses, as well as disease stabilization in 11 of 15 patients [153]. Tumor dosimetry also was exceptionally high in several patients, with six patients receiving >2,000 cGy to at least one lesion and several

lesions even exceeded 5,000 cGy. To circumvent dose-limiting hematologic toxicity, the other trial used myeloablative doses of ^{131}I-mMN-14 F(ab)$_2$ with autologous stem cell support [155]. This trial adopted a similar design that was being used successfully for treating non-Hodgkin lymphoma with high-dose ^{131}I-labeled mMAb that based the treatment dose on organ dosimetry [156, 157]. Administered activity for the therapeutic doses started at a level that would deliver 900 cGy to the kidneys (and not to exceed 1,200 cGy to lungs and liver), and then progressed to a 1,200 cGy renal-dose level. Twelve patients were enrolled, with some patients experiencing nondose-limiting gastrointestinal and cardiac toxicity. There was one partial response for 1 year, one minor response and ten with stabilization of disease for 1–16 months. Thus, while there were anecdotal responses in a select number of patients, clinical studies with the higher affinity ^{131}I-labeled mMN-14 anti-CEA antibody still did not produce sufficient evidence of clinically meaningful responses, even when the activity was escalated with the aid hematological support measures. However, with excellent tumor localization properties, the MN-14 antibody was humanized to reduce immunogenicity. Initial testing showed excellent targeting [158] (e.g., Fig. 13.2), and a Phase I trial in advanced CRC patients determined the MTD for ^{131}I-hMN-14 IgG (labetuzumab) to be 40 mCi/m^2, but no objective responses were observed [159].

Since most initial testing is performed in patients with advanced disease, clinical studies turned to investigating antibodies labeled with ^{90}Y, a radionuclide with no gamma emissions for imaging, but with a strong beta-emission (2.27 MeV, 64 h half-life) that can penetrate more deeply in tissues than ^{131}I [108, 160]. However, unlike ^{131}I-MAb treatments that had required patients to be hospitalized for prolonged periods of time, patients could be treated with ^{90}Y-MAbs on an outpatient basis. Although patient-release criteria have been relaxed in the USA [161], ^{131}I-MAbs still require close oversight, particularly outside the USA [162–164]. ^{90}Y lacks a gamma emission, and thus, its biodistribution is most often determined with the same product labeled with ^{111}In.

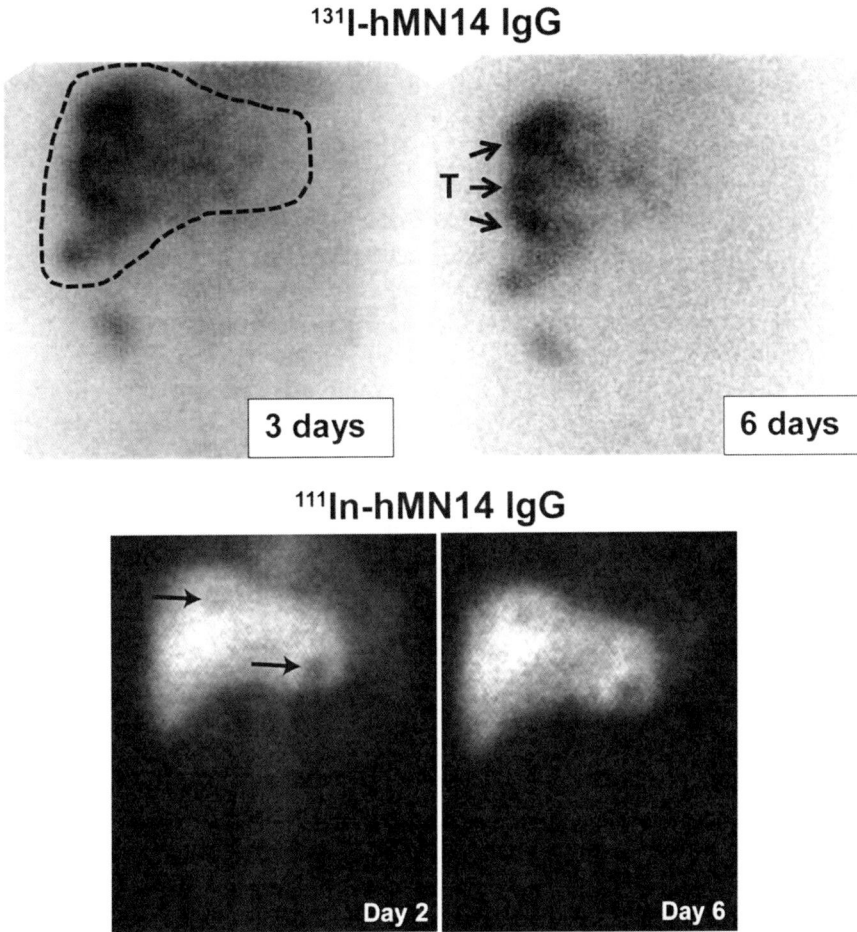

Fig. 13.2 Example of targeting with second-generation and humanized anti-CEACAM5 IgG (labetuzumab). Anterior planar images that illustrate the targeting of hepatic metastases in a patient with colorectal cancer (CRC) at 72 h and 144 h after receiving 8.8 mCi of ^{131}I-hMN-14 IgG. The radioactivity in the tumor bed [*arrows* show several tumor (T) lesions present in the liver] is retained while the activity in the uninvolved hepatic tissue is cleared (*dashed* region of interest outlines the liver). Figures reprinted from reference [159] with permission. The *bottom* two photographs are an example of targeting with ^{111}In-hMN-14 IgG in a CRC patient with two hepatic metastases shown by the *arrows* as photopenic areas. Note also that the uptake in the normal liver remains high over time

Early adoption of ^{90}Y-MAbs faced a number of issues, in terms of isotope supply and availability, but also stable binding of ^{90}Y to the antibody. For example, preclinical studies with ^{90}Y-labeled cyclic-anhydride DTPA-conjugated NP-2 reported selective therapeutic responses in mice with just 50 µCi of the labeled IgG compared to an irrelevant IgG, but higher doses were too toxic [165]. The responses with the ^{90}Y-antibody were not as impressive as those found in separate studies using ^{131}I-NP-4, leading us to speculate that ^{90}Y-labeled antibodies might not be suitable therapeutics. However, this experience reflected the use of the first generation cyclic anhydride DTPA as the ^{90}Y-chelating agent, which later studies confirmed was not sufficiently stable for the bone-seeking ^{90}Y [166–169]. Subsequent studies found other DTPA derivatives were more suitable for ^{90}Y-antibody therapy [170], as well as macrocyclic chelating agents, most notably DOTA (1,4,7,10-tetraazacyclodo-decane-N,N′,N″,N‴-tetraacetic acid) [171–174].

One study found a ^{90}Y-labeled antibody prepared using the macrocyclic DOTA derivative 2-IT-BAD had less bone uptake and higher tolerance in mice than one of the preferred DTPA derivatives (MX-DTPA) [175]. We also found conjugates prepared with DOTA were more stable than with MX-DTPA [175].

[90]Y and other radiometal-labeled conjugates often were found to have longer retention in tumors than ^{131}I-labeled antibodies, particularly when the antibody was actively internalized [176–178]. Unfortunately, this retention also occurs in normal tissues that are involved with the removal of the antibody from the body (e.g., liver and to some degree the spleen for IgG). Hepatic uptake and retention was more problematic with antibodies that bound to antigens found in the blood, since the immune complexes would be deposited in the liver. Biodistribution studies also indicated that antibody Fab' fragments would not be suitable for therapy, because renal retention of ^{90}Y-Fab' was as much as tenfold higher than for the tumor [170].

Wong et al. reported the first clinical RAIT trial in CRC examining a high-affinity, ^{90}Y-labeled chimeric T84.66 anti-CEACAM5 IgG [179]. Patients were given 5 mg of the antibody conjugated with a stable isothiocyanatobenzyl-DTPA derivative that was radiolabeled first with ^{111}In for imaging, and then starting 1 week later, they were eligible for receiving the therapeutic dose of the ^{90}Y-DTPA cT84.66, also with 5 mg of the antibody. Patients received an infusion of DTPA after the antibody injection in an effort to scavenge any ^{90}Y that might be liberated from the conjugated antibody. The trial started at 5 mCi/m², but patients could receive up to three cycles of treatment at 6-week intervals. Up to this point, there had been considerable preclinical and even some clinical experience that illustrated differences between the biodistribution of [131]I- and ^{111}In-labeled anti-CEA antibodies [180–188]. Therefore, it was not surprising in this first therapy trial that some patients had more rapid blood clearance associated with increased hepatic uptake that correlated with plasma CEA. Also, some hepatic lesions were photopenic, a consequence of higher uptake in the liver than the

tumor with the radiometal-labeled antibody. The full trial results with the ^{90}Y-cT84.66 IgG found dose-limiting toxicity at 22 mCi/m², again finding hematological toxicity to be dose-limiting, despite high uptake in the liver [189]. Only three patients received repeated treatments. The investigators concluded that patients with excessive hepatic involvement should not be considered for enrollment because of high hepatic uptake and rapid blood clearance. Dosimetry estimated tumors received 8.7–55.2 cGy/mCi. No objective responses were observed, but as in the earlier studies with ^{131}I-labeled antibodies, some patients had significant shrinkage in select lesions. Based on in vitro data supporting superior stability with ^{111}In and ^{90}Y compared to the previous DTPA conjugate [190], a later study examined the same antibody conjugated with DOTA. In this study, dose-limiting hematologic toxicity occurred at 16 mCi/m², again using DTPA infusions after the ^{90}Y-MAb injection to scavenge [90]Y [191]. In comparing these results to their previous study, they noted that each conjugate had the same clearance kinetics and considered their tolerances to be similar. Tumor doses ranged from 4.4 to as high as 569 cGy/mCi, but still no clinically relevant antitumor responses were observed, albeit five lesions ranging from 2 to 7.5 cm in diameter decreased 25–47%. They also reported antichimeric antibody responses hampered efforts to repeat the treatment.

Other Monoclonal Antibodies

Many other antibodies to CEA have provided additional insightful preclinical and clinical data, but there are too many to review their individual contributions in this chapter (e.g., F6 as mentioned above, ZCE025 [182, 187, 192], COL-1 [193–195], Mab 35 [142, 196], C110 [186], A5B7 [197–201], rch24 [202], 38S1 [203–205], F33-104 [206, 207], CL58 [208], and A10 [209]). However, there also have been a number of other MAbs that bind to CRC that have paralleled and enriched the preclinical and clinical experiences of RAIT in colon cancer that we will mention briefly.

One of the earliest non-CEA antibodies to be studied was 17-1A (anti-EpCam) and 19-9 mMAbs (anti-CA19-9), initially focusing on targeting studies in animals [210, 211] and some imaging trials in patients [212, 213]. Although MAb 19-9 was never developed for therapy, the antigen, CA19-9, remains an important tumor marker for pancreatic cancer [214–217]. MAb 17-1A went on to be used primarily as an unconjugated antibody for the treatment of gastrointestinal cancers rather than as a radioconjugate [218–223]. Nevertheless, there were some early preclinical and a limited number of clinical studies. One such application focused on the possible use of ^{125}I-labeled 17-1A as one of the earliest antibody-targeted Auger-emitting therapeutics. 17-1A was selected specifically for this application because it internalized and was translocated to the nucleus [176, 224–226]. Advanced CRC patients received as much as 250 mCi of ^{125}I-chimeric 17-1A in 2–3 doses given over 4–8 days. No severe toxicity was reported in a 6-week follow-up period, but neither were there any objective responses. Another antibody, MAb 425 that binds to the epithelial growth factor receptor (EGFR), was also radiolabeled with ^{125}I for RAIT, but it was used primarily to treat brain tumors [227]. With the later development of other nonradiolabeled anti-EGFR antibodies, cetuximab and panitumumab, which have been used successfully to treat colon cancer, perhaps an anti-EGFR radioconjugate should be studied in CRC in the future [228–230].

One of the more extensively studied non-CEA antibodies has been directed to TAG-72 (tumor-associated glycoprotein-72). In its first reporting, the murine antibody, B72.3, was noted for its long retention in the tumor, with initial studies finding that the radioiodinated antibody's uptake in the tumor was elevated at the same level for 19 days [231]. The first FDA-approved antibody-based imaging agent was developed with this antibody [232, 233], as well as the initial studies with radioguided surgery [234].

Therapeutic studies with the ^{131}I-labeled B72.3 mMAb in nude mice bearing human colonic cancer xenografts showed the expected ability to arrest tumor growth [235]. From these first studies, a plethora of preclinical and some clinical studies were undertaken [236–240], but studies quickly turned to a second generation, higher affinity, anti-TAG 72 antibody, CC49, that was ultimately humanized [241–246]. Like the previous studies with the higher affinity anti-CEA antibody, where tumor uptake improved in xenograft models, so too did the second-generation CC49 anti-TAG-72 antibody enhance targeting [239, 244]. Clinical studies in CRC certainly attested to the excellent targeting with this antibody, even showing a preference for the CC49 antibody over the first generation B72.3, not because of a difference in tumor uptake, but because the former cleared more quickly from the blood [247, 248]. However, even when given at myeloablative doses as high as 300 mCi/m^2 (using posttreatment hematologic support), there was insufficient evidence of therapeutic responses with the ^{131}I-murine CC49, leading investigators to suggest that a high-energy beta emitter, such as ^{90}Y, might be better suited for treatments involving advanced metastatic disease [249]. However, when a Phase I therapy trial using ^{90}Y-CC49 escalated to as high as 0.5 mCi/kg with hematopoietic support failed to obtain any objective responses, the investigators concluded that tumor doses were suboptimal and liver uptake was too high for additional studies to be performed [250]. It should be noted that like CEA, TAG-72 is found in the serum, and thus immune complexes were deposited in the liver. Unlike ^{131}I-MAbs, where the radioactivity would be eliminated quickly from the liver, the radioactivity of radiometal-labeled MAbs was retained at a high level.

Preclinical studies indicated that the combination of gamma-interferon with RAIT, using the ^{90}Y-CC49 antibody, improved therapeutic responses based on the interferon's ability to upregulate TAG-72 (and CEA) production by cells [251, 252], but clinical trials with ^{131}I-CC49 plus interferon in colon cancer, as well as breast cancer, concluded that the combination did not have the desired enhanced therapeutic effect [253, 254]. Investigators also performed a Phase II trial combining the ^{131}I-CC49 antibody with an ^{131}I-anti-CEA antibody (COL-1) and gamma-interferon in anticipation that targeting two antigens that were both upregulated in the presence of gamma-interferon would enhance uptake (quantitatively and more uniformly); however, encouraging responses were not observed [195].

We developed and tested clinically another antibody, Mu-9, that also bound to a mucin-associated antigen similar to a polyclonal antibody that was called colon-specific antigen-p (CSAp) [255]. This antibody also had exceptionally high uptake and long retention in xenograft models, providing excellent therapeutic responses [141, 144, 256]. ^{131}I-Mu-9 IgG and F(ab')$_2$ fragments localized known lesions well in patients with advanced colorectal and pancreatic cancer and, importantly, did not form complexes in the blood, suggesting the epitope was present only in the tumors [257]. However, tumor dosimetry was not substantially better than seen with anti-CEA antibodies, so this antibody was not developed further.

A33 is another antibody/antigen that is highly expressed in CRCs that has been reported extensively in preclinical and clinical settings [258–260]. The first clinical trial with mMAb A33 found the ^{131}I-IgG targeted lesions in 19 of 20 patients, with good uptake and tumor–nontumor ratios; however, there was uptake in the intestine that, at the time, the investigators could not determine if it was specific localization [261]. A Phase I/II therapy trial with ^{131}I-A33 in advanced CRC patients determined the MTD to be 75 mCi/m^2, but as with other RAIT trials, no major objective responses were observed [262]. Because this antibody also internalized with deposition near the nucleus [263], a Phase I/II trial using an ^{125}I-labeled A33 IgG also was examined [264]. Even at doses up to 350 mCi/m^2, dose-limiting toxicity was not observed, but major objective responses were lacking, albeit the investigators thought it was significant that patients receiving various forms of chemotherapy after ^{125}I-A33 treatment had robust antitumor responses.

The development of A33 continued, with other studies examining combinations with chemotherapy and external beam therapy, and more recent studies have focused on the possible use with an alpha-emitter for therapy, or also for PET imaging [265–271]. Scott et al. [272] reported

the initial biodistribution/imaging studies with ^{131}I-hA33, which showed favorable tumor targeting properties, but they also confirmed earlier findings with the mA33, showing that the antibody localized to the large intestine with a changing pattern over time. The turnover time was consistent with that of normal colonocytes, suggesting the uptake was cellular and not in the stool. A Phase I therapy trial with ^{131}I-hA33 found patients could tolerate up to 40 mCi/m^2. Hematologic and not GI toxicity was dose-limiting; however, as in trials with other ^{131}I-labeled antibodies in advanced CRC, no significant responses occurred [273]. In addition, a clinical trial evaluating the unconjugated hA33 also found the CDRs of the antibody were immunogenic, with 8 of 11 patients given 4-week cycles of the antibody developing an antiidiotype response [274]. Thus, the future clinical utility of this particular clone of hA33 is uncertain. However, PET-imaging studies in patients given [124]I-humanized A33 IgG were reported recently, showing excellent tumor localization several days after injection [275].

Another antibody worth mentioning is F19, which does not bind to tumor cells, but instead is directed against a surface glycoprotein (FAP, fibroblast activation protein) found in stromal tissues [276]. The antibody raised interest initially for its potential to be combined with antibodies that selectively target cancer cells. This dual-targeting approach might allow a more homogeneous distribution of radioactivity in the tumor. Indeed, many tumors, particularly pancreatic cancer, have extensive stroma that may hinder the ability of radiolabeled antibodies to deliver cytotoxic radiation effectively in all tumor pockets. This antibody was first shown to target hepatic metastases of CRC patients [277, 278]. It was later humanized (sibrotuzumab; BIBH-1) and examined in an unconjugated form, where weekly injections of 100 mg over 12 weeks failed to show any partial or complete responses [279]. Two phase-I therapy trials using ^{131}I-BIBH-1 or F19 are listed as completed in Clinicaltrials.gov, but the results of these trials have not been reported.

Other Constructs

Early in the development of RAIT, investigators were examining how to reduce red marrow exposure with antibody fragments, as well as second antibody and extracorporeal removal of circulating IgG [136, 139, 280–286]. Second antibody clearance methods were effective in removing the radiolabeled antibody from the blood, but this procedure was only useful with radioiodinated antibodies, because radiometal-labeled antibodies would be trapped in high concentrations in the liver. Extracorporeal removal eliminates the formation of immune complexes in vivo, but it still requires the radiolabeled antibody to remain in the blood for 1–2 days to optimize tumor uptake,

during which time a substantial portion of the total radiation exposure to the red marrow occurs. Thus, the most commonly investigated method has been to create antibody fragments [287, 288] or engineered antibodies that have altered pharmacokinetic properties (Fig. 13.3). The first engineered antibody to be studied was the single chain Fv (scFv), a ~25-kD protein that fused the variable heavy and variable light regions of an antibody into a single polypeptide sequence using a peptide linker [289–293]. These structures cleared from the blood very rapidly, and localized very quickly in tumors with good penetration [291, 293]. Their rapid targeting and clearance were ideal for imaging, but their accelerated clearance and monovalent binding proved to be an Achilles heel, since their tumor uptake

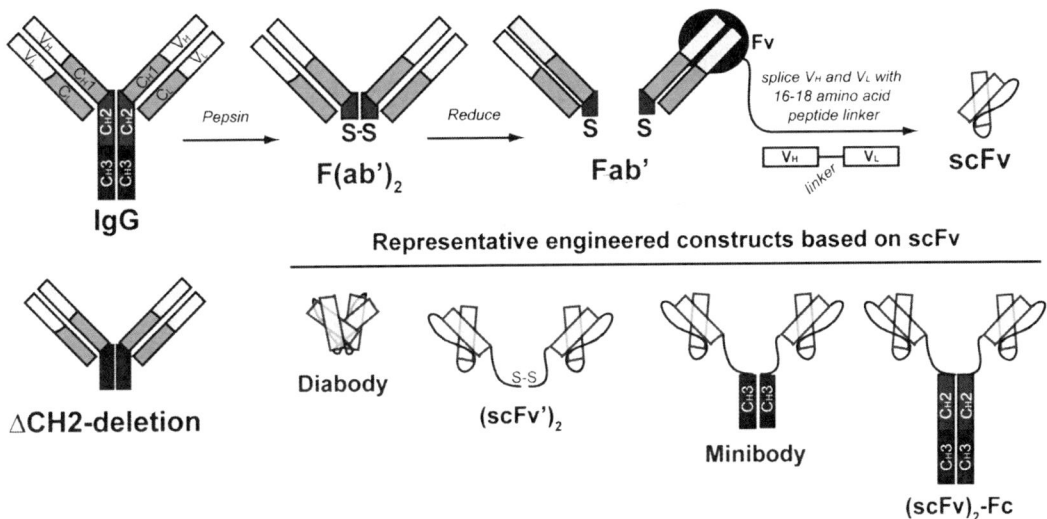

Fig. 13.3 Different forms of immunoglobulins used for targeting CRCs preclinically and clinically. IgG (~150 kD) is the most commonly used immunoglobulin isotype studied. Early studies prepared fragments by enzymatically removing most of the Fc-portion of the IgG (CH2 and CH3 domains). The two arms of the F(ab')$_2$ (~100 kD) are held together by disulfide bonds between cysteine residues in the heavy chains, which can be released by suitable reduction conditions to form the monovalent binding Fab' fragment (~50 kD). Molecular engineering studies found that if the CH2 domains on the heavy chains were deleted, the immunoglobulin would still self-assemble to form what was termed as the delta CH2 deletion construct, which had accelerated clearance from the blood while retaining divalent binding to antigen [307]. Molecular engineering further reduced the size of the antigen-binding

fragment by splicing the genetic sequences of the variable heavy (VH) and variable light (VL) domains into a linear sequence using a short peptide linker [290]. The resulting monovalent-binding construct, known as a single-chain Fv (scFv) has served as a building block for many other structures. Single-chain Fv's often self-anneal, particularly when the linker length is shortened to form divalent-binding diabodies [295], but other noncovalently bound structures known as (scFv)$_2$ have been reported [301]. By adding another peptide chain with a terminal cysteine, one can form covalently linked divalent (scFv')$_2$ structures [297, 298]. Others have tethered 2 scFvs to the CH3 domain of the heavy chain to form a minibody [302], or to the full Fc-portion, which is genetically modified to remove the FcRn-binding sites to alter the pharmacokinetic behavior of this structure [303] was low and retention short, making them less attractive for therapeutic applications [294].

A number of other constructs based on scFvs have been reported [295–298]. For example, Batra and his colleagues reported the formation of divalent and tetravalent CC49 scFv-based constructs [299–301]. When radiolabeled with ^{99m}Tc, both the 60-kD divalent and 120-kD tetravalent constructs had favorable localization properties in human colonic tumor xenografts 6 h post injection, with the tetravalent form providing nearly 2.5-fold higher tumor uptake with acceptable tumor–nontumor ratios [299]. For therapeutic applications, studies in xenograft-bearing nude mice given the tetravalent form or the IgG of CC49 labeled with ^{177}Lu showed similar tumor uptake but more rapid blood clearance, suggesting this form may be suitable for therapy, yet there was higher renal retention with the engineered fragment. Wu and her colleagues also have examined a number of different constructs [302]. Some of their more recent constructs were made from the anti-CEA T84.66 antibody and include 2 scFv fused with a genetically modified Fc fragment, which removed the neonatal-receptor binding sequences, thereby affecting the pharmacokinetic behavior [301, 303–306]. An extensive review of the targeting behavior of various mutated forms labeled with ^{111}In or ^{125}I revealed a preference for an ^{131}I-scFv-Fc over a ^{90}Y-labeled product, which this testing further suggested would not be any better than the anti-CEA IgG [305].

These modified scFv products were predated by another engineered antibody that had the CH2 domain of the IgG removed (delta-CH2-deletion). This section of the IgG most often contains carbohydrates and a portion of the neonatal receptor binding site, both being responsible for the extended serum half-life of IgGs [303, 307–311]. This form of engineered protein retained the divalent binding of the IgG to enhance retention, but had a shortened clearance time, similar to a F(ab')$_2$ fragment, making it at the time of its discovery a more attractive molecule for therapy than the scFv [312–314]. There have been a few reports in patients over the past several years with the radioiodinated humanized CC49[delta] CH2 (IDEC-159), showing that it does clear

more quickly than the IgG [315–317]. A more recent report in five CRC patients given ^{111}In-hCC49[delta]CH2 showed that the fragment had a shorter median effective beta half-life in the blood of 38 h compared to 50 h that was reported from clinical studies with the CC49 antibody [318]; however, radiation dose estimates to the red marrow for the IgG and fragment form were not significantly different. Nevertheless, tumor dosimetry suggested a twofold improvement in tumor/blood ratios. It is uncertain whether this agent will be evaluated further, since the trial listed on Clinicaltrials.gov (NCT00102024) was terminated in 2010 and no new trials are listed.

Improving RAIT'S Efficacy

Human colonic tumor xenografts have almost universally shown good responses to a single treatment with a radiolabeled antibody, and from a pure drug-discovery perspective, early preclinical studies showed RAIT was better than conventional 5-FU/leucovorin in 5/8 human colonic cancer xenografts and equally effective in the other three xenografts [319]. However, clinically, the results have been disappointing, with no evidence of objective responses, but there has been some evidence of disease shrinkage or stabilization reported in a number of trials, indicating that RAIT is active. Thus, RAIT can have an effect, but in the situations in which it has been tested, it has not provided sufficient evidence supporting additional clinical testing in most solid tumors. However, in CRC, the combination of earlier detection leading to extended survival with just surgical intervention in stage I/II, and more effective chemotherapeutic regimens for stage III CRCs, there remains an urgent need for developing effective treatments for patients with metastatic (stage IV) disease. There have been preclinical and clinical studies focusing on combining RAIT with external beam radiation therapy in patients with unresectable hepatic metastases [103, 150], but this approach has not moved forward. Since most chemotherapeutic agents used in treating gastrointestinal cancer have some ability to enhance sensitivity to radiation, it is not surprising that preclinical studies have found combinations with chemotherapy can enhance responses, as well as agents that affect tumor vasculature [199, 269, 320–326]. Again, there have been early clinical trials exploring the possibility for various combination approaches, but the first results of these trials did not appear to be any better than those with RAIT alone [327–330].

Perhaps there are lessons to learn from the clinical experience with RAIT in lymphoma. Although there is clear evidence in B-cell lymphomas (specifically follicular types) that RAIT produces significant objective responses and enhances disease-free survival, even in this indication RAIT has not been widely accepted. However, because RAIT is better tolerated than most chemotherapy regimens, and at least in lymphoma, only a single treatment is effective compared to months of repeated chemotherapy injections, at least RAIT is being given a chance in a frontline setting [331, 332]. One of the more promising developments has been the introduction of RAIT as part of a consolidation regimen given to lymphoma patients after they receive their initial chemotherapy ± antibody treatment [77, 78]. In this latter experience, the major bulk of the disease is reduced first with chemotherapy. Thus, RAIT is given after there has been a partial response (i.e., more in the context of treating "minimal" residual disease), and because a number of patients experience a complete response to the primary therapy, the consolidation is given more in the context of an adjuvant setting. Importantly, unlike external beam therapy that is localized, RAIT is systemic, and therefore capable of eradicating cancer cells disseminated throughout the body.

As mentioned earlier, there is ample evidence in preclinical models that RAIT has superior activity in a setting of minimal disease or even as an adjuvant therapy. Because RAIT has not been effective in advanced disease, interest in pursuing RAIT for stage IV CRC has faded. However, in patients with hepatic metastases, where R0 resection is indicated, these patients do have an improved survival, with data suggesting one-third of the patients can survive 5 years, and nearly 25% for 10 years [22, 23]. However, at least 60% of the patients who have curative resection will have a recurrence, with 85% recurring within the first 30 months [21]. While a debate over the value of adjuvant chemotherapy continues, this indication affords RAIT an excellent opportunity to assume an important role in the treatment of disseminated CRC in an adjuvant setting.

This concept has been examined in a number of studies in xenograft models [333–335], but Behr et al. were the first to explore this approach clinically [336, 337]. The initial clinical trial included primarily CRC patients with ≤3.0 cm lesions that were given escalating doses of ^{131}I-hMN-14 IgG. The MTD was determined to be 60 mCi/m^2 [336], and in a subsequent report, 3 of the 19 assessable patients showed a partial response, and 8 had minor responses [337]. They also reported the first results in 9 patients who were treated after having a curative hepatic resection, finding 7/9 patients were disease-free up to 36 months (one relapsing after 6 months and another after 30 months). Liersch et al. followed these promising results with a Phase II trial examining patients after salvage R0 resection of hepatic metastases, using a single 40–60 mCi/m^2 treatment of ^{131}I-hMN-14 anti-CEACAM5 IgG (labetuzumab) [338, 339]. In their first report of 23 patients with a median follow-up of 64 months, 51% of the patients were still alive, with a median overall survival of 68 months [338]. A subsequent report updated the findings after a median follow-up of 91 months. At that time, the median survival was 58 months, but they compared this to a contemporaneous group of patients seen at the same institution that had a liver resection without RAIT, finding this group's median survival to be only 31 months (51-month median follow-up for the controls). These results were very encouraging and showed for the first time in CRC that RAIT potentially could have a role in managing stage IV disease, justifying consideration for a randomized controlled study.

A Different Approach: Pretargeting

Pretargeting is the name given to several multistep procedures that separate the antibody-targeting step from the targeting of the radionuclide (refer to Chap. 20). The first pretargeting experience was with an anti-CEA pretargeting system for localizing CRCs. This approach utilized an anti-CEA Fab' fragment chemically coupled to another Fab' fragment that bound a chelate loaded with a radiometal (a derivative of EDTA for binding[111]In) [340, 341]. All pretargeting procedures start with the administration of the primary antibody-targeting agent, such as the Fab' × Fab' bispecific antibody (bsMAb) used in this first study. After giving sufficient time for the antibody to localize in the tumor and clear from the blood and tissues, the chelate loaded with the radiometal was given. Chelated radiometals clear very quickly and efficiently from the body, and thus with this approach, tumor visualization was observed within a few hours of the radiolabeled chelate's injection. The initial effort was significant because it allowed the use of ^{111}In to disclose metastatic colon cancer in the liver, whereas metastatic sites in the liver would be revealed most often as photopenic areas with ^{111}In-labeled anti-CEA IgG [340].

The original technology was improved with the discovery that by joining to two haptens (i.e., chelates) together, tumor uptake of the radiolabeled divalent-hapten would be enhanced [342]. After establishing appropriate pretargeting conditions with this new improvement [343], efforts were pursued with the anti-CEA bsMAb using a divalent (In)DTPA-Tyr[^{131}I]-Lys peptide for therapy. Preclinical studies showed uptake in human colon cancer xenografts could rival that of a directly radiolabeled F(ab')$_2$, but with less activity in normal tissues [344, 345]. Clinical trials with this anti-CEA bsMAb pretargeting procedure and the ^{131}I-hapten-peptide were open to all patients with advanced CEA-producing tumors [346–349], but a special emphasis was placed on enrolling patients with medullary thyroid cancer, since there was no accepted treatment for this indication. A retrospective analysis of the collective experience with this anti-CEA pretargeting system in medullary thyroid cancer revealed a subset of patients with rapidly rising serum calcitonin (tumor marker for this indication) who had a poor prognosis had improved survival [350]. The investigators speculated that this may be have been related to eradication of micrometastatic

disease, since they also found medullary thyroid cancer patients frequently had bone marrow involvement, which also explained why dose-limiting hematological toxicity was lower than in patients with other CEA-producing tumors [348].

Another pretargeting procedure was examined in advanced CRC, but this method utilized a primary targeting agent composed of the NR-LU-10 IgG (now known to bind EpCam) conjugated to streptavidin, which was used capture ^{90}Y-biotin [351, 352]. The procedure was first optimized in a diverse population of EpCam-expressing cancers [353], giving various amounts of the conjugate several days to localize in the tumor before a clearing agent was given and determining the MTD. The clearing agent was essential to the success of this method, because the affinity between streptavidin and biotin is so high (10^{-15} M compared to antibodies that are usually 10^{-9} M), residual conjugate in the blood would have captured the radiolabeled biotin before it reached the tumor. The clearing agent contained biotin to bind and block the streptavidin portion of the conjugate and galactose residues so that the complex would be quickly removed by the liver. Within 6–24 h, the ^{90}Y-biotin was given. In the Phase II trial performed exclusively in CRC patients, doses of 110 mCi/m^2 of the ^{90}Y-biotin were given. There were two partial responses and four stable disease in the 25 patients treated. The dose-limiting toxicity of this particular system was gastrointestinal, because the NR-LU-10 conjugate bound to the large intestine, but rising serum creatinine levels in patients who survived more than 3 months suggested renal toxicity was occurring. Tumor dosimetry in two patients found a lung mass received 479 cGy and a liver mass received 2,885 cGy. This same pretargeting procedure was later examined using a molecularly engineered multi-scFv-streptavidin fusion protein and substituting the CC49 anti-TAG-72 antibody for NR-LU-10. Dosimetry estimates in several patients suggested tumor doses might meet or exceed 5,000 cGy if patients were able to tolerate an administered activity that would deliver ~2,000 cGy to the kidneys [354, 355]. However, the immunogenicity of the streptavidin in these types of conjugates/constructs likely contributed to the decision not to pursue this procedure for therapy.

Our group is continuing with the development and testing of a new bsMAb pretargeting system using a humanized recombinant bsMAb and a ^{90}Y/^{177}Lu-labeled hapten-peptide [356]. Preclinical studies have shown encouraging results alone, but also in combination with gemcitabine in models of human pancreatic cancer or even with an antibody-SN-38 conjugate [357–359]. Clinical studies are now underway.

Summary and Future Directions

The collective clinical experiences in advanced CRC have indicated that RAIT alone cannot provide sufficient benefit to warrant further consideration in advanced disease. However, future studies with antibody-targeted radionuclides should not be dismissed. As mentioned earlier, the clinical trial reported by Liersch et al. [338, 339] for treating patients who undergo a curative hepatic resection is perhaps the most encouraging to pursue, and all preclinical studies suggest this is the most likely setting where RAIT should provide optimal benefit; namely, in an adjuvant setting. Thus, based on their encouraging results, consideration to expand this trial into a randomized Phase II/III is warranted.

In future clinical trials, there are chemotherapeutic agents that could be added to the overall treatment regimen that might enhance the overall survival. Many of the standard chemotherapeutics used in colorectal or GI malignancies have some radiosensitization capability [360–366], and there have been a number of preclinical studies showing combinations with various chemotherapeutic agents can enhance RAIT or pretargeted RAIT (e.g., [320, 367–380]). In a trial examining RAIT in advanced pancreatic cancer, low-dose gemcitabine (200 mg/m^2) could be given weekly in conjunction with fractionated ^{90}Y-hPAM4 (clivatuzumab) [381, 382]. This trial utilizes subtherapeutic amounts of the chemotherapeutic agent in combination with RAIT, but in lymphoma, RAIT is now being given as part of an overall therapeutic regimen that includes full-dose chemotherapy and RAIT [78]. Thus, as more data are generated that confirm RAIT does not preclude a patient from receiving subsequent chemotherapy, or that RAIT can be tolerated at its full dose when patients are not so heavily pretreated with other myelosuppressive therapies, we may begin to see RAIT integrated into future regimens. Indeed, in preclinical testing, we also found an antibody-SN-38 drug conjugate and a ^{90}Y-IgG could be co-administered, with each given at therapeutically effective doses [359]. In fact, the drug conjugate was so nontoxic at therapeutically active doses, it could be given together with the MTD of the ^{90}Y-antibody treatment with no additional toxicity.

We also should not discount the possibility of using RAIT with unlabeled antibodies. There is no question that in B-cell lymphomas, the addition of the excess anti-CD20 IgG, which itself is very effective in follicular lymphoma, potentiates the overall response to the radiolabeled anti-CD20 antibody [114]. It could be argued that in solid tumors, RAIT has had a lackluster performance because most of the antibodies used for these treatments do not have antitumor activity by themselves. However, it is not necessary, and perhaps not recommended, to use a therapeutically active unconjugated antibody as a radioimmunoconjugate. Radiolabeled antibodies are intended to deliver radiation to tumor cells, and as such, their specific activity should be reasonably high, allowing as many molecules that localize in the tumor to harbor the radionuclide. Thus, the amount of antibody given as a radioimmunoconjugate should be relatively small. Naturally, there are situations where additional antibody protein is necessary to improve biodistribution, but overall, the protein dose given with the radioconjugate should be minimized. Since many unconjugated antibodies are given at much higher doses and repetitively, the radioconjugate and unconjugated therapeutic antibody can be decoupled, or perhaps even better, different targets can be utilized without concern for competitive binding.

Cetuximab and bevacizumab are commonly used in CRC, and at least cetuximab has been examined fairly extensively in combination with radiation and other chemotherapeutic agents for response potentiation [383–392]. Bevacizumab has also been used in combination therapy, including radiation, in CRC [393–396], and Salaun et al. [397] reported the addition of bevacizumab to RAIT improved responses in mice bearing human MTC xenografts.

Thus, additional clinical trials with RAIT in patients with stage IV CRC who have hepatic resections should be pursued. Certainly an examination of RAIT alone will be required prior to testing it in combination with other agents. If current studies show improved efficacy and reduced toxicity with bsMAb-pretargeted radionuclides, this may become the paradigm of future RAIT trials.

References

1. Jemal A, Siegel R, Xu J, Ward E. Cancer statistics, 2010. CA Cancer J Clin. 2010;60:277–300.
2. Jemal A, Bray F, Center MM, Ferlay J, Ward E, Forman D. Global cancer statistics. CA Cancer J Clin. 2011;61:69–90.
3. Howlader N, Noone AM, Krapcho M, Neyman N, Aminou R, Waldron W, et al. SEER cancer statistics review, 1975–2008. 2011. http://seer.cancer.gov/csr/1975_2008/.
4. Lombardi L, Morelli F, Cinieri S, Santini D, Silvestris N, Fazio N, et al. Adjuvant colon cancer chemotherapy: where we are and where we'll go. Cancer Treat Rev. 2010;36 Suppl 3:S34–41.
5. Lubezky N, Geva R, Shmueli E, Nakache R, Klausner JM, Figer A, et al. Is there a survival benefit to neoadjuvant versus adjuvant chemotherapy, combined with surgery for resectable colorectal liver metastases? World J Surg. 2009;33:1028–34.
6. Jonker DJ, Spithoff K, Maroun J. Adjuvant systemic chemotherapy for stage II and III colon cancer after complete resection: an updated practice guideline. Clin Oncol (R Coll Radiol). 2011;23:314–22.
7. Sato H, Maeda K, Sugihara K, Mochizuki H, Kotake K, Teramoto T, et al. High-risk stage II colon cancer after curative resection. J Surg Oncol. 2011;104:45–52.
8. Chua TC, Saxena A, Liauw W, Kokandi A, Morris DL. Systematic review of randomized and nonrandomized trials of the clinical response and outcomes of neoadjuvant systemic chemotherapy for resectable colorectal liver metastases. Ann Surg Oncol. 2010;17:492–501.
9. Engstrom PF. Systemic therapy for advanced or metastatic colorectal cancer: National Comprehensive Cancer Network guidelines for combining anti-vascular endothelial growth factor and anti-epidermal growth factor receptor monoclonal antibodies with chemotherapy. Pharmacotherapy. 2008;28:18S–22.
10. Engstrom PF, Arnoletti JP, Benson III AB, Chen YJ, Choti MA, Cooper HS, et al. NCCN clinical practice guidelines in oncology: colon cancer. J Natl Compr Canc Netw. 2009;7:778–831.
11. Tol J, Punt CJ. Monoclonal antibodies in the treatment of metastatic colorectal cancer: a review. Clin Ther. 2010;32:437–53.
12. Saltz LB. Adjuvant therapy for colon cancer. Surg Oncol Clin N Am. 2010;19:819–27.
13. Catenacci DV, Kozloff M, Kindler HL, Polite B. Personalized colon cancer care in 2010. Semin Oncol. 2011;38:284–308.
14. de Gramont A, Chibaudel B, Bachet JB, Larsen AK, Tournigand C, Louvet C, et al. From chemotherapy to targeted therapy in adjuvant treatment for stage III colon cancer. Semin Oncol. 2011;38:521–32.
15. Allegra CJ, Yothers G, O'Connell MJ, Sharif S, Petrelli NJ, Colangelo LH, et al. Phase III trial assessing bevacizumab in stages II and III carcinoma of the colon: results of NSABP protocol C-08. J Clin Oncol. 2011;29:11–6.
16. Dotan E, Cohen SJ. Challenges in the management of stage II colon cancer. Semin Oncol. 2011;38:511–20.
17. Kelley RK, Van Bebber SL, Phillips KA, Venook AP. Personalized medicine and oncology practice guidelines: a case study of contemporary biomarkers in colorectal cancer. J Natl Compr Canc Netw. 2011;9:13–25.
18. Minsky BD. Unique considerations in the patient with rectal cancer. Semin Oncol. 2011;38:542–51.
19. Van Loon K, Venook AP. Adjuvant treatment of colon cancer: what is next? Curr Opin Oncol. 2011;23:403–9.
20. Edwards MS, Chadda SD, Zhao Z, Barber BL, Sykes DP. A systematic review of treatment guidelines for metastatic colorectal cancer. Colorectal Dis. 2012;14:e31–47.
21. McLoughlin JM, Jensen EH, Malafa M. Resection of colorectal liver metastases: current perspectives. Cancer Control. 2006;13:32–41.
22. Rees M, Tekkis PP, Welsh FK, O'Rourke T, John TG. Evaluation of long-term survival after hepatic resection for metastatic colorectal cancer: a multifactorial model of 929 patients. Ann Surg. 2008;247:125–35.
23. Welsh FK, Tekkis PP, O'Rourke T, John TG, Rees M. Quantification of risk of a positive (R1) resection margin following hepatic resection for metastatic colorectal cancer: an aid to clinical decision-making. Surg Oncol. 2008;17:3–13.
24. Mayo SC, Pawlik TM. Current management of colorectal hepatic metastasis. Expert Rev Gastroenterol Hepatol. 2009;3:131–44.
25. Robertson DJ, Stukel TA, Gottlieb DJ, Sutherland JM, Fisher ES. Survival after hepatic resection of colorectal cancer metastases: a national experience. Cancer. 2009;115:752–9.
26. Kemeny N. The management of resectable and unresectable liver metastases from colorectal cancer. Curr Opin Oncol. 2010;22:364–73.

27. Yang AD, Brouquet A, Vauthey JN. Extending limits of resection for metastatic colorectal cancer: risk benefit ratio. J Surg Oncol. 2010;102:996–1001.

28. Davies JM, Goldberg RM. Treatment of metastatic colorectal cancer. Semin Oncol. 2011;38:552–60.

29. Swan PJ, Welsh FK, Chandrakumaran K, Rees M. Long-term survival following delayed presentation and resection of colorectal liver metastases. Br J Surg. 2011;98:1309–17.

30. Labianca R, Fossati R, Zaniboni A, Torri V, Marsoni S, Nitti D, et al. Randomized trial of intraportal and/or systemic adjuvant chemotherapy in patients with colon carcinoma. J Natl Cancer Inst. 2004;96:750–8.

31. Wang P, Chen Z, Huang WX, Liu LM. Current preventive treatment for recurrence after curative hepatectomy for liver metastases of colorectal carcinoma: a literature review of randomized control trials. World J Gastroenterol. 2005;11:3817–22.

32. Parks R, Gonen M, Kemeny N, Jarnagin W, D'Angelica M, DeMatteo R, et al. Adjuvant chemotherapy improves survival after resection of hepatic colorectal metastases: analysis of data from two continents. J Am Coll Surg. 2007;204:753–61.

33. Gravalos C, Garcia-Escobar I, Garcia-Alfonso P, Cassinello J, Malon D, Carrato A. Adjuvant chemotherapy for stages II, III and IV of colon cancer. Clin Transl Oncol. 2009;11:526–33.

34. Kemeny NE, Jarnagin WR, Capanu M, Fong Y, Gewirtz AN, Dematteo RP, et al. Randomized phase II trial of adjuvant hepatic arterial infusion and systemic chemotherapy with or without bevacizumab in patients with resected hepatic metastases from colorectal cancer. J Clin Oncol. 2011;29:884–9.

35. Power DG, Kemeny NE. Role of adjuvant therapy after resection of colorectal cancer liver metastases. J Clin Oncol. 2010;28:2300–9.

36. Snoeren N, Voest EE, Bergman AM, Dalesio O, Verheul HM, Tollenaar RA, et al. A randomized two arm phase III study in patients post radical resection of liver metastases of colorectal cancer to investigate bevacizumab in combination with capecitabine plus oxaliplatin (CAPOX) vs CAPOX alone as adjuvant treatment. BMC Cancer. 2010;10:545.

37. Eng C. The evolving role of monoclonal antibodies in colorectal cancer: early presumptions and impact on clinical trial development. Oncologist. 2010;15:73–84.

38. Ocvirk J, Brodowicz T, Wrba F, Ciuleanu TE, Kurteva G, Beslija S, et al. Cetuximab plus FOLFOX6 or FOLFIRI in metastatic colorectal cancer: CECOG trial. World J Gastroenterol. 2010;16:3133–43.

39. Saltz LB, Clarke S, Diaz-Rubio E, Scheithauer W, Figer A, Wong R, et al. Bevacizumab in combination with oxaliplatin-based chemotherapy as first-line therapy in metastatic colorectal cancer: a randomized phase III study. J Clin Oncol. 2008;26:2013–9.

40. Van Cutsem E, Kohne CH, Hitre E, Zaluski J, Chang Chien CR, Makhson A, et al. Cetuximab and chemotherapy as initial treatment for metastatic colorectal cancer. N Engl J Med. 2009;360:1408–17.

41. Van Cutsem E, Kohne CH, Lang I, Folprecht G, Nowacki MP, Cascinu S, et al. Cetuximab plus irinotecan, fluorouracil, and leucovorin as first-line treatment for metastatic colorectal cancer: updated analysis of overall survival according to tumor KRAS and BRAF mutation status. J Clin Oncol. 2011;29: 2011–9.

42. Peeters M, Price TJ, Cervantes A, Sobrero AF, Ducreux M, Hotko Y, et al. Randomized phase III study of panitumumab with fluorouracil, leucovorin, and irinotecan (FOLFIRI) compared with FOLFIRI alone as second-line treatment in patients with metastatic colorectal cancer. J Clin Oncol. 2010;28:4706–13.

43. Peeters M, Cohn A, Kohne CH, Douillard JY. Panitumumab in combination with cytotoxic chemotherapy for the treatment of metastatic colorectal carcinoma. Clin Colorectal Cancer. 2012;11:14–23.

44. Alberts SR, Sargent DJ, Smyrk TC, Shields AF, Chan E, Goldberg RM, et al. Adjuvant mFOLFOX6 with or without cetuxiumab (Cmab) in KRAS wild-type (WT) patients (pts) with resected stage III colon cancer (CC): results from NCCTG Intergroup Phase III Trial N0147. J Clin Oncol. 2010;28:18s:abst CRA3507.

45. Goldberg RM, Sargent DJ, Thibodeau SN, Mahoney MR, Shields AF, Chan E, et al. Adjuvant mFOLFOX6 plus or minus cetuximab (Cmab) in patients (pts) with KRAS mutant (m) resected stage III colon cancer (CC): NCCTG Intergroup Phase III Trial N0147. J Clin Oncol. 2010;28(15s):abstr 3508.

46. Murthy R, Nunez R, Szklaruk J, Erwin W, Madoff DC, Gupta S, et al. Yttrium-90 microsphere therapy for hepatic malignancy: devices, indications, technical considerations, and potential complications. Radiographics. 2005;25 Suppl 1:S41–55.

47. Gulec SA, Mesoloras G, Stabin M. Dosimetric techniques in ^{90}Y-microsphere therapy of liver cancer: The MIRD equations for dose calculations. J Nucl Med. 2006;47:1209–11.

48. Gulec SA, Mesoloras G, Dezarn WA, McNeillie P, Kennedy AS. Safety and efficacy of Y-90 microsphere treatment in patients with primary and metastatic liver cancer: the tumor selectivity of the treatment as a function of tumor to liver flow ratio. J Transl Med. 2007;5:15.

49. Sharma RA, Van Hazel GA, Morgan B, Berry DP, Blanshard K, Price D, et al. Radioembolization of liver metastases from colorectal cancer using yttrium-90 microspheres with concomitant systemic oxaliplatin, fluorouracil, and leucovorin chemotherapy. J Clin Oncol. 2007;25:1099–106.

50. Van De Wiele C, Defreyne L, Peeters M, Lambert B. Yttrium-90 labelled resin microspheres for treatment of primary and secondary malignant liver tumors. Q J Nucl Med Mol Imaging. 2009;53:317–24.

51. Ahmadzadehfar H, Biersack HJ, Ezziddin S. Radioembolization of liver tumors with yttrium-90 microspheres. Semin Nucl Med. 2010;40:105–21.

52. Sangro B, Carpanese L, Cianni R, Golfieri R, Gasparini D, Ezziddin S, et al. Survival after Yttrium-90 resin microsphere radioembolization of

hepatocellular carcinoma across barcelona clinic liver cancer stages: a European evaluation. Hepatology. 2011;54:868–78.

53. Sangro B, Inarrairaegui M, Bilbao JI. Radioembolization for hepatocellular carcinoma. J Hepatol. 2012;56:464–73.

54. Gray B, Van Hazel G, Hope M, Burton M, Moroz P, Anderson J, et al. Randomised trial of SIR-Spheres plus chemotherapy vs. chemotherapy alone for treating patients with liver metastases from primary large bowel cancer. Ann Oncol. 2001;12:1711–20.

55. Hendlisz A, Van den Eynde M, Peeters M, Maleux G, Lambert B, Vannoote J, et al. Phase III trial comparing protracted intravenous fluorouracil infusion alone or with yttrium-90 resin microspheres radioembolization for liver-limited metastatic colorectal cancer refractory to standard chemotherapy. J Clin Oncol. 2010;28:3687–94.

56. Van Hazel G, Blackwell A, Anderson J, Price D, Moroz P, Bower G, et al. Randomised phase 2 trial of SIR-Spheres plus fluorouracil/leucovorin chemotherapy versus fluorouracil/leucovorin chemotherapy alone in advanced colorectal cancer. J Surg Oncol. 2004;88:78–85.

57. Sharma RA, Wasan HS, Love SB, Dutton S, Stokes JC, Smith JL. FOXFIRE: a phase III clinical trial of chemo-radio-embolisation as first-line treatment of liver metastases in patients with colorectal cancer. Clin Oncol (R Coll Radiol). 2008;20:261–3.

58. Nakajo M, Kobayashi H, Shimabukuro K, Shirono K, Sakata H, Taguchi M, et al. Biodistribution and in vivo kinetics of iodine-131 lipiodol infused via the hepatic artery of patients with hepatic cancer. J Nucl Med. 1988;29:1066–77.

59. Novell R, Hilson A, Hobbs K. Ablation of recurrent primary liver cancer using ^{131}I-lipiodol. Postgrad Med J. 1991;67:393–5.

60. Al-Mufti RA, Pedley RB, Marshall D, Begent RH, Hilson A, Winslet MC, et al. In vitro assessment of Lipiodol-targeted radiotherapy for liver and colorectal cancer cell lines. Br J Cancer. 1999;79:1665–71.

61. Brans B, De Winter F, Defreyne L, Troisi R, Vanlangenhove P, Van Vlierberghe H, et al. The antitumoral activity of neoadjuvant intra-arterial ^{131}I-lipiodol treatment for hepatocellular carcinoma: a pilot study. Cancer Biother Radiopharm. 2001;16: 333–8.

62. Rindani RB, Hugh TJ, Roche J, Roach PJ, Smith RC. [131]I lipiodol therapy for unresectable hepatocellular carcinoma. ANZ J Surg. 2002;72:210–4.

63. Garin E, Rakotonirina H, Lejeune F, Denizot B, Roux J, Noiret N, et al. Effect of a [188]Re-SSS lipiodol/^{131}I-lipiodol mixture, [188]Re-SSS lipiodol alone or ^{131}I-lipiodol alone on the survival of rats with hepatocellular carcinoma. Nucl Med Commun. 2006;27: 363–9.

64. Raoul JL, Boucher E, Olivie D, Guillygomarc'h A, Boudjema K, Garin E. Association of cisplatin and intra-arterial injection of ^{131}I-lipiodol in treatment of hepatocellular carcinoma: results of phase II trial. Int J Radiat Oncol Biol Phys. 2006;64:745–50.

65. Oyen WJ, Bodei L, Giammarile F, Maecke HR, Tennvall J, Luster M, et al. Targeted therapy in nuclear medicine–current status and future prospects. Ann Oncol. 2007;18:1782–92.

66. Bretagne JF, Raoul JL, Bourguet P, Duvauferrier R, Deugnier Y, Faroux R, et al. Hepatic artery injection of I-131-labeled lipiodol. Part II. Preliminary results of therapeutic use in patients with hepatocellular carcinoma and liver metastases. Radiology. 1988; 168:547–50.

67. Lau WY, Lai EC, Lau SH. The current role of neoadjuvant/adjuvant/chemoprevention therapy in partial hepatectomy for hepatocellular carcinoma: a systematic review. Hepatobiliary Pancreat Dis Int. 2009;8:124–33.

68. Giammarile F, Bodei L, Chiesa C, Flux G, Forrer F, Kraeber-Bodere F, et al. EANM procedure guideline for the treatment of liver cancer and liver metastases with intra-arterial radioactive compounds. Eur J Nucl Med Mol Imaging. 2011;38:1393–406.

69. Saclarides TJ, Szeluga D, Staren ED. Neuroendocrine cancers of the colon and rectum. Results of a ten-year experience. Dis Colon Rectum. 1994;37:635–42.

70. Bernick PE, Klimstra DS, Shia J, Minsky B, Saltz L, Shi W, et al. Neuroendocrine carcinomas of the colon and rectum. Dis Colon Rectum. 2004;47:163–9.

71. Nisa L, Savelli G, Giubbini R. Yttrium-90 DOTATOC therapy in GEP-NET and other SST2 expressing tumors: a selected review. Ann Nucl Med. 2011;25:75–85.

72. Pfeifer AK, Gregersen T, Gronbaek H, Hansen CP, Muller-Brand J, Herskind Bruun K, et al. Peptide receptor radionuclide therapy with ^{90}Y-DOTATOC and ^{177}Lu-DOTATOC in advanced neuroendocrine tumors: results from a Danish cohort treated in Switzerland. Neuroendocrinology. 2011;93:189–96.

73. Imhof A, Brunner P, Marincek N, Briel M, Schindler C, Rasch H, et al. Response, survival, and long-term toxicity after therapy with the radiolabeled somatostatin analogue [^{90}Y-DOTA]-TOC in metastasized neuroendocrine cancers. J Clin Oncol. 2011;29: 2416–23.

74. Basu B, Sirohi B, Corrie P. Systemic therapy for neuroendocrine tumours of gastroenteropancreatic origin. Endocr Relat Cancer. 2010;17:R75–90.

75. Ramage JK, Ahmed A, Ardill J, Bax N, Breen DJ, Caplin ME, et al. Guidelines for the management of gastroenteropancreatic neuroendocrine (including carcinoid) tumours (NETs). Gut. 2012;61:6–32.

76. Goldsmith SJ. Radioimmunotherapy of lymphoma: Bexxar and Zevalin. Semin Nucl Med. 2010;40: 122–35.

77. Hagemeister FB. Maintenance and consolidation strategies in non-Hodgkin's lymphoma: a review of the data. Curr Oncol Rep. 2010;12:395–401.

78. Morschhauser F, Dreyling M, Rohatiner A, Hagemeister F, Bischof Delaloye A. Rationale for consolidation to improve progression-free survival in patients with non-Hodgkin's lymphoma: a review of the evidence. Oncologist. 2009;14 Suppl 2:17–29.

79. Behr TM, Behe MP. Radioimmunotherapy versus traditional, nontargeted forms of systemic cancer

treatment. Expert Rev Anticancer Ther. 2001;1: 501–5.

80. Koppe MJ, Bleichrodt RP, Oyen WJ, Boerman OC. Radioimmunotherapy and colorectal cancer. Br J Surg. 2005;92:264–76.

81. Wong JYC, Williams LE, Yazaki PJ. Radioimmunotherapy of colorectal cancer. In: Spear TW, editor. Targeted radionuclide therapy. Philadelphia: Lippincott Williams and Wilkins; 2011. p. 321–51.

82. Goldenberg DM, Gaffar SA, Bennett SJ, Beach JL. Experimental radioimmunotherapy of a xenografted human colonic tumor (GW-39) producing carcinoembryonic antigen. Cancer Res. 1981;41:4354–60.

83. Order SE, Klein JL, Ettinger D, Alderson P, Siegelman S, Leichner P. Use of isotopic immunoglobulin in therapy. Cancer Res. 1980;40:3001–7.

84. Order SE, Klein JL, Leichner PK. Antiferritin IgG antibody for isotopic cancer therapy. Oncology. 1981;38:154–60.

85. Leichner PK, Klein JL, Garrison JB, Jenkins RE, Nickoloff EL, Ettinger DS, et al. Dosimetry of ^{131}I-labeled anti-ferritin in hepatoma: a model for radioimmunoglobulin dosimetry. Int J Radiat Oncol Biol Phys. 1981;7:323–33.

86. Ettinger DS, Order SE, Wharam MD, Parker MK, Klein JL, Leichner PK. Phase I-II study of isotopic immunoglobulin therapy for primary liver cancer. Cancer Treat Rep. 1982;66:289–97.

87. Order SE. Monoclonal antibodies: potential role in radiation therapy and oncology. Int J Radiat Oncol Biol Phys. 1982;8:1193–201.

88. Leichner PK, Klein JL, Siegelman SS, Ettinger DS, Order SE. Dosimetry of ^{131}I-labeled antiferritin in hepatoma: specific activities in the tumor and liver. Cancer Treat Rep. 1983;67:647–58.

89. Primus FJ, Wang RH, Goldenberg DM, Hansen HJ. Localization of human GW-39 tumors in hamsters by radiolabeled heterospecific antibody to carcinoembryonic antigen. Cancer Res. 1973;33:2977–82.

90. Goldenberg DM, Preston DF, Primus FJ, Hansen HJ. Photoscan localization of GW-39 tumors in hamsters using radiolabeled anticarcinoembryonic antigen immunoglobulin G. Cancer Res. 1974;34:1–9.

91. Jain RK. Therapeutic implications of tumor physiology. Curr Opin Oncol. 1991;3:1105–8.

92. Jain RK. Transport of molecules, particles, and cells in solid tumors. Annu Rev Biomed Eng. 1999;1:241–63.

93. Thurber GM, Schmidt MM, Wittrup KD. Factors determining antibody distribution in tumors. Trends Pharmacol Sci. 2008;29:57–61.

94. Primus FJ, Macdonald R, Goldenberg DM, Hansen HJ. Localization of GW-39 human tumors in hamsters by affinity-purified antibody to carcinoembryonic antigen. Cancer Res. 1977;37:1544–7.

95. Wessels BW, Rogus RD. Radionuclide selection and model absorbed dose calculations for radiolabeled tumor associated antibodies. Med Phys. 1984; 11:638–45.

96. Wessels BW, Vessella RL, Palme 2nd DF, Berkopec JM, Smith GK, Bradley EW. Radiobiological comparison of external beam irradiation and radioimmu-

97. Buchsbaum DJ, ten Haken RK, Heidorn DB, Lawrence TS, Glatfelter AA, Terry VH, et al. A comparison of ^{131}I-labeled monoclonal antibody 17-1A treatment to external beam irradiation on the growth of LS174T human colon carcinoma xenografts. Int J Radiat Oncol Biol Phys. 1990;18:1033–41.

98. Wessels BW, Yorke ED, Bradley EW. Dosimetry of heterogeneous uptake of radiolabeled antibody for radioimmunotherapy. Front Radiat Ther Oncol. 1990;24:104–8.

99. Fowler JF. Radiobiological aspects of low dose rates in radioimmunotherapy. Int J Radiat Oncol Biol Phys. 1990;18:1261–9.

100. Wong JY, Williams LE, Demidecki AJ, Wessels BW, Yan XW. Radiobiologic studies comparing Yttrium-90 irradiation and external beam irradiation in vitro. Int J Radiat Oncol Biol Phys. 1991;20: 715–22.

101. Fujimori K, Fisher DR, Weinstein JN. Integrated microscopic-macroscopic pharmacology of monoclonal antibody radioconjugates: the radiation dose distribution. Cancer Res. 1991;51:4821–7.

102. Knox SJ, Goris ML, Wessels BW. Overview of animal studies comparing radioimmunotherapy with dose equivalent external beam irradiation. Radiother Oncol. 1992;23:111–7.

103. Buras RR, Wong JY, Kuhn JA, Beatty BG, Williams LE, Wanek PM, et al. Comparison of radioimmunotherapy and external beam radiotherapy in colon cancer xenografts. Int J Radiat Oncol Biol Phys. 1993;25:473–9.

104. Yorke ED, Williams LE, Demidecki AJ, Heidorn DB, Roberson PL, Wessels BW. Multicellular dosimetry for beta-emitting radionuclides: autoradiography, thermoluminescent dosimetry and three-dimensional dose calculations. Med Phys. 1993;20:543–50.

105. Langmuir VK, Fowler JF, Knox SJ, Wessels BW, Sutherland RM, Wong JY. Radiobiology of radiolabeled antibody therapy as applied to tumor dosimetry. Med Phys. 1993;20:601–10.

106. Humm JL, Chin LM. A model of cell inactivation by alpha-particle internal emitters. Radiat Res. 1993;134:143–50.

107. Roeske JC, Chen GT, Brill AB. Dosimetry of intraperitoneally administered radiolabeled antibodies. Med Phys. 1993;20:593–600.

108. Howell RW, Goddu SM, Rao DV. Application of the linear-quadratic model to radioimmunotherapy: further support for the advantage of longer-lived radionuclides. J Nucl Med. 1994;35:1861–9.

109. Hui TE, Fisher DR, Kuhn JA, Williams LE, Nourigat C, Badger CC, et al. A mouse model for calculating cross-organ beta doses from yttrium-90-labeled immunoconjugates. Cancer. 1994;73:951–7.

110. Roberson PL, Heidorn DB, Kessler ML, Ten Haken RK, Buchsbaum DJ. Three-dimensional reconstruction of monoclonal antibody uptake in tumor and calculation of beta dose-rate nonuniformity. Cancer. 1994;73:912–8.

111. Roberson PL, Buchsbaum DJ. Reconciliation of tumor dose response to external beam radiotherapy versus radioimmunotherapy with 131-iodine-labeled antibody for a colon cancer model. Cancer Res. 1995;55:5811s–6.

112. Ning S, Trisler K, Wessels BW, Knox SJ. Radiobiologic studies of radioimmunotherapy and external beam radiotherapy in vitro and in vivo in human renal cell carcinoma xenografts. Cancer. 1997;80:2519–28.

113. Barendswaard EC, O'Donoghue JA, Larson SM, Tschmelitsch J, Welt S, Finn RD, et al. 131I radioimmunotherapy and fractionated external beam radiotherapy: comparative effectiveness in a human tumor xenograft. J Nucl Med. 1999;40:1764–8.

114. Hernandez MC, Knox SJ. Radiobiology of radioimmunotherapy with 90Y ibritumomab tiuxetan (Zevalin). Semin Oncol. 2003;30:6–10.

115. Sharkey RM, Primus FJ, Shochat D, Goldenberg DM. Comparison of tumor targeting of mouse monoclonal and goat polyclonal antibodies to carcinoembryonic antigen in the GW-39 human tumor-hamster host model. Cancer Res. 1988;48:1823–8.

116. Primus FJ, Freeman JW, Goldenberg DM. Immunological heterogeneity of carcinoembryonic antigen: purification from meconium of an antigen related to carcinoembryonic antigen. Cancer Res. 1983;43:679–85.

117. Primus FJ, Kuhns WJ, Goldenberg DM. Immunological heterogeneity of carcinoembryonic antigen: immunohistochemical detection of carcinoembryonic antigen determinants in colonic tumors with monoclonal antibodies. Cancer Res. 1983;43:693–701.

118. Primus FJ, Newell KD, Blue A, Goldenberg DM. Immunological heterogeneity of carcinoembryonic antigen: antigenic determinants on carcinoembryonic antigen distinguished by monoclonal antibodies. Cancer Res. 1983;43:686–92.

119. Hansen HJ, Goldenberg DM, Newman ES, Grebenau R, Sharkey RM. Characterization of second-generation monoclonal antibodies against carcinoembryonic antigen. Cancer. 1993;71:3478–85.

120. Sharkey RM, Goldenberg DM, Goldenberg H, Lee RE, Ballance C, Pawlyk D, et al. Murine monoclonal antibodies against carcinoembryonic antigen: immunological, pharmacokinetic, and targeting properties in humans. Cancer Res. 1990;50:2823–31.

121. Goldenberg DM, Primus FJ, Ford EH, Brennan K, Goldenberg H. Monoclonal antibodies to CEA: use in cancer radioimmunodetection. J Nucl Med. 1986;27:897.

122. Primus FJ, Bennett SJ, Kim EE, DeLand FH, Zahn MC, Goldenberg DM. Circulating immune complexes in cancer patients receiving goat radiolocalizing antibodies to carcinoembryonic antigen. Cancer Res. 1980;40:497–501.

123. Beauchemin N, Draber P, Dveksler G, Gold P, Gray-Owen S, Grunert F, et al. Redefined nomenclature for members of the carcinoembryonic antigen family. Exp Cell Res. 1999;252:243–9.

124. Hammarstrom S, Shively JE, Paxton RJ, Beatty BG, Larsson A, Ghosh R, et al. Antigenic sites in carcinoembryonic antigen. Cancer Res. 1989;49:4852–8.

125. Moffat Jr FL, Pinsky CM, Hammershaimb L, Petrelli NJ, Patt YZ, Whaley FS, et al. Clinical utility of external immunoscintigraphy with the IMMU-4 technetium-99 m Fab' antibody fragment in patients undergoing surgery for carcinoma of the colon and rectum: results of a pivotal, phase III trial. The Immunomedics Study Group. J Clin Oncol. 1996;14:2295–305.

126. Goldenberg DM. Perspectives on oncologic imaging with radiolabeled antibodies. Cancer. 1997;80:2431–5.

127. Behr TM, Sharkey RM, Juweid ME, Dunn RM, Vagg RC, Ying Z, et al. Phase I/II clinical radioimmunotherapy with an iodine-131-labeled anti-carcinoembryonic antigen murine monoclonal antibody IgG. J Nucl Med. 1997;38:858–70.

128. Sharkey RM, Pykett MJ, Siegel JA, Alger EA, Primus FJ, Goldenberg DM. Radioimmunotherapy of the GW-39 human colonic tumor xenograft with 131I-labeled murine monoclonal antibody to carcinoembryonic antigen. Cancer Res. 1987;47:5672–7.

129. Sharkey RM, Weadock KS, Natale A, Haywood L, Aninipot R, Blumenthal RD, et al. Successful radioimmunotherapy for lung metastasis of human colonic cancer in nude mice. J Natl Cancer Inst. 1991;83:627–32.

130. Siegel JA, Pawlyk DA, Lee RE, Sasso NL, Horowitz JA, Sharkey RM, et al. Tumor, red marrow, and organ dosimetry for 131I-labeled anti-carcinoembryonic antigen monoclonal antibody. Cancer Res. 1990;50:1039s–42.

131. Behr TM, Sharkey RM, Juweid MI, Dunn RM, Ying Z, Zhang CH, et al. Factors influencing the pharmacokinetics, dosimetry, and diagnostic accuracy of radioimmunodetection and radioimmunotherapy of carcinoembryonic antigen-expressing tumors. Cancer Res. 1996;56:1805–16.

132. Boerman OC, Sharkey RM, Blumenthal RD, Aninipot RL, Goldenberg DM. The presence of a concomitant bulky tumor can decrease the uptake and therapeutic efficacy of radiolabeled antibodies in small tumors. Int J Cancer. 1992;51:470–5.

133. Fujimori K, Covell DG, Fletcher JE, Weinstein JN. A modeling analysis of monoclonal antibody percolation through tumors: a binding-site barrier. J Nucl Med. 1990;31:1191–8.

134. Boerman OC, Sharkey RM, Wong GY, Blumenthal RD, Aninipot RL, Goldenberg DM. Influence of antibody protein dose on therapeutic efficacy of radioiodinated antibodies in nude mice bearing GW-39 human tumor. Cancer Immunol Immunother. 1992;35:127–34.

135. Saga T, Neumann RD, Heya T, Sato J, Kinuya S, Le N, et al. Targeting cancer micrometastases with monoclonal antibodies: a binding-site barrier. Proc Natl Acad Sci U S A. 1995;92:8999–9003.

136. Sharkey RM, Primus FJ, Goldenberg DM. Second antibody clearance of radiolabeled antibody in cancer radioimmunodetection. Proc Natl Acad Sci U S A. 1984;81:2843–6.

137. Goldenberg DM, Sharkey RM, Ford E. Anti-antibody enhancement of iodine-131 anti-CEA radioimmunodetection in experimental and clinical studies. J Nucl Med. 1987;28:1604–10.

138. Begent RH, Bagshawe KD, Pedley RB, Searle F, Ledermann JA, Green AJ, et al. Use of second antibody in radioimmunotherapy. NCI Monogr. 1987;3:59–61.

139. Pedley RB, Dale R, Boden JA, Begent RH, Keep PA, Green AJ. The effect of second antibody clearance on the distribution and dosimetry of radiolabelled anti-CEA antibody in a human colonic tumor xenograft model. Int J Cancer. 1989;43:713–8.

140. Sharkey RM, Boerman OC, Natale A, Pawlyk D, Monestier M, Losman MJ, et al. Enhanced clearance of radiolabeled murine monoclonal antibody by a syngeneic anti-idiotype antibody in tumor-bearing nude mice. Int J Cancer. 1992;51:266–73.

141. Blumenthal RD, Sharkey RM, Kashi R, Goldenberg DM. Comparison of therapeutic efficacy and host toxicity of two different 131I-labelled antibodies and their fragments in the GW-39 colonic cancer xenograft model. Int J Cancer. 1989;44:292–300.

142. Buchegger F, Pfister C, Fournier K, Prevel F, Schreyer M, Carrel S, et al. Ablation of human colon carcinoma in nude mice by 131I-labeled monoclonal anti-carcinoembryonic antigen antibody F(ab')2 fragments. J Clin Invest. 1989;83:1449–56.

143. Buchegger F, Pelegrin A, Delaloye B, Bischof-Delaloye A, Mach JP. Iodine-131-labeled MAb F(ab')2 fragments are more efficient and less toxic than intact anti-CEA antibodies in radioimmunotherapy of large human colon carcinoma grafted in nude mice. J Nucl Med. 1990;31:1035–44.

144. Blumenthal RD, Sharkey RM, Haywood L, Natale AM, Wong GY, Siegel JA, et al. Targeted therapy of athymic mice bearing GW-39 human colonic cancer micrometastases with 131I-labeled monoclonal antibodies. Cancer Res. 1992;52:6036–44.

145. Pedley RB, Boden JA, Boden R, Dale R, Begent RH. Comparative radioimmunotherapy using intact or F(ab')2 fragments of 131I anti-CEA antibody in a colonic xenograft model. Br J Cancer. 1993;68:69–73.

146. Juweid ME, Sharkey RM, Behr T, Swayne LC, Dunn R, Siegel J, et al. Radioimmunotherapy of patients with small-volume tumors using iodine-131-labeled anti-CEA monoclonal antibody (ab')2. J Nucl Med. 1996;37:1504–10.

147. Ychou M, Pelegrin A, Faurous P, Robert B, Saccavini JC, Guerreau D, et al. Phase-I/II radio-immunotherapy study with Iodine-131-labeled anti-CEA monoclonal antibody F6 F(ab')2 in patients with non-resectable liver metastases from colorectal cancer. Int J Cancer. 1998;75:615–9.

148. Buchegger F, Allal AS, Roth A, Papazyan JP, Dupertuis Y, Mirimanoff RO, et al. Combined radioimmunotherapy and radiotherapy of liver metastases from colorectal cancer: a feasibility study. Anticancer Res. 2000;20:1889–96.

149. Buchegger F, Gillet M, Doenz F, Vogel CA, Achtari C, Mach JP, et al. Biodistribution of anti-CEA F(ab')2 fragments after intra-arterial and intravenous injection in patients with liver metastases due to colorectal carcinoma. Nucl Med Commun. 1996;17:500–3.

150. Buchegger F, Roth A, Allal A, Dupertuis YM, Slosman DO, Delaloye AB, et al. Radioimmunotherapy of colorectal cancer liver metastases: combination with radiotherapy. Ann N Y Acad Sci. 2000;910:263–9.

151. Juweid M, Sharkey RM, Alavi A, Swayne LC, Herskovic T, Hanley D, et al. Regression of advanced refractory ovarian cancer treated with iodine-131-labeled anti-CEA monoclonal antibody. J Nucl Med. 1997;38:257–60.

152. Juweid M, Swayne LC, Sharkey RM, Dunn R, Rubin AD, Herskovic T, et al. Prospects of radioimmunotherapy in epithelial ovarian cancer: results with iodine-131-labeled murine and humanized MN-14 anti-carcinoembryonic antigen monoclonal antibodies. Gynecol Oncol. 1997;67:259–71.

153. Juweid ME, Hajjar G, Swayne LC, Sharkey RM, Suleiman S, Herskovic T, et al. Phase I/II trial of 131I-MN-14F(ab)2 anti-carcinoembryonic antigen monoclonal antibody in the treatment of patients with metastatic medullary thyroid carcinoma. Cancer. 1999;85:1828–42.

154. Juweid M, Sharkey RM, Behr T, Swayne LC, Herskovic T, Pereira M, et al. Radioimmunotherapy of medullary thyroid cancer with iodine-131-labeled anti-CEA antibodies. J Nucl Med. 1996;37:905–11.

155. Juweid ME, Hajjar G, Stein R, Sharkey RM, Herskovic T, Swayne LC, et al. Initial experience with high-dose radioimmunotherapy of metastatic medullary thyroid cancer using 131I-MN-14 F(ab)2 anti-carcinoembryonic antigen MAb and AHSCR. J Nucl Med. 2000;41:93–103.

156. Bernstein ID, Eary JF, Badger CC, Press OW, Appelbaum FR, Martin PJ, et al. High dose radiolabeled antibody therapy of lymphoma. Cancer Res. 1990;50:1017s–21.

157. Press OW, Eary JF, Appelbaum FR, Martin PJ, Badger CC, Nelp WB, et al. Radiolabeled-antibody therapy of B-cell lymphoma with autologous bone marrow support. N Engl J Med. 1993;329:1219–24.

158. Sharkey RM, Juweid M, Shevitz J, Behr T, Dunn R, Swayne LC, et al. Evaluation of a complementarity-determining region-grafted (humanized) anti-carcinoembryonic antigen monoclonal antibody in preclinical and clinical studies. Cancer Res. 1995;55:5935s–45.

159. Hajjar G, Sharkey RM, Burton J, Zhang CH, Yeldell D, Matthies A, et al. Phase I radioimmunotherapy trial with iodine-131-labeled humanized MN-14 anti-carcinoembryonic antigen monoclonal antibody in patients with metastatic gastrointestinal and colorectal cancer. Clin Colorectal Cancer. 2002;2:31–42.

160. Humm JL. Dosimetric aspects of radiolabeled antibodies for tumor therapy. J Nucl Med. 1986;27:1490–7.

161. Siegel JA. Revised Nuclear Regulatory Commission regulations for release of patients administered radioactive materials: outpatient iodine-131 anti-B1 therapy. J Nucl Med. 1998;39:28S–33.

162. Beckers C. Regulations and policies on radioiodine 131I therapy in Europe. Thyroid. 1997;7:221–4.

163. Grigsby PW, Siegel BA, Baker S, Eichling JO. Radiation exposure from outpatient radioactive iodine 131I therapy for thyroid carcinoma. JAMA. 2000;283:2272–4.

164. Wrixon AD. New ICRP recommendations. J Radiol Prot. 2008;28:161–8.

165. Sharkey RM, Kaltovich FA, Shih LB, Fand I, Govelitz G, Goldenberg DM. Radioimmunotherapy of human colonic cancer xenografts with 90Y labeled monoclonal antibodies to carcinoembryonic antigen. Cancer Res. 1988;48:3270–5.

166. Sharkey RM, Motta-Hennessy C, Gansow OA, Brechbiel MW, Fand I, Griffiths GL, et al. Selection of a DTPA chelate conjugate for monoclonal antibody targeting to a human colonic tumor in nude mice. Int J Cancer. 1990;46:79–85.

167. Fand I, Sharkey RM, Goldenberg DM. Use of whole-body autoradiography in cancer targeting with radiolabeled antibodies. Cancer Res. 1990;50:885s–91.

168. Gansow OA, Brechbiel MW, Mirzadeh S, Colcher D, Roselli M. Chelates and antibodies: current methods and new directions. Cancer Treat Res. 1990;51:153–71.

169. Roselli M, Schlom J, Gansow OA, Raubitschek A, Mirzadeh S, Brechbiel MW, et al. Comparative biodistributions of yttrium- and indium-labeled monoclonal antibody B72.3 in athymic mice bearing human colon carcinoma xenografts. J Nucl Med. 1989;30:672–82.

170. Sharkey RM, Motta-Hennessy C, Pawlyk D, Siegel JA, Goldenberg DM. Biodistribution and radiation dose estimates for yttrium- and iodine-labeled monoclonal antibody IgG and fragments in nude mice bearing human colonic tumor xenografts. Cancer Res. 1990;50:2330–6.

171. Deshpande SV, DeNardo SJ, Kukis DL, Moi MK, McCall MJ, DeNardo GL, et al. Yttrium-90-labeled monoclonal antibody for therapy: labeling by a new macrocyclic bifunctional chelating agent. J Nucl Med. 1990;31:473–9.

172. Meares CF, Moi MK, Diril H, Kukis DL, McCall MJ, Deshpande SV, et al. Macrocyclic chelates of radiometals for diagnosis and therapy. Br J Cancer Suppl. 1990;10:21–6.

173. Moi MK, DeNardo SJ, Meares CF. Stable bifunctional chelates of metals used in radiotherapy. Cancer Res. 1990;50:789s–93.

174. Subramanian R, Meares CF. Bifunctional chelating agents for radiometal-labeled monoclonal antibodies. Cancer Treat Res. 1990;51:183–99.

175. DeNardo GL, Kroger LA, DeNardo SJ, Miers LA, Salako Q, Kukis DL, et al. Comparative toxicity studies of yttrium-90 MX-DTPA and 2-IT-BAD conjugated monoclonal antibody (BrE-3). Cancer. 1994;73:1012–22.

176. Buchsbaum DJ, Lawrence TS, Roberson PL, Heidorn DB, Ten Haken RK, Steplewski Z. Comparison of 131I- and 90Y-labeled monoclonal antibody 17-1A for treatment of human colon cancer xenografts. Int J Radiat Oncol Biol Phys. 1993;25:629–38.

177. Kyriakos RJ, Shih LB, Ong GL, Patel K, Goldenberg DM, Mattes MJ. The fate of antibodies bound to the surface of tumor cells in vitro. Cancer Res. 1992;52:835–42.

178. Mattes MJ, Griffiths GL, Diril H, Goldenberg DM, Ong GL, Shih LB. Processing of antibody-radioisotope conjugates after binding to the surface of tumor cells. Cancer. 1994;73:787–93.

179. Wong JY, Williams LE, Yamauchi DM, Odom-Maryon T, Esteban JM, Neumaier M, et al. Initial experience evaluating 90yttrium-radiolabeled anti-carcinoembryonic antigen chimeric T84.66 in a phase I radioimmunotherapy trial. Cancer Res. 1995;55:5929s–34.

180. Fairweather DS, Bradwell AR, Dykes PW, Vaughan AT, Watson-James SF, Chandler S. Improved tumour localisation using indium-111 labelled antibodies. Br Med J (Clin Res Ed). 1983;287:167–70.

181. Abdel-Nabi HH, Schwartz AN, Goldfogel G, Ortman-Nabi JA, Matsuoka DM, Unger MW, et al. Colorectal tumors: scintigraphy with In-111 anti-CEA monoclonal antibody and correlation with surgical, histopathologic, and immunohistochemical findings. Radiology. 1988;166:747–52.

182. Halpern SE, Haindl W, Beauregard J, Hagan P, Clutter M, Amox D, et al. Scintigraphy with In-111-labeled monoclonal antitumor antibodies: kinetics, biodistribution, and tumor detection. Radiology. 1988;168:529–36.

183. Patt YZ, Lamki LM, Haynie TP, Unger MW, Rosenblum MG, Shirkhoda A, et al. Improved tumor localization with increasing dose of indium-111-labeled anti-carcinoembryonic antigen monoclonal antibody ZCE-025 in metastatic colorectal cancer. J Clin Oncol. 1988;6:1220–30.

184. Andrew SM, Perkins AC, Pimm MV, Baldwin RW. A comparison of iodine and indium labelled anti CEA intact antibody, F(ab)2 and Fab fragments by imaging tumour xenografts. Eur J Nucl Med. 1988;13:598–604.

185. Wong JY, Williams LE, Hill LR, Paxton RJ, Beatty BG, Shively JE, et al. The effects of tumor mass, tumor age, and external beam radiation on tumor-specific antibody uptake. Int J Radiat Oncol Biol Phys. 1989;16:715–20.

186. Divgi CR, McDermott K, Johnson DK, Schnobrich KE, Finn RD, Cohen AM, et al. Detection of hepatic metastases from colorectal carcinoma using indium-111 (111In) labeled monoclonal antibody (mAb): MSKCC experience with mAb 111In-C110. Int J Rad Appl Instrum B. 1991;18:705–10.

187. Patt YZ, Podoloff DA, Curley S, Smith R, Badhkamkar VA, Lamki LM, et al. Monoclonal antibody imaging in patients with colorectal cancer and increasing levels of serum carcinoembryonic antigen. Experience with ZCE-025 and IMMU-4

monoclonal antibodies and proposed directions for clinical trials. Cancer. 1993;71:4293–7.

188. Wong JY, Thomas GE, Yamauchi D, Williams LE, Odom-Maryon TL, Liu A, et al. Clinical evaluation of indium-111-labeled chimeric anti-CEA monoclonal antibody. J Nucl Med. 1997;38:1951–9.

189. Wong JYC, Chu DZ, Yamauchi DM, Williams LE, Liu A, Wilczynski S, et al. A phase I radioimmunotherapy trial evaluating 90yttrium-labeled anti-carcinoembryonic antigen (CEA) chimeric T84.66 in patients with metastatic CEA-producing malignancies. Clin Cancer Res. 2000;6:3855–63.

190. Lewis MR, Raubitschek A, Shively JE. A facile, water-soluble method for modification of proteins with DOTA. Use of elevated temperature and optimized pH to achieve high specific activity and high chelate stability in radiolabeled immunoconjugates. Bioconj Chem. 1994;5:565–76.

191. Wong JY, Chu DZ, Williams LE, Liu A, Zhan J, Yamauchi DM, et al. A phase I trial of 90Y-DOTA-anti-CEA chimeric T84.66 (cT84.66) radioimmunotherapy in patients with metastatic CEA-producing malignancies. Cancer Biother Radiopharm. 2006;21:88–100.

192. Fagnani R, Halpern S, Hagan M. Altered pharmacokinetic and tumour localization properties of Fab' fragments of a murine monoclonal anti-CEA antibody by covalent modification with low molecular weight dextran. Nucl Med Commun. 1995;16:362–9.

193. Siler K, Eggensperger D, Hand PH, Milenic DE, Miller LS, Houchens DP, et al. Therapeutic efficacy of a high-affinity anticarcinoembryonic antigen monoclonal antibody (COL-1). Biotechnol Ther. 1993;4:163–81.

194. Yu B, Carrasquillo J, Milenic D, Chung Y, Perentesis P, Feuerestein I, et al. Phase I trial of iodine 131-labeled COL-1 in patients with gastrointestinal malignancies: influence of serum carcinoembryonic antigen and tumor bulk on pharmacokinetics. J Clin Oncol. 1996;14:1798–809.

195. Meredith RF, Khazaeli MB, Plott WE, Grizzle WE, Liu T, Schlom J, et al. Phase II study of dual 131I-labeled monoclonal antibody therapy with interferon in patients with metastatic colorectal cancer. Clin Cancer Res. 1996;2:1811–8.

196. Delaloye AB, Delaloye B, Buchegger F, Vogel CA, Gillet M, Mach JP, et al. Comparison of copper-67- and iodine-125-labeled anti-CEA monoclonal antibody biodistribution in patients with colorectal tumors. J Nucl Med. 1997;38:847–53.

197. Boxer GM, Begent RH, Kelly AM, Southall PJ, Blair SB, Theodorou NA, et al. Factors influencing variability of localisation of antibodies to carcinoembryonic antigen (CEA) in patients with colorectal carcinoma–implications for radioimmunotherapy. Br J Cancer. 1992;65:825–31.

198. Lane DM, Eagle KF, Begent RH, Hope-Stone LD, Green AJ, Casey JL, et al. Radioimmunotherapy of metastatic colorectal tumours with iodine-131-labelled antibody to carcinoembryonic antigen: phase

I/II study with comparative biodistribution of intact and F(ab')2 antibodies. Br J Cancer. 1994;70:521–5.

199. Pedley RB, Begent RH, Boden JA, Boxer GM, Boden R, Keep PA. Enhancement of radioimmunotherapy by drugs modifying tumour blood flow in a colonic xenograft model. Int J Cancer. 1994;57:830–5.

200. Delgado C, Pedley RB, Herraez A, Boden R, Boden JA, Keep PA, et al. Enhanced tumour specificity of an anti-carcinoembrionic antigen Fab' fragment by poly(ethylene glycol) (PEG) modification. Br J Cancer. 1996;73:175–82.

201. Casey JL, Pedley RB, King DJ, Green AJ, Yarranton GT, Begent RH. Dosimetric evaluation and radioimmunotherapy of anti-tumour multivalent Fab' fragments. Br J Cancer. 1999;81:972–80.

202. Lu QJ, Bian GX, Chen YY, Zhang M, Guo SM, Wen LQ. Radioimmunotherapy of carcinoma of colon with 131I-labeled recombinant chimeric monoclonal antibodies to carcinoembryonic antigen. Acta Pharmacol Sin. 2005;26:1259–64.

203. Sundin A, Enblad P, Ahlstrom H, Carlsson J, Maripuu E, Hedin A. Radioimmunolocalization of human colonic cancer xenografts; aspects of extensive purification of monoclonal anti-CEA-antibodies. Int J Rad Appl Instrum B. 1991;18:891–9.

204. Mahteme H, Lovqvist A, Graf W, Lundqvist H, Carlsson J, Sundin A. Adjuvant 131I-anti-CEA-antibody radioimmunotherapy inhibits the development of experimental colonic carcinoma liver metastases. Anticancer Res. 1998;18:843–8.

205. Mahteme H, Sundin A, Larsson B, Khamis H, Arow K, Graf W. 5-FU uptake in peritoneal metastases after pretreatment with radioimmunotherapy or vasoconstriction: an autoradiographic study in the rat. Anticancer Res. 2005;25:917–22.

206. Watanabe N, Oriuchi N, Endo K, Inoue T, Kuroki M, Matsuoka Y, et al. CaNa2EDTA for improvement of radioimmunodetection and radioimmunotherapy with 111In and 90Y-DTPA-anti-CEA MAbs in nude mice bearing human colorectal cancer. J Nucl Med. 2000;41:337–44.

207. Saga T, Sakahara H, Nakamoto Y, Sato N, Zhao S, Iida Y, et al. Radioimmunotherapy for liver micrometastases in mice: pharmacokinetics, dose estimation, and long-term effect. Jpn J Cancer Res. 1999;90:342–8.

208. Liu Z, Jin C, Yu Z, Zhang J, Liu Y, Zhao H, et al. Radioimmunotherapy of human colon cancer xenografts with 131I-labeled anti-CEA monoclonal antibody. Bioconjug Chem. 2010;21:314–8.

209. Kamigaki T, Ajiki T, Yamamoto M, Kuroda Y. Enhancement of tumor uptakes by stabilized Fab homo-oligomers of a chimeric monoclonal antibody against carcinoembryonic antigen. Int J Oncol. 1999;14:139–44.

210. Herlyn D, Powe J, Alavi A, Mattis JA, Herlyn M, Ernst C, et al. Radioimmunodetection of human tumor xenografts by monoclonal antibodies. Cancer Res. 1983;43:2731–5.

211. Douillard JY, Chatal JF, Saccavini JC, Curtet C, Kremer M, Peuvrel P, et al. Pharmacokinetic study of radiolabeled anti-colorectal carcinoma monoclonal antibodies in tumor-bearing nude mice. Eur J Nucl Med. 1985;11:107–13.

212. Chatal JF, Saccavini JC, Fumoleau P, Douillard JY, Curtet C, Kremer M, et al. Immunoscintigraphy of colon carcinoma. J Nucl Med. 1984;25:307–14.

213. Mach JP, Chatal JF, Lumbroso JD, Buchegger F, Forni M, Ritschard J, et al. Tumor localization in patients by radiolabeled monoclonal antibodies against colon carcinoma. Cancer Res. 1983;43: 5593–600.

214. Malesci A, Tommasini MA, Bocchia P, Zerbi A, Beretta E, Vecchi M, et al. Differential diagnosis of pancreatic cancer and chronic pancreatitis by a monoclonal antibody detecting a new cancer-associated antigen (CA 19-9). Ric Clin Lab. 1984;14: 303–6.

215. Steinberg W. The clinical utility of the CA 19-9 tumor-associated antigen. Am J Gastroenterol. 1990;85:350–5.

216. Barton JG, Bois JP, Sarr MG, Wood CM, Qin R, Thomsen KM, et al. Predictive and prognostic value of CA 19-9 in resected pancreatic adenocarcinoma. J Gastrointest Surg. 2009;13:2050–8.

217. Buxbaum JL, Eloubeidi MA. Molecular and clinical markers of pancreas cancer. JOP. 2010;11:536–44.

218. Douillard JY, Le Mevel B, Curtet C, Vignoud J, Chatal JF, Koprowski H. Immunotherapy of gastrointestinal cancer with monoclonal antibodies. Med Oncol Tumor Pharmacother. 1986;3:141–6.

219. Herlyn D, Lubeck M, Sears H, Koprowski H. Specific detection of anti-idiotypic immune responses in cancer patients treated with murine monoclonal antibody. J Immunol Methods. 1985;85: 27–38.

220. Sears HF, Herlyn D, Steplewski Z, Koprowski H. Effects of monoclonal antibody immunotherapy on patients with gastrointestinal adenocarcinoma. J Biol Response Mod. 1984;3:138–50.

221. Paul AR, Engstrom PF, Weiner LM, Steplewski Z, Koprowski H. Treatment of advanced measurable or evaluable pancreatic carcinoma with 17-1A murine monoclonal antibody alone or in combination with 5-fluorouracil, adriamycin and mitomycin (FAM). Hybridoma. 1986;5 Suppl 1:S171–4.

222. Sindelar WF, Maher MM, Herlyn D, Sears HF, Steplewski Z, Koprowski H. Trial of therapy with monoclonal antibody 17-1A in pancreatic carcinoma: preliminary results. Hybridoma. 1986;5 Suppl 1:S125–32.

223. Verrill H, Goldberg M, Rosenbaum R, Abbott R, Simunovic L, Steplewski Z, et al. Clinical trial of Wistar Institute 17-1A monoclonal antibody in patients with advanced gastrointestinal adenocarcinoma: a preliminary report. Hybridoma. 1986;5 Suppl 1:S175–83.

224. Buchsbaum DJ, Brubaker PG, Hanna DE, Glatfelter AA, Terry VH, Guilbault DM, et al. Comparative

225. Meredith RF, Khazaeli MB, Plott WE, Spencer SA, Wheeler RH, Brady LW, et al. Initial clinical evaluation of iodine-125-labeled chimeric 17-1A for metastatic colon cancer. J Nucl Med. 1995;36:2229–33.

226. Meredith RF, LoBuglio AF, Plott WE, Orr RA, Brezovich IA, Russell CD, et al. Pharmacokinetics, immune response, and biodistribution of iodine-131-labeled chimeric mouse/human IgG1k 17-1A monoclonal antibody. J Nucl Med. 1991;32:1162–8.

227. Brady LW, Miyamoto C, Woo DV, Rackover M, Emrich J, Bender H, et al. Malignant astrocytomas treated with iodine-125 labeled monoclonal antibody 425 against epidermal growth factor receptor: a phase II trial. Int J Radiat Oncol Biol Phys. 1992;22:225–30.

228. Wong KJ, Baidoo KE, Nayak TK, Garmestani K, Brechbiel MW, Milenic DE. In vitro and in vivo preclinical analysis of a F(ab')2 fragment of panitumumab for molecular imaging and therapy of HER1 positive cancers. EJNMMI Res. 2011;1:1.

229. Milenic DE, Brady ED, Garmestani K, Albert PS, Abdulla A, Brechbiel MW. Improved efficacy of alpha-particle-targeted radiation therapy: dual targeting of human epidermal growth factor receptor-2 and tumor-associated glycoprotein 72. Cancer. 2010;116:1059–66.

230. Ray GL, Baidoo KE, Wong KJ, Williams M, Garmestani K, Brechbiel MW, et al. Preclinical evaluation of a monoclonal antibody targeting the epidermal growth factor receptor as a radioimmunodiagnostic and radioimmunotherapeutic agent. Br J Pharmacol. 2009;157:1541–8.

231. Colcher D, Keenan AM, Larson SM, Schlom J. Prolonged binding of a radiolabeled monoclonal antibody (B72.3) used for the in situ radioimmunodetection of human colon carcinoma xenografts. Cancer Res. 1984;44:5744–51.

232. Abdel-Nabi HH, Doerr RJ. Multicenter clinical trials of monoclonal antibody B72.3-GYK-DTPA 111In (111In-CYT-103; OncoScint CR103) in patients with colorectal carcinoma. Targeted Diagn Ther. 1992;6:73–88.

233. Doerr RJ, Abdel-Nabi H, Krag D, Mitchell E. Radiolabeled antibody imaging in the management of colorectal cancer. Results of a multicenter clinical study. Ann Surg. 1991;214:118–24.

234. Povoski SP, Neff RL, Mojzisik CM, O'Malley DM, Hinkle GH, Hall NC, et al. A comprehensive overview of radioguided surgery using gamma detection probe technology. World J Surg Oncol. 2009;7:11.

235. Esteban JM, Schlom J, Mornex F, Colcher D. Radioimmunotherapy of athymic mice bearing human colon carcinomas with monoclonal antibody B72.3: histological and autoradiographic study of effects on tumors and normal organs. Eur J Cancer Clin Oncol. 1987;23:643–55.

binding and preclinical localization and therapy studies with radiolabeled human chimeric and murine 17-1A monoclonal antibodies. Cancer Res. 1990;50:993s–9.

236. Colcher DM, Milenic DE, Schlom J. Generation and characterization of monoclonal antibody B72.3. Experimental and preclinical studies. Targeted Diagn Ther. 1992;6:23–44.
237. Meredith RF, Khazaeli MB, Plott WE, Saleh MN, Liu T, Allen LF, et al. Phase I trial of iodine-131-chimeric B72.3 (human IgG4) in metastatic colorectal cancer. J Nucl Med. 1992;33:23–9.
238. Colcher D, Carrasquillo JA, Esteban JM, Sugarbaker P, Reynolds JC, Siler K, et al. Radiolabeled monoclonal antibody B72.3 localization in metastatic lesions of colorectal cancer patients. Int J Rad Appl Instrum B. 1987;14:251–62.
239. Colcher D, Minelli MF, Roselli M, Muraro R, Simpson-Milenic D, Schlom J. Radioimmunolocalization of human carcinoma xenografts with B72.3 second generation monoclonal antibodies. Cancer Res. 1988;48:4597–603.
240. Schlom J, Colcher D, Roselli M, Carrasquillo JA, Reynolds JC, Larson SM, et al. Tumor targeting with monoclonal antibody B72.3. Int J Rad Appl Instrum B. 1989;16:137–42.
241. Muraro R, Kuroki M, Wunderlich D, Poole DJ, Colcher D, Thor A, et al. Generation and characterization of B72.3 second generation monoclonal antibodies reactive with the tumor-associated glycoprotein 72 antigen. Cancer Res. 1988;48:4588–96.
242. Hanisch FG, Uhlenbruck G, Egge H, Peter-Katalinic J. A B72.3 second-generation-monoclonal antibody (CC49) defines the mucin-carried carbohydrate epitope Gal beta(1-3) [NeuAc alpha(2-6)]GalNAc. Biol Chem Hoppe Seyler. 1989;370:21–6.
243. Molinolo A, Simpson JF, Thor A, Schlom J. Enhanced tumor binding using immunohistochemical analyses by second generation anti-tumor-associated glycoprotein 72 monoclonal antibodies versus monoclonal antibody B72.3 in human tissue. Cancer Res. 1990;50:1291–8.
244. Schlom J, Eggensperger D, Colcher D, Molinolo A, Houchens D, Miller LS, et al. Therapeutic advantage of high-affinity anticarcinoma radioimmunoconjugates. Cancer Res. 1992;52:1067–72.
245. Kashmiri SV, Iwahashi M, Tamura M, Padlan EA, Milenic DE, Schlom J. Development of a minimally immunogenic variant of humanized anti-carcinoma monoclonal antibody CC49. Crit Rev Oncol Hematol. 2001;38:3–16.
246. Kashmiri SV, Shu L, Padlan EA, Milenic DE, Schlom J, Hand PH. Generation, characterization, and in vivo studies of humanized anticarcinoma antibody CC49. Hybridoma. 1995;14:461–73.
247. Divgi CR, Scott AM, Dantis L, Capitelli P, Siler K, Hilton S, et al. Phase I radioimmunotherapy trial with iodine-131-CC49 in metastatic colon carcinoma. J Nucl Med. 1995;36:586–92.
248. Divgi CR, Scott AM, McDermott K, Fallone PS, Hilton S, Siler K, et al. Clinical comparison of radiolocalization of two monoclonal antibodies (mAbs) against the TAG-72 antigen. Nucl Med Biol. 1994;21:9–15.
249. Tempero M, Leichner P, Dalrymple G, Harrison K, Augustine S, Schlam J, et al. High-dose therapy with iodine-131-labeled monoclonal antibody CC49 in patients with gastrointestinal cancers: a phase I trial. J Clin Oncol. 1997;15:1518–28.
250. Tempero M, Leichner P, Baranowska-Kortylewicz J, Harrison K, Augustine S, Schlom J, et al. High-dose therapy with 90Yttrium-labeled monoclonal antibody CC49: a phase I trial. Clin Cancer Res. 2000;6:3095–102.
251. Greiner JW, Guadagni F, Roselli M, Ullmann CD, Nieroda C, Schlom J. Improved experimental radioimmunotherapy of colon xenografts by combining 131I-CC49 and interferon-gamma. Dis Colon Rectum. 1994;37:S100–5.
252. Greiner JW, Ullmann CD, Nieroda C, Qi CF, Eggensperger D, Shimada S, et al. Improved radioimmunotherapeutic efficacy of an anticarcinoma monoclonal antibody (131I-CC49) when given in combination with gamma-interferon. Cancer Res. 1993;53:600–8.
253. Triozzi PL, Kim JA, Martin Jr EW, Colcher D, Heffelfinger M, Rucker R. Clinical and immunologic effects of monoclonal antibody CC49 and interleukin-2 in patients with metastatic colorectal cancer. Hybridoma. 1997;16:147–51.
254. Macey DJ, Grant EJ, Kasi L, Rosenblum MG, Zhang HZ, Katz RL, et al. Effect of recombinant alpha-interferon on pharmacokinetics, biodistribution, toxicity, and efficacy of 131I-labeled monoclonal antibody CC49 in breast cancer: a phase II trial. Clin Cancer Res. 1997;3:1547–55.
255. Nocera MA, Shochat D, Primus FJ, Krupey J, Jespersen DL, Goldenberg DM. Representation of epitopes on colon-specific antigen-p defined by monoclonal antibodies. J Natl Cancer Inst. 1987;79:943–8.
256. Sharkey RM, Gold DV, Aninipot R, Vagg R, Ballance C, Newman ES, et al. Comparison of tumor targeting in nude mice by murine monoclonal antibodies directed against different human colorectal cancer antigens. Cancer Res. 1990;50:828s–34.
257. Sharkey RM, Goldenberg DM, Vagg R, Pawlyk D, Wong GY, Siegel JA, et al. Phase I clinical evaluation of a new murine monoclonal antibody (Mu-9) against colon-specific antigen-p for targeting gastrointestinal carcinomas. Cancer. 1994;73:864–77.
258. Heath JK, White SJ, Johnstone CN, Catimel B, Simpson RJ, Moritz RL, et al. The human A33 antigen is a transmembrane glycoprotein and a novel member of the immunoglobulin superfamily. Proc Natl Acad Sci U S A. 1997;94:469–74.
259. Sakamoto J, Kojima H, Kato J, Hamashima H, Suzuki H. Organ-specific expression of the intestinal epithelium-related antigen A33, a cell surface target for antibody-based imaging and treatment in gastrointestinal cancer. Cancer Chemother Pharmacol. 2000;46 Suppl:S27–32.
260. Ritter G, Cohen LS, Nice EC, Catimel B, Burgess AW, Moritz RL, et al. Characterization of posttranslational modifications of human A33 antigen, a novel

palmitoylated surface glycoprotein of human gastro-intestinal epithelium. Biochem Biophys Res Commun. 1997;236:682–6.

261. Welt S, Divgi CR, Real FX, Yeh SD, Garin-Chesa P, Finstad CL, et al. Quantitative analysis of antibody localization in human metastatic colon cancer: a phase I study of monoclonal antibody A33. J Clin Oncol. 1990;8:1894–906.

262. Welt S, Divgi CR, Kemeny N, Finn RD, Scott AM, Graham M, et al. Phase I/II study of iodine 131-labeled monoclonal antibody A33 in patients with advanced colon cancer. J Clin Oncol. 1994;12:1561–71.

263. Daghighian F, Barendswaard E, Welt S, Humm J, Scott A, Willingham MC, et al. Enhancement of radiation dose to the nucleus by vesicular internalization of iodine-125-labeled A33 monoclonal antibody. J Nucl Med. 1996;37:1052–7.

264. Welt S, Scott AM, Divgi CR, Kemeny NE, Finn RD, Daghighian F, et al. Phase I/II study of iodine 125-labeled monoclonal antibody A33 in patients with advanced colon cancer. J Clin Oncol. 1996; 14:1787–97.

265. Barendswaard EC, Humm JL, O'Donoghue JA, Sgouros G, Finn RD, Scott AM, et al. Relative therapeutic efficacy of 125I- and 131I-labeled monoclonal antibody A33 in a human colon cancer xenograft. J Nucl Med. 2001;42:1251–6.

266. Barendswaard EC, Scott AM, Divgi CR, Williams Jr C, Coplan K, Riedel E, et al. Rapid and specific targeting of monoclonal antibody A33 to a colon cancer xenograft in nude mice. Int J Oncol. 1998;12: 45–53.

267. Lee FT, Hall C, Rigopoulos A, Zweit J, Pathmaraj K, O'Keefe GJ, et al. Immuno-PET of human colon xenograft- bearing BALB/c nude mice using 124I-CDR-grafted humanized A33 monoclonal antibody. J Nucl Med. 2001;42:764–9.

268. Ruan S, O'Donoghue JA, Larson SM, Finn RD, Jungbluth A, Welt S, et al. Optimizing the sequence of combination therapy with radiolabeled antibodies and fractionated external beam. J Nucl Med. 2000;41:1905–12.

269. Tschmelitsch J, Barendswaard E, Williams Jr C, Yao TJ, Cohen AM, Old LJ, et al. Enhanced antitumor activity of combination radioimmunotherapy (131I-labeled monoclonal antibody A33) with chemotherapy (fluorouracil). Cancer Res. 1997;57:2181–6.

270. Almqvist Y, Orlova A, Sjostrom A, Jensen HJ, Lundqvist H, Sundin A, et al. In vitro characterization of 211At-labeled antibody A33-a potential therapeutic agent against metastatic colorectal carcinoma. Cancer Biother Radiopharm. 2005;20:514–23.

271. Almqvist Y, Steffen AC, Lundqvist H, Jensen H, Tolmachev V, Sundin A. Biodistribution of 211At-labeled humanized monoclonal antibody A33. Cancer Biother Radiopharm. 2007;22:480–7.

272. Scott AM, Lee FT, Jones R, Hopkins W, MacGregor D, Cebon JS, et al. A phase I trial of humanized monoclonal antibody A33 in patients with colorectal carcinoma:

biodistribution, pharmacokinetics, and quantitative tumor uptake. Clin Cancer Res. 2005;11:4810–7.

273. Chong G, Lee FT, Hopkins W, Tebbutt N, Cebon JS, Mountain AJ, et al. Phase I trial of 131I-huA33 in patients with advanced colorectal carcinoma. Clin Cancer Res. 2005;11:4818–26.

274. Welt S, Ritter G, Williams Jr C, Cohen LS, John M, Jungbluth A, et al. Phase I study of anticolon cancer humanized antibody A33. Clin Cancer Res. 2003;9:1338–46.

275. Carrasquillo JA, Pandit-Taskar N, O'Donoghue JA, Humm JL, Zanzonico P, Smith-Jones PM, et al. 124I-huA33 antibody PET of colorectal cancer. J Nucl Med. 2011;52:1173–80.

276. Garin-Chesa P, Old LJ, Rettig WJ. Cell surface glycoprotein of reactive stromal fibroblasts as a potential antibody target in human epithelial cancers. Proc Natl Acad Sci U S A. 1990;87:7235–9.

277. Welt S, Divgi CR, Scott AM, Garin-Chesa P, Finn RD, Graham M, et al. Antibody targeting in metastatic colon cancer: a phase I study of monoclonal antibody F19 against a cell-surface protein of reactive tumor stromal fibroblasts. J Clin Oncol. 1994;12:1193–203.

278. Scott AM, Wiseman G, Welt S, Adjei A, Lee FT, Hopkins W, et al. A Phase I dose-escalation study of sibrotuzumab in patients with advanced or metastatic fibroblast activation protein-positive cancer. Clin Cancer Res. 2003;9:1639–47.

279. Hofheinz RD, al-Batran SE, Hartmann F, Hartung G, Jager D, Renner C, et al. Stromal antigen targeting by a humanised monoclonal antibody: an early phase II trial of sibrotuzumab in patients with metastatic colorectal cancer. Onkologie. 2003;26:44–8.

280. Wahl RL, Parker CW, Philpott GW. Improved radioimaging and tumor localization with monoclonal F(ab')2. J Nucl Med. 1983;24:316–25.

281. Sharkey RM, Blumenthal RD, Hansen HJ, Goldenberg DM. Biological considerations for radioimmunotherapy. Cancer Res. 1990;50:964s–9.

282. Goldenberg DM, Blumenthal RD, Sharkey RM. Biological and clinical perspectives of cancer imaging and therapy with radiolabeled antibodies. Semin Cancer Biol. 1990;1:217–25.

283. Garkavij M, Tennvall J, Strand SE, Norrgren K, Nilsson R, Lindgren L, et al. Improving radioimmunotargeting of tumors. Variation in the amount of L6 MAb administered, combined with an immunoadsorption system (ECIA). Acta Oncol. 1993;32:853–9.

284. Hartmann C, Bloedow DC, Dienhart DG, Kasliwal R, Johnson TK, Gonzalez R, et al. A pharmacokinetic model describing the removal of circulating radiolabeled antibody by extracorporeal immunoadsorption. J Pharmacokinet Biopharm. 1991; 19:385–403.

285. Martensson L, Nilsson R, Ohlsson T, Sjogren HO, Strand SE, Tennvall J. Improved tumor targeting and decreased normal tissue accumulation through extracorporeal affinity adsorption in a two-step pretargeting strategy. Clin Cancer Res. 2007;13:5572s–6.

286. Martensson L, Nilsson R, Ohlsson T, Sjogren HO, Strand SE, Tennvall J. Reduced myelotoxicity with sustained tumor concentration of radioimmunoconjugates in rats after extracorporeal depletion. J Nucl Med. 2007;48:269–76.

287. Covell DG, Barbet J, Holton OD, Black CD, Parker RJ, Weinstein JN. Pharmacokinetics of monoclonal immunoglobulin G1, F(ab')2, and Fab' in mice. Cancer Res. 1986;46:3969–78.

288. Holton III OD, Black CD, Parker RJ, Covell DG, Barbet J, Sieber SM, et al. Biodistribution of monoclonal IgG1, F(ab')2, and Fab' in mice after intravenous injection. Comparison between anti-B cell (anti-Lyb8.2) and irrelevant (MOPC-21) antibodies. J Immunol. 1987;139:3041–9.

289. Huston JS, Levinson D, Mudgett-Hunter M, Tai MS, Novotny J, Margolies MN, et al. Protein engineering of antibody binding sites: recovery of specific activity in an anti-digoxin single-chain Fv analogue produced in Escherichia coli. Proc Natl Acad Sci U S A. 1988;85:5879–83.

290. Bird RE, Hardman KD, Jacobson JW, Johnson S, Kaufman BM, Lee SM, et al. Single-chain antigen-binding proteins. Science. 1988;242:423–6.

291. Colcher D, Bird R, Roselli M, Hardman KD, Johnson S, Pope S, et al. In vivo tumor targeting of a recombinant single-chain antigen-binding protein. J Natl Cancer Inst. 1990;82:1191–7.

292. Schlom J, Milenic DE, Roselli M, Colcher D, Bird R, Johnson S, et al. New concepts in monoclonal antibody based radioimmunodiagnosis and radioimmunotherapy of carcinoma. Int J Rad Appl Instrum B. 1991;18:425–35.

293. Milenic DE, Yokota T, Filpula DR, Finkelman MA, Dodd SW, Wood JF, et al. Construction, binding properties, metabolism, and tumor targeting of a single-chain Fv derived from the pancarcinoma monoclonal antibody CC49. Cancer Res. 1991; 51:6363–71.

294. Colcher D, Pavlinkova G, Beresford G, Booth BJ, Choudhury A, Batra SK. Pharmacokinetics and biodistribution of genetically-engineered antibodies. Q J Nucl Med. 1998;42:225–41.

295. Holliger P, Prospero T, Winter G. "Diabodies": small bivalent and bispecific antibody fragments. Proc Natl Acad Sci U S A. 1993;90:6444–8.

296. Pluckthun A, Pack P. New protein engineering approaches to multivalent and bispecific antibody fragments. Immunotechnology. 1997;3:83–105.

297. King DJ, Turner A, Farnsworth AP, Adair JR, Owens RJ, Pedley RB, et al. Improved tumor targeting with chemically cross-linked recombinant antibody fragments. Cancer Res. 1994;54:6176–85.

298. Wang D, Berven E, Li Q, Uckun F, Kersey JH. Optimization of conditions for formation and analysis of anti-CD19 FVS191 single-chain Fv homodimer (scFv')2. Bioconj Chem. 1997;8:64–70.

299. Goel A, Baranowska-Kortylewicz J, Hinrichs SH, Wisecarver J, Pavlinkova G, Augustine S, et al. 99mTc-labeled divalent and tetravalent CC49 single-chain Fv's: novel imaging agents for rapid in vivo localization of human colon carcinoma. J Nucl Med. 2001;42:1519–27.

300. Chauhan SC, Jain M, Moore ED, Wittel UA, Li J, Gwilt PR, et al. Pharmacokinetics and biodistribution of 177Lu-labeled multivalent single-chain Fv construct of the pancarcinoma monoclonal antibody CC49. Eur J Nucl Med Mol Imaging. 2005;32:264–73.

301. Wittel UA, Jain M, Goel A, Chauhan SC, Colcher D, Batra SK. The in vivo characteristics of genetically engineered divalent and tetravalent single-chain antibody constructs. Nucl Med Biol. 2005;32: 157–64.

302. Hu S, Shively L, Raubitschek A, Sherman M, Williams LE, Wong JY, et al. Minibody: a novel engineered anti-carcinoembryonic antigen antibody fragment (single-chain Fv-CH3) which exhibits rapid, high-level targeting of xenografts. Cancer Res. 1996;56:3055–61.

303. Kenanova V, Olafsen T, Crow DM, Sundaresan G, Subbarayan M, Carter NH, et al. Tailoring the pharmacokinetics and positron emission tomography imaging properties of anti-carcinoembryonic antigen single-chain Fv-Fc antibody fragments. Cancer Res. 2005;65:622–31.

304. Kenanova VE, Olafsen T, Salazar FB, Williams LE, Knowles S, Wu AM. Tuning the serum persistence of human serum albumin domain III: diabody fusion proteins. Protein Eng Des Sel. 2010;23:789–98.

305. Kenanova V, Olafsen T, Williams LE, Ruel NH, Longmate J, Yazaki PJ, et al. Radioiodinated versus radiometal-labeled anti-carcinoembryonic antigen single-chain Fv-Fc antibody fragments: optimal pharmacokinetics for therapy. Cancer Res. 2007;67: 718–26.

306. Olafsen T, Kenanova VE, Wu AM. Tunable pharmacokinetics: modifying the in vivo half-life of antibodies by directed mutagenesis of the Fc fragment. Nat Protoc. 2006;1:2048–60.

307. Mueller BM, Reisfeld RA, Gillies SD. Serum half-life and tumor localization of a chimeric antibody deleted of the CH2 domain and directed against the disialoganglioside GD2. Proc Natl Acad Sci U S A. 1990;87:5702–5.

308. Ghetie V, Hubbard JG, Kim JK, Tsen MF, Lee Y, Ward ES. Abnormally short serum half-lives of IgG in beta 2-microglobulin-deficient mice. Eur J Immunol. 1996;26:690–6.

309. Ober RJ, Radu CG, Ghetie V, Ward ES. Differences in promiscuity for antibody-FcRn interactions across species: implications for therapeutic antibodies. Int Immunol. 2001;13:1551–9.

310. Hinton PR, Johlfs MG, Xiong JM, Hanestad K, Ong KC, Bullock C, et al. Engineered human IgG antibodies with longer serum half-lives in primates. J Biol Chem. 2004;279:6213–6.

311. Dumont JA, Low SC, Peters RT, Bitonti AJ. Monomeric Fc fusions: impact on pharmacokinetic and biological activity of protein therapeutics. BioDrugs. 2006;20:151–60.

312. Slavin-Chiorini DC, Horan Hand PH, Kashmiri SV, Calvo B, Zaremba S, Schlom J. Biologic properties of a CH2 domain-deleted recombinant immunoglobulin. Int J Cancer. 1993;53:97–103.

313. Slavin-Chiorini DC, Kashmiri SV, Schlom J, Calvo B, Shu LM, Schott ME, et al. Biological properties of chimeric domain-deleted anticarcinoma immunoglobulins. Cancer Res. 1995;55:5957s–67.

314. Slavin-Chiorini DC, Kashmiri SV, Lee HS, Milenic DE, Poole DJ, Bernon E, et al. A CDR-grafted (humanized) domain-deleted antitumor antibody. Cancer Biother Radiopharm. 1997;12:305–16.

315. Agnese DM, Abdessalam SF, Burak Jr WE, Arnold MW, Soble D, Hinkle GH, et al. Pilot study using a humanized CC49 monoclonal antibody (HuCC49DeltaCH2) to localize recurrent colorectal carcinoma. Ann Surg Oncol. 2004;11:197–202.

316. Forero A, Meredith RF, Khazaeli MB, Carpenter DM, Shen S, Thornton J, et al. A novel monoclonal antibody design for radioimmunotherapy. Cancer Biother Radiopharm. 2003;18:751–9.

317. Xiao J, Horst S, Hinkle G, Cao X, Kocak E, Fang J, et al. Pharmacokinetics and clinical evaluation of 125I-radiolabeled humanized CC49 monoclonal antibody (HuCC49deltaCH2) in recurrent and metastatic colorectal cancer patients. Cancer Biother Radiopharm. 2005;20:16–26.

318. Shen S, Forero A, Meredith RF, LoBuglio AF. Biodistribution and dosimetry of In-111/Y-90-HuCC49DeltaCh2 (IDEC-159) in patients with metastatic colorectal adenocarcinoma. Cancer Biother Radiopharm. 2011;26:127–33.

319. Blumenthal RD, Sharkey RM, Natale AM, Kashi R, Wong G, Goldenberg DM. Comparison of equitoxic radioimmunotherapy and chemotherapy in the treatment of human colonic cancer xenografts. Cancer Res. 1994;54:142–51.

320. Chalandon Y, Mach JP, Pelegrin A, Folli S, Buchegger F. Combined radioimmunotherapy and chemotherapy of human colon carcinoma grafted in nude mice, advantages and limitations. Anticancer Res. 1992;12:1131–9.

321. Remmenga SW, Colcher D, Gansow O, Pippen CG, Raubitschek A. Continuous infusion chemotherapy as a radiation-enhancing agent for yttrium-90-radiolabeled monoclonal antibody therapy of a human tumor xenograft. Gynecol Oncol. 1994;55:115–22.

322. Kinuya S, Yokoyama K, Konishi S, Hiramatsu T, Watanabe N, Shuke N, et al. Enhanced efficacy of radioimmunotherapy combined with systemic chemotherapy and local hyperthermia in xenograft model. Jpn J Cancer Res. 2000;91:573–8.

323. Blumenthal RD, Taylor A, Osorio L, Ochakovskaya R, Raleigh JA, Papadopoulou M, et al. Optimizing the use of combined radioimmunotherapy and hypoxic cytotoxin therapy as a function of tumor hypoxia. Int J Cancer. 2001;94:564–71.

324. Pedley RB, Hill SA, Boxer GM, Flynn AA, Boden R, Watson R, et al. Eradication of colorectal xenografts by combined radioimmunotherapy and combretastatin a-4 3-O-phosphate. Cancer Res. 2001;61:4716–22.

325. Kinuya S, Kawashima A, Yokoyama K, Kudo M, Kasahara Y, Watanabe N, et al. Anti-angiogenic therapy and radioimmunotherapy in colon cancer xenografts. Eur J Nucl Med. 2001;28:1306–12.

326. Kinuya S, Yokoyama K, Koshida K, Mori H, Shiba K, Watanabe N, et al. Improved survival of mice bearing liver metastases of colon cancer cells treated with a combination of radioimmunotherapy and antiangiogenic therapy. Eur J Nucl Med Mol Imaging. 2004;31:981–5.

327. Meyer T, Gaya AM, Dancey G, Stratford MR, Othman S, Sharma SK, et al. A phase I trial of radioimmunotherapy with 131I-A5B7 anti-CEA antibody in combination with combretastatin-A4-phosphate in advanced gastrointestinal carcinomas. Clin Cancer Res. 2009;15:4484–92.

328. Mittal BB, Zimmer MA, Sathiaseelan V, Benson 3rd AB, Mittal RR, Dutta S, et al. Phase I/II trial of combined 131I anti-CEA monoclonal antibody and hyperthermia in patients with advanced colorectal adenocarcinoma. Cancer. 1996;78:1861–70.

329. Shibata S, Raubitschek A, Leong L, Koczywas M, Williams L, Zhan J, et al. A phase I study of a combination of yttrium-90-labeled anti-carcinoembryonic antigen (CEA) antibody and gemcitabine in patients with CEA-producing advanced malignancies. Clin Cancer Res. 2009;15:2935–41.

330. Wong JY, Shibata S, Williams LE, Kwok CS, Liu A, Chu DZ, et al. A Phase I trial of 90Y-anti-carcinoembryonic antigen chimeric T84.66 radioimmunotherapy with 5-fluorouracil in patients with metastatic colorectal cancer. Clin Cancer Res. 2003;9:5842–52.

331. Fisher RI, Kaminski MS, Wahl RL, Knox SJ, Zelenetz AD, Vose JM, et al. Tositumomab and iodine-131 tositumomab produces durable complete remissions in a subset of heavily pretreated patients with low-grade and transformed non-Hodgkin's lymphomas. J Clin Oncol. 2005;23:7565–73.

332. Kaminski MS, Tuck M, Estes J, Kolstad A, Ross CW, Zasadny K, et al. 131I-tositumomab therapy as initial treatment for follicular lymphoma. N Engl J Med. 2005;352:441–9.

333. de Jong GM, Bleichrodt RP, Eek A, Oyen WJ, Boerman OC, Hendriks T. Experimental study of radioimmunotherapy versus chemotherapy for colorectal cancer. Br J Surg. 2011;98:436–41.

334. de Jong GM, Hendriks T, Eek A, Oyen WJ, Nagtegaal ID, Bleichrodt RP, et al. Adjuvant radioimmunotherapy improves survival of rats after resection of colorectal liver metastases. Ann Surg. 2011;253:336–41.

335. Koppe MJ, Hendriks T, Boerman OC, Oyen WJ, Bleichrodt RP. Radioimmunotherapy is an effective adjuvant treatment after cytoreductive surgery of experimental colonic peritoneal carcinomatosis. J Nucl Med. 2006;47:1867–74.

336. Behr TM, Salib AL, Liersch T, Behe M, Angerstein C, Blumenthal RD, et al. Radioimmunotherapy of small volume disease of colorectal cancer metastatic to the liver: preclinical evaluation in comparison to standard chemotherapy and initial results of a phase I clinical study. Clin Cancer Res. 1999;5:3232s–42.

337. Behr TM, Liersch T, Greiner-Bechert L, Griesinger F, Behe M, Markus PM, et al. Radioimmunotherapy of small-volume disease of metastatic colorectal cancer. Cancer. 2002;94:1373–81.

338. Liersch T, Meller J, Kulle B, Behr TM, Markus P, Langer C, et al. Phase II trial of carcinoembryonic antigen radioimmunotherapy with 131I-labetuzumab after salvage resection of colorectal metastases in the liver: five-year safety and efficacy results. J Clin Oncol. 2005;23:6763–70.

339. Liersch T, Meller J, Bittrich M, Kulle B, Becker H, Goldenberg DM. Update of carcinoembryonic antigen radioimmunotherapy with 131I-labetuzumab after salvage resection of colorectal liver metastases: comparison of outcome to a contemporaneous control group. Ann Surg Oncol. 2007;14:2577–90.

340. Stickney DR, Anderson LD, Slater JB, Ahlem CN, Kirk GA, Schweighardt SA, et al. Bifunctional antibody: a binary radiopharmaceutical delivery system for imaging colorectal carcinoma. Cancer Res. 1991;51:6650–5.

341. Stickney DR, Slater JB, Kirk GA, Ahlem CN, Chang CH, Frincke JM. Bifunctional antibody: ZCE/CHA 111indium-BLEDTA-IV clinical imaging in colorectal carcinoma. Antibody Immunoconjug Radiopharm. 1989;2:1–13.

342. Le Doussal JM, Martin M, Gautherot E, Delaage M, Barbet J. In vitro and in vivo targeting of radiolabeled monovalent and divalent haptens with dual specificity monoclonal antibody conjugates: enhanced divalent hapten affinity for cell-bound antibody conjugate. J Nucl Med. 1989;30:1358–66.

343. Chetanneau A, Barbet J, Peltier P, Le Doussal JM, Gruaz-Guyon A, Bernard AM, et al. Pretargetted imaging of colorectal cancer recurrences using an 111In-labelled bivalent hapten and a bispecific antibody conjugate. Nucl Med Commun. 1994;15:972–80.

344. Gautherot E, Le Doussal JM, Bouhou J, Manetti C, Martin M, Rouvier E, et al. Delivery of therapeutic doses of radioiodine using bispecific antibody-targeted bivalent haptens. J Nucl Med. 1998; 39:1937–43.

345. Gautherot E, Rouvier E, Daniel L, Loucif E, Bouhou J, Manetti C, et al. Pretargeted radioimmunotherapy of human colorectal xenografts with bispecific antibody and 131I-labeled bivalent hapten. J Nucl Med. 2000;41:480–7.

346. Kraeber-Bodere F, Bardet S, Hoefnagel CA, Vieira MR, Vuillez JP, Murat A, et al. Radioimmunotherapy in medullary thyroid cancer using bispecific antibody and iodine 131-labeled bivalent hapten: preliminary results of a phase I/II clinical trial. Clin Cancer Res. 1999;5:3190s–8.

347. Kraeber-Bodere F, Faivre-Chauvet A, Ferrer L, Vuillez JP, Brard PY, Rousseau C, et al. Pharmacokinetics and dosimetry studies for optimization of anti-carcinoembryonic antigen x anti-hapten bispecific antibody-mediated pretargeting of Iodine-131-labeled hapten in a phase I radioimmunotherapy trial. Clin Cancer Res. 2003;9:3973S–81.

348. Kraeber-Bodere F, Rousseau C, Bodet-Milin C, Ferrer L, Faivre-Chauvet A, Campion L, et al. Targeting, toxicity, and efficacy of 2-step, pretargeted radioimmunotherapy using a chimeric bispecific antibody and 131I-labeled bivalent hapten in a phase I optimization clinical trial. J Nucl Med. 2006;47:247–55.

349. Kraeber-Bodere F, Salaun PY, Oudoux A, Goldenberg DM, Chatal JF, Barbet J. Pretargeted radioimmunotherapy in rapidly progressing, metastatic, medullary thyroid cancer. Cancer. 2010;116:1118–25.

350. Chatal JF, Campion L, Kraeber-Bodere F, Bardet S, Vuillez JP, Charbonnel B, et al. Survival improvement in patients with medullary thyroid carcinoma who undergo pretargeted anti-carcinoembryonic-antigen radioimmunotherapy: a collaborative study with the French Endocrine Tumor Group. J Clin Oncol. 2006;24:1705–11.

351. Knox SJ, Goris ML, Tempero M, Weiden PL, Gentner L, Breitz H, et al. Phase II trial of yttrium-90-DOTA-biotin pretargeted by NR-LU-10 antibody/streptavidin in patients with metastatic colon cancer. Clin Cancer Res. 2000;6:406–14.

352. Breitz HB, Fisher DR, Goris ML, Knox S, Ratliff B, Murtha AD, et al. Radiation absorbed dose estimation for 90Y-DOTA-biotin with pretargeted NR-LU-10/streptavidin. Cancer Biother Radiopharm. 1999;14:381–95.

353. Breitz HB, Weiden PL, Beaumier PL, Axworthy DB, Seiler C, Su FM, et al. Clinical optimization of pretargeted radioimmunotherapy with antibody-streptavidin conjugate and 90Y-DOTA-biotin. J Nucl Med. 2000;41:131–40.

354. Forero-Torres A, Shen S, Breitz H, Sims RB, Axworthy DB, Khazaeli MB, et al. Pretargeted radioimmunotherapy (RIT) with a novel anti-TAG-72 fusion protein. Cancer Biother Radiopharm. 2005;20:379–90.

355. Shen S, Forero A, LoBuglio AF, Breitz H, Khazaeli MB, Fisher DR, et al. Patient-specific dosimetry of pretargeted radioimmunotherapy using CC49 fusion protein in patients with gastrointestinal malignancies. J Nucl Med. 2005;46:642–51.

356. Sharkey RM, Rossi EA, McBride WJ, Chang CH, Goldenberg DM. Recombinant bispecific monoclonal antibodies prepared by the dock-and-lock strategy for pretargeted radioimmunotherapy. Semin Nucl Med. 2010;40:190–203.

357. Karacay H, Brard PY, Sharkey RM, Chang CH, Rossi EA, McBride WJ, et al. Therapeutic advantage of pretargeted radioimmunotherapy using a recombinant bispecific antibody in a human colon cancer xenograft. Clin Cancer Res. 2005;11:7879–85.

358. Karacay H, Sharkey RM, Gold DV, Ragland DR, McBride WJ, Rossi EA, et al. Pretargeted radioimmunotherapy of pancreatic cancer xenografts: TF10-90Y-IMP-288 alone and combined with gemcitabine. J Nucl Med. 2009;50:2008–16.

359. Sharkey RM, Karacay H, Govindan SV, Goldenberg DM. Combination radioimmunotherapy and chemoimmunotherapy involving different or the same targets improves therapy of human pancreatic carcinoma xenograft models. Mol Cancer Ther. 2011;10:1072–81.

360. Lawrence TS. Radiation sensitizers and targeted therapies. Oncology (Williston Park). 2003;17:23–8.

361. Girdhani S, Bhosle SM, Thulsidas SA, Kumar A, Mishra KP. Potential of radiosensitizing agents in cancer chemo-radiotherapy. J Cancer Res Ther. 2005;1:129–31.

362. Shewach DS, Lawrence TS. Antimetabolite radiosensitizers. J Clin Oncol. 2007;25:4043–50.

363. Hermann RM, Rave-Frank M, Pradier O. Combining radiation with oxaliplatin: a review of experimental results. Cancer Radiother. 2008;12:61–7.

364. Morgan MA, Parsels LA, Maybaum J, Lawrence TS. Improving gemcitabine-mediated radiosensitization using molecularly targeted therapy: a review. Clin Cancer Res. 2008;14:6744–50.

365. Karar J, Maity A. Modulating the tumor microenvironment to increase radiation responsiveness. Cancer Biol Ther. 2009;8:1994–2001.

366. Illum H. Irinotecan and radiosensitization in rectal cancer. Anticancer Drugs. 2011;22:324–9.

367. Graves SS, Dearstyne E, Lin Y, Zuo Y, Sanderson J, Schultz J, et al. Combination therapy with pretarget CC49 radioimmunotherapy and gemcitabine prolongs tumor doubling time in a murine xenograft model of colon cancer more effectively than either monotherapy. Clin Cancer Res. 2003;9:3712–21.

368. Kraeber-Bodere F, Sai-Maurel C, Campion L, Faivre-Chauvet A, Mirallie E, Cherel M, et al. Enhanced antitumor activity of combined pretargeted radioimmunotherapy and paclitaxel in medullary thyroid cancer xenograft. Mol Cancer Ther. 2002;1:267–74.

369. Al-Ejeh F, Darby JM, Brown MP. Chemotherapy synergizes with radioimmunotherapy targeting La autoantigen in tumors. PLoS One. 2009;4:e4630.

370. Blumenthal RD, Leone E, Goldenberg DM, Rodriguez M, Modrak D. An in vitro model to optimize dose scheduling of multimodal radioimmunotherapy and chemotherapy: effects of p53 expression. Int J Cancer. 2004;108:293–300.

371. Burke PA, DeNardo SJ, Miers LA, Kukis DL, DeNardo GL. Combined modality radioimmunotherapy. Promise and peril. Cancer. 2002;94:1320–31.

372. Crow DM, Williams L, Colcher D, Wong JY, Raubitschek A, Shively JE. Combined radioimmunotherapy and chemotherapy of breast tumors with Y-90-labeled anti-Her2 and anti-CEA antibodies with taxol. Bioconj Chem. 2005;16:1117–25.

373. DeNardo SJ, Kroger LA, Lamborn KR, Miers LA, O'Donnell RT, Kukis DL, et al. Importance of temporal relationships in combined modality radioimmunotherapy of breast carcinoma. Cancer. 1997;80:2583–90.

374. Gold DV, Modrak DE, Schutsky K, Cardillo TM. Combined 90Yttrium-DOTA-labeled PAM4 antibody radioimmunotherapy and gemcitabine radiosensitization for the treatment of a human pancreatic cancer xenograft. Int J Cancer. 2004;109:618–26.

375. Gold DV, Schutsky K, Modrak D, Cardillo TM. Low-dose radioimmunotherapy (90Y-PAM4) combined with gemcitabine for the treatment of experimental pancreatic cancer. Clin Cancer Res. 2003;9:3929S–37.

376. Kinuya S, Yokoyama K, Tega H, Hiramatsu T, Konishi S, Watanabe N, et al. Efficacy, toxicity and mode of interaction of combination radioimmunotherapy with 5-fluorouracil in colon cancer xenografts. J Cancer Res Clin Oncol. 1999;125:630–6.

377. Li XF, Kinuya S, Yokoyama K, Koshida K, Mori H, Shiba K, et al. Benefits of combined radioimmunotherapy and anti-angiogenic therapy in a liver metastasis model of human colon cancer cells. Eur J Nucl Med Mol Imaging. 2002;29:1669–74.

378. O'Donnell RT, DeNardo SJ, Miers LA, Lamborn KR, Kukis DL, DeNardo GL, et al. Combined modality radioimmunotherapy for human prostate cancer xenografts with taxanes and 90yttrium-DOTA-peptide-ChL6. Prostate. 2002;50:27–37.

379. Roffler SR, Chan J, Yeh MY. Potentiation of radioimmunotherapy by inhibition of topoisomerase I. Cancer Res. 1994;54:1276–85.

380. Santos O, Pant KD, Blank EW, Ceriani RL. 5-Iododeoxyuridine increases the efficacy of the radioimmunotherapy of human tumors growing in nude mice. J Nucl Med. 1992;33:1530–4.

381. Ocean AJ, Guarino MJ, Pennington KL, Montero AJ, Bekaii-Saab T, Gulec SA, et al. Activity of fractionated radioimmunotherapy with clivatuzumab tetraxetan combined with low-dose gemcitabine (Gem) in advanced pancreatic cancer (APC). J Clin Oncol. 2011;29:abstr 240.

382. Ocean AJ, Pennington KL, Guarino MJ, Sheikh A, Bekaii-Saab T, Serafini AN, et al. Fractionated radioimmunotherapy with 90Y-clivatuzumab tetraxetan (90Y-hPAM4) and low-dose gemcitabine is active in advanced pancreatic cancer: a Phase I trial. Cancer. 2012 (Epub ahead of print) doi: 10.1002/cncr 27592.

383. van Gog FB, Brakenhoff RH, Stigter-van Walsum M, Snow GB, van Dongen GA. Perspectives of combined radioimmunotherapy and anti-EGFR antibody therapy for the treatment of residual head and neck cancer. Int J Cancer. 1998;77:13–8.

384. Saleh MN, Raisch KP, Stackhouse MA, Grizzle WE, Bonner JA, Mayo MS, et al. Combined modality therapy of A431 human epidermoid cancer using anti-EGFr antibody C225 and radiation. Cancer Biother Radiopharm. 1999;14:451–63.

385. Buchsbaum DJ, Bonner JA, Grizzle WE, Stackhouse MA, Carpenter M, Hicklin DJ, et al. Treatment of pancreatic cancer xenografts with Erbitux (IMC-C225) anti-EGFR antibody, gemcitabine, and radiation. Int J Radiat Oncol Biol Phys. 2002;54: 1180–93.

386. Bonner JA, Buchsbaum DJ, Russo SM, Fiveash JB, Trummell HQ, Curiel DT, et al. Anti-EGFR-mediated radiosensitization as a result of augmented EGFR expression. Int J Radiat Oncol Biol Phys. 2004;59:2–10.

387. Macarulla T, Ramos FJ, Elez E, Capdevila J, Peralta S, Tabernero J. Update on novel strategies to optimize cetuximab therapy in patients with metastatic colorectal cancer. Clin Colorectal Cancer. 2008;7: 300–8.

388. Gerber DE, Choy H. Cetuximab in combination therapy: from bench to clinic. Cancer Metastasis Rev. 2010;29:171–80.

389. Pini S, Pinto C, Angelelli B, Giampalma E, Blotta A, Di Fabio F, et al. Multimodal sequential approach in colorectal cancer liver metastases: hepatic resection after yttrium-90 selective internal radiation therapy and cetuximab rescue treatment. Tumori. 2010;96:157–9.

390. Glynne-Jones R, Mawdsley S, Harrison M. Antiepidermal growth factor receptor radiosensitizers in rectal cancer. Anticancer Drugs. 2011;22: 330–40.

391. Arnoletti JP, Frolov A, Eloubeidi M, Keene K, Posey J, Wood T, et al. A phase I study evaluating the role of the anti-epidermal growth factor receptor (EGFR) antibody cetuximab as a radiosensitizer with chemoradiation for locally advanced pancreatic cancer. Cancer Chemother Pharmacol. 2011;67:891–7.

392. Haggblad Sahlberg S, Spiegelberg D, Lennartsson J, Nygren P, Glimelius B, Stenerlow B. The effect of a dimeric Affibody molecule (ZEGFR:1907)2 targeting EGFR in combination with radiation in colon cancer cell lines. Int J Oncol. 2012;40:176–84.

393. Zhu AX, Willett CG. Chemotherapeutic and biologic agents as radiosensitizers in rectal cancer. Semin Radiat Oncol. 2003;13:454–68.

394. Hosein PJ, Rocha-Lima CM. Role of combined-modality therapy in the management of locally advanced rectal cancer. Clin Colorectal Cancer. 2008;7:369–75.

395. Koukourakis MI, Giatromanolaki A, Sheldon H, Buffa FM, Kouklakis G, Ragoussis I, et al. Phase I/II trial of bevacizumab and radiotherapy for locally advanced inoperable colorectal cancer: vasculature-independent radiosensitizing effect of bevacizumab. Clin Cancer Res. 2009;15:7069–76.

396. Willett CG, Duda DG, Ancukiewicz M, Shah M, Czito BG, Bentley R, et al. A safety and survival analysis of neoadjuvant bevacizumab with standard chemoradiation in a phase I/II study compared with standard chemoradiation in locally advanced rectal cancer. Oncologist. 2010;15:845–51.

397. Salaun PY, Bodet-Milin C, Frampas E, Oudoux A, Sai-Maurel C, Faivre-Chauvet A, et al. Toxicity and efficacy of combined radioimmunotherapy and bevacizumab in a mouse model of medullary thyroid carcinoma. Cancer. 2010;116:1053–8.

Radioimmunotherapy of Pancreatic Adenocarcinoma

14

David M. Goldenberg, William A. Wegener,
David V. Gold, and Robert M. Sharkey

Introduction

The Problem

This chapter reviews the problems and prospects for the treatment of pancreatic ductal adenocarcinoma (PDAC), which is the principal type of pancreatic cancer, and the potential role for targeted radionuclide therapy in its management. Most articles begin by characterizing this tumor as "devastating," "challenging," or other descriptors of the morbid statistics indicating that it has the worst 1- and 5-year survival of any cancer. Pancreatic adenocarcinoma's dismal outlook is reflected by the estimated 37,660 deaths from an estimated 44,030 new cases in the USA in 2011 [1]. Because early clinical features are nonspecific,

most patients present with surgically unresectable locally advanced or metastatic disease [1], emphasizing its poor prognosis. Indeed, pancreatic adenocarcinoma represents the fourth highest cause of cancer deaths in the USA. On an international scale, the incidence is 213,000 annually [2]. Long-term survival is very poor, with a 5-year survival rate of 0.4% [3] to 6% [1]. Resection is the only potential for cure, where survival beyond 10 years is described in 5% of patients [4]. However, only about 10% of patients are eligible for complete resection [5].

Biology and Etiology

The biology and etiology of PDAC has been the subject of several reviews, most recently by Hidalgo [6]. There are both environmental (tobacco use), comorbidities (diabetes or chronic pancreatitis), and familial factors (families affected with four or more members have a 57-fold higher risk than unaffected families) [7]. The genetics of PDAC reveal that this is a very heterogeneous neoplasm; in one study, an average of 63 genetic changes, mostly point mutations, were noted in each tumor [8]. Nevertheless, it has been observed that all patients with PDAC carry one or more of four genetic defects, with almost all having activating mutations in the KRAS2 oncogene, inactivation of the CDKN2A gene, and an abnormal TP53 gene in 50–75% of tumors [9]. Although many pathways seem to be involved, there do not appear to be key mutations in any one [6].

D.M. Goldenberg, Sc.D., M.D.
IBC Pharmaceuticals, Inc. and Immunomedics, Inc,
Morris Plains, NJ, USA

Garden State Cancer Center, Center for Molecular
Medicine and Immunology, 300 The American Road,
Morris Plains, NJ, USA
e-mail: dmg.gscancer@att.net

W.A. Wegener, M.D., Ph.D.
Clinical Research, Immunomedics, Inc.,
300 The American Road, Morris Plains, NJ 07950, USA
e-mail: bwegener@immunomedics.com

D.V. Gold, Ph.D. • R.M. Sharkey, Ph.D. (✉)
Center for Molecular Medicine and Immunology
and the Garden State Cancer Center,
300 The American Road, Morris Plains, NJ 07950, USA
e-mail: dvgold@gscancer.org; rmsharkey@gscancer.org

C. Aktolun and S.J. Goldsmith (eds.), *Nuclear Medicine Therapy: Principles and Clinical Applications*,
DOI 10.1007/978-1-4614-4021-5_14, © Springer Science+Business Media New York 2013

Biology and Etiology of PDAC

- Environmental (tobacco use)
- Comorbidities (diabetes or chronic pancreatitis)
- Familial factors
- Genetic defects

(in almost all)

Activating mutations in the *KRAS2* oncogene,

Inactivation of the *CDKN2A* gene (in 50–75% of tumors),

Abnormal *TP53* gene

Pathogenesis

The pathogenesis of this tumor may help explain its ominous course because of late clinical manifestations. Most tumors develop in the head of the pancreas, where they cause cholestasis, as well as nausea and abdominal pain or discomfort, but possibly also duodenal obstruction or bleeding. Pancreatic duct obstruction may result in pancreatitis, as well as dsyglycemia, thus raising the concern of PDAC in patients with acute pancreatitis or new-onset diabetes. Other more general symptoms include weight loss, anorexia, and asthenia. Clinically, such patients may present with hepatomegaly, jaundice, ascites, peripheral lymphadenopathy, and wasting.

Diagnosis

Diagnostic procedures include contrast-enhanced, helical computed tomography, followed by ^{18}F-fluorodeoxglucose (FDG) positron-emission tomography (PET) and/or endoscopic ultrasonography if the CT results are equivocal. Endoscopic retrograde cholangiopancreatography (ERCP) is also used to disclose the anatomy for ductal brushing or lavage to capture cells for pathological examination.

Immunology and Immunoassay

Unfortunately, there is no biomarker that is diagnostic for PDAC. However, carbohydrate antigen 19–9 (CA19-9) can be used to monitor disease activity, such as therapeutic response and early recurrence [10–13]. Since it is not specific for pancreatic cancer, and is not produced in about 10% of patients not producing blood group Lewis antigens A or B, its role as a screening or diagnostic test is limited. A number of other biomarkers have been studied [14], but only the recently described PAM4 immunoassay appears to offer a high specificity for PDAC, and thus can be combined with CA19-9 to afford improved sensitivity and specificity for diagnosis [15]. This could be very important, since early detection is generally considered as a major requirement to alter the dismal outcome of most patients now being diagnosed with advanced disease. Therefore, we describe the PAM4 assay results in more detail, especially since the target antigen is being studied both for diagnostic imaging and for therapy.

The PAM4-antigen is a mucin-glycoprotein, originally isolated by hot phenol–water partition-extraction of a xenografted human pancreatic carcinoma, followed by molecular sieve and hydroxyapatite chromatography. It was then employed as an immunogen to develop a murine monoclonal antibody, PAM4 [16]. By immunohistology, PAM4 was reactive with 54/61 (89%) PDAC specimens. Normal pancreatic tissues, including ducts, ductules, acini, and islet cells, were negative [16, 17]. An enzyme immunoassay (ELISA) was developed with PAM4 as the capture reagent and a polyclonal anti-mucin IgG used as a probe. Analyses of aqueous extracts derived from normal adult tissues provided support for the immunohistology data. It was found that PAM4 identifies a biomarker that is highly specific for pancreatic adenocarcinoma.

The PAM4 ELISA test was developed to detect elevated titers of this mucin antigen in the blood of patients with PDAC. Hence, it was evaluated in a variety of serum specimens from disease-free volunteers as well as patients with pancreatic and other cancers, as well as benign diseases, particularly chronic pancreatitis [15, 17, 18]. The primary conclusion was that the PAM4-immunoassay is able to identify >85% of patients with stage 2 or higher disease, but also approximately two-thirds of early, stage-1, PDAC patients, and does so with a high discriminatory power with respect to benign pancreatic diseases. There are only a few reports that describe the use of a noninvasive biomarker assay to detect stage-1 disease, and the majority of these discuss the performance characteristics of CA19-9 [19–21]. The sensitivity reported for CA19-9 in stage-1 PDAC ranges from 40 to 64%, with our results showing a similar detection rate of 58%. However, the specificity reported for CA19-9 in the literature [22–24] is considerably lower than reported for the PAM4-antigen, as is also the case for the paired study performed by us, particularly with respect to discrimination of PDAC and chronic pancreatitis [15].

These findings also suggest that the PAM4-antigen is not expressed by pancreatic tumors originating from nonepithelial tissues. However, the PAM4-antigen is expressed and released by extrahepatic biliary and periampullary adenocarcinomas [15]. Detection of these cancers, although rare (approximately 3,500 new cases/year altogether in the USA), is likely to prove of clinical value, with follow-up imaging studies providing confirmation of tumor mass and location. That these cancers express the PAM4-antigen and are detectable by the PAM4-immunoassay was not unexpected, considering that these tissues are derived from closely related structures in early embryonic development. Indeed, many of the reported biomarkers for PDAC are reactive with these tumors as well. The limited expression of PAM4 in a control colon cancer group confirms prior serum assay and immunohistochemical studies suggesting that the PAM4-antigen has limited elevation with other gastrointestinal and nongastrointestinal cancers [15–18, 25].

Without regard to the limitations of the CA19-9 assay (as mentioned, the CA19-9 assay is not useful in Lewis antigen-negative patients and may be affected by serum bilirubin levels), we determined that a combined PAM4 and CA19-9 biomarker assay would provide a superior detection and diagnostic tool than either assay alone [15]. Overall sensitivity was improved without loss of specificity. The results suggest that a combination of PAM4 and CA19-9 biomarker analyses could provide for the improved detection of PDAC, and a rationale for proceeding to diagnostic imaging methods to confirm and identify sites of disease.

Finally, the ability of the PAM4-immunoassay to discriminate PDAC (and adjacent carcinomas) from benign disease of the pancreas and, in particular, the discrimination of PDAC and chronic pancreatitis, is worthy of mention. In a prior study, a discordance was reported between the PAM4-antigen levels in the serum of patients with chronic pancreatitis and immunohistochemical data on a separate group of patients with chronic pancreatitis [18]. Of 30 tissue specimens evaluated, one invasive PDAC and one large PanIN-2-3 lesion (in separate specimens) were identified by use of PAM4, whereas the surrounding acinar ductal metaplasia and inflamed tissue were negative.

In a follow-up blind study [26], tissue sections of PDAC (N=14), chronic pancreatitis (N=32), serous cystadenomas (N=15) and benign, nonmucinous cystic lesions of the pancreas (N=19) were evaluated for expression of the PAM4-biomarker. The PAM4-biomarker was present in 79% (11/14) invasive PDAC, but only weakly labeled 1/15 serous cystadenomas, and 1/19 benign nonmucinous cystic lesions. PAM4 labeled 19% (6/32) of chronic pancreatitis specimens; however, PAM4 reactivity was restricted to the PanIN precursor lesions associated with chronic pancreatitis. Inflamed tissue was negative in all cases [26].

The biological and clinical significance of a positive PAM4 result in patients diagnosed with chronic pancreatitis is of considerable interest. The results suggest that chronic pancreatitis patients with PAM4-positive serum have pancreatic neoplasia [26] and should be provided with follow-up clinical investigation. Further, these data suggest that the specificity and sensitivity of the PAM4-assay itself may be considerably higher than is indicated in the above discussion.

Therapeutic Options

Surgical Resection is the only therapy that offers the prospect of cure or significant long-term survival. Long-term survival (>10 years) has been achieved in 5% of patients with resected PDAC [4], and in cases where completed resection of cancers of the head of the pancreas having both lymph nodes and resection margins negative, a 5-year survival rate of 41% has been reported [27]. The operative procedures for those with resectable disease may be pancreatoduodenectomy (Whipple procedure), distal pancreatectomy, or total pancreatectomy, removing at least 12–15 lymph nodes and achieving tumor-free margins. A recent extensive analysis of surgical outcome based on various prognostic indicators indicated that age, carcinoembryonic antigen (CEA)- and CA19-9 serum levels, preoperative insulin-dependent diabetes mellitus, T-, N-, M-, R-, G-tumor classification, advanced disease, and lymph node ratio were all significant in a univariate analysis [28]. However, only 10–20% of PDAC patients are candidates for total resection [5, 29], and the outcome in these patients with putative early cancer is not good; about 85% of these patients relapse and die [30, 31]. Therefore, postoperative (adjuvant) *chemotherapy* has been studied, showing improvement in progression-free and overall survival; however, the increases were not significant, with a median survival of 20–23 months (reviewed by [6, 32, 33]).

In patients with locally advanced (stage III) disease, the outcome is much better than in those with metastatic (stage IV) disease. It is almost four decades since studies in patients with unresectable pancreatic cancer showed that 5-fluorouracil prolonged median survival to 9 or 10 months when given in combination with external radiation therapy [34]. The 2010 National Comprehensive Cancer Network (NCCN) guidelines suggest that *chemotherapy combined with external irradiation* (*chemoradiation*) is the conventional standard for the treatment of unresectable, locally advanced PDAC [35]. However, the specifics of which chemotherapy regimens and in what sequence with radiation is still being debated.

The NCCN recommends fractionated doses totaling 50–60 Gy combined with 5-fluorouracil, together with CT simulation and 3D treatment planning. It is stated that systemic chemotherapy followed by chemoradiation is the recommended option for patients with unresectable disease, no metastases, and good performance status [35]. A recent trial comparing full-dose gemcitabine with radiation therapy compared to 5-fluorouracil with radiation for locally advanced pancreas cancer was significantly better for the former combination (overall survival 12.5 vs. 10.2 months; 51% vs. 34% at 1 year; 12% vs. 0% at 3 years; 7% vs. 0% at 5 years, respectively; all $P=0.04$) [36]. There was also no difference in side effects, rates of distant metastasis, or subsequent hospitalization between the groups. Other trials had already shown an advantage of gemcitabine+radiation over gemcitabine alone in this patient population (11.1 vs. 9.2 months for the combination vs. gemcitabine alone; one-side $P=0.017$) [37].

Despite more than 30 new agents studied in the past 15 years, systemic therapy options for metastatic disease have been largely disappointing. In particular, the overall median survival remains 9–12 months with a 5-year survival rate of only 3% [38]. Historically, response rates surpassing 15% have been reproducibly reported only with 5-fluorouracil and mitomycin C, but response duration lasts only months, with no clear improvement in median survival, and combination therapy has rarely proven superior to single agent treatments [39]. Gemcitabine is the only drug to show greater efficacy than fluorouracil in patients with advanced pancreatic cancer [40]. Patients treated with gemcitabine have a median survival of about 6 months and a 1-year survival rate of about 20%. In previously untreated patients, gemcitabine modestly improved median survival (5.7 months) vs. 5-fluorouracil (4.4 months) and demonstrated a 23.8% clinical benefit response (composite measure of pain, performance status and weight) vs. 4.8% with 5-fluorouracil [40]. As such, gemcitabine is indicated for locally advanced or metastatic disease and has become standard palliative treatment for unresectable disease. Gemcitabine has been combined with many different cytotoxic drugs and even biologicals, but with mostly disappointing results [41]. In particular, random-ized Phase III trials in patients with advanced disease have shown little improvement in median survival compared with gemcitabine alone, when gemcitabine is combined with 5-fluorouracil (6.7 vs. 5.4 months, respectively), capecitabine (7.4 vs. 6.0 months, respectively), and erlotinib (6.2 vs. 5.9 months, respectively) [42–44]. Clearly there remains an unmet medical need to develop more effective treatments for this deadly disease.

At present, only gemcitabine alone or com-bined with erlotinib are approved therapies for patients with metastatic PDAC [45, 46]. The NCCN guidelines suggest the combination of a fluoropyrimidine with gemcitabine as a reason-able therapy option for PDAC patients with meta-static disease and a good performance status [35]. These also recommend gemcitabine–erlotinib combination therapy, as approved by FDA. More recent studies with other combinations are inter-esting and appear to offer improved survival results. FOLFIRINOX (5-fluorouracil, leuco-vorin, irinotecan, and oxaliplatin) was compared to gemcitabine in a randomized trial of 342 patients [47]. The median overall survival was 11.1 months in the FOLFIRONOX group com-pared to 6.8 months in those who received stan-dard gemcitabine ($P<0.001$), with a median progression-free survival of 6.4 and 3.3 months, respectively. FOLFIRINOX was also superior in the objective response rate: 31.6% vs. 9.4% ($P<0.001$); however, more adverse effects were in the FOLFIRINOX group, where 46% of patients had grade 3 and 4 neutropenia and 5.4% had grade 3 and 4 febrile neutropenia, despite 42.5% receiving G-CSF support. Also, at 6 months, this group showed a degradation of qual-ity of life in 31% of patients compared to 66% in the gemcitabine group ($P<0.001$). Despite such encouraging results, a few concerns raise the question whether or not this approach will become the new standard therapy for this patient population [48, 49]. First, the trial was selective, since only 39% had primary cancers of the pan-creas head, whereas about two-thirds usually present with this location, possibly requiring biliary stents. Second, this regimen required infusional pump therapy and central catheters, and patients with a good performance status (ECOG 0–1). Third, the median number of treat-ment cycles administered was 30 (range, 1–47) for FOLFIRINOX and 6 (range, 1–26) in the gemcitabine group ($P<0.001$), confirming that these patients had a relatively good performance status. Whether all of the components of this four-drug therapy are required also needs to be addressed in future studies. Nevertheless, these survival and response results appear to be the best reported in stage IV PDAC patients.

The combination of gemcitabine with an albu-min-bound formulation of paclitaxel particles, *nab*-paclitaxel, also has been reported to be active in patients with advanced PDAC who had no prior therapy for metastatic disease [50]. A phase I/II trial was completed and reported recently, whereby standard gemcitabine combined with 125 mg/m^2 *nab*-paclitaxel was found to be the weekly maximal tolerated doses (MTD). A median of 6 (range 1–24) cycles was given, and this produced a median progression-free sur-vival of 7.9 months, a median overall survival of 12.2 months, a 1-year survival of 48%, a response rate of 48%, and a disease control rate (PR + stable disease) of 68%. In terms of adverse effects, the dose-limiting toxicities (DLTs) were sepsis and neutropenia, with the most common events being anemia, leucopenia, neutropenia, thrombocytopenia, fatigue, alopecia, sensory neuropathy, and nausea, most being grades 1 and 2. The most common grade 3 nonhematological toxicities were fatigue (21%) and sensory neu-ropathy (15%). The overall survival of more than 1 year appears to be the highest of any investiga-tional therapy in this patient population, so it will be interesting to learn if this is confirmed in the ongoing phase III randomized trial.

Radioimmunotherapy

Radiolabeled Anti-CEA Antibody

Numerous antibodies and radionuclides have been studied in pancreatic cancer models, both alone and also as part of an effort to treat gastrointestinal cancers over the past 30 years. Some of these efforts have been summarized in Chap. 13 by Sharkey and Goldenberg devoted to colorectal cancer, including an extensive discussion of the development, problems and prospects of radioimmunotherapy as well as in a more recent review [51]. Suffice it to say that antibodies against CEA and TAG-72, as examples of the most frequently studied targets clinically [52–55], and the use of beta- and alpha-emitters [52, 53, 55–58] clinically or preclinically, has been extensively studied. However, few studies were undertaken in PDAC patients, and those that were did not encourage further development with the radionuclides or antibodies used [54, 55].

Perhaps an exception is the use of CEA-targeting antibodies, as discussed in the chapter on colorectal cancer (Chap. 13 Sharkey and Goldenberg). As part of the clinical studies of radioimmunotherapy in gastrointestinal cancer patients, the murine anti-CEA antibody, NP-4, radiolabeled with ^{131}I was evaluated. [52, 53] Behr et al. reported that of the 7 pancreatic cancer patients studied in this phase I/II trial of 57 gastrointestinal cancer patients, one with liver metastases showed a partial response within 2 months, which converted to a complete response by 3 months post therapy (Fig. 14.1) [52]. This disease-free response continued for a year before a liver relapse was observed. Five months later, or 17 months from the initial radioimmunotherapy, the patient died of endocarditis following an aortic valve replacement.

Radiolabeled Antibody Combined with Gemcitabine

Since the standard drug used in pancreatic cancer therapy, gemcitabine, is a radiosensitizing agent, and has been pursued in combination with radiation in diverse clinical trials [59], it was considered for combination studies with radioimmunotherapy. The combination of a drug with radiation is certainly more complex than the combination of two drugs, since it involves two modalities delivered differently, as well as interactions between them. Indeed, in vitro studies have shown that gemcitabine enhances the effects of radiation in killing cells, even at nontoxic doses of gemcitabine [59]. In vivo radiosensitization studies administered gemcitabine prior to radiation, with the shortest interval being the most effective, and with weekly dosing less damaging to normal tissues than dosing twice weekly [59].

Radiolabeled PAM4

Thus, radiation delivered by an antibody that targets pancreatic cancer could provide a better alternative for combining gemcitabine with radiation, both in terms of safety and efficacy. Most pancreatic cancers are mucin-producing adenocarcinomas [34], and PAM4 is an antibody produced against a mucin glycoprotein isolated from xenografted human pancreatic cancer, as discussed above. Initial characterization studies showed PAM4 reacted with approximately 85% of pancreatic cancers [16], and that the radiolabeled antibody specifically targeted xenografted human pancreatic cancers in athymic nude mice [60, 61], while an initial immunosctintigraphic study demonstrated specific targeting in patients with pancreatic cancer subsequently confirmed at surgery [62, 63]. In tumor-bearing animals, Gold and coworkers reported that PAM4 radiolabeled with I-131 or Y-90 had growth-inhibitory effects against pancreatic cancer xenografts, that radiolabeled PAM4 is more potent than gemcitabine when compared at MTD, and that combining radiolabeled PAM4 with gemcitabine further increased antitumor activity and survival [62, 64, 65].

Radiolabeled Humanized PAM4 (hPAM4): Clivatuzumab

Based on these findings, PAM4 was humanized (hPAM4, or clivatuzumab) for clinical development, and a DOTA-conjugated hPAM4 was developed for improved stability of radiolabeling

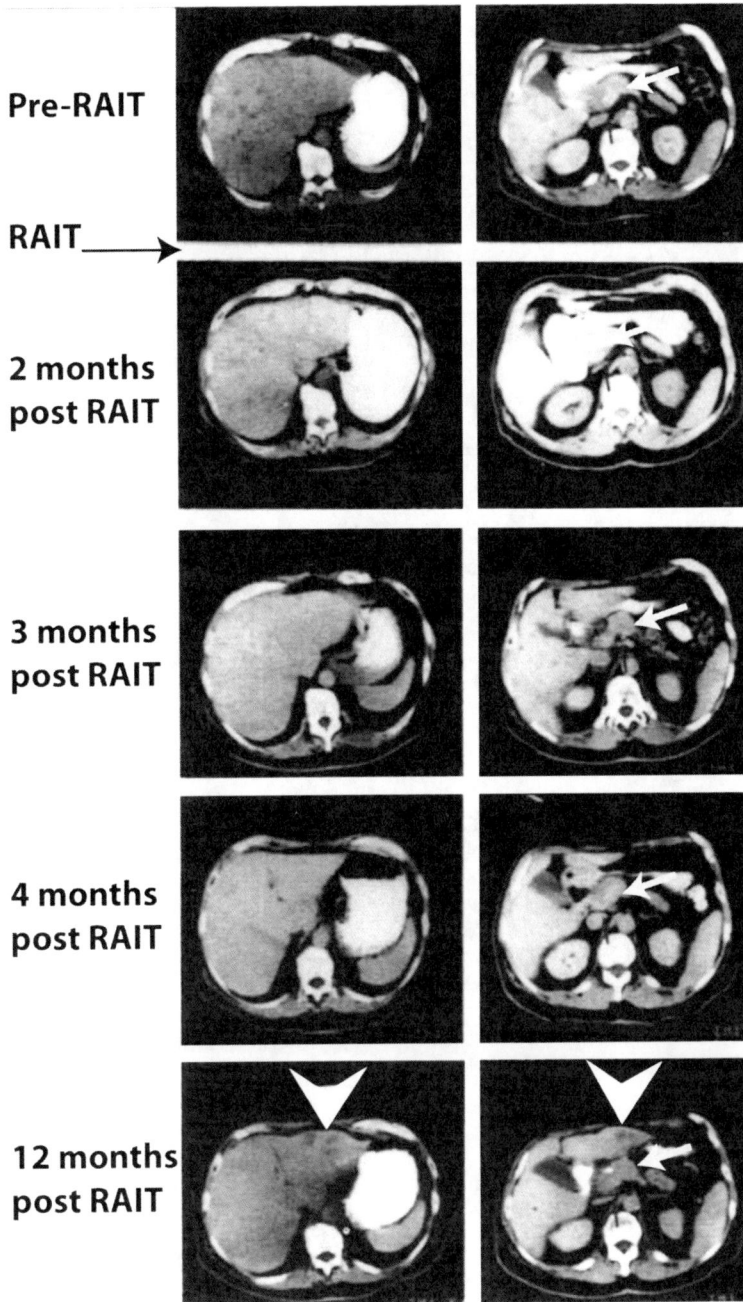

Fig. 14.1 Abdominal CT of a 66-year-old man with pancreatic cancer metastatic to the liver who was treated with a single dose of ^{131}I-NP-4 anti-CEACAM5 IgG (146 mCi). The baseline CT shows multiple small liver metastases and the primary in the pancreatic head (*white arrow*). The treatment led to a complete disappearance of all liver lesions in the 4-month follow-up scan, whereas the primary lesion remained unchanged. This status was maintained until the 12-month scan revealed new lesions in the left hepatic lobe (*white arrowhead*) (reproduced with permission from Behr et al. [52])

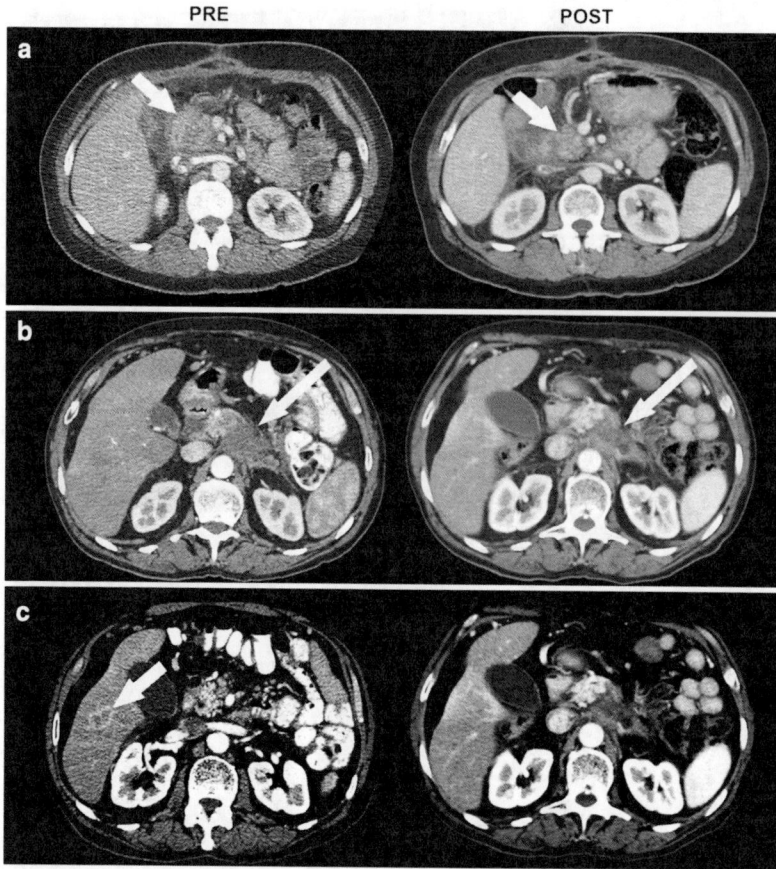

Fig. 14.2 Examples of partial responses in two patients treated with a single dose of ^{90}Y-hPAM4 IgG. Computed tomography image examples before (PRE) and 4 weeks after treatment with ^{90}Y-hPAM4 (POST). (**a**) A 63-year old female with locally advanced pancreatic cancer previously treated with gemcitabine and external radiation therapy with a 6.3 mass in the head of the pancreas at study entry reduced to 3.0 cm after therapy (*arrows*). (**b**, **c**) A 70-year old male previously treated with 5FU, gemcitabine, and external radiation therapy with a 4.5 cm mass in the body of the pancreas at study entry reduced to 3.3-cm after therapy (**b**; *arrows*) and 2.3-cm lesion in the liver (**c**, *Pre; arrow*) no longer measurable after therapy (reproduced with permission from Gulec et al. [67])

with ^{90}Y (^{90}Y clivatuzumab tetraxetan from Immunomedics, Inc.) [66]. The first clinical trial of ^{90}Y-hPAM4 was a single-agent dose-escalation trial in patients with unresectable locally advanced or metastatic disease most of whom had failed 5-fluorouracil, gemcitabine or other standard therapies [67]. The MTD of a single dose was found to be 20 mCi/m^2. Several patients had objective evidence of tumor shrinkage (Fig. 14.2). However, since this involved only a single administration of radioimmunotherapy, it is not surprising that all patients progressed rapidly.

^{90}Y; hPAM4 Fractionated Radioimmunotherapy and Combination with Gemcitabine

Given the refractory nature of advanced pancreatic cancer and based on the above considerations, the clinical development plans for ^{90}Y-hPAM4 anticipated a fractionated radioimmunotherapy dosing schedule in combination with gemcitabine administered at radiosensitizing dose levels. This was based on the hypothesis that fractionated radioimmunotherapy is more tolerable than single-dose radiotherapy, based on the experience with external beam irradiation delivered conventionally in multiple fractionated doses and our own experience with fractionated radioimmunotherapy using a different antibody in non-Hodgkin lymphoma, for which very high doses of ^{90}Y were tolerated vs. single-dose MTD values [68].

Our second hypothesis was that noncytotoxic doses of gemcitabine can potentiate the radiation effects of ^{90}Y-PAM4 to sites of pancreatic cancer, if there is an increased uptake ratio of the latter in cancer as compared to normal tissues, as suggested in the animal studies of Gold et al. [65]. Both gemcitabine and ^{90}Y-PAM4 are associated with hematological toxicity, and in order to decrease toxicities to normal tissues, gemcitabine was administered at least 1–2 days after radioimmunotherapy, since by then much of the radioactivity would have cleared background tissues.

In the first clinical study of fractionated radioimmunotherapy [69], only treatment-naïve patients were eligible to better ensure adequate bone marrow reserve and further decrease the degree of hematologic toxicity experienced. All patients received 1 or more 4-week treatment cycles, with gemcitabine given once-weekly for 4 weeks, and ^{90}Y-hPAM4 given once-weekly for the last 3 weeks. Initially, 42 patients were enrolled to determine the MTD for the 3 weekly ^{90}Y doses for the first treatment cycle when given in combination with 4 weekly low doses of 200 mg/m^2 gemcitabine, since this was on the lower side of once-weekly doses found to be acceptable for use with conventional radiotherapy [59]. The initial ^{90}Y dose was selected as 6.5 mCi/m^2 per infusion, since the 3 weekly doses would result in a total cumulative dose of 19.5 mCi/m^2, nearly equivalent to the MTD of 20 mCi/m^2 determined in the previous study for a single dose administration. These patients also received any retreatment cycles at the same ^{90}Y-dose as their first cycle. Hematologic suppression was the main toxicity, and while all severe cytopenias were reversible after cycle 1, several patients at weekly doses of 12 mCi/m^2 or higher had prolonged severe thrombocytopenia after cycle 2. This portion of the study established 12 mCi/m^2 as the MTD for the weekly ^{90}Y doses

for cycle 1 and also concluded that a lower weekly ^{90}Y dose would then be needed for retreatment.

Subsequently, 58 patients were enrolled, receiving a 12 mCi/m^2 weekly ^{90}Y dose for cycle 1, but given lower ^{90}Y doses with repeated treatment cycles. Several patients retreated at 9 mCi/m^2 had DLTs with prolonged thrombocytopenia, albeit at Grade 2–3 levels and not transfusion-dependent. However, all five patients who received cycle 2 at a 6.5 mCi/m^2 ^{90}Y dose level had readily reversible cytopenias and none encountered any DLTs. As such, 6.5 mCi/m^2 was selected for retreatment following a first cycle administered at 12 mCi/m^2. This portion of the study also evaluated higher weekly×4 doses of gemcitabine up to the standard dose of 1,000 mg/m^2. While there was no substantial increase in toxicity, there appeared to be no advantage to higher gemcitabine doses with fractionated radioimmunotherapy, since there was also no apparent increased efficacy.

The main toxicity in the prior study of fractionated radioimmunotherapy was Grade 3–4 thrombocytopenia and neutropenia, which in most cases was transient and resolved rapidly. As such, it is not surprising that there were no major treatment-related bleeding events in that study and minor bleeding was infrequent. Serious infections requiring IV antibiotics did occur, including bacteremia/sepsis (7%); febrile neutropenia (4%); ascending cholangitis (one with liver abscesses, 3%); pneumonia (2%); and splenic abscess, peritonitis, cellulitis, and urinary tract infection (1% each). However, low rates of these events are expected in this population, since all patients had undergone one or more prior invasive procedures (surgical or needle biopsies, biliary or gastrointestinal stenting, attempted curative surgical resections) and, except for the abscesses which took longer to disappear, the infections resolved promptly under appropriate IV antibiotic coverage. Thus, it does not appear that the transient neutropenia substantially facilitated or exacerbated infections but this remains to be determined in a controlled trial setting. As such, a fractionated radioimmunotherapy regimen with 12 mCi/m^2 ^{90}Y-hPAM4×3 plus 200 mg/m^2×4 gemcitabine for cycle 1 and

Table 14.1 Evaluation of treatment response in phase I/II clinical trial with fractionated ^{90}Y-clivatuzumab tetraxetan and gemcitabine (20 mg/m^2) (reproduced with permission from Ocean et al. [69])

CT (best response)[a]

	N	Disease control (CR + PR + SD)		PR		SD	
Overall	38	22	(58%)	6	(16%)	16	(42%)
Dose level: 1	4	3	(75%)	1	(25%)	2	(50%)
2	12	5	(42%)	1	(8%)	4	(33%)
3	17	12	(71%)	3	(18%)	9	(53%)
4	5	2	(40%)	1	(20%)	1	(20%)

FDG-PET (best response to first treatment cycle)[b]

	N	All index lesions >25% decrease[c]		Maximum lesion >50% decrease[d]	
Overall	25	13	(52%)	9	(36%)
Dose level: 1	2	2	(100%)	2	(100%)
2	7	1	(14%)	0	(0%)
3	11	7	(64%)	4	(36%)
4	5	3	(60%)	3	(60%)

PR (partial response), SD (stable disease), CR (complete response), SUV (standardized uptake value)
[a] Best response achieved (RECIST 1.0): no patient achieved a CR. All PRs occurred in patients with stage IV disease
[b] Twenty-five patients with positive baseline PET studies and ≥ posttreatment PET study prior to receiving any retreatment
[c] Each index lesion SUV decreased >25% from baseline
[d] The lesion with highest pretreatment SUV (19 pancreatic primaries, 6 hepatic metastases) decreased >50% from baseline

6.5 mCi/m^2 ^{90}Y-hPAM4 × 3 plus 200 mg/m^2 × 4 gemcitabine for cycle 2 has been selected for further clinical development in the first-line setting.

Of the 38 patients treated in the first trial of fractionated radioimmunotherapy, CT-based evaluations showed partial responses by RECIST criteria and stabilization for all dose levels (Table 14.1). The overall disease control rate (CR + PR + SD, N = 22) was 58%, with 6 patients (16%) having PRs (all stage IV) and 16 (42%) with stabilization as best response. All five stage-III patients had stable disease, and 52% of stage-IV patients had PR in 6/17 and SD in 11/17.

Twenty-five treated patients had positive baseline FDG-PET studies. Standard uptake values (SUVs) were obtained for all index lesions, and responses were based on decreases of >25% from baseline for all index lesions or >50% for just the baseline lesion with maximal SUV value. PET-SUV decreased at all dose levels, with overall response rates of 52% (all index lesions) and 36% (maximal baseline lesion only) (Table 14.1). PET responses to treatment are shown in Fig. 14.3.

Immunotherapy Trials

- Radiolabeled Anti-CEA Antibody
- 131-I NP-4 (a murine anti-CEA antibody)
- 131-I PAM4
- 90-Y PAM4
- Radiolabeled PAM4 combined gemcitabine (a radiosensitizing agent)
- 90-Y clivatuzumab (DOTA) tetraxetan (a humanized PAM4)
- 90-Y-hPAM4 fractionated radioimmunotherapy
- 90-Y-hPAM4 fractionated radioimmunotherapy in combination with gemcitabine

Kaplan-Meier estimated overall survival (OS) curves are given in Fig. 14.4. For all patients, there was a median OS of 7.7 months (95% CI: 5.6–9.6) with 58% (22/38) surviving ≥6 months

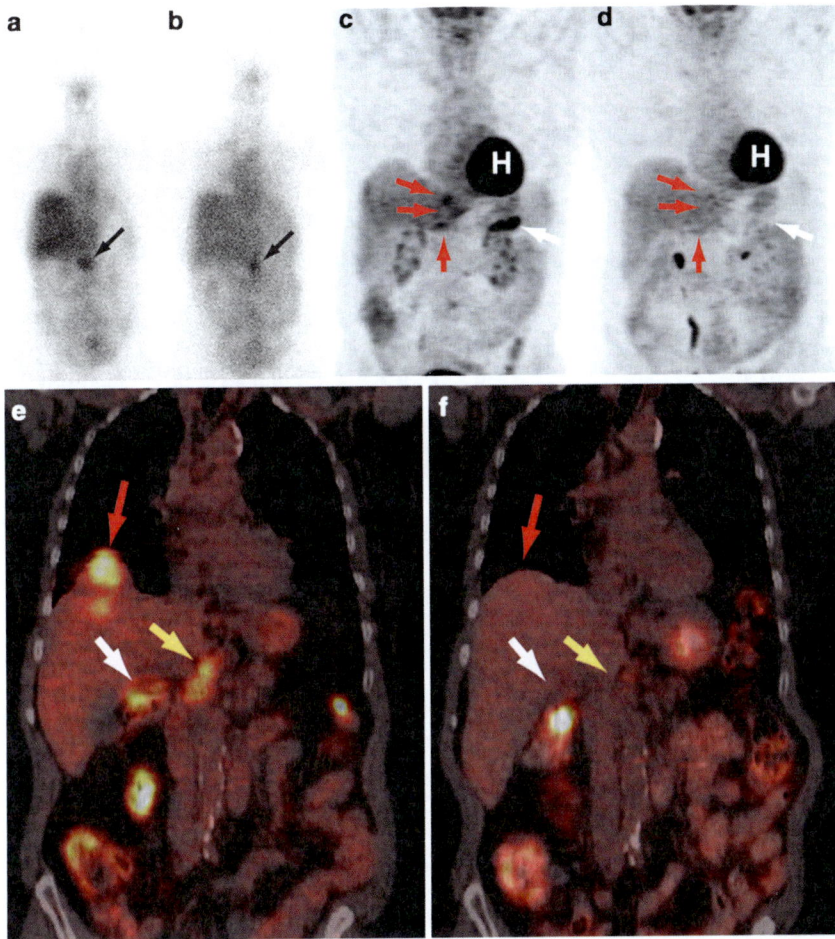

Fig. 14.3 Examples of targeting (^{111}In-hPAM4 IgG) and responses in patients given fractionated ^{90}Y-hPAM4 IgG (^{90}Y-clivatuzumab tetraxetan) with gemcitabine. (**a**, **b**) Anterior planar ^{111}In-hPAM4 images from one patient receiving two treatment cycles, both at 3×12.0 mCi/m^2. The uptake seen at the site of the known primary pancreatic mass (*arrows*) demonstrates how the antibody delivers the radiation dose directly to the tumor. In (**a**), the pancreatic mass, initially measured as 3.7×2.6-cm, received 39 Gy in the first cycle. In (**b**), after decreasing to 1.8×2.9-cm, the pancreatic mass received 44 Gy in the second cycle. The patient's disease remained stable until 8 weeks after the second treatment cycle, at which time disease progression occurred outside the pancreatic bed with the finding of new omental lesions. (**c**, **d**) PET-FDG imaging prior to treatment (**c**) shows uptake in primary pancreatic tail mass (*white arrow*) and in three left-lobe liver metastases (*red arrows*) that are no longer seen 4 weeks after treatment (*right*). Serum CA19-9 titers decreased from 1,297 at study entry to 77 at 4 weeks after treatment. (**e**, **f**) PET-FDG imaging prior to treatment (**e**) shows uptake in primary pancreatic mass (*yellow arrow*), portacaval lymph nodes (*white arrow*), and in a large hepatic mass extending from the dome of the liver (*red arrow*) that is no longer seen 4 weeks after treatment (**f**) (reproduced with permission from Ocean et al. [69])

[26 % (10/38) ≥1 year]. Of the repeated cycle group, 46 % (6/13) were alive at ≥1 year. The median OS was 6.0 months (95 % CI: 5.2–8.0) for 33 stage-IV patients; the five stage-III patients had a median OS of 19.6 months (95 % CI: 7.9–24.3). The patients ($N = 22$) treated at the two highest dose levels (12.0 and 15.0 mCi/m$^2 \times 3$) had a median OS of 8.0 months (95 % CI: 5.6–9.8); 3 patients were still alive at 21–25 months. In terms of the effect of retreatment, 46 % (6/13) survived ≥1 year and had a median OS of 11.8 months (95 % CI: 8.0–13.5), compared to 5.4 months (95 % CI: 3.0–8.0), $P < 0.034$ by log-rank, for the 25 patients having only one treatment cycle. In terms of results by disease stage for those receiving repeated cycles, three

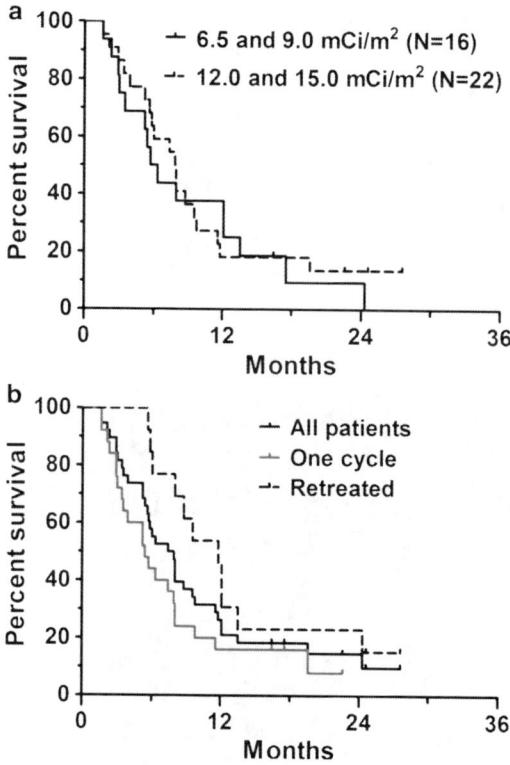

Fig. 14.4 Kaplan-Meier estimates of overall survival for all 38 treated patients. (**a**) Results at the two highest dose levels (12.0 and 15.0 mCi/m^2 × 3) compared to results at the two lowest dose levels (6.5 and 9.0 mCi/m^2 × 3). (**b**) Results for all patients and for patients who were retreated compared to those who received only a single cycle (reproduced with permission from Ocean et al. [69])

including fractionated radioimmunotherapy, did confirm these assumptions and provide a potential paradigm for future radioimmunotherapy trials in other solid tumors.

> **Advantages of Combination Fractionated Radioimmunotherapy**
>
> • Radioimmunotherapy fractionation may be more potent with less myelosuppression than a single dose administration
> • The combination of radioimmunotherapy with low-dose, 200 mg/m^2, gemcitabine could potentiate the therapy without increasing toxicity
> • Repeated cycles would be more potent than single therapy cycles

Fractionated radioimmunotherapy was tolerated well, and after completing this treatment, 20 of 38 patients proceeded to receive various regimens of chemotherapy in the course of their later therapy, despite the dose-related myelosuppression induced with radioimmunotherapy. Thus, combined radioimmunotherapy plus chemotherapy did not preclude subsequent treatments.

with stage-III disease had a median overall survival of 24.3 months, while the remaining 10 had a median survival of 10.7 months.

Based on our prior study with radioimmunotherapy alone, where several patients had transient responses by CT [67], our hypotheses for the combination, fractionated study were (a) radioimmunotherapy fractionation may be more potent with less myelosuppression than a single dose administration, (b) the combination of radioimmunotherapy with low-dose, 200 mg/m^2, gemcitabine could potentiate the therapy without increasing toxicity, and (c) repeated cycles would be more potent than single therapy cycles. The results of the trial of combination radioimmunotherapy + gemcitabine,

Conclusion

These radioimmunotherapy studies show encouraging therapeutic activity and survival results, particularly at higher dose levels and in patients receiving more than one treatment cycle of low-dose gemcitabine plus radioimmunotherapy. The study also confirmed the hypotheses that fractionated dosing can result in better tolerability of higher cumulative radiation doses than a single radioimmunotherapy application, and that low-dose gemcitabine can be combined with repeated cycles of radioimmunotherapy without compromising anticancer activity. Importantly, this combination did not preclude patients from receiving subsequent chemotherapy in the course of their disease. Hence, additional, randomized control trials are being planned to confirm these initial observations.

Future Prospects

The demonstration of objective responses as well as an indication of a survival benefit in advanced PDAC when a radioimmunoconjugate is combined with low doses of a radiosensitizing drug that is used in the treatment of this neoplasm is most encouraging for undertaking further studies involving radioimmunotherapy + chemotherapy, especially in cancers where chemotherapy and traditional treatment approaches have been inadequate, such as pancreatic carcinoma. Whether

the PAM4 agent combined with other chemotherapeutic agents or combination of drugs, or even another antibody, can be more effective needs to be evaluated, as well as the combination of radioimmunotherapy + chemotherapy in other stages of PDAC, such as in second- and third-line, as well as in adjuvant (post R0 and R1 resections) settings. This concept is of course applicable to other solid tumors where a reasonably specific antibody for radionuclide targeting is available, as discussed already in the chapter on colorectal cancer (Chap. 13 Sharkey and Goldenberg). Also discussed in that chapter is the application of radioimmunotherapy by pretargeting methods, which have shown improved tumor-to-normal signal ratios in prior studies [70, 71], and which is in clinical evaluation in colorectal cancer patients [72]. Pretargeting has also been applied

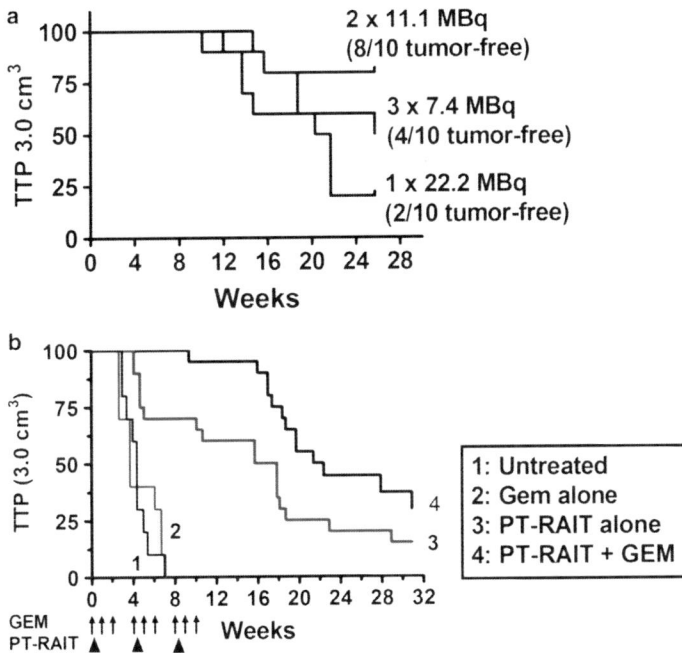

Fig. 14.5 (**a**) Comparative efficacies of a single dose of pretargeted radioimmunotherapy vs. the same dose split into 2 or 3 fractions, each given 1 week apart. Animals were given the hPAM4-based tri-Fab bispecific antibody (TF10) that binds to the pancreatic mucin divalently and monovalently to the hapten-peptide IMP288 radiolabeled with ^{90}Y. Animals received TF10 16 h before each injection of the ^{90}Y-IMP288. The data show fractionated

treatments improve responses over the single dose (no significant survival advantage for two or three doses). (**b**) Fractionated pretargeted radioimmunotherapy using the TF10/^{90}Y-hapten-peptide given monthly for 3 months and combined with gemcitabine given in 3-weekly fractions each month. The combination with gemcitabine improves the response. Data were reported previously by Karacay et al. [74]

with PAM4 bispecific antibody constructs, and has shown very encouraging therapeutic responses in animal xenografts models, especially when combined with gemcitabine [73, 74], as illustrated in Fig. 14.5 of an experimental study. Since the specific PDAC targeting of PAM4 has been demonstrated clinically and the pretargeting method appears to be a next-generation methodology for improving radioimmunotherapy based on preclinical and initial clinical studies [72, 75], it is reasonable to conjecture that this may be an opportunity to improve radioimmunotherapy plus chemotherapy even further.

Yet another potential approach is the combination of PAM4 radioimmunotherapy with other antibody-based therapies, such as an antibody–drug conjugate (ADC). In a preclinical study, we have shown that an anti-Trop-2 antibody conjugated with the active form of irinotecan, SN-38, can enhance the antitumor effects of ^{90}Y-PAM4 as compared to either agent alone [76]. Although the anti-Trop-2 antibody is not specific for pancreatic adenocarcinoma, having a broad reactivity with solid tumors [77–79], the specificity of PAM4 provides a combination of interest for pancreatic cancer therapy. Indeed, combining an ADC with radioimmunotherapy may be more rational to improve the therapeutic index than just adding a cytotoxic drug to the regimen. However, these prospects need to await clinical validation.

Acknowledgements The PAM4 in vitro assay research has been supported in part by grants to DVG from the National Cancer Institute (CA096924), the Horizon Foundation of New Jersey, The Canale Fund, and The Turpin Foundation. We are grateful to the many patients and clinical investigators who participated in the radioimmunotherapy trials described herein.

References

1. Siegel R, Ward E, Brawley O, Jemal A. Cancer statistics, 2011: the impact of eliminating socioeconomic and racial disparities on premature cancer deaths. CA Cancer J Clin. 2011;61:212–36.
2. Koorstra JB, Hustinx SR, Offerhaus GJ, Maitra A. Pancreatic carcinogenesis. Pancreatology. 2008; 8:110–25.
3. Bramhall SR, Neoptolemos JP. Advances in diagnosis and treatment of pancreatic cancer. Gastroenterologist. 1995;3:301–10.
4. Ferrone CR, Brennan MF, Gonen M, et al. Pancreatic adenocarcinoma: the actual 5-year survivors. J Gastrointest Surg. 2008;12:701–6.
5. Sener SF, Fremgen A, Menck HR, Winchester DP. Pancreatic cancer: a report of treatment and survival trends for 100,313 patients diagnosed from 1985–1995, using the National Cancer Database. J Am Coll Surg. 1999;189:1–7.
6. Hidalgo M. Pancreatic cancer. N Engl J Med. 2010;362:1605–17.
7. Tersmette AC, Petersen GM, Offerhaus GJ, et al. Increased risk of incident pancreatic cancer among first-degree relatives of patients with familial pancreatic cancer. Clin Cancer Res. 2001;7:738–44.
8. Jones S, Zhang X, Parsons DW, et al. Core signaling pathways in human pancreatic cancers revealed by global genomic analyses. Science. 2008;321:1801–6.
9. Maitra A, Hruban RH. Pancreatic cancer. Annu Rev Pathol. 2008;3:157–88.
10. Berger AC, Garcia Jr M, Hoffman JP, et al. Postresection CA 19–9 predicts overall survival in patients with pancreatic cancer treated with adjuvant chemoradiation: a prospective validation by RTOG 9704. J Clin Oncol. 2008;26:5918–22.
11. Ferrone CR, Finkelstein DM, Thayer SP, Muzikansky A, Fernandez-del Castillo C, Warshaw AL. Perioperative CA19-9 levels can predict stage and survival in patients with resectable pancreatic adenocarcinoma. J Clin Oncol. 2006;24:2897–902.
12. Hess V, Glimelius B, Grawe P, et al. CA 19–9 tumour-marker response to chemotherapy in patients with advanced pancreatic cancer enrolled in a randomised controlled trial. Lancet Oncol. 2008;9:132–8.
13. Ko AH, Hwang J, Venook AP, Abbruzzese JL, Bergsland EK, Tempero MA. Serum CA19-9 response as a surrogate for clinical outcome in patients receiving fixed-dose rate gemcitabine for advanced pancreatic cancer. Br J Cancer. 2005;93:195–9.
14. Harsha HC, Kandasamy K, Ranganathan P, et al. A compendium of potential biomarkers of pancreatic cancer. PLoS Med. 2009;6:e1000046.
15. Gold DV, Gaedcke J, Ghadimi BM, et al. PAM4 immunoassay alone and in combination with CA19-9 for the detection of early-stage pancreatic adenocarcinoma. Cancer. 2012 (in press).
16. Gold DV, Lew K, Maliniak R, Hernandez M, Cardillo T. Characterization of monoclonal antibody PAM4 reactive with a pancreatic cancer mucin. Int J Cancer. 1994;57:204–10.
17. Gold DV, Modrak DE, Ying Z, Cardillo TM, Sharkey RM, Goldenberg DM. New MUC1 serum immunoassay differentiates pancreatic cancer from pancreatitis. J Clin Oncol. 2006;24:252–8.
18. Gold DV, Goggins M, Modrak DE, et al. Detection of early-stage pancreatic adenocarcinoma. Cancer Epidemiol Biomarkers Prev. 2010;19:2786–94.

19. Maestranzi S, Przemioslo R, Mitchell H, Sherwood RA. The effect of benign and malignant liver disease on the tumour markers CA19-9 and CEA. Ann Clin Biochem. 1998;35:99–103.
20. Marrelli D, Caruso S, Pedrazzani C, et al. CA19-9 serum levels in obstructive jaundice: clinical value in benign and malignant conditions. Am J Surg. 2009;198:333–9.
21. Safi F, Schlosser W, Kolb G, Beger HG. Diagnostic value of CA 19–9 in patients with pancreatic cancer and nonspecific gastrointestinal symptoms. J Gastrointest Surg. 1997;1:106–12.
22. Ballehaninna UK, Chamberlain RS. The clinical utility of serum CA19-9 in the diagnosis, prognosis and management of pancreatic adenocarcinoma: an evidence based appraisal. J Gastrointest Oncol. 2012;3:105–109.
23. Singh S, Tang SJ, Sreenarasimhaiah J, Lara LF, Siddiqui A. The clinical utility and limitations of serum carbohydrate antigen (CA19-9) as a diagnostic tool for pancreatic cancer and cholangiocarcinoma. Dig Dis Sci. 2011;56:2491–6.
24. Steinberg W. The clinical utility of the CA 19–9 tumor-associated antigen. Am J Gastroenterol. 1990;85:350–5.
25. Gold DV, Karanjawala Z, Modrak DE, Goldenberg DM, Hruban RH. PAM4-reactive MUC1 is a biomarker for early pancreatic adenocarcinoma. Clin Cancer Res. 2007;13:7380–7.
26. Shi C, Goldenberg DM, Gold DV. Use of the monoclonal antibody PAM4 to differentiate pancreatic ductal adenocarcinoma (PDAC) from chronic pancreatitis and benign nonmucinous cysts of the pancreas. J Clin Oncol. 2012; 30(Suppl 4):Abstract 188.
27. Cameron JL, Riall TS, Coleman J, Belcher KA. One thousand consecutive pancreaticoduodenectomies. Ann Surg. 2006;244:10–5.
28. Hartwig W, Hackert T, Hinz U, et al. Pancreatic cancer surgery in the new millennium: better prediction of outcome. Ann Surg. 2011;254:311–9.
29. Ghaneh P, Costello E, Neoptolemos JP. Biology and management of pancreatic cancer. Gut. 2007;56:1134–52.
30. Conlon KC, Klimstra DS, Brennan MF. Long-term survival after curative resection for pancreatic ductal adenocarcinoma. Clinicopathologic analysis of 5-year survivors. Ann Surg. 1996;223:273–9.
31. Sohn TA, Yeo CJ, Cameron JL, et al. Pancreaticoduodenectomy: role of interventional radiologists in managing patients and complications. J Gastrointest Surg. 2003;7:209–19.
32. Neoptolemos JP, Stocken DD, Bassi C, et al. Adjuvant chemotherapy with fluorouracil plus folinic acid vs gemcitabine following pancreatic cancer resection: a randomized controlled trial. JAMA. 2010;304:1073–81.
33. O'Reilly EM. Refinement of adjuvant therapy for pancreatic cancer. JAMA. 2010;304:1124–5.
34. Moertel CG, Childs Jr DS, Reitemeier RJ, Colby Jr MY, Holbrook MA. Combined 5-fluorouracil and supervoltage radiation therapy of locally unresectable gastrointestinal cancer. Lancet. 1969;2:865–7.
35. Tempero M, Arnoletti JP, Behrman S, et al. Pancreatic adenocarcinoma. NCCN Clin Pract Guidel Oncol. 2010;v.2.2010. [http://www.nccn.org].
36. Huang J, Robertson JM, Margolis J, et al. Long-term results of full-dose gemcitabine with radiation therapy compared to 5-fluorouracil with radiation therapy for locally advanced pancreas cancer. Radiother Oncol. 2011;99:114–9.
37. Loehrer Sr PJ, Feng Y, Cardenes H, et al. Gemcitabine alone versus gemcitabine plus radiotherapy in patients with locally advanced pancreatic cancer: an Eastern Cooperative Oncology Group trial. J Clin Oncol. 2011;29:4105–12.
38. Brower ST, Benson III AB, Myerson RJ, Hoff PM. Pancreatic, neuroendocrine GI, and adrenal cancers. In: Pazdur R, Coia LR, Hoskins WJ, Wagman LD, editors. Cancer management: a multidisciplinary approach. 5th ed. Melville: PRR Publishing; 2001. p. 227–53.
39. Douglass Jr HO, Kim SY, Meropol NJ. Neoplasms of the exocrine pancreas. In: Holland JF, Frei EI, editors. Cancer Medicine. 4th ed. Baltimore: Williams & Wilkins; 1997. p. 1989–2017.
40. Burris 3rd HA, Moore MJ, Andersen J, et al. Improvements in survival and clinical benefit with gemcitabine as first-line therapy for patients with advanced pancreas cancer: a randomized trial. J Clin Oncol. 1997;15:2403–13.
41. Van Cutsem E, Verslype C, Grusenmeyer PA. Lessons learned in the management of advanced pancreatic cancer. J Clin Oncol. 2007;25:1949–52.
42. Berlin JD, Catalano P, Thomas JP, Kugler JW, Haller DG, Benson 3rd AB. Phase III study of gemcitabine in combination with fluorouracil versus gemcitabine alone in patients with advanced pancreatic carcinoma: Eastern Cooperative Oncology Group Trial E2297. J Clin Oncol. 2002;20:3270–5.
43. Cunningham D, Chau I, Stocken DD, et al. Phase III randomized comparison of gemcitabine versus gemcitabine plus capecitabine in patients with advanced pancreatic cancer. J Clin Oncol. 2009;27:5513–8.
44. Moore MJ, Goldstein D, Hamm J, et al. Erlotinib plus gemcitabine compared with gemcitabine alone in patients with advanced pancreatic cancer: a phase III trial of the National Cancer Institute of Canada Clinical Trials Group. J Clin Oncol. 2007;25:1960–6.
45. Conroy T, Gavoille C, Adenis A. Metastatic pancreatic cancer: old drugs, new paradigms. Curr Opin Oncol. 2011;23:390–5.
46. Castellanos E, Berlin J, Cardin DB. Current treatment options for pancreatic carcinoma. Curr Oncol Rep. 2011;13:195–205.
47. Conroy T, Desseigne F, Ychou M, et al. FOLFIRINOX versus gemcitabine for metastatic pancreatic cancer. N Engl J Med. 2011;364:1817–25.
48. Kim R. FOLFIRINOX: a new standard treatment for advanced pancreatic cancer? Lancet Oncol. 2011;12:8–9.

49. Ko AH. FOLFIRINOX: a small step or a great leap forward? J Clin Oncol. 2011;29:3727–9.

50. Von Hoff DD, Ramanathan RK, Borad MJ, et al. Gemcitabine plus *nab*-paclitaxel is an active regimen in patients with advanced pancreatic cancer: a phase I/II trial. J Clin Oncol. 2011;29:4548–54.

51. Sharkey RM, Goldenberg DM. Cancer radioimmunotherapy. Immunotherapy. 2011;3:349–70.

52. Behr TM, Sharkey RM, Juweid ME, et al. Phase I/II clinical radioimmunotherapy with an iodine-131-labeled anti-carcinoembryonic antigen murine monoclonal antibody IgG. J Nucl Med. 1997;38:858–70.

53. Hajjar G, Sharkey RM, Burton J, et al. Phase I radioimmunotherapy trial with iodine-131-labeled humanized MN-14 anti-carcinoembryonic antigen monoclonal antibody in patients with metastatic gastrointestinal and colorectal cancer. Clin Colorectal Cancer. 2002;2:31–42.

54. Sultana A, Shore S, Raraty MG, et al. Randomised Phase I/II trial assessing the safety and efficacy of radiolabelled anti-carcinoembryonic antigen I-131 KAb201 antibodies given intra-arterially or intravenously in patients with unresectable pancreatic adenocarcinoma. BMC Cancer. 2009;9:66.

55. Tempero M, Leichner P, Baranowska-Kortylewicz J, et al. High-dose therapy with ⁹⁰yttrium-labeled monoclonal antibody CC49: a phase I trial. Clin Cancer Res. 2000;6:3095–102.

56. Gold DV, Modrak DE, Schutsky K, Cardillo TM. Combined ⁹⁰Yttrium-DOTA-labeled PAM4 antibody radioimmunotherapy and gemcitabine radiosensitization for the treatment of a human pancreatic cancer xenograft. Int J Cancer. 2004;109:618–26.

57. Milenic D, Garmestani K, Dadachova E, et al. Radioimmunotherapy of human colon carcinoma xenografts using a ²¹³Bi-labeled domain-deleted humanized monoclonal antibody. Cancer Biother Radiopharm. 2004;19:135–47.

58. Qu CF, Songl YJ, Rizvi SM, et al. In vivo and in vitro inhibition of pancreatic cancer growth by targeted alpha therapy using ²¹³Bi-CHX.A"-C595. Cancer Biol Ther. 2005;4:848–53.

59. Pauwels B, Korst AE, Lardon F, Vermorken JB. Combined modality therapy of gemcitabine and radiation. Oncologist. 2005;10:34–51.

60. Alisauskus R, Wong GY, Gold DV. Initial studies of monoclonal antibody PAM4 targeting to xenografted orthotopic pancreatic cancer. Cancer Res. 1995;55:5743s–8.

61. Gold DV, Alisauskas R, Sharkey RM. Targeting of xenografted pancreatic cancer with a new monoclonal antibody, PAM4. Cancer Res. 1995;55:1105–10.

62. Gold DV, Cardillo T, Goldenberg DM, Sharkey RM. Localization of pancreatic cancer with radiolabeled monoclonal antibody PAM4. Crit Rev Oncol Hematol. 2001;39:147–54.

63. Mariani G, Molea N, Bacciardi D, et al. Initial tumor targeting, biodistribution, and pharmacokinetic evaluation of the monoclonal antibody PAM4 in patients with pancreatic cancer. Cancer Res. 1995;55:5911s–5.

64. Gold DV, Cardillo T, Vardi Y, Blumenthal R. Radioimmunotherapy of experimental pancreatic cancer with ¹³¹I-labeled monoclonal antibody PAM4. Int J Cancer. 1997;71:660–7.

65. Gold DV, Schutsky K, Modrak D, Cardillo TM. Low-dose radioimmunotherapy (⁹⁰Y-PAM4) combined with gemcitabine for the treatment of experimental pancreatic cancer. Clin Cancer Res. 2003;9:3929S–37.

66. Griffiths GL, Govindan SV, Sharkey RM, Fisher DR, Goldenberg DM. ⁹⁰Y-DOTA-hLL2: an agent for radioimmunotherapy of non-Hodgkin's lymphoma. J Nucl Med. 2003;44:77–84.

67. Gulec SA, Cohen SJ, Pennington KL, et al. Treatment of advanced pancreatic carcinoma with ⁹⁰Y-clivatuzumab tetraxetan: a phase I single-dose escalation trial. Clin Cancer Res. 2011;17:4091–100.

68. Morschhauser F, Kraeber-Bodere F, Wegener WA, et al. High rates of durable responses with anti-CD22 fractionated radioimmunotherapy: results of a multicenter, phase I/II study in non-Hodgkin's lymphoma. J Clin Oncol. 2010;28:3709–16.

69. Ocean AJ, Pennington KL, Guarino MJ, et al. Fractionated radioimmunotherapy with ⁹⁰Y-clivatuzumab tetraxetan (⁹⁰Y-hPAM4) and low-dose gemcitabine is active in advanced pancreatic cancer: a Phase I trial. Cancer. 2012; Epub ahead of print [doi: 10.1002/cncr.27592].

70. Goldenberg DM, Chatal JF, Barbet J, Boerman O, Sharkey RM. Cancer imaging and therapy with bispecific antibody pretargeting. Update Cancer Ther. 2007;2:19–31.

71. Goldenberg DM, Sharkey RM, Paganelli G, Barbet J, Chatal JF. Antibody pretargeting advances cancer radioimmunodetection and radioimmunotherapy. J Clin Oncol. 2006;24:823–34.

72. Schoffelen R, Boerman OC, van der Graff WT, et al. Phase I clinical study of the feasibility of pretargeted radioimmunotherapy (PT-RAIT) in patients with colorectal cancer (CRC): first results. J Nucl Med. 2011;52:107p (abstr 358).

73. Gold DV, Goldenberg DM, Karacay H, et al. A novel bispecific, trivalent antibody construct for targeting pancreatic carcinoma. Cancer Res. 2008;68:4819–26.

74. Karacay H, Sharkey RM, Gold DV, et al. Pretargeted radioimmunotherapy of pancreatic cancer xenografts: TF10-90Y-IMP-288 alone and combined with gemcitabine. J Nucl Med. 2009;50:2008–16.

75. Chatal JF, Campion L, Kraeber-Bodere F, et al. Survival improvement in patients with medullary thyroid carcinoma who undergo pretargeted anti-carcinoembryonic-antigen radioimmunotherapy: a collaborative study with the French Endocrine Tumor Group. J Clin Oncol. 2006;24:1705–11.

76. Sharkey RM, Karacay H, Govindan SV, Goldenberg DM. Combination radioimmunotherapy and chemoimmunotherapy involving different or the same targets

improves therapy of human pancreatic carcinoma xenograft models. Mol Cancer Ther. 2011;10:1072–81.
77. Stein R, Basu A, Chen S, Shih LB, Goldenberg DM.
Specificity and properties of MAb RS7-3G11 and the
antigen defined by this pancarcinoma monoclonal
antibody. Int J Cancer. 1993;55:938–46.
78. Stein R, Basu A, Goldenberg DM, Lloyd KO, Mattes
MJ. Characterization of cluster 13: the epithelial/

carcinoma antigen recognized by MAb RS7. Int J
Cancer Suppl. 1994;8:98–102.
79. Cardillo TM, Govindan SV, Sharkey RM, Trisal P,
Goldenberg DM. Humanized anti-Trop-2 IgG-SN-38
conjugate for effective treatment of diverse epithelial
cancers: preclinical studies in human cancer xenograft
models and monkeys. Clin Cancer Res. 2011;17:
3157–69.

Radioimmunotherapy of Renal Cell Carcinoma

15

Chaitanya Divgi

Introduction

There are estimated to be 60,920 new cases of renal carcinoma in the United States in 2011, with an associated annual mortality of 13,120 [1]. On presentation, approximately 70% of renal cortical tumors are confined to the kidney and 30% either present with, or later develop, metastatic disease [2]. The majority of cases (70%) are now discovered incidentally during the course of a cross-sectional imaging procedure obtained for other purposes [3]. The median tumor size is approximately 4 cm, well within safe limits for partial nephrectomy when technically feasible. Recent data demonstrate that 50–70% represent the more aggressive conventional clear cell carcinoma [4].

Characterization of histology and pathological features (i.e., T stage) can guide appropriate follow-up and entry into clinical trials. For patients with localized renal cortical tumors treated surgically, postoperative nomograms have been constructed that are effective in predicting long-term survival based on a combination of clinical and pathological features [5, 6]. Although

benign, indolent, and malignant renal cortical tumors all can display growth over time, metastatic potential is intrinsic to the histological subtype. Approximately 90% of patients who either present with or later develop metastatic renal cancer have the conventional clear cell histological subtype [7]. The clear cell renal cancer phenotype is associated with aggressive behavior and has the greatest metastatic potential of all renal malignancies [8].

Numerous relatively safe molecular therapies for ccRCC have been developed, and this has transformed the natural course of the disease. The most promising agents have been those that inhibit tyrosine kinase, particularly the small molecules sunitinib and sorafenib [9]. Moreover, inhibitors of the mammalian target of rapamycin (mTOR) have also been shown to prolong survival of patients with metastatic ccRCC [10].

Monoclonal antibody G250, both in its murine form and in its chimeric form (cG250, girentuximab), binds with carbonic anhydrase-IX (CA-IX), a cell surface antigen highly expressed in the vast majority of clear cell renal cell cancers [11]. Normal tissue expression is limited to biliary canaliculi and gastric epithelium, but not the normal kidney or other benign and malignant renal neoplasms [12]. This antibody has been extensively studied as a clinical therapeutic and diagnostic agent in ccRCC. The antibody has been labeled with both radioiodine and radiometals [13], and has been used in Phase 1/2 trials, initially in its murine form [14, 15]. These studies

C. Divgi, M.D. (✉)
Department of Radiology, PET/Nuclear Medicine
Division Columbia University, 722 W 168 Street R-114,
New York, NY 10032, USA
e-mail: crdivgi@columbia.edu

C. Aktolun and S.J. Goldsmith (eds.), *Nuclear Medicine Therapy: Principles and Clinical Applications*,
DOI 10.1007/978-1-4614-4021-5_15, © Springer Science+Business Media New York 2013

made it clear that the murine antibody was immunogenic, precluding multiple administrations. Consequently, a chimeric antibody, cG250, was developed [16] and is currently being evaluated as both an immunotherapeutic agent [17] and a radioimmunotherapy, labeled with iodine-131 [18–20] or a radiometal (yttrium-90 and lutetium-177) [21].

Murine G250 (mG250)

The laboratory of Dr. Lloyd Old pioneered the systematic development of antibodies targeting solid tumors. The initial human studies were carried out in a pre-surgical population [22]. Escalating mass amounts of antibody were administered to patients scheduled for surgical resection of their primary malignancy. A fixed amount of radiolabeled antibody was co-administered, and detailed pharmacokinetic and imaging analyses carried out preoperatively, with microscopic examination of resected tumor for standard histology, immunohistochemistry, and autoradiography. These studies helped establish blood clearance and normal tissue biodistribution, with correlation of uptake to features of the cancer phenotype, particularly tumor antigen presence and distribution. In all studies, immunogenicity of xenogeneic protein was assessed by serum human anti-mouse antibody (HAMA) measurement.

The first-in-human study [14] with ^{131}I-labeled murine G250 followed this pattern. Patients with renal cancer scheduled for surgical resection received escalating mass amounts of murine G250, and serial serum samples and planar whole-body images were obtained. Surgical specimens were assessed for histology and immunohistochemistry as well as autoradiography. The study demonstrated that (a) saturation of antigen sites in the liver (presumably the bile ducts) occurred at doses of 10 mg or greater; (b) antibody targeting closely paralleled antigen distribution, and (c) tumor uptake of antibody a week after administration was among the highest seen in any solid tumor.

Based on these promising initial results, the therapeutic potential of the antibody was tested in a Phase 1/2 setting in patients with metastatic ccRCC. Escalating amounts of iodine-131 labeled to a fixed total amount (10 mg) of murine G250 were administered to cohorts of three to six patients, following a classical Phase 1 dose escalation design [15, 23]. At the maximum tolerated dose (MTD) of ^{131}I-mG250 (90 mCi/m^2), an additional 9 (for a total of 15) patients were studied. Transient elevation of hepatic enzymes was observed in all patients; this was mild, asymptomatic, and self-limiting, and not related to amount of radioactivity. The murine antibody was immunogenic, though there were no associated symptoms. Dose-limiting toxicity was hematopoietic, with nadir occurring between 4 and 6 weeks after therapy administration; the MTD was determined to be 90 mCi/m^2 ^{131}I. Targeting to all metastatic disease was uniformly good (Fig. 15.1). There were, however, no responses although almost half of the treated patients' disease was stable.

It was concluded that the lack of responses seen in this Phase 1/2 study demonstrated that single agent ^{131}I-mG250 was ineffective at least as a single therapeutic administration—by standard evaluation parameters of response in the therapy of metastatic ccRCC. The immunogenicity of the murine protein precluded repeat administration. The excellent targeting and the stable disease population, however, suggested that repeat therapies of a non-immunogenic G250 may have promise in metastatic ccRCC therapy. The development of chimeric G250 (cG250) enabled exploration of this hypothesis.

Chimeric G250 (cG250, Girentuximab)

The initial clinical trials with cG250 were carried out in pre-surgical patients with ccRCC, and followed a pattern identical to the initial trial with mG250 [16]. Results were very similar too. Targeting was excellent; hepatic uptake was saturated at doses >5 mg. Serum clearance

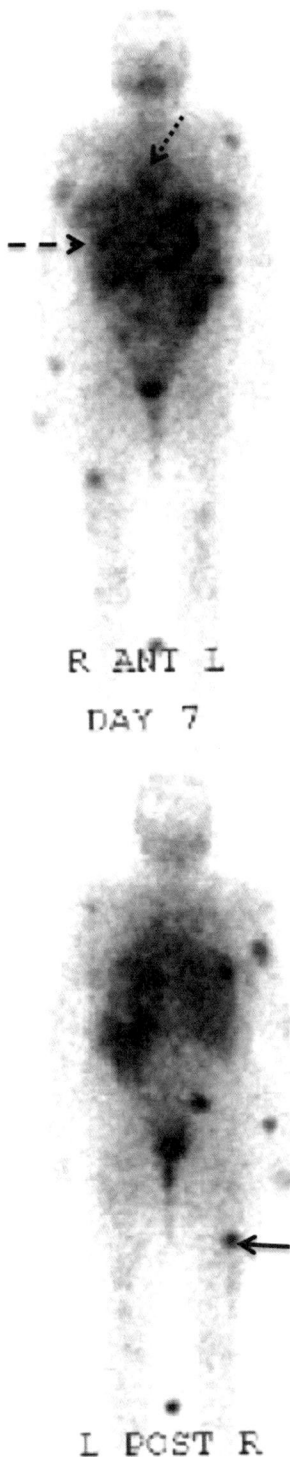

Fig. 15.1 Anterior and posterior whole body images a week after 75 mCi/m^2 ^{131}I-labeled murine G250 in a patient with metastatic ccRCC. There is excellent targeting to metastatic lesions in the bone (*solid arrow*), liver (*dashed arrow*) and nodes (*dotted arrow*)

characteristics were comparable as well. As anticipated, immunogenicity of the protein was strikingly less, with human anti-chimeric antibody (HACA) present in low titers in only 2 of the 16 patients studied. These promising results led the way to further exploration of ^{131}I-cG250 as a radioimmunotherapeutic agent.

Close collaboration between the investigators at Memorial Sloan-Kettering Cancer Center (MSKCC) at New York in the United States, and Radboud University at Nijmegen in the Netherlands, permitted parallel trial design and conduct. The New York group carried out a Phase 1 study [19] with multiple infusions of ^{131}I-cG250 based on a novel fractionated design, with radiation absorbed dose to the whole body (measured based on the clearance kinetics of a "scout" infusion of 185 MBq/5 mg ^{131}I-cG250) being escalated in groups of three to six patients (Fig. 15.2). The group at Nijmegen carried out a classical Phase 1 study with ^{131}I-cG250 [19–21], with escalating amounts of radioactivity (1,665–2,775 MBq ^{131}I) administered after an initial "scout" infusion of 222 MBq/5 mg ^{131}I-cG250. Patients were reevaluated with another scout dose 3 months after the initial treatment, and retreated when appropriate.

These studies, particularly when taken together, shed light on several key elements of radioimmunotherapy in solid tumors in general, and ccRCC in particular [24]. Radioimmunotherapy was well tolerated and generally safe. Kinetics of a therapeutic administration of radioimmunotherapy could be predicted by a scout infusion. External imaging permitted assessment of tumor dosimetry, while serial measurements of blood radioactivity permitted quantification of whole body and marrow radiation absorbed dose. Both studies also showed that targeting to tumor was comparable with the scout and therapeutic infusions, during the first treatment course. Both showed that hematopoietic toxicity was dose-limiting and self-limiting. There was no major treatment response by RECIST criteria following the first treatment course. There were in fact no major responses even in those patients who received multiple treatment courses. There appeared to be a progression-free survival advantage to radioimmunotherapy.

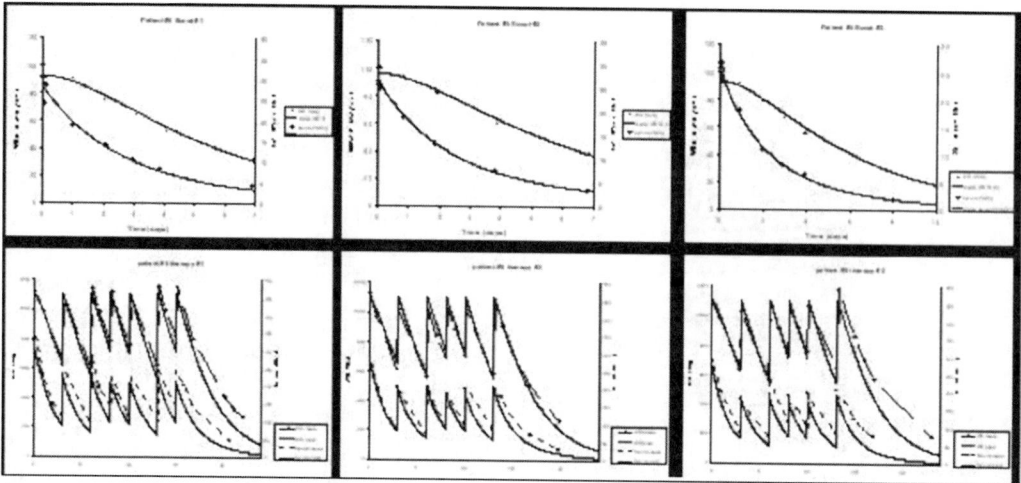

Fig. 15.2 Patient with metastatic ccRC who was treated over a year with three courses of fractionated radioimmunotherapy with ^{131}I-labeled chimeric G250. A whole body dose of 0.5 Gy was calculated based on scout doses (*upper panel*), with excellent reproducibility between predicted and measured clearance curves of the multiple therapies (*lower panel*). The whole body clearance is depicted as *solid curves* and the serum clearance as *dashed curves*

Both studies also demonstrated that changes in serum kinetics were predictive of an immune response, with a clear relationship between more rapid clearance (with usually lack of tumor targeting) and an HACA response. There were, however, major differences in immunogenicity, allowing for the limitations of trial design. A fractionated schema was much less likely to be immunogenic (2 of 15 patients) than a schema where there was a 3-month or greater interval between treatments (8 of 27 patients). It thus appeared that a shorter interval between administrations of xenogeneic protein was more likely to result in tolerance, while longer intervals resulted in an immune response.

> ### Principles of Radioimmunotherapy of Clear Cell Renal Cell
>
> - High Metastatic potential [8].
> - Uniform tumor expression of CA-9 [14, 15].
> - Antibody: cG250, girentuximab [17].
> - Radionuclides: I-131, Y-90, Lu-177 [18, 21].

Future Considerations with Radiolabeled cG250 Therapy

[131]I-cG250 is an ideal radiolabeled antibody for therapy for many reasons. The nuclide is understood well, having been the backbone of Nuclear Medicine for decades. Any radioactive iodine that dissociates from the antibody is cleared rapidly by concomitant oral administration of stable iodide and additional thyroid blockade when appropriate. [131]I has a relatively "soft" beta-minus emission, limiting radiation dose to contiguous normal tissue. Its gamma emissions, while of relatively high energy, nonetheless permit external imaging and quantification. Attachment of radioiodine to protein is easily accomplished by established direct iodination methods.

Iodinated antibodies, however, suffer from disadvantages, particularly when the antibody undergoes cellular internalization into lysosomes. This usually results in prompt dehalogenation of the radioiodinated antibody with rapid clearance of the (now unbound) radioactivity. Studies have demonstrated that in internalizing systems, radiometal-labeled antibodies accumulate to a greater extent in tumor than do radioiodinated antibodies

[25, 26]. While there is no convincing evidence that the cG250/CA-IX complex internalizes, the observation, both in patients [27] and in preclinical experiments [13], that radiometal-labeled cG250 accumulated to a greater extent than did ^{131}I-cG250, spurred the clinical evaluation of radiometal-labeled cG250 for the treatment of metastatic ccRCC.

Phase 1 studies with radiometal-labeled cG250 are under way. As with prior clinical trials, these were also initiated both at Radboud University and at MSKCC, with escalating amounts of Lutetium-177 cG250 at the former and Yttrium-90 labeled cG250 at the latter. In both trials, the initial imaging study is carried out with Indium-111 labeled cG250. Preliminary results [21] have demonstrated that ^{111}In-cG250 imaging can predict radiation dose and hematopoietic toxicity of ^{177}Lu-cG250, and suggest that ^{177}Lu-cG250 may have a better therapeutic window than ^{90}Y-cG250.

Therapeutic options for metastatic ccRCC have changed considerably since the initial explorations with radiolabeled G250 began. There are an increasing number of tyrosine kinase inhibitors (TKi) with therapeutic promise [9], and other agents, including mTOR inhibitors, are being approved for use [10]. Moreover, it is becoming clear that solid tumor radioimmunotherapy will be most useful in small volume disease, with an inverse correlation between tumor mass and absorbed dose being observed [21]. Radioimmunotherapy will therefore be most promising as part of a multi-modality therapy strategy. In this context, the timing of radiolabeled cG250 administration is crucial. This will be determined, of course, based on antigen expression.

Preclinical studies have suggested that CA-IX expression begins to decrease soon after initiation of TKi therapy; Oosterwijk-Wakka and her colleagues demonstrated [28], in xenograft models, that antibody uptake begins to decrease soon after TKi administration, resuming, especially at the tumor periphery, after discontinuation. It is unclear how these observations translate into effective clinical trial design. Perhaps the radiolabeled antibody should be given first, to maximize tumor uptake, and also perhaps to change what appear to be cytostatic therapies into a tumoricidal combination. The consequent effect, however, on toxicity is uncertain, since hematopoietic toxicity after radioimmunotherapy is delayed and thus be additive to TKi myelotoxicity. Nevertheless, it is clear that radioimmunotherapy will need to be one component of a multi-modality therapy strategy, and such preclinical studies will need to address these issues to aid in intelligent clinical trial design.

Conclusion

Renal cancer is typically thought of as an aggressive, radio-resistant cancer. Systemic chemotherapy has also been largely ineffective in this disease. Immunotherapy for renal cancer has been shown to be effective, particularly therapy with high doses of interleukin-2. This spurred the exploration of less toxic immunotherapy, and led to the development of antibodies that target cell surface antigens over-expressed in renal cancer.

The incidence of renal cancer has changed over the decades, with more and more renal malignancies being detected serendipitously during abdominal imaging for other conditions, with consequently a greater fraction of benign and small tumors. Along with a decrease in median size of renal neoplasm (permitting curative surgery and decreasing the likelihood of metastatic disease) has been an increase in effective molecular therapies with very acceptable toxicity profiles. This has led to a decrease in the need for and study of toxic systemic therapies, including chemotherapy and radioimmunotherapy.

It is clear now that the renal cancer with the greatest propensity to metastasis, and hence the only renal cancer for which aggressive systemic therapies may be warranted, is the clear cell phenotype. Carbonic anhydrase-IX is a cell surface antigen over-expressed in the vast majority of clear cell renal cancers, and G250 is an antibody that has been radiolabeled and extensively studied as a therapeutic (and diagnostic) agent in clear cell renal cell cancer (ccRCC). Murine and chimeric antibody G250 has been investigated in initial studies, and there are ongoing studies with girentuximab for radionuclide therapy of ccRCC. Chimeric G250 has low immunogenic potential, and radiolabeled cG250 has considerable potential in the therapy of metastatic ccRCC. Advances in the molecular therapy of ccRCC necessitate careful evaluation of the role and nature of radiolabeled cG250 therapy in a multi-modality therapeutic strategy.

Acknowledgement This chapter is dedicated to the memory of Lloyd J. Old, whose seminal observations on the nature and potential of monoclonal antibodies in cancer treatment have influenced the development of cG250 in renal cancer diagnosis and therapy.

References

1. American Cancer Society. Cancer facts & figures 2011. Atlanta: American Cancer Society; 2011.
2. National Comprehensive Cancer Network Clinical Practice Guidelines in Oncology—Kidney Cancer. Version 2.2011;NCCN.org.
3. Berland LL, Silverman SG, Gore RM, et al. Managing incidental findings on abdominal CT: white paper of the ACR incidental findings committee. J Am Coll Radiol. 2010;7(10):754–73.
4. Linehan WM, Walther MM, Zbar B. The genetic basis of cancer of the kidney. J Urol. 2003;170:2163–72.
5. Kattan MW, Reuter V, Motzer RJ, et al. A postoperative prognostic nomogram for renal cell. J Urol. 2001;166:63–7.
6. Sorbellini M, Kattan MW, Snyder ME, et al. A postoperative prognostic nomogram predicting recurrence for patients with conventional clear cell renal cell carcinoma. J Urol. 2005;173:48–51.
7. Motzer RJ, Bacik J, Mariani T, et al. Treatment outcome and survival associated with metastatic renal cell carcinoma of non-clear cell histology. J Clin Oncol. 2002;20:2376–81.
8. Cheville JC, Lohse CM, Zincke H, et al. Comparisons of outcome and prognostic features among histologic subtypes of renal cell carcinoma. Am J Surg Pathol. 2003;27:612–24.
9. Motzer RJ, Bukowski RM. Targeted therapy for metastatic renal cell carcinoma. J Clin Oncol. 2006;24:5601–8.
10. Cho DC, Atkins MB. Future directions in renal cell carcinoma: 2011 and beyond. Hematol Oncol Clin North Am. 2011;25(4):917–35.
11. Oosterwijk E, Ruiter DJ, Hoedemaeker PJ, et al. Monoclonal antibody G 250 recognizes a determinant present in renal-cell carcinoma and absent from normal kidney. Int J Cancer. 1986;38:489–94.
12. Oosterwijk E, Divgi CR, Brouwers A, et al. Monoclonal antibody-based therapy for renal cell carcinoma. Urol Clin North Am. 2003;30(3):623–31.
13. Brouwers AH, van Eerd JE, Frielink C, et al. Optimization of radioimmunotherapy of renal cell carcinoma: labeling of monoclonal antibody cG250 with 131I, 90Y, 177Lu, or 186Re. J Nucl Med. 2004;45:327–37.
14. Oosterwijk E, Bander NH, Divgi CR, et al. Antibody localization in human renal cell carcinoma: a phase I study of monoclonal antibody G250. J Clin Oncol. 1993;11:738–50.
15. Divgi CR, Bander NH, Scott AM, et al. Phase I/II radioimmunotherapy trial with iodine-131-labeled monoclonal antibody G250 in metastatic renal cell carcinoma. Clin Cancer Res. 1998;4:2729–39.
16. Steffens MG, Boerman OC, Oosterwijk-Wakka JC, et al. Targeting of renal cell carcinoma with iodine-131-labeled chimeric monoclonal antibody G250. J Clin Oncol. 1997;15:1529–37.
17. Stillebroer AB, Mulders PF, Boerman OC, Oyen WJ, Oosterwijk E. Carbonic anhydrase IX in renal cell carcinoma: implications for prognosis, diagnosis, and therapy. Eur Urol. 2010;58:75–83.
18. Divgi CR, O'Donoghue JA, Welt S, et al. Phase I clinical trial with fractionated radioimmunotherapy using 131I-labeled chimeric G250 in metastatic renal cancer. J Nucl Med. 2004;45:1412–21.
19. Steffens MG, Boerman OC, de Mulder PH, et al. Phase I radioimmunotherapy of metastatic renal cell carcinoma with 131I-labeled chimeric monoclonal antibody G250. Clin Cancer Res. 1999;5(10 Suppl):3268s–74s.
20. Brouwers AH, Mulders PF, de Mulder PH, et al. Lack of efficacy of two consecutive treatments of radioimmunotherapy with 131I-cG250 in patients with metastasized clear cell renal cell carcinoma. J Clin Oncol. 2005;23:6540–8.
21. Stillebroer AB, Zegers CM, Boerman OC, et al. Dosimetric analysis of 177Lu-cG250 radioimmunotherapy in renal cell carcinoma patients: correlation with myelotoxicity and pretherapeutic absorbed dose predictions based on 111In-cG250 imaging. J Nucl Med. 2012;53:82–9.
22. Welt S, Divgi CR, Real FX, et al. Quantitative analysis of antibody localization in human metastatic colon cancer: a phase I study of monoclonal antibody A33. J Clin Oncol. 1990;8:1894–906.
23. Loh A, Sgouros G, O'Donoghue JA, et al. Pharmacokinetic model of iodine-131-G250 antibody in renal cell carcinoma patients. J Nucl Med. 1998;39(3):484–9.
24. Brouwers AH, Buijs WC, Mulders PF, et al. Radioimmunotherapy with [131I]cG250 in patients with metastasized renal cell cancer: dosimetric analysis and immunologic response. Clin Cancer Res. 2005;11(19 Pt 2):7178s–86s.
25. Carrasquillo JA, Bunn Jr PA, Keenan AM, et al. Radioimmunodetection of cutaneous T-cell lymphoma with 111In-labeled T101 monoclonal antibody. N Engl J Med. 1986;315:673–80.

26. Clarke K, Lee FT, Brechbiel MW, Smyth FE, Old LJ, Scott AM. In vivo biodistribution of a humanized anti-Lewis Y monoclonal antibody (hu3S193) in MCF-7 xenografted BALB/c nude mice. Cancer Res. 2000;60:4804–11.

27. Brouwers AH, Buijs WC, Oosterwijk E, et al. Targeting of metastatic renal cell carcinoma with the chimeric monoclonal antibody G250 labeled with (131)I or (111)In: an intrapatient comparison. Clin Cancer Res. 2003;9(10 Pt 2):3953S–60S.

28. Oosterwijk-Wakka JC, Kats-Ugurlu G, Leenders WP, et al. Effect of tyrosine kinase inhibitor treatment of renal cell carcinoma on the accumulation of carbonic anhydrase IX-specific chimeric monoclonal antibody cG250. BJU Int. 2011;107: 118–25.

Radioimmunotherapy of Prostate Carcinoma

16

Stanley J. Goldsmith, Scott T. Tagawa,
Shankar Vallabhajosula, Anastasia Nikolopoulou,
Irina Lipai, David M. Nanus, and Neil H. Bander

Introduction

Prostate cancer accounts for 25% of the newly diagnosed cancers among men in developed countries. With the availability of serum Prostate Specific Antigen (PSA) determinations, many patients present early with limited disease but a significant percent will experience recurrences and will eventually die from disseminated disease. Initial evaluation of the extent of disease is rendered difficult by the biology of the disease involving micrometastases in bone marrow and lymph nodes that are often too small to detect in the early stages of the disease with currently available methods. Even when a rising PSA suggests that there is residual disease, the multifocal nature of metastatic prostate carcinoma renders surgical and external beam radiation therapy of little value after treatment of the primary tumor. Whereas androgen deprivation is transiently effective as therapy for as long as 12–18 months in some patients, it is not curative. Subsequent use of chemotherapy is transiently beneficial in a subset of patients but progression of disease is inevitable. Hence, prostate carcinoma represents a distinct challenge and opportunity for radioimmunotherapy based upon selective targeting of tumor sites by an immunoglobulin to which a radioactive atom has been attached, thus serving as a vehicle for targeted radiotherapy.

Radioimmunotherapy

Radioimmunotherapy is based upon several elements:
- Identification of an antigen that is expressed on tumor tissue, either uniquely or to a significantly greater degree than in other tissues.
- Development of an antibody with sufficient specificity and affinity to serve as a delivery vehicle.

S.J. Goldsmith, M.D. (✉)
Division of Nuclear Medicine and Molecular Imaging,
New York-Presbyterian Hospital, Weill College of
Medicine of Cornell University, NY, USA

S. Vallabhajosula, Ph.D. • A. Nikolopoulou, Ph.D.
I. Lipai, M.S., C.N.M.T.
Division of Nuclear Medicine and Molecular Imaging,
New York-Presbyterian Hospital-Weill Cornell Medical
Center, Weill Cornell Medical College,
525 E 68th Street, Starr 2-21, New York, NY, USA
e-mail: sjg2002@med.cornell.edu

S.T. Tagawa, M.D. • D.M. Nanus, M.D., Ph.D.
Division of Hematology and Oncology, Deane Prostate
Health and Research Center, New York-Presbyterian
Hospital-Weill Cornell Medical Center, Weill Cornell
Medical College, New York, NY, USA

N.H. Bander, M.D.
Department of Urology, New York-Presbyterian
Hospital-Weill Cornell Medical Center, Weill Cornell
Medical College, 525 E 68th Street, New York, NY, USA

C. Aktolun and S.J. Goldsmith (eds.), *Nuclear Medicine Therapy: Principles and Clinical Applications*,
DOI 10.1007/978-1-4614-4021-5_16, © Springer Science+Business Media New York 2013

- Identification of a radionuclide with an emission that will deliver an effective radiation absorbed dose.
- Chemistry that provides convenient stable binding of the radionuclide to the antibody.

The goal of radioimmunotherapy is to deliver a therapeutic radiation dose to the targeted tumor tissue with minimal irradiation of normal tissues in proximity to disseminated tumor foci and to tissues that receive exposure while the radiolabeled antibody is circulating in the serum.

Since 1995, a team consisting of physicians, scientists, technologists, and nurses in the Division of Nuclear Medicine and Molecular Imaging of the Department of Radiology, in the Division of Hematology-Oncology of the Department of Medicine, and the Department of Urology at the Weill Cornell Medical College have proceeded in a stepwise manner to develop and evaluate a radiolabeled antibody as an agent for the treatment of metastatic prostate carcinoma. This review will document the procedures and observations to date and provide a template for further investigations.

Requirements for Development of a Radioimmunotherapy

- Tumor expression of antigen, unique, or to a greater degree than other tissues
- Monoclonal antibody with appropriate specificity and affinity
- Linker chemistry that provides stable binding of radionuclide to antibody
- Radionuclide with physical properties compatible with antibody pharmacokinetics and tumor biology

Prostate Specific Membrane Antigen

Prostate specific membrane antigen (PSMA) is a membrane protein expressed on prostate epithelial cells. It is upregulated on virtually all prostate carcinoma and not shed into the circulation [1–7]. Recent studies have demonstrated low levels of PSMA expression in the small intestine, proximal renal tubules, and salivary glands [0.01–1.0% compared to expression on prostatic cells] as well as by vascular endothelial cells of various other solid tumors [5, 6]. PSMA is a complex molecule with an extracellular, transmembrane, and intracellular portion (Fig. 16.1). This structure is probably significant and the basis for its enzymatic function but the precise physiologic function of PSMA in prostate tumor biology is uncertain. PSMA expression increases progressively in higher grade cancers, metastatic disease, and hormone-refractory prostate cancer [3, 4, 8, 9].

A variety of antibodies have been developed to PSMA. In 1998, capromab (7E11/CYT-356), a murine monoclonal IgG1 that binds to the intracellular portion of PSMA was labeled with Indium-111 [^{111}In] and developed as a prostate carcinoma imaging agent. It was approved by the FDA in the United States and has been marketed as *Prostascint®* [Cytogen, Inc.] to evaluate extent of disease in high-risk patients presenting with Gleason scores of 7 or more and in patients with rising PSA following prostatectomy. At the time of *Prostascint®'s* introduction, the procedure involved obtaining planar images on the day of administration and again 3–5 days later. The initial images were used to provide mapping of the activity in vascular structures and bone marrow for comparison with the later images. Subsequently, the technique evolved to obtain SPECT of the pelvis. More recently, SPECT/CT has been used with further improvement in overall accuracy [10–12]. Transaxial SPECT images have been fused with separately acquired CT images for radiation treatment planning [13, 14]. Nevertheless, the agent has not found widespread acceptance in the urologic oncology community and efforts to utilize this antibody as a radioimmunotherapy agent have been unsatisfactory [15, 16]. Since 7E11 preferentially recognizes the intracellular portion of the PSMA molecule, it is likely that localization depends upon the presence of necrotic cells. This conclusion is supported by observations in cell suspensions in which there is no demonstrable binding in viable LnCaP cells but binding is demonstrated when cells are exposed to toxic or membranolytic

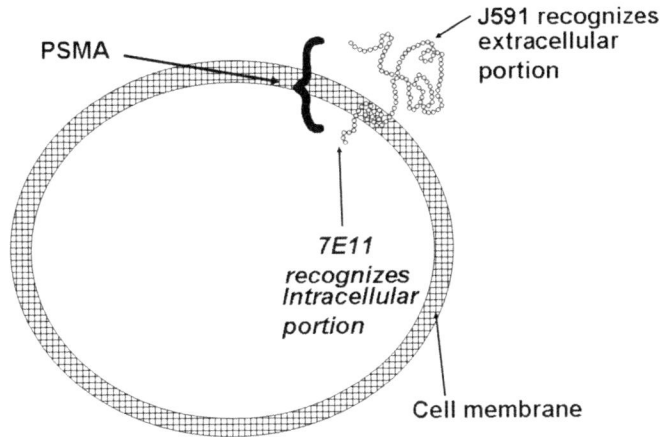

PSMA

J591 recognizes
extracellular
portion

*7E11
recognizes
Intracellular
portion*

Cell membrane

Non-Permeabilized   Permeabilized

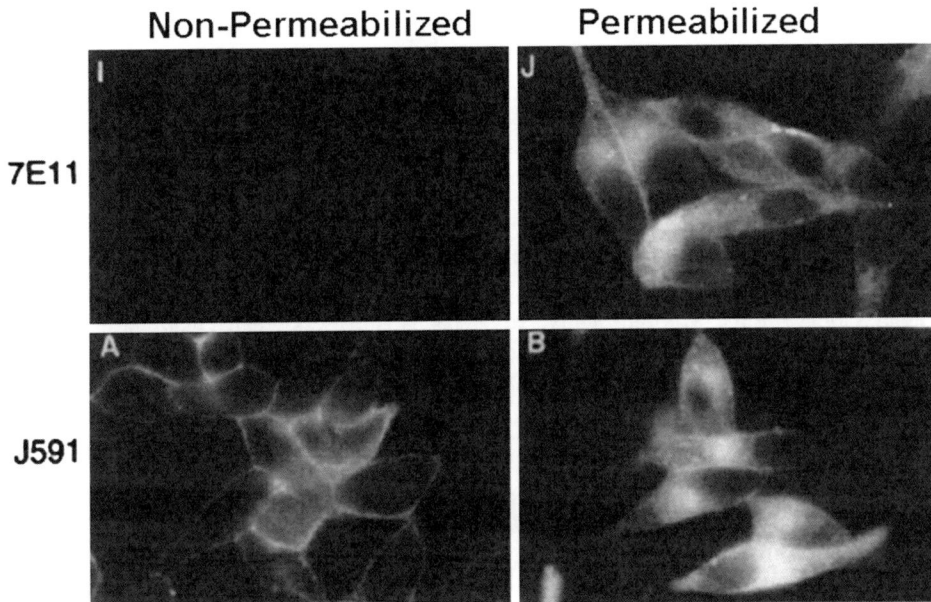

7E11

J591

Fig. 16.2 Immuno-fluorescent stain demonstrating antibody binding of J591 to intact LnCaP cells and no binding of 7E11 which recognizes only the intra-cellular epitope. Antibodies are large molecules which do not permeate intact cell membranes. When the cells are permeabilized, the 7E11 antibody gains access to the epitope. Radioimmunotherapy is directed against viable (nonpermeabilized) tumor cells [18]

reagents (Fig. 16.2) [17]. Although it is likely that some necrosis is present in even relatively small tumor foci, this is a suboptimal basis for localization of a therapeutic agent, the purpose of which is to destroy viable tumor.

Subsequently, other monoclonal antibodies were developed [18]. Our group has pursued an antibody identified as J591 which had a high degree of affinity for viable prostate ca cells [LnCaP] that express PSMA in cell suspensions, animal models of human prostate carcinoma, and other human tumors [18]. After binding to the external epitope of PSMA, the membrane evaginates with internalization on the antigen-antibody complex.

Preclinical Studies

Although absolute evidence of utility in human disease requires clinical studies, the LnCaP suspensions were used in preclinical studies to quantify and compare immunoreactivity of radiolabeled preparations and to select the appropriate radionuclide for clinical trials as a therapeutic agent. The physical properties and labeling chemistry of [131]iodine [^{131}I], [90]yttrium [^{90}Y], and [177]lutetium [^{177}Lu] were reviewed (Table 16.1). [131]Iodine, of course, had been used for the treatment of thyroid carcinoma and as a label in earlier radioimmunotherapy trials. There was considerable experience with radioiodine labeling techniques and high specific activity ^{131}I was readily available and relatively inexpensive. [90]Y might be thought to be the preferred radionuclide for therapy because of the greater β energy with consequently longer range in tissue. The short half-life of ^{90}Y may be also viewed as a potential advantageous feature because of the possible dose rate effect (greater radiobiologic effect of radiation dose delivered at shorter interval). In the 1990s, ^{177}Lu became available (courtesy of the Missouri University Research Reactor (MURR)). [177]Lu, like ^{90}Y, is a radiometal. Although the chemistry of ^{177}Lu and ^{90}Y is somewhat similar, the physical properties (physical half-life, β energy, and accompanying γ emission) of ^{177}Lu were more similar to ^{131}I than to [90]Y (Table 16.1). While not as convenient as iodination techniques, methods to prepare chemically stable radiometal labeled immunoglobulins have been developed. The DOTA (1,4,7,10-tetra aza cyclo dodecane-1,4,7,10-tetra acetic acid) complex is covalently bound to the immunoglobulin. This moiety (DOTA-IgG) has a high affinity for both ^{177}Lu and ^{90}Y and is readily labeled with either of these radiometals as well as with [111]In. ^{111}In-DOTA-J591 is useful to provide a gamma emitting radiometal labeled version of the antibody complex in order to obtain pharmacokinetic, imaging, and biodistribution data without exposing subjects to any beta component.

Initially, studies were performed to evaluate the affinity of murine J591 to LnCaP cells and the stability of the bound radiolabeled immunoglobulins. [111]In DOTA-J591 was used as a surrogate for the radiometals to evaluate binding to LnCaP cell suspensions and imaging in intact animals. Although J591 binds to an external epitope of PSMA, the epitope-antibody complex is internalized and likely digested in the intracellular environment. Despite intracellular digestion of the intact radiometal-DOTA-J591 complex, ^{111}In DOTA-J591 demonstrated high cellular retention of 90–95% of the radioactivity with minimal washout of radioactivity. The intracellular half-life was greater than 500 h. By contrast, although the iodinated form of the antibody had excellent affinity for the PSMA-expressing tumors, the ^{131}I label was observed to wash out of the cells. Hence, subsequent evaluations of therapeutic effects were limited to the radiometals ^{177}Lu and [90]Y. Significant antitumor responses were observed in LNCaP xenograft tumor bearing nude mice and a dose response relationship was observed

Table 16.1 Beta emitting radionuclides for therapy

	[131]I	[90]Y	[177]Lu
Physical half-life (days)	8.05	2.67	6.7
β^- particles (MeV)			
Max	0.61	2.280	0.497
Average	0.20	0.935	0.149
Range in tissue (mm)			
Max	2.4	12.0	2.20
Average	0.4	2.7	0.25
Gamma emission (MeV)	0.364 (81%)	None	0.113 (7%)
			0.208 (11%)
Equilibrium dose constant (rad.g/h)			
β^- radiation	0.389	1.9886	0.314
Gamma	0.815	None	0.075

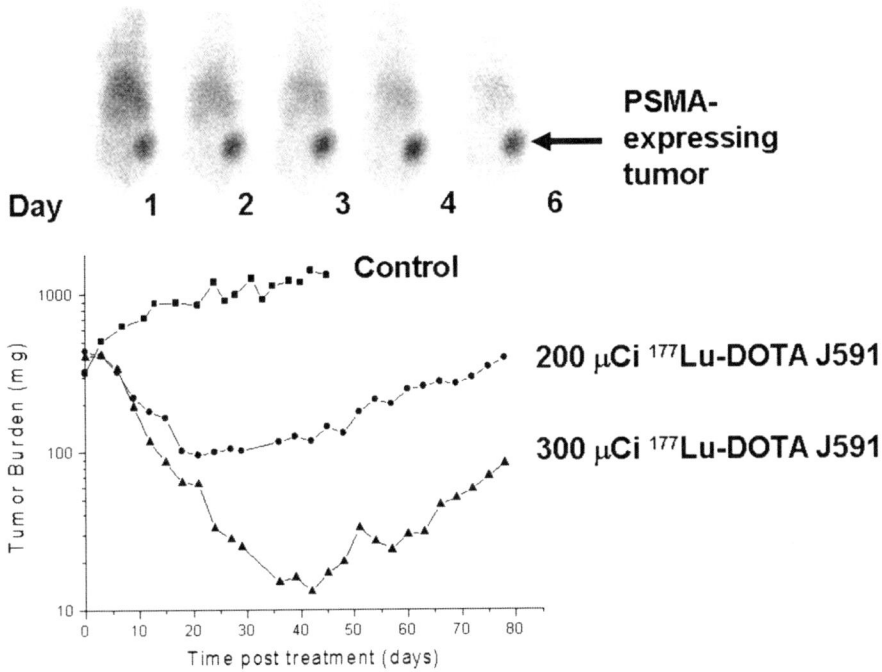

Fig. 16.3 Dose response antitumor effect of ^{177}Lu-J591 in nude mice nearing human prostate ca xenografts that express PSMA [19]

(Fig. 16.3). Higher cumulative doses of either ^{90}Y or ^{177}Lu were possible using fractionated dosing (multiple sub-Maximum Tolerated Dose (MTD)) rather than a single MTD dose. Median survival of the animals improved threefold for fractionated ^{90}Y-muJ591 therapy vs. control (150 vs. 52 days). With fractionated doses of ^{177}Lu-muJ591, >80% of the mice were cured [19].

Clinical Studies

To prepare for the possibility that patients might receive more than a single exposure to the antibody, and also anticipating that patients may have had prior exposure to murine antigens, the J591 antibody was re-engineered to replace the murine backbone with an equivalent human IgG sequence without disturbing the immuno-recognition portion of the J591 [Biovation, Ltd. (Aberdeen, UK)]. This modified preparation, huJ591, was subsequently covalently linked to as many as six DOTA molecules per IgG molecule without loss of reactivity.

Following approval by the FDA and Medical Center IRB, initial studies were performed in humans to determine the safety and effect on biodistribution of incremental amounts of the humanized antibody using ^{111}In DOTA-J591. Repetitive dosing was well tolerated up to 500 mg without the development of a human antihumanized (de-immunized) antibody (HAHA) response or evidence of dose-limiting toxicity (DLT); the MTD was not reached [20]. Monoclonal antibody targeting to normal tissues was not observed but significant uptake of the radiolabel was seen in the liver, typical of radiometal labeled immunoglobulin biodistribution patterns (Fig. 16.4). The liver activity diminishes with increasing dose of antibody but a considerable fraction of the injected dose appears in the liver. Increasing the amount of antibody infused results in longer plasma clearance times (i.e., slower plasma clearance) [21, 22]. These data demonstrated that relatively low amounts of total immunoglobulin, in the order of 20 mg, were sufficient to minimize hepatic uptake and maximize plasma circulation time. Accordingly, a decision was made to use a

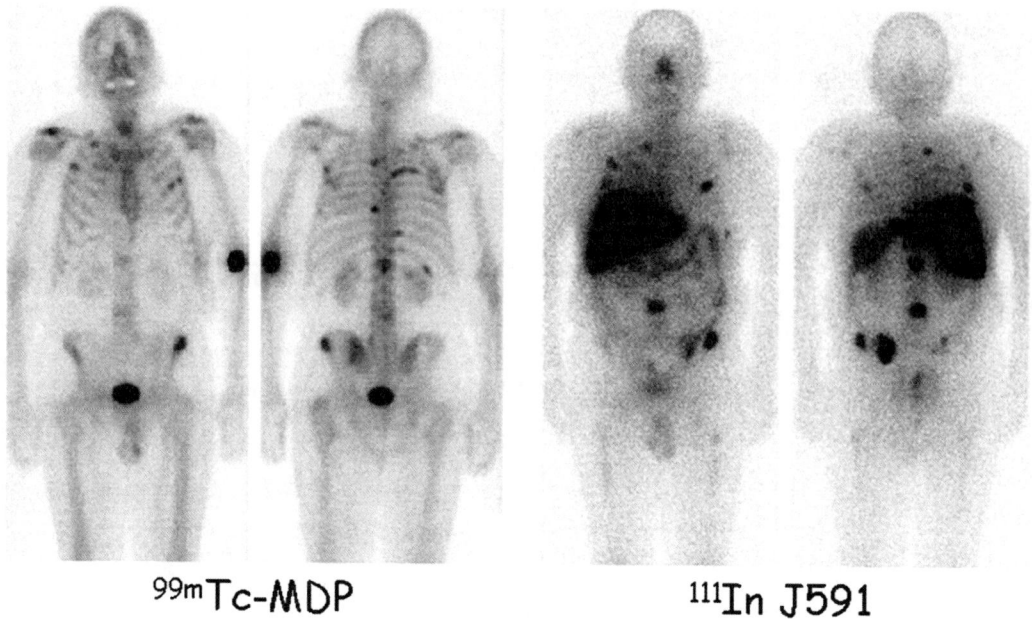

^{99m}Tc-MDP ^{111}In J591

Fig. 16.4 Planar anterior and posterior ^{99m}Tc-MDP bone scans and ^{111}In-DOTA-J591 scans in a patient with prostate carcinoma and bone metastases demonstrating targeting of osseous metastases. At some sites, targeting is less successful which may indicate that tumor is no longer viable. Nevertheless, the radiolabeled antibody targets some sites that are not seen on the radionuclide bone scan

total of 20 mg of the J591 antibody in all clinical studies.

While the nude mouse xenograft model using inplanted LnCaP cells demonstrated a dose response antitumoral effect for both ^{90}Y and ^{177}Lu, the contrasting physical properties (most notable the β particle energy and physical half-lives) represented a perplexing issue (Table 16.1). From a regulatory point of view (and to a degree, on an ethical basis), however, it would be desirable to demonstrate efficacy in patients with measureable disease where depending upon uniformity of distribution within tumor masses, ^{90}Y would be expected to be more effective. In all likelihood, however, the lower energy β particle of ^{177}Lu might be more effective and less toxic in addressing micrometastases in the bone marrow [22, 23].

Initially, two independent phase I clinical trials were performed using either ^{90}Y DOTA-J591 or ^{177}Lu DOTA-J591 in patients with castrate-resistant prostate cancer [24–27]. The primary objectives of these trials were to define the MTDs of the isotopes as well as to further define dosimetry, pharmacokinetics, and potential appearance of human antihuman antibodies

(HAHA) as the radiolabeled DOTA conjugate has some immunogenic potential despite replacement of most of the murine IgG backbone with human IgG. In those trials, antitumor responses were a secondary endpoint.

The protocol design and entry criteria of the two trials were identical. Eligibility criteria included histologically confirmed prostate cancer and evidence of progressing recurrent or metastatic disease defined by at least three serially rising PSAs and/or imaging evidence of tumor. Other criteria included the usual requirements: an absolute neutrophil count (ANC) $\geq 2.0 \times 10^9$/L, platelet count $\geq 150 \times 10^9$/L. Patients were excluded if they had had prior radiation therapy encompassing >25% of the skeleton or prior treatment with ^{89}Strontium or ^{153}Samarium as well as other standard laboratory exclusion criteria [24–27]. Since all prostate cancers at presentation are PSMA-positive, PSMA expression on tissue samples was not required. DLT in both the ^{90}Y and ^{177}Lu DOTA-J591 trials was defined as severe thrombocytopenia (platelet <10 $\times 10^9$/L) and/or grade 4 neutropenia (ANC <0.5 $\times 10^9$) for greater than 5 days or other toxicity consisting of grade ≥ 3 nonhematologic toxicity that could reasonably be attributable to radiolabeled J591. Consistent with the usual Phase 1 clinical trial design, three patients were evaluated at each dose level; if 1 of 3 experienced a grade 3 or 4 DLT, up to an additional three patients would be evaluated at that level. If a second patient experienced a DLT, no additional doses were administered at that level and the prior dosing level was designated as the MTD.

^{90}Y-DOTA-J591

In the ^{90}Y-J591 phase I trial, patients received an initial 185 MBq (5 mCi) dose of ^{111}In-J591 (20 mg) for pharmacokinetic and biodistribution (imaging) studies [26]. One week later, the patients received a dose of ^{90}Y-J591 based on prior published experience with ^{90}Y labeled antibodies. Twenty-nine subjects were entered at incremental dose levels of 185, 370, 555, 650, and 740 MBq/m^2 (5, 10, 15, 17.5, and 20 mCi/m^2). Patients were eligible for up to three retreatments if platelet and neutrophil recovery were satisfactory. Four patients were re-treated. Dose-limiting toxicity occurred at 740 MBq/m^2 (20 mCi/m^2). Two patients experienced severe thrombocytopenia with nonlife-threatening bleeding episodes requiring platelet transfusions. Accordingly, the 650 MBq/m^2 (17.5 mCi/m^2) dose level was determined to be the MTD for ^{90}Y-DOTA-J591. Among the 29 patients, 19 had bone lesions and 13 patients had soft tissue lesions. On pretreatment imaging during the week following the ^{111}In-DOTA-J591 tracer, 17 of 19 (89%) patients with bone lesions and 9 of 13 (69%) with soft tissue lesions were accurately targeted; overall targeting sensitivity of 81% (26 of 32). Two patients treated at the 740 MBq/m^2 (20 mCi/m^2) dose level exhibited 85 and 70% declines in PSA lasting 8 and 8.6 months prior to returning to pretreatment values. In addition, these two patients had objective measurable disease responses with 90 and 40% decrease in the size of pelvic and retroperitoneal lymphadenopathy. Both patients were castrate resistant with lymph node-only disease and had not received prior chemotherapy. The second patient was re-treated with ^{90}Y-J591

on day 119. An additional six patients experienced PSA stabilization by week 12.

^{177}Lu-DOTA-J591

Since the β energy of ^{177}Lu was lower than ^{90}Y, it was decided that the ^{177}Lu-J591 phase I trial could be safely initiated at the 370 MBq (10 mCi)/m^2 level [27]. In this trial, 35 patients received ^{177}Lu-DOTA-J591 with doses ranging from 370 MBq (10 mCi)/m^2 to 2.8 GBq (75 mCi)/m^2 following the previously described trial design. Of the three patients at the 2.8 GBq (75 mCi)/m^2 dose level, one experienced dose-limiting (grade 4) thrombocytopenia; the remaining two patients experienced grade 3 thrombocytopenia. All three patients experienced grade 4 neutropenia; one of which was of 6 days duration. At the prior dose level of 2.6 GBq (70 mCi)/m^2, two of six patients had transient grade 4 neutropenia, not meeting the definition of DLT. One of these patients had grade 4 thrombocytopenia. Hence, the 2.6 GBq (70 mCi)/m^2 dose level was determined to be the MTD. Thirty of thirty-five patients had well-defined metastatic disease on diagnostic imaging prior to radioimmunotherapy. These known sites of metastatic disease were successfully imaged using the γ emission of the ^{177}Lu. All 35 patients in this trial had abnormal, rising PSAs and 7 patients had measurable disease. None of the seven patients with measurable disease had an objective tumor response, nor $\geq 50\%$ PSA decline suggesting that the lower energy β emission of ^{177}Lu may not be effective in patients with measurable disease on CT or MRI. Fourteen of thirty-five patients had progressive disease (PSA increase of $\geq 25\%$) after treatment while 21 of 35 patients had evidence of a radiobiologic effect. Sixteen patients had PSA stabilization for 28 days or longer. The median duration of PSA stabilization was 60 days with a range of 28–601+ days. Four patients had $\geq 50\%$ PSA decline lasting from 3 to 8 months [27]. No HAHA responses were detected.

For a variety of reasons, it was necessary to concentrate resources on only one of the two radionuclides and ^{177}Lu was chosen for further evaluation even though metastatic castrate-resistant prostate carcinoma (CRPC) patients with bulky disease (the population most readily accessible) are likely a suboptimal patient population to initially assess the utility of ^{177}Lu-DOTA-J591. The ^{177}Lu labeled antibody to the external epitope of PSMA would be expected to be a better match for subsequent trials in patients with biochemical evidence of disease as well as potential adjuvant use rather than treatment of bulky disease.

Phase II Trial of ^{177}Lu-J591 for Metastatic CRPC

Following determination of 2.6 GBq/m² as the MTD, a phase II trial was planned to evaluate clinical efficacy and potential toxicity in a larger group of patients [28]. Based upon concerns for patient safety, however, the FDA required that an additional group of patients be evaluated at a slightly lower dose [2.4 GBq (65 mCi)/m²]. Accordingly, the Phase 2 trial consisted of 2 cohorts: cohort 1, 15 patients at 2.4 GBq (65 mCi)/m² and cohort 2,

17 patients at 2.6 GBq (70 mCi)/m². Whole-body planar imaging of the ^{177}Lu-DOTA-J591 was performed to evaluate biodistribution and assess tumor targeting. The primary endpoint was PSA and/or measurable disease response; the secondary endpoint was toxicity. Excellent targeting of known sites of prostate cancer metastases was observed in 30/32 (94%) of patients (Fig. 16.5). Three patients achieved PSA declines of >50% and nine patients (28%) experienced at least 30% decline in PSA. PSA decline of ≥30% in PSA is associated with survival benefits [29, 30]. Of the 15 subjects receiving 2.4 GBq (65 mCi)/m², 7 of 15 (26%) had a PSA decline and 2 of 15 (13%) achieved a 30% PSA decline. Of the 17 subjects receiving 2.6 GBq (70 mCi)/m², 12 (71%) had a PSA decline and 7 (47%) had ≥30% decrease in PSA (Fig. 16.5). Since significant decline in PSA was observed more frequently in the 2.6 GBq (70 mCi)/m² cohort, the results suggest a dose response relationship.

A platelet nadir less than 25×10^9/L occurred in 42% of patients, 9 of whom required 1–4

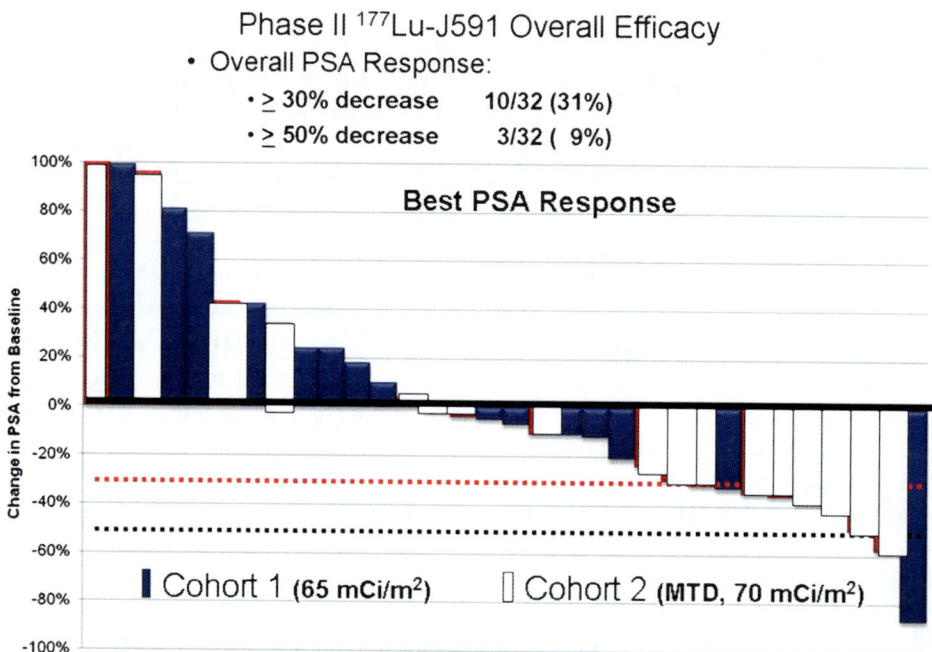

Fig. 16.5 So-called "waterfall plot" of PSA response to ^{177}Lu-J591 in a Phase II study involving 32 patients. Although a previous phase I study had demonstrated that the maximum tolerated dose was 70 mCi/m², the initial 15 patients in this phase II study received 65 mC/m² to further assess safety. Characteristic of studies involving various degrees of tumor burden and tumor aggressiveness, there is a range of responses. Most of the PSA declines >30% (*dotted line*) were in the group that received the 70 mCi/m² dose [43]

platelet transfusions (median=2). Twenty-nine of 32 patients recovered normal platelet counts; the course of the remaining 3 patients was complicated by rapidly progressive disease with bone marrow involvement. Neutropenia $\leq 0.5 \times 10^9$/L occurred in 27% of patients, six of whom received brief therapy with growth factors. All 32 patients had normal neutrophil recovery, and no patient experienced febrile neutropenia. No significant nonhematologic toxicity was observed [28].

In summary, the Phase 2 experience suggested that despite the many variables amongst patients in terms of tumor burden, tumor size, location, and perfusion in addition to the uncharacterized tumor biology at the time of radioimmunotherapy, there was a dose response, in that in general more patients receiving 2.6 GBq (70 mCi)/m^2 responded more vigorously based on decline in PSA than those receiving the slightly lower 2.4 GBq (65 mCi)/m^2 dose.

Nevertheless, the responses in each group varied considerably. This led to a reconsideration of the potential significance of assessing the degree of targeting (fractional dose delivery) to account at least in part for these differences. Although imaging of the radiolabeled antiPSMA antibody tumor uptake was not a primary objective of any of these protocols, a retrospective analysis of the ^{177}Lu-DOTA-J591 images obtained approximately 3 days after infusion was performed based upon visual scoring of uptake compared to lesions identified on skeletal scintigraphy. Twenty-two bone scans were available for comparison. A score from 0 to 3 was assigned as follows: 0=undetectable ^{177}Lu localization; 1=faint activity at sites of known disease; 2=vigorous activity but < liver activity; 3=activity equivalent to liver activity. Four of nine patients scored as 0 or 1 had either stable PSA or at least a significant decline compared to 10 of 13 patients scored as 2 or 3 (Fig. 16.6) [29]. These findings

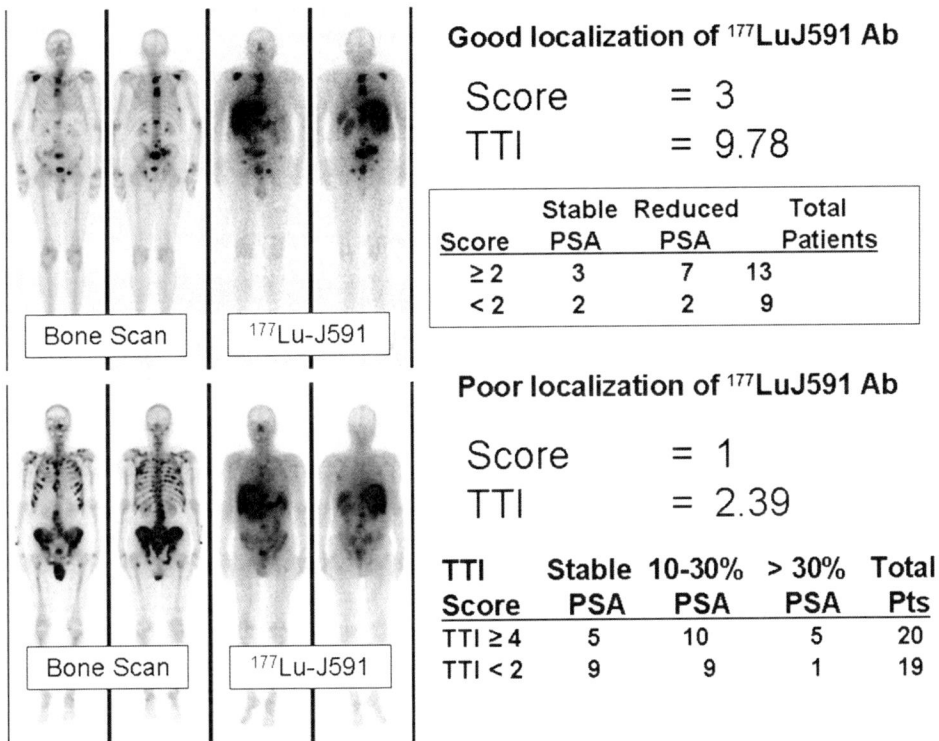

Good localization of ^{177}LuJ591 Ab

Score   = 3
TTI   = 9.78

Score	Stable PSA	Reduced PSA	Total Patients
≥2	3	7	13
<2	2	2	9

Poor localization of ^{177}LuJ591 Ab

Score   = 1
TTI   = 2.39

TTI Score	Stable PSA	10-30% PSA	> 30% PSA	Total Pts
TTI ≥ 4	5	10	5	20
TTI < 2	9	9	1	19

Fig. 16.6 Correlation of PSA response with an improvised method to quantify targeting by comparing ^{177}Lu-J591 images to lesions identified on bone scintigraphy (reference [29]). In general, improved targeting correlated with better responses. Since bone scintigraphy does not assess soft tissue involvement, the utility of this approach is limited to assessing the targeting to osseous metastases [29]

suggested that for patients with an identifiable lesion, an antitumor response as evidenced by stabilization or a decline in serum PSA is related to the vigor of radiolabeled antibody targeting. The problem is complicated, however, by the difficulty in the assessment of tumor burden, extra-osseous as well as micrometastases. Good results in terms of a biochemical response might be expected in individuals without evidence of targeting since micrometastases might not be identified by any of the imaging modalities employed. This assessment of the relationship of tumor targeting, tumor burden, and evidence of response is ongoing.

Clinical Protocols for Evaluation of a Potential Radioimmunotherapy Agent

- Preclinical Assessment of Specificity and Affinity
- Cell Suspensions; Tissue Sections
- Animal Models of Human Tumors
- Phase 1
  - Evaluation of Carrier Effect [Total Protein]
  - Dose Escalation—Identification of MTD
  - Safety Assessment as primary endpoint
- Phase 2
  - Limited Clinical Efficacy at MTD; continued monitoring of safety
- Phase 3
  - Large Clinical Trial per protocol with defined eligibility criteria, endpoints

---

Summary of Completed Trials

In summary, the ^{90}Y labeled J591 Phase 1 trial and the ^{177}Lu-J591 Phase 1 and 2 trials provided evidence that radiolabeled humanized J591 is well tolerated and nonimmunogenic. Radiolabeled J591 effectively targets prostate cancer metastases and results in significant (>30%) decline in PSA values in a subset of patients, all of whom

had entered an aggressive phase of their disease. Dosing of both ^{177}Lu-J591 and ^{90}Y-J591 is limited by reversible and manageable myelosuppression with little nonhematologic toxicity. Patients with metastatic CRPC tolerate anti-PSMA radioimmunotherapy either prior to or after chemotherapy and no long-term effects on bone marrow function have been seen. It was concluded that radioimmunotherapy of CRPC has antitumor effects but even when effective—as measured by either reduction in size of lesions on CT examination or decline in PSA—the disease inevitably progresses.

On-Going Trials

Based on the evidence that targeted radionuclide therapy employing DOTA-J591 as a targeting vehicle did indeed demonstrate antitumor efficacy, several alternative strategies were designed:

1. Explore further whether the degree of targeting of visualizable lesions is predictive of a therapeutic effect.
2. Dose fractionation—evaluate whether repeat dosing at lower dose levels is more advantageous in terms of greater tumor response and less hematologic toxicity [30–32].
3. Combine radioimmunotherapy with best-available, radiosensitizing chemotherapy [33–38].
4. Conduct separate trials in patients at risk for relapse including rising PSA but without demonstrable tumor on diagnostic imaging [39, 40].
5. Pretargeting strategy-involving development of a bi-specific antibody with (at least) one "arm" directed toward the specific epitope and another arm available to bind a carrier molecule that has been radiolabeled and is infused after localization of the bi-specific synthetic immunoglobulin. The molecule carrying the radiolabel is smaller in molecular weight and hence would be cleared more rapidly from the circulation (renal excretion), reducing bone marrow radiation exposure. This approach has been under investigation for years in other tumor systems [41].

Dose Fractionation

A phase I dose escalation trial has been performed to evaluate fractionated doses of ^{177}Lu-J591 administered 2 weeks apart in men with progressive metastatic castrate-resistant prostate cancer. The design of the trial involves cohorts of three patients beginning with a dose of 740 MBq (20 mCi)/m^2 × 2 with subsequent groups of three patients receiving incremental doses of 185 MBq (5 mCi)/m^2 per dose per three patient cohort. The primary endpoint is to determine DLT and the cumulative MTD of fractionated ^{177}Lu-J591 RIT with pharmacokinetics and dosimetry and secondary endpoints of efficacy. DLT is defined as severe thrombocytopenia (platelet count <15 or need for >3 platelet transfusions in 30 days), grade 4 neutropenia, febrile neutropenia, or grade >2 nonhematologic toxicity.

In the initial 28 patients, the median age was 73 years (range 55–86), median baseline PSA 44.7 ng/mL (2–766). Twenty-five of 28 (88%) had bone metastases and 11 (38%) had extraosseous visceral metastases (lung, liver). All patients had progressed after 1–4 hormonal therapies and 47% progressed on 1–4 lines of chemotherapy including docetaxel. Despite cumulative doses exceeding the single-dose MTD (70 mCi/m^2, a dose at which 41% require platelet transfusions), during the dose escalation phase of the multidose regimen, only six patients receiving up to a total dose of 90 mCi/m^2 experienced grade 4 thrombocytopenia (two requiring a transfusion). Three patients experienced grade 4 neutropenia without fever or growth factor intervention. Grade >1 nonhematologic toxicity was rare.

The MTD for the multidose regimen without growth factor is 40 mCi/m^2 × 2. No transfusions were needed at this dose [42]. By planar imaging, accurate targeting of known sites of prostate carcinoma metastases was seen in 82.4%. Including expansion cohorts, 50% overall experienced PSA declines, with 10 of 18 experiencing PSA decline at the currently recommended Phase 2 doses. Twelve of thirteen patients with baseline and follow-up circulating tumor cell counts (Cell Search methodology) had virtual elimination of circulating tumor cells. Median survival is 25.3 months

[95% CI 15.3, 35.3]. In contrast to previous trials with single doses of ^{177}Lu-DOTA-J591, the principle toxicity was leukopenia. The leukopenia was relatively mild and could be managed clinically with granulocyte colony stimulating factor (GCSF) and antibiotics if necessary. As this is not an unusual component in the management of patients with advanced tumors, and since it was observed that the tumors were sensitive to radiation and small increments near the previously encountered MTD in the single dose trial had had a significant effect, it is planned at this time to enroll a small cohort of patients at 45 mCi/m^2 × 2, a level 5 mCi/m^2 above the initially defined MTD for the fractionated dose regimen [42].

Chemo-Radioimmunotherapy

A Phase 1 trial has begun to evaluate the radiosensitizing, tumor bulk-reducing taxane drug docetaxel (75 mg/m^2) every 21 days and prednisone with two doses of ^{177}Lu-J591 in an escalating dose scheme in men with metastatic CRPC who will also be assessed for targeting potential with whole body and SPECT imaging follow ^{111}In-DOTA-J591 infusion prior to initiation of the therapy phase of the protocol.

Treatment of Biochemical Failure

Based upon acceptable toxicity and demonstrated antitumor activity, a multicenter randomized phase II trial in castrate nonmetastatic biochemically progressive disease began accrual recently in which the primary objective is to prevent or delay radiographically evident metastatic disease. Patients with biochemical relapse (elevated absolute PSA and/or rapid doubling time) after local therapy and initial hormonal therapy (testosterone level <50) but no identifiable tumor by traditional imaging procedure will be included. Patients will be randomized to ketoconazole and hydrocortisone with a single infusion of ^{177}Lu-J591 or trace-labeled ^{111}In-J591 (i.e., placebo). Radiolabeled J591 imaging will also be obtained using either the ^{111}In or ^{177}Lu signal. This challenging protocol requires long-term follow-up of large numbers of patients. A Power analysis indicated that 140 patients are needed to detect a 25% absolute difference in progression of disease to the point where it is demonstrable radiographically; hence the initiation of a multicenter trial. This protocol addresses patients with biochemical evidence of relapse and no identifiable source which is perhaps the most common problem confronting urologists and oncologists who are managing patients with this diagnosis. At this time, the trial is ongoing and results are not yet available.

Conclusion

Radioimmunotherapy of prostate carcinoma targeting PSMA is well tolerated and antitumor activity has been demonstrated. Multiple clinical trials are underway to improve patient selection and specific therapeutic protocol designs for the several clinical scenarios experienced by men who develop prostate carcinoma, some of which may be more suitable to radioimmunotherapy than others.

Acknowledgement Research Support: Prostate Cancer Foundation, Department of Defense, National Institutes of Health, David H. Koch Foundation, Yablans Family Foundation.

References

1. Horoszewicz JS, Kawinski E, Murphy GP. Monoclonal antibodies to a new antigenic marker in epithelial prostatic cells and serum of prostatic cancer patients. Anticancer Res. 1987;7:927–35.
2. Israeli RS, Powell CT, Fair WR, Heston WD. Molecular cloning of a complementary DNA encoding a prostate-specific membrane antigen. Cancer Res. 1993;53:227–30.
3. Israeli RS, Powell CT, Corr JG, Fair WR, Heston WD. Expression of the prostate-specific membrane antigen. Cancer Res. 1994;54:1807–11.
4. Wright GL, Haley C, Beckett ML, Schellhammer PF. Expression of prostate-specific membrane antigen in normal, benign, and malignant prostate tissues. Urol Oncol. 1995;1:18–28.
5. Troyer JK, Beckett ML, Wright Jr GL. Detection and characterization of the prostate-specific membrane antigen (PSMA) in tissue extracts and body fluids. Int J Cancer. 1995;62:552–8.
6. Sokoloff RL, Norton KC, Gasior CL, Marker KM, Grauer LS. A dual-monoclonal sandwich assay for prostate-specific membrane antigen: levels in tissues, seminal fluid and urine. Prostate. 2000;43:150–7.
7. Bostwick DG, Pacelli A, Blute M, Roche P, Murphy GP. Prostate specific membrane antigen expression in prostatic intraepithelial neoplasia and adenocarcinoma: a study of 184 cases. Cancer. 1998;82:2256–61.
8. Wright Jr GL, Grob BM, Haley C, et al. Upregulation of prostate-specific membrane antigen after androgen-deprivation therapy. Urology. 1996;48:326–34.
9. Sweat SD, Pacelli A, Murphy GP, Bostwick DG. Prostate-specific membrane antigen expression is greatest in prostate adenocarcinoma and lymph node metastases. Urology. 1998;52:637–40.
10. Bartley S, Alazraki NP, Goldsmith SJ. SPECT/CT imaging for prostate cancer. In: Israel O, Goldsmith SJ, editors. Hybrid SPECT/CT imaging in clinical practice. New York: Taylor & Francis; 2006. p. 141–56.
11. Kahn D, Williams RD, Manyak MJ, et al. 111Indium-capromab pendetide in the evaluation of patients with residual or recurrent prostate cancer after radical prostatectomy. The ProstaScint study group. J Urol. 1998;159:2041–6.
12. Kahn D, Williams RD, Haseman MK, Reed NL, Miller SJ, Gerstbrein J. Radioimmunoscintigraphy with In-111-labeled capromab pendetide predicts prostate cancer response to salvage radiotherapy after failed radical prostatectomy. J Clin Oncol. 1998;16:284–9.
13. Jani AB, Spelbray D, Hamilton R, et al. Impact of radioimmunoscintigraphy on definition of clinical target volume after prostatectomy. J Nucl Med. 2004; 45:238–46.
14. Jani AB, Blend MJ, Hamilton R, et al. Influence of radioimmunoscintigraphy on post prostatectomy radiotherapy treatment decision making. J Nucl Med. 2004;45:571–8.
15. Kahn D, Austin JC, Maguire RT, Miller SJ, Gerstbrein J, Williams RD. A phase II study of [90Y] yttrium-capromab pendetide in the treatment of men with prostate cancer recurrence following radical prostatectomy. Cancer Biother Radiopharm. 1999;14:99–111.
16. Deb N, Goris M, Trisler K, et al. Treatment of hormone-refractory prostate cancer with 90Y-CYT-356 monoclonal antibody. Clin Cancer Res. 1996;2:1289–97.
17. Smith-Jones PM, Vallabhajosula S, Goldsmith SJ, et al. In vitro characterization of radiolabeled monoclonal antibodies specific for the extracellular domain of prostate-specific membrane antigen. Cancer Res. 2000;60:5237–43.
18. Liu H, Moy P, Kim S, et al. Monoclonal antibodies to the extracellular domain of prostate-specific membrane antigen also react with tumor vascular endothelium. Cancer Res. 1997;57:3629–34.
19. Smith-Jones PM, Vallabhajosula S, Navarro V, Bastidas D, Goldsmith SJ, Bander NH. Radiolabeled monoclonal antibodies specific to the extracellular domain of prostate-specific membrane antigen: preclinical studies in nude mice bearing LNCaP human prostate tumor. J Nucl Med. 2003;44:610–7.

20. Bander NH, Nanus D, Bremer S, et al. Phase I clinical trial targeting a monoclonal antibody (mAb) to the extracellular domain of prostate specific membrane antigen (PSMAext) in patients with hormone-independent prostate cancer. Proc Am Soc Clin Oncol. 2000;19:Abstr 1872.

21. Bander NH, Nanus D, Goldstein S, et al. Phase I trial of humanized monoclonal antibody (mAb) to prostate specific membrane antigen/extracellular domain (PSMAext). Proc Am Soc Clin Oncol. 2001;20: Abstr 722.

22. Vallabhajosula S, Goldsmith SJ, Hamacher KA, et al. Prediction of myelotoxicity based on bone marrow radiation-absorbed dose: radioimmunotherapy studies using ^{90}Y- and ^{177}Lu-labeled J591 antibodies specific for prostate-specific membrane antigen. J Nucl Med. 2005;46:850–8.

23. O'Donohue JA, Bardies M, Wheldon TE. Relationship between tumor size and curability for uniformly targeted therapy with beta-emitting radionuclides. J Nucl Med. 1995;36:1902–9.

24. Vallabhajosula S, Goldsmith SJ, Kostakoglu L, Milowsky MI, Nanus DM, Bander NH. Radioimmunotherapy of prostate cancer using 90Y- and ^{177}Lu-labeled J591 monoclonal antibodies: effect of multiple treatments on myelotoxicity. Clin Cancer Res. 2005;11:7195s–200.

25. Vallabhajosula S, Kuji I, Hamacher KA, et al. Pharmacokinetics and biodistribution of ^{111}In- and ^{177}Lu-labeled J591 antibody specific for prostate-specific membrane antigen: prediction of ^{90}Y-J591 radiation dosimetry based on ^{111}In or ^{177}Lu. J Nucl Med. 2005;46:634–41.

26. Milowsky MI, Nanus DM, Kostakoglu L, Vallabhajosula S, Goldsmith SJ, Bander NH. Phase I trial of yttrium-90-labeled anti-prostate-specific membrane antigen monoclonal antibody J591 for androgen-independent prostate cancer. J Clin Oncol. 2004; 22:2522–31.

27. Bander NH, Milowsky MI, Nanus DM, Kostakoglu L, Vallabhajosula S, Goldsmith SJ. Phase I trial of ^{177}lutetium-labeled J591, a monoclonal antibody to prostate-specific membrane antigen, in patients with androgen-independent prostate cancer. J Clin Oncol. 2005;23:4591–601.

28. Tagawa ST, Milowsky MI, Morris M, et al. Phase II trial of ^{177}Lutetium radiolabeled anti-prostate-specific membrane antigen (PSMA) monoclonal antibody J591 (^{177}Lu-J591) in patients with metastatic castrate-resistant prostate cancer (metCRPC). J Clin Oncol. 2008;26:284s; Abstr 5140.

29. Hynecek R, Goldsmith SJ, Vallabahajosula S, Nanus D, Tagawa ST, Bander NH. 177Lu-J591 monoclonal antibody (lu-J591) therapy in metastatic castrate resistant prostate cancer (metCRPC): correlation of antibody-tumor targeting and treatment response. J Nucl Med. 2008;49:144P.

30. DeNardo GL, Schlom J, Buchsbaum DJ, et al. Rationales, evidence, and design considerations for fractionated radioimmunotherapy. Cancer. 2002;94: 1332–48.

31. O'Donoghue JA, Sgouros G, Divgi CR, Humm JL. Single-dose versus fractionated radioimmunotherapy: model comparisons for uniform tumor dosimetry. J Nucl Med. 2000;41:538–47.

32. DeNardo GL, DeNardo SJ, Lamborn KR, et al. Low-dose, fractionated radioimmunotherapy for B-cell malignancies using 131I-lym-1 antibody. Cancer Biother Radiopharm. 1998;13:239–54.

33. Choy H, Rodriguez FF, Koester S, Hilsenbeck S, Von Hoff DD. Investigation of taxol as a potential radiation sensitizer. Cancer. 1993;71:3774–8.

34. Tishler RB, Schiff PB, Geard CR, Hall EJ. Taxol: a novel radiation sensitizer. Int J Radiat Oncol Biol Phys. 1992;22:613–7.

35. Hennequin C, Giocanti N, Favaudon V. Interaction of ionizing radiation with paclitaxel (taxol) and docetaxel (taxotere) in HeLa and SQ20B cells. Cancer Res. 1996;56:1842–50.

36. O'Donnell RT, DeNardo SJ, Miers LA, et al. Combined modality radioimmunotherapy for human prostate cancer xenografts with taxanes and ^{90}yttrium-DOTA-peptide-ChL6. Prostate. 2002;50:27–37.

37. Richman CM, Denardo SJ, O'Donnell RT, et al. High-dose radioimmunotherapy combined with fixed, low-dose paclitaxel in metastatic prostate and breast cancer by using a MUC-1 monoclonal antibody, m170, linked to indium-111/yttrium-90 via a cathepsin cleavable linker with cyclosporine to prevent human anti-mouse antibody. Clin Cancer Res. 2005;11:5920–7.

38. Kelly MP, Lee FT, Smyth FE, Brechbiel MW, Scott AM. Enhanced efficacy of ^{90}Y-radiolabeled anti-Lewis Y humanized monoclonal antibody hu3S193 and paclitaxel combined-modality radioimmunotherapy in a breast cancer model. J Nucl Med. 2006;47:716–25.

39. Moul JW. Prostate specific antigen only progression of prostate cancer. J Urol. 2000;163:1632–42.

40. Scher HI, Eisenberger M, D'Amico AV, et al. Eligibility and outcomes reporting guidelines for clinical trials for patients in the state of a rising prostate-specific antigen: recommendations from the prostate-specific antigen working group. J Clin Oncol. 2004;22:537–56.

41. Sharkey RM, Rossi EA, McBride WJ, et al. Recombinant bispecific monoclonal antibodies prepared by the Dock-and-Lock strategy for pretargeted radioimmunotherapy. Semin Nucl Med. 2010;40: 190–203.

42. Tagawa ST, Vallabhajosula S, Akhtar NH, Osborne J, et al. Phase I trial of fractionated-dose ^{177}Lutetium radiolabeled anti-prostate-specific membrane antigen monoclonal antibody J591 (^{177}Lu-J591) in patients with metastatic castration-resistant prostate cancer (metCRPC). AACR Annual Meeting; 2012; Abstract # 748.

Part II

Radionuclide Therapy of Benign Diseases

Radioiodine Therapy of Benign Thyroid Diseases: Graves' Disease, Plummer's Disease, Non-toxic Goiter and Nodules

17

Cumali Aktolun and Muammer Urhan

Introduction

Thyroid diseases are common in all parts of the world. Hormonal disorders of thyroid gland negatively affect whole metabolism, and cause various health problems while goiter and nodules can cause local, compressive symptoms. Once a correct diagnosis is made, a definitive treatment protocol should be initiated. Medications, surgery, and radioactive iodine are currently the most widely available options. Each treatment option has its own advantages, disadvantages, and limitations. This chapter focuses on the role of radioiodine therapy of benign thyroid diseases. Pertinent information is also provided on the basics of thyroid diseases, thyroid medication, and surgery.

Thyroid, Diseases, and Diagnostic Tools

The thyroid is a hormone secreting gland located superficially in the anterior part of the neck with close proximity to the trachea, larynx, vocal cords,

carotid arteries, jugular veins, recurrent laryngeal nerves, and esophagus. There are two functional cell groups in the thyroid gland: thyrocytes that produce thyroxine (T4) and triiodothyronine (T3), and parafollicular cells (C-cells) that secrete another hormone called calcitonin. The term "thyroid hormones" in this text refers to T3 and T4 only, and does not include calcitonin. At the cellular level, the active form of thyroid hormones is T3; its effects are prompt and short-lived, and these characteristics are therefore exploited in Nuclear Medicine practice during thyroid cancer management.

Acquired benign thyroid diseases include hormonal disorders, goiter, nodules, inflammation, and infection. Prevalence of goiter and thyroid nodules, despite widespread use of iodinated salt, is about 35 % in moderately iodine-deficient countries. The prevalence of hyperthyroidism in the United States is about 1.2 %. Diagnosis of benign diseases is based on the findings on palpation, thyroid ultrasonography, scintigraphy, radioiodine uptake test, fine needle aspiration biopsy, and laboratory tests.

Thyroid ultrasonography using high frequency transducers gives detailed morphological information including the size, volume, and parenchymal echo pattern of the gland, the presence, location, number, vascularity, capsule, size, and internal echo pattern of the nodule and the presence or absence of calcification. It has high spatial resolution; it can detect nodules as small as 1 mm in diameter.

17

C. Aktolun, M.D., M.Sc. (✉)
Tirocenter Nuclear Medicine Center, Istanbul, Turkey
e-mail: aktolun@aktolun.com

M. Urhan, M.D.
Nuclear Medicine Service, GATA Haydarpasa
Teaching Hospital, Istanbul, Turkey
e-mail: muammerurhan@yahoo.com

C. Aktolun and S.J. Goldsmith (eds.), *Nuclear Medicine Therapy: Principles and Clinical Applications*, DOI 10.1007/978-1-4614-4021-5_17, © Springer Science+Business Media New York 2013

Thyroid scintigraphy (thyroid scan) is an essential tool to obtain functional information about the whole gland and also the nodules(s). It is not the ideal tool for the detection of nodules as most of the nodules are normoactive, and the spatial resolution of scintigraphy is much lower than ultrasonography. Although hypoactive (cold) nodules have a higher risk of malignancy, both normoactive and hyperactive nodules also have about a 5 % risk of malignancy. Correlation of ultrasonographic and scintigraphic findings is useful to reveal the functional status and morphological characteristics of the gland and the nodules, if present.

The choice of radiopharmaceutical used for scintigraphy is associated with regional differences mainly due to supply and logistics. Iodine-123 (I-123) is commonly used in North America while technetium-99m (Tc-99m) pertechnetate is preferred in the rest of the world. I-123 has the advantage of giving more physiologic information, which can be exploited in the differentiation of etiologies in thyrotoxicosis.

There is always more than one therapeutic option for almost every patient with benign thyroid diseases. Each option has advantages and disadvantages. The final therapeutic decision should be made after ensuring that the patient is given sufficient, detailed, and comprehensive information about the choices. The priorities, preferences, and wishes of the patients should be respected and given sufficient importance at the decision-making process.

Radioactive Iodine Treatment (RAIT)

Iodine is an essential element for the production of thyroid hormones. Its uptake is regulated by sodium iodide symporter (NIS). Thyroid stimulating hormone (TSH) and amount of available iodine have significant effects on the regulation of iodine uptake through NIS. Radioiodine follows the same metabolic pathway as the "cold" iodine within the thyroid gland. It is rapidly and totally absorbed from the gastrointestinal system,

Table 17.1 Physical characteristics of iodine-131

Physical half-life	8.1 Days
γ Photons	Energy (keV)
Principal γ photon	364
Other γ photons	637
	284
	80
β Particle energy	Energy (MeV)
Average energy	0.192
Maximum energy	0.61
Mean path range	0.4 mm

concentrated in the thyroid gland, oxidized and organified by thyrocytes.

Iodine-131 (I-131) emits β particles and γ photons, and is the only radionuclide used for treatment purposes in thyroid diseases (Table 17.1). I-131 is a β-emitting radionuclide with a physical half-life of 8.1 days; a principal γ ray of 364 keV; and a principal β particle with a maximum energy of 0.61 MeV, an average energy of 0.192 MeV, and a mean range in tissue of 0.4 mm. The β particle energy of I-131 is exploited for therapy, while its γ photons are used for imaging and uptake studies.

In benign thyroid diseases, radioactive iodine treatment (RAIT) is a safe, reliable, and cost-effective tool, and currently utilized in three major clinical situations:

- Treatment of diffuse toxic goiter (Graves' disease)
- Treatment of toxic multinodular goiter and toxic adenomas (Plummer's disease)
- Treatment (volume reduction) of non-toxic goiter and nodules

Hyperthyroidism

Hyperthyroidism is a clinical entity that results from abnormally high synthesis and secretion of thyroid hormones (T3 and T4). Thyrotoxicosis is also used as a synonym but there is a difference between these two definitions (i.e., thyrotoxicosis refers to a clinical condition due to increased thyroid hormone levels of any cause

Table 17.2 Etiology of thyrotoxicosis

Thyroid diseases (hyperthyroidism)
Graves disease (Basedow Graves disease)
Toxic multinodular goiter
Solitary toxic adenoma
Subacute thyroiditis
TSH secreting pituitary adenoma (hyperthyroidism)
Metastatic follicular thyroid carcinoma
Excessive iodine (hyperthyroidism)
Exogenous thyroid hormone
Trophoblastic disease
Struma ovarii

Laboratory in Patients with Subclinical Thyroid Disease

Subclinical hyperthyroidism
 T3: Normal
 T4: Normal
 TSH: Low/suppressed
Subclinical hypothyroidism
 T3: Normal
 T4: Normal
 TSH: Increased

including ingestion of excessive amount of thyroid hormones while hyperthyroidism is due to increased synthesis and secretion of thyroid hormones by a hyperfunctioning thyroid gland or thyroid nodules) (Table 17.2). Thyrotoxicosis affects multiple tissues and organs in the body causing various complaints, clinical signs, and symptoms. The typical laboratory triad of "overt hyperthyroidism" includes increased level of free T4 and T3 and decreased (suppressed) level of TSH. As a general rule, the amount of T3 secreted from the hyperfunctioning gland or thyroid nodules is higher than T4.

Three main causes of hyperthyroidism include *Graves' disease, toxic multinodular goiter,* and *toxic adenoma* (Table 17.2). RAIT is used for the treatment of hyperthyroidism. Other causes of thyrotoxicosis including thyroiditis, high iodine intake, high dose of thyroxin ingestion, TSH producing pituitary adenoma, trophoblastic disease, struma ovarii, and metastatic follicular carcinoma require different treatment methods and thus should be definitely excluded before making a decision about RAIT administration for the treatment of hyperthyroidism.

There is another clinical entity called *subclinical hyperthyroidism*, in which both T4 and T3 levels are within normal range but TSH is suppressed or undetectable. In most cases, subclinical hyperthyroidism occurs in patients with normal thyroid morphology ultrasonographically and scintigraphically, but it can also occur in patients with large goiters and functioning or nonfunctioning nodules.

Table 17.3 Common complaints in thyrotoxicosis

Heat intolerance
Weight loss
Nervousness
Palpitations
Fatigue, weakness
Diarrhea
Increased respiration
Tremor
Hyperactivity
Increased appetite
Menstrual irregularities

Heat intolerance, weight loss, nervousness, and palpitations are cardinal complaints for patients with hyperthyroidism regardless of the underlying cause. Fatigue, weakness, diarrhea, increased respiration, tremor, hyperactivity, increased appetite, and menstrual irregularities are also seen in the majority of patients (Table 17.3).

These complaints are more sudden and severe in Graves' disease than other causes of thyrotoxicosis. The cardiac complaints, symptoms, and signs seen in patients with hyperthyroidism are mainly due to increased adrenergic stimulation. The severity of complaints, signs, and symptoms are not strongly correlated with the level of elevation of thyroid hormones. Hyperthyroidism causes significant changes to the basal metabolic rate, cardiovascular hemodynamics, and neurophysiological function [1, 2]. If untreated, hyperthyroidism can cause osteoporosis, atrial fibrillation, embolic events, heart failure, and death.

a   b

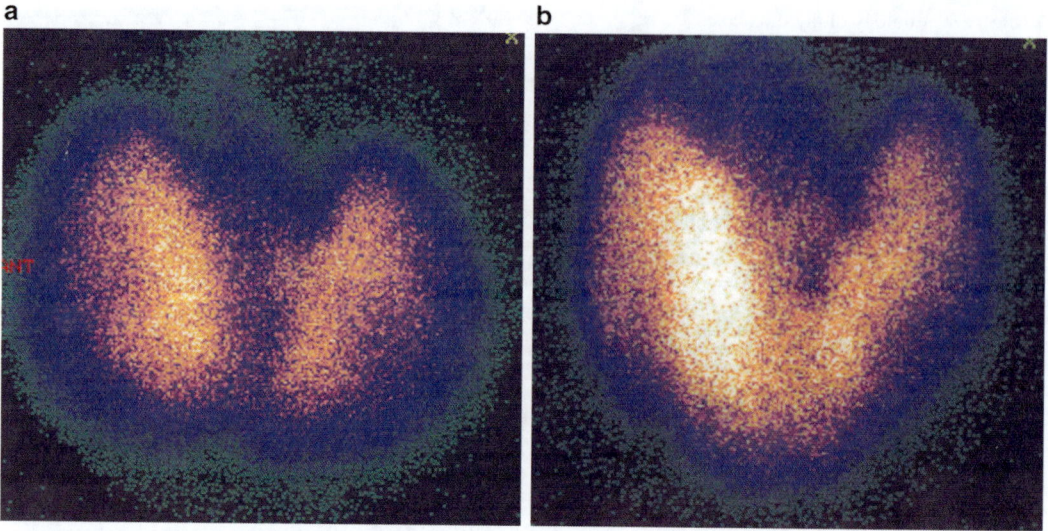

Fig. 17.1 Scintigraphic pattern of Graves' disease: increased parenchymal uptake in a globally hyperfunctioning thyroid gland and decreased background activity. Thyroid gland is enlarged in both patients (**a**, **b**)

Graves' Disease

Graves' disease is also called Basedow disease, Basedow Graves' disease, or Graves' hyperthyroidism. It is mainly an autoimmune disease with significant systemic effects. Smoking is thought by some to trigger several underlying mechanisms. Thyroid autoantibodies are increased in most of the patients. Thyroid autoantibodies include anti-thyroglobulin antibody (anti-tg ab), anti-peroxidase antibody (anti-tpo ab), and anti-TSH receptor antibody, the latter being the most important one in the differential diagnosis of Graves' disease. These autoantibodies play a significant role in the processes leading to hyperfunctioning of thyroid gland and also attack other organs and tissues including eyes (thyroid ophthalmopathy).

The typical laboratory findings consist of high serum levels of T4 and T3, low/suppressed TSH, anti-TSH receptor antibody in Graves disease', and high levels of anti-tg and anti-tpo antibodies in thyroiditis-associated Graves' hyperthyroidism. Iodine uptake studies and diagnostic thyroid scans (both I-123 and Tc-99m pertechnetate scans) reveal globally increased radionuclide uptake in the thyroid gland (hyperfunctioning) and decreased background activity (Fig. 17.1; Tables 17.4 and 17.5).

Table 17.4 RAI uptake test results in hyperthyroid patients

Uptake result	Etiology
Increased uptake	Graves disease
	TSH secreting pituitary adenoma
Moderately increased	Toxic adenoma
Normal uptake	Toxic multinodular goiter
Decreased uptake	Subacute thyroiditis
	Excessive iodine intake
	Exogeneous thyroid hormone

Toxic Multinodular Goiter and Toxic Adenoma

The term "Plummer's disease" is used for either of these entities. The terminology "toxic nodules" and "thyroid autonomy" are also used to refer this clinical situation. In toxic multinodular goiter, there are more than one hyperfunctioning nodule (hyperactive nodule on scintigraphy) within the enlarged thyroid gland (hyperactive nodules in goiter). The term toxic adenoma is, however, a solitary hyperfunctioning nodule in the thyroid gland. The nodules in both cases function autonomously without the control of feedback mechanism, and produce thyroid hormones independently of TSH. TSH receptor stimulating autoantibodies are absent and are not

Table 17.5 Tc-99m/I-123 scintigraphic pattern in thyrotoxicosis

Scintigraphic pattern	Etiology
Homogeneous hyperactive/hyperfunctioning gland (globally increased uptake in the thyroid) with lack of background activity	Graves' disease
Multiple foci of increased uptake in a heterogeneous, enlarged gland with decreased background activity	Toxic multinodular goiter
Focally increased uptake with suppression in the rest of the gland with lack of background activity	Toxic adenoma
Diffusely decreased thyroid uptake with increased background activity	Subacute thyroiditis
Increased or normal homogeneous uptake	TSH secreting pituitary adenoma
Decreased uptake/totally suppressed gland with increased background activity	Excessive iodine intake
	Exogenous thyroid hormone

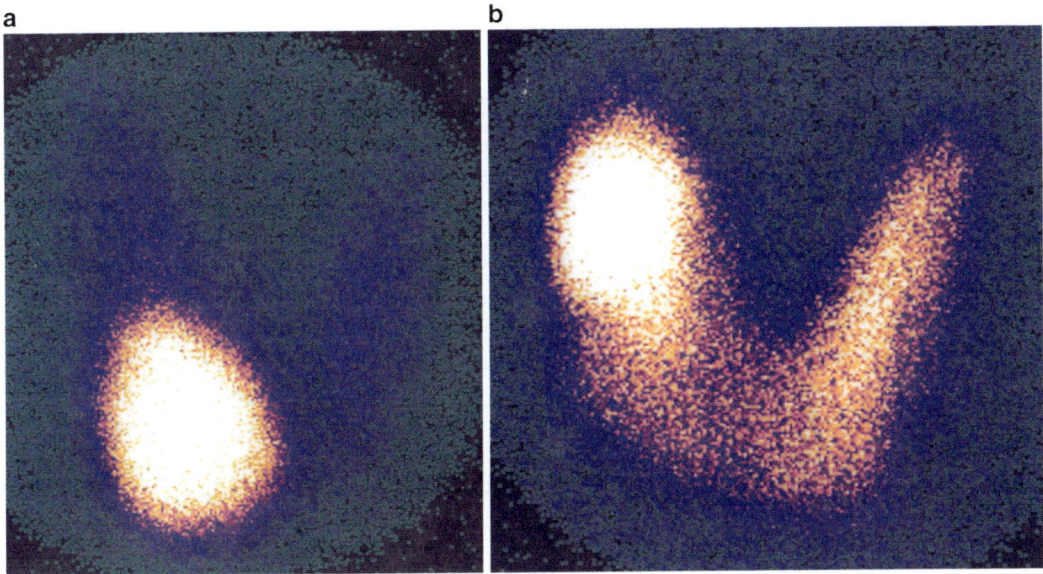

Fig. 17.2 Scintigraphic appearance of toxic adenoma. (**a**) Focally increased circumscribed uptake in the hyperfunctioning (hyperactive, *hot*) autonomous nodule in the lower pole of the right lobe and parenchymal suppression (significantly decreased or almost absent radionuclide uptake) in non-nodular thyroid tissue (TSH: < 0.005 mIU/L). (**b**) Hyperfunctioning nodule in the upper pole of the right lobe and moderately decreased but not totally suppressed uptake in non-nodular thyroid parenchyma (TSH: 0.2 mIU/L). Decreased background activity is evident on both scans

the cause of hyperfunctioning of thyrocytes in these nodules. These nodules secrete excessive amounts of T3 and T4 causing overt or subclinical hyperthyroidism.

This type of hyperthyroidism is common in iodine-deficient regions and countries. The prevalence of toxic nodular goiter and toxic adenoma increases with age. Toxic nodules are associated with somatic mutations of thyroid hormone-regulating genes. Hyperfunctioning nodules escape the normal thyroid-hypophysis-hypothalamus feedback mechanism, and function autonomously causing suppression of radionuclide uptake in the rest of thyroid parenchyma (thyroid autonomy). Typical scintigraphic pattern consists of increased, focal circumscribed uptake in the hyperfunctioning nodules (hyperactive nodules, *hot* nodules), parenchymal suppression (decreased or absent radionuclide uptake) in non-nodular thyroid tissue and decreased background activity (Fig. 17.2). If these nodules remain untreated for a long time and the nodule(s) are large enough, secondary atrophy of the non-nodular thyroid tissue can be seen, possibly due to suppressed TSH for a long time.

The clinical signs and symptoms of hyperthyroidism seen in patients with toxic multinodular goiter and toxic adenomas are generally less severe than Graves' disease. In some patients with hyperfunctioning nodules, serum T4 levels can be normal, T3 high, and TSH suppressed; this is called "T3-toxicosis." This condition is generally seen as an early sign of the autonomous thyroid nodular disease.

Hyperactive nodules incidentally detected on thyroid scan without clinical and laboratory signs and symptoms of hyperthyroidism are not uncommon. Serum thyroid hormones and TSH levels can be normal in a significant number of patients with hyperfunctioning nodules. These patients can also be treated with radioiodine.

Non-toxic Goiters and Nodules

Goiter is the global enlargement of thyroid gland. It is also called thyroid hyperplasia. It is generally in the form of diffuse hyperplasia but can contain nodules in diffusely hyperplasic parenchyma: diffuse goiter or nodular or multinodular goiter. This clinical entity is common in iodine-deficient regions, but can be seen in other parts of the world without iodine deficiency.

Patients are generally euthyroid, but it is not uncommon to see hypothyroid or subclinical hypothyroid patients with non-toxic goiter and nodules. Subclinical hyperthyroidism can also develop at a later stage in a euthyroid patient when the gland becomes larger. Some of the normoactive nodules may convert to hyperactive nodules in long term.

Patients are generally asymptomatic, but when the gland is large enough, it can cause local mechanical compressive symptoms and cosmetic concerns (Fig. 17.3). Scintigraphic pattern consists of inhomogeneous activity distribution in an enlarged thyroid gland. If there is accompanying hypothyroidism, scintigraphic uptake can be higher due to increased TSH (Fig. 17.4).

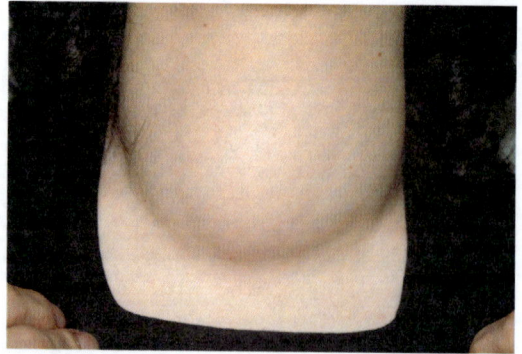

Fig. 17.3 Picture of a patient with large non-toxic multinodular goiter causing compressive symptoms and cosmetic concerns

Treatment Options for Graves' Disease

Anti-thyroid drugs (methimazole, carbimazole, propylthiouracil) in combination with β-blockers are used to maintain euthyroid status. They are used in high doses in the first few weeks to control hyperthyroidism, and then reduced according to the serum levels of T4, T3, and TSH. Graves' disease cannot be cured permanently with these drugs, but they temporarily reduce thyroid hormone synthesis and render the patient euthyroid for a period of time until spontaneous remission. They should not be used for a period longer than 1 year. If hyperthyroidism persists or relapse occurs after 1 year, RAIT or surgery should be performed.

After discontinuation of anti-thyroid drugs, relapse should be expected, and depends on the *patient's age* (relapse is seen in a shorter interval in younger patients), *volume of the thyroid gland* (relapse or persistence of hyperthyroidism is more frequent in larger goiter), and serum levels of *autoantibodies* (high serum levels of antibodies pose a risk of early relapse and persistence). Significant side-effects include reduction in low white counts (agranulocytosis can be seen) and increase in liver transaminase enzymes (FDA recently issued an alert regarding multiple cases of fulminant hepatic necrosis due to propylthiouracil use) [3].

Surgery reveals a permanent result and involves in removing almost all of the thyroid tissue (near total thyroidectomy). The end-result

a

b

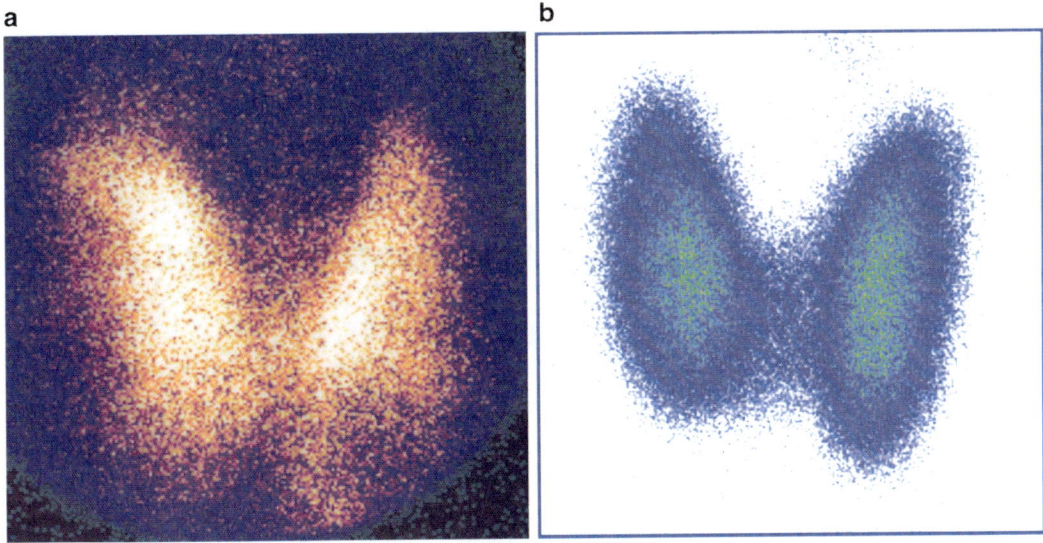

Fig. 17.4 Scintigraphic appearance non-toxic goiter. (**a**) Heterogeneous distribution of Tc-99m pertechnetate in a euthyroid patient with an enlarged thyroid gland. (**b**) Homogeneously increased uptake in a patient with an enlarged thyroid gland and subclinical hypothyroidism

is generally hypothyroidism requiring rapid initiation of thyroxin supplementation. Although in experienced hands the risk is low, *recurrent laryngeal nerve injury, accidental removal of parathyroid glands, bleeding, and anesthetic risk* are the significant (but rare) side-effects associated with surgery [4–8]. It has, however, the advantage of removing incidental malignancies (microcarcinomas). If there is a suspicious nodule in the thyroid, fine needle aspiration biopsy is required to exclude malignancy before RAIT. Normoactive or hypoactive nodules and malignancy are not uncommon clinical conditions in patients with Graves' disease, actually probability of malignancy in patients with Graves' disease is higher than most of other benign thyroid diseases for the treatment of Graves' disease [9]. Surgery is more widely performed in Europe, probably due to strict regulations restricting the use of sufficiently high activity of radioiodine on out-patient basis and the requirement of hospitalization.

RAIT in Graves' Disease

The main aim of RAIT is to stop production and secretion of thyroid hormones permanently rendering the patient hypothyroid. Some practi-tioners aim to achieve euthyroidism and to avoid the subsequent hypothyroidism mainly using lower activities of radioiodine but this effort usually results in persistence of hyperthyroidism or relapse. The aim of RAIT has therefore been controversial, but the American Thyroid Association has clearly defined in its 2011 guidelines this aim as "to render the patient hypothyroid."

Since thyroid gland is enlarged in most of the patients with Graves' disease, volume reduction is another merit of radioiodine treatment (Fig. 17.5). The decrease in serum levels of autoantibodies in long term following RAIT is also helpful in stabilizing the clinical symptoms of the patients and improvement of thyroid eye disease, if present [10].

RAIT can be administered in hyperthyroid patients of all ages including children [11]. It should not be used in pregnant or breastfeeding/lactating women. In Europe, it is almost a constant rule to administer RAIT after the use of anti-thyroid medications for 1 year. If hyperthyroidism persists or relapse occurs after 1 year despite good compliance of patients with the anti-thyroid drugs regimen, radioiodine or surgery is then indicated. In North America, however, RAIT is generally the primary tool for treatment of Graves' disease. It is used at an earlier stage than in Europe.

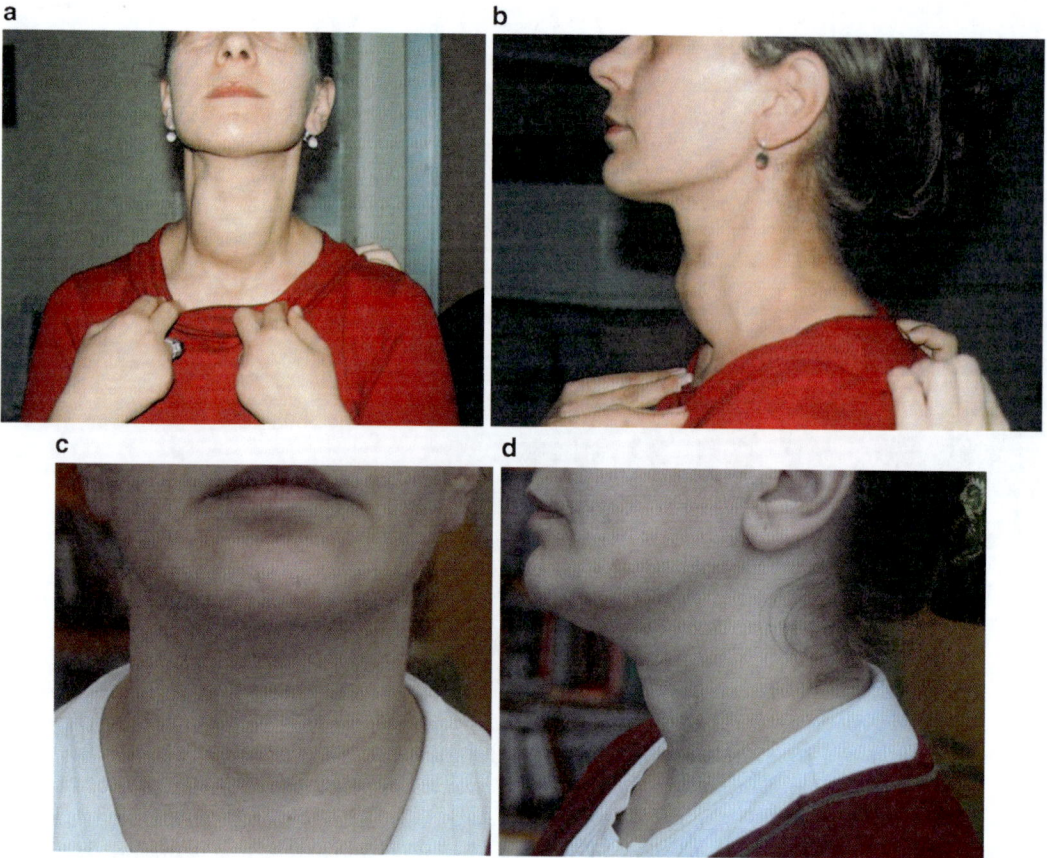

Fig. 17.5 Graves' disease treated with RAIT in a 31-year-old woman. (**a**, **b**) Pictures of patient's neck; front and left lateral views before RAIT in 2003. (**c**, **d**) Pictures of patient's neck; front and lateral views after RAIT in 2011, representing "*radiosurgical effect*" of RAIT

As a general rule, if the patients have *large goiter*, at a *young age* and/or the *high autoantibodies*, the decision to use RAIT can be made earlier since these patients have higher risk of persistence of hyperthyroid status and earlier relapse [12].

of experienced thyroid surgeon, contraindication and allergy to anti-thyroid drugs. Patients, who prefer RAIT, give priority to the prompt, permanent control of hyperthyroidism and avoidance of surgery and side-effects of anti-thyroid drugs.

Risks of Failure for RAIT
• Very large goiter (larger than 200 gr)
• Young age
• High thyroid autoantibodies

RAIT Is Used as the First Choice If One of the Clinical Situations Given Below Is Noted in Patient's History
• Surgical risk due to comorbidities
• Previous external irradiation of neck
• Previous thyroid or neck surge ry
• Absence of experienced thyroid surgeon
• Contraindication or allergy to anti-thyroid drugs

RAIT can be the sole modality of treatment for patients with increased *surgical risk due to comorbidities; previous external irradiation of neck, previous thyroid or neck surgery; absence*

Treatment Options for Toxic Multinodular Goiter and Toxic Adenoma

The possibility of malignancy should be definitely excluded before any treatment is initiated in patients with toxic nodules. Fine needle aspiration under ultrasonographic guidance is the most reliable method for this purpose.

Anti-thyroid drugs (methimazole) are rarely preferred in these patients. If chosen, it can be used for a short term until a decision is made for a definitive treatment with radioiodine or surgery. Either short- or long-term use of anti-thyroid drugs will not cure the main pathology (i.e., the hyperfunctioning nodules), but may alleviate the hyperthyroid symptoms and complaints of the patient temporarily, particularly when combined with β receptor blockers. Anti-thyroid drugs can be used for long term only if the patients are not eligible for surgery or RAIT.

Surgery should be the first-line treatment for these patients if there is a suspicion of malignancy. Also, if the nodules are large enough to cause local compressive symptoms, surgery is preferred even in the absence of malignancy because the shrinkage of large nodules takes a long time after RAIT. In addition, it should be noted that nodules larger than 100–120 mL are difficult to treat with radioiodine and frequently require re-treatment [13–15]. The surgical methods consist of selectively removing the hyperfunctioning nodule (i.e. enucleation), lobectomy or isthmusectomy for solitary toxic nodules or subtotal thyroidectomy or near total thyroidectomy or total thyroidectomy for toxic multinodular goiter depending on the number, size, and location of the nodules and the volume of the goiter [16–19]. But, recurrence of hyperfunctioning autonomic nodules in long term is more frequent than RAIT (10–12 % vs. 2–5 %), when significant amount of thyroid tissue is left in the thyroid bed in surgical operation (e.g., enucleation). On the other hand, enucleation results in hypothyroidism much less frequently than RAIT. Surgery is also associated with significant side-effects and complications including laryngeal nerve injury and accidental removal of parathyroid glands. Hypothyroidism is rapid and thyroxin dependency after near total or total thyroidectomy is 100 %. Hypothyroidism is less severe after subtotal thyroidectomy (usually T3 and T4 levels are normal, TSH is high subclinical hypothyroidism), but thyroxin supplementation is still needed in these patients.

Radioiodine Treatment in Toxic Multinodular Goiter and Toxic Adenomas

Focal uptake in the nodule(s) and relative or complete suppression in the rest of the thyroid parenchyma (autonomy) are typical finding on thyroid scintigraphy in the presence of TSH suppression, and constitute the base of the decision for RAIT in patients with toxic multinodular goiter and toxic adenoma (Fig. 17.6). The goals of RAIT are to achieve euthyroidism and volume reduction, although hypothyroidism is inevitable in some (contrary to Graves' disease, not all) of the patients. If TSH is suppressed at the time of RAIT, the non-nodular parenchyma is relatively protected, but, due to *"cross-fire effect"* from the radioiodine accumulated in the hyperfunctioning nodule(s), the suppressed non-nodular parenchyma also absorbs significant amount of radiation resulting in temporary or permanent hypothyroidism.

If the hyperfunctioning autonomous nodule exists for a long time, the non-nodular thyroid tissue develops secondary atrophy, most probably due to long-term TSH suppression secondary to high amount of thyroid hormones secreted from this hyperfunctioning nodule. It is not uncommon to see during long-term follow-up the increase in volume and the recovery of function in the "normal," non-nodular parenchyma due to increasing TSH after the ablation of hyperfunctioning nodule with RAIT (Fig. 17.7).

There is no consensus on the threshold volume of an autonomic nodule for the patient to receive RAIT.

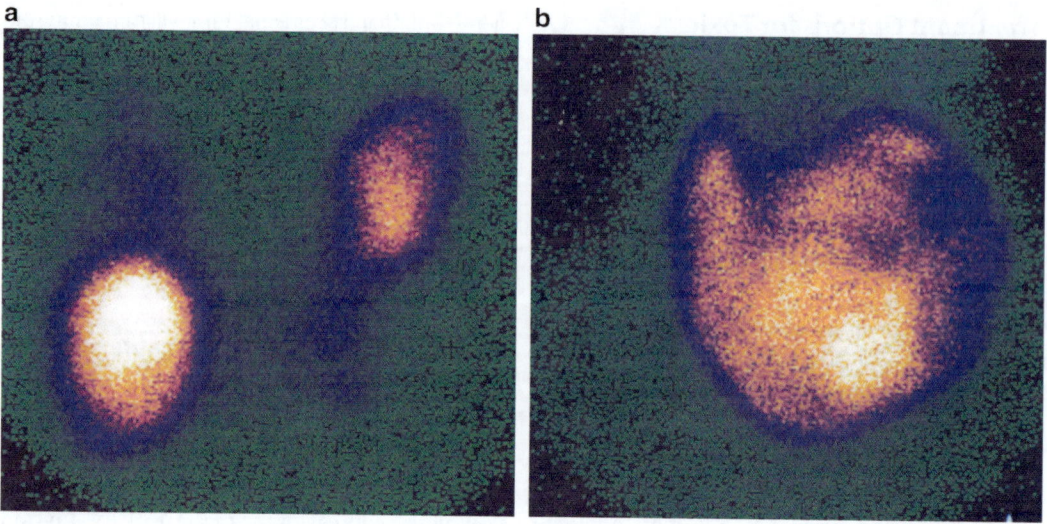

Fig. 17.6 Plummer's disease. (**a**) Tc-99m pertechnetate thyroid scan showing two foci of increased uptake in the lower pole of the right lobe and the upper pole of the left lobe corresponding to two autonomous toxic nodules in a 56-year-old man with subclinical hyperthyroidism (thyroid scan was performed as a part of diagnostic work-up of atrial fibrillation). (**b**) Thyroid scan in a 63-year-old hyperthyroid man with a large autonomous hyperactive nodule (toxic adenoma) in the left lobe of the thyroid. Non-nodular thyroid tissue in the ipsilateral and contralateral lobes and isthmus is totally suppressed in both patients. Note the absence of background activity on both scans. Right lobe and isthmus were almost totally atrophied on ultrasonographic examination (data not shown)

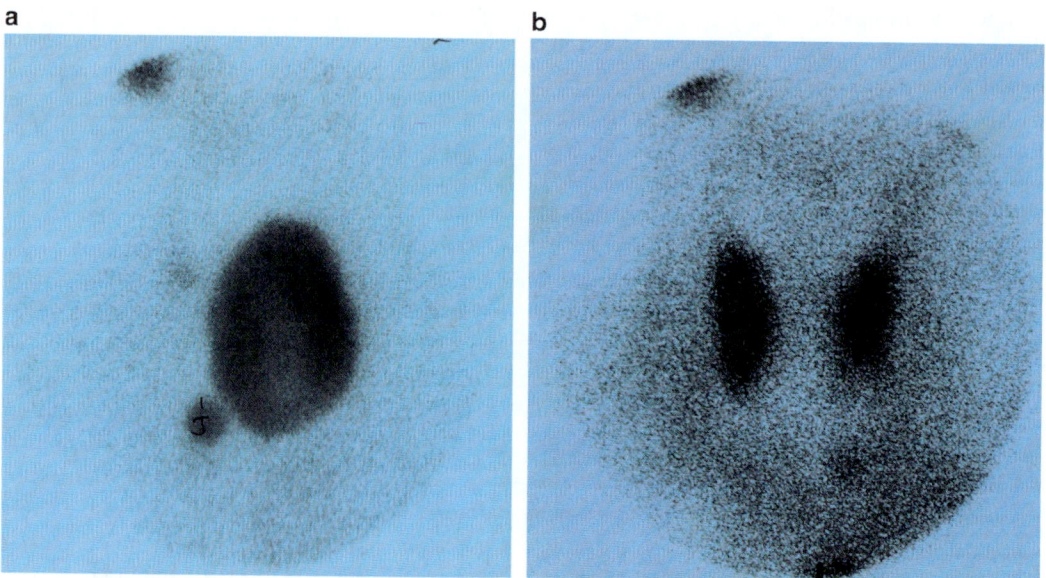

Fig. 17.7 Toxic adenoma treated with 23 mCi (851 MBq) I-131 in a 52-year-old hyperthyroid woman. (**a**) Thyroid scan before RAIT shows a hyperactive autonomous nodule in the left lobe and total suppression in the rest of the gland and lack of background activity. (**b**) Thyroid scan taken 11 months after RAIT shows total disappearance of functional uptake in the nodule which showed moderate shrinkage on ultrasonography (data not shown) and recovery of functional uptake in non-nodular thyroid tissue in right and left lobes. The shrinkage of the adenoma as a response to RAIT was moderate on ultrasonography but the functional response was maximum both in the adenoma (disappearance) and the non-nodular thyroid tissue (recovery)

a

b

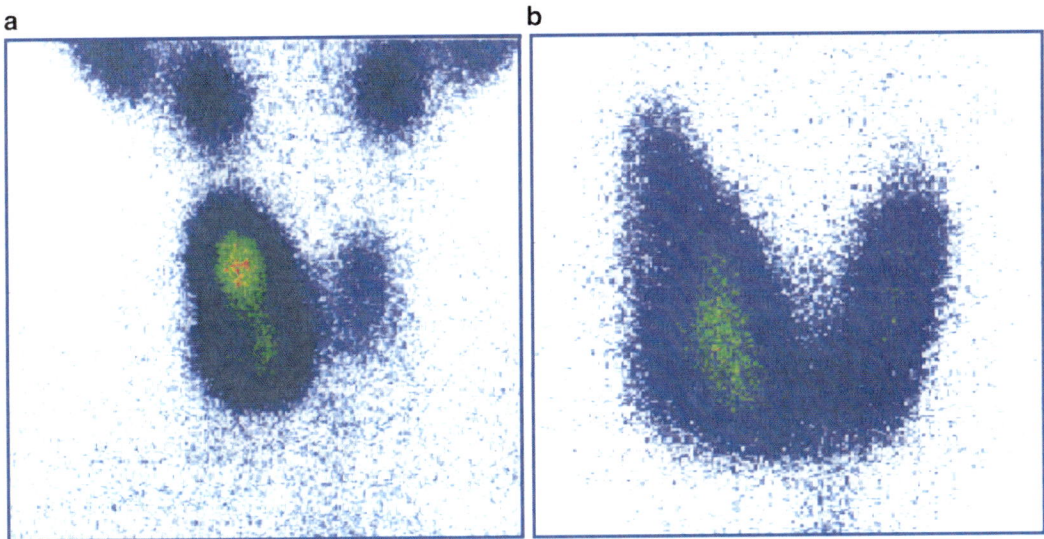

Fig. 17.8 Toxic adenoma in the right lobe in a 71-year-old hyperthyroid woman treated with 19 mCi (703 MBq) I-131. (**a**) Thyroid scan before RAIT showing thyroid autonomy in the right lobe and significant suppression and atrophy in the left lobe. (**b**) Thyroid scan performed 18 months after RAIT showing significant decrease in the nodular uptake in the right lobe and functional recovery in the extra-nodular thyroid tissue both in right and left lobe. Note the moderate increase in the size of the left lobe

An excessive amount of "cold" iodine intake in a patient with mildly hyperfunctioning nodule may cause a diagnostic challenge as TSH is suppressed in these patients, and thyroid scintigraphy shows suppression in the whole gland causing false-negative results. Thyroid scintigraphy should be repeated in these patients after a 2-week low iodine diet (Fig. 17.9).

It is not uncommon to detect hyperfunctioning nodule(s) and coexistent normoactive and/or hypoactive nodules in the same patient. After definite exclusion of malignancy in all nodules through fine needle aspiration biopsy, the hyperfunctioning nodules in these patients can be treated by RAIT. Presence of coexistent normoactive and/or hypoactive nodules is not thus a contraindication for RAIT of hyperfunctioning nodules.

Although use of low-dose anti-thyroid drugs before RAIT is advised by some reports to avoid the risk of hyperthyroidism [20], our recommendation is otherwise as a suppressed level of TSH is always more protective for non-nodular thyroid tissue and anti-thyroid drugs usually cause some increase in serum TSH level. Increased level of TSH as a result of anti-thyroid drug use causes higher uptake of radioiodine in the non-nodular thyroid tissue. The clinical control of hyperthyroidism should be done through the use of β receptor blockers if worsening of thyroid status is a strong possibility and in the presence of cardiac risks, particularly in patients older than 60 years. The thyroid autoantibodies are generally not increased in patients with Plummer's disease, but may be increased after RAIT.

Compared to the Graves' disease thyroid, a higher radiation absorbed dose is needed to achieve a satisfactory clinical response and/or "ablation" of hyperfunctioning nodules. Although higher activity of radioiodine is used for RAIT in Plummer's disease, the rate of post-RAIT hypothyroidism is lower in comparison to Graves's disease because the remainder of the thyroid gland is suppressed and thus protected at the time of RAIT. The expected therapeutic results are disappearance of hyperthyroidism, shrinkage of hyperfunctioning nodules, and recovery of "suppressed" non-nodular thyroid tissue. The evidence of recovery from suppression is the visualization of non-nodular thyroid tissue on post-treatment thyroid scan (Fig. 17.8).

Thyroid autoantibodies can be elevated in patients with multiple hyperfunctioning nodules after RAIT probably due to entering of significant amount of antigenic fragments from destructed thyrocytes into systemic circulation while some argue that this may be due to preexistent or coexistent Graves' disease [21].

The probability of hypothyroidism following RAIT depends on the radiation absorbed dose and the recovery of non-nodular thyroid tissue. It can be as low as 3–5 % in 1 year, but it can rise to 65–70 % in long term [13–15, 22–25]. Long-term follow-up is therefore important after RAIT for the detection of hypothyroidism in time [26].

Treatment Options for Non-toxic Goiter and Nodules

"Cold" iodine has been used alone to treat goiter without nodules, and is still used in some parts of the world. TSH suppression using *thyroxin* tablets is the most commonly used treatment modality to control the enlargement of thyroid gland. None of these choices result in definite control of thyroid enlargement and volume reduction in the long term, and they may also be associated with side-effects.

Surgery is commonly used if there is a suspicion of malignancy, cytological diagnosis of follicular neoplasia, very large gland, presence of one or more benign hypoactive nodules, and the presence of compressive signs. It has the advantage of allowing histologic examination, which may incidentally discover microcarcinomas. It is the most radical method of volume reduction but has the risk of serious side-effects including laryngeal nerve injury resulting in vocal cord paralysis and hypoparathyroidism. Thyroxin replacement is needed in almost all of the patients as currently the most preferred surgical technique is the removal of most of the thyroid tissue removed by surgery (near total thyroidectomy). If the amount of tissue is limited, recurrence is high requiring second surgical intervention, which carries much higher risk of side-effects including laryngeal nerve injury and vocal cord paralysis.

RAIT in Non-toxic Goiter and Nodules

The main aim of RAIT in these patients is to relieve compressive symptoms by volume reduction in the enlarged thyroid gland and/or nodules. If the patient has recurrence of goiter with or without nodules after surgical treatment, RAIT is the treatment of choice as second surgery has about tenfold higher risk of laryngeal nerve injury and vocal cord paralysis [27, 28]. Also, in patients with coexistent cardiac disease, diabetes, and similar risks, which make anesthesia and surgery more risky, RAIT should be preferred as the first-line treatment. RAIT is less commonly used in this group of patients than those with Graves' or Plummer's disease. In some countries, it is not yet an absolute indication for RAIT.

If there is any nodule larger than 1 cm, fine needle aspiration biopsy should be carried out and the presence of malignancy be definitively excluded before RAIT.

Since the uptake is not as high as Graves' disease, the patients should be given a strict iodine deficiency diet at least for 2 weeks before RAIT (Fig. 17.9). Hypothyroidism is not uncommon in these patients, and thus very high uptake mimicking Graves' disease can be seen due to high TSH (Fig. 17.10). Thyroxin supplement should be discontinued in these patients 2–3 weeks before RAIT. Although high TSH levels result in higher uptake as most of the thyroid tissue is "normoactive" or has a mixed hypoactive and normoactive appearance on thyroid scan, the avidity for radioiodine is not as high as that seen in Graves' disease or Plummer's disease (Fig. 17.11). It is not uncommon to see relatively low uptake, mostly due to a partly suppressed TSH level in patients with large thyroid gland. Recombinant TSH can be used in these patients to increase TSH level and radioiodine uptake, allowing the use of lower amount of radioactivity [29, 30].

If the thyroid is extremely voluminous, a larger amount of radioiodine activity should be given. If the amount of activity is high and the volume of thyroid gland is very large, the total activity can be divided [31]. Each treatment session should be at least 3 months apart from each other.

a

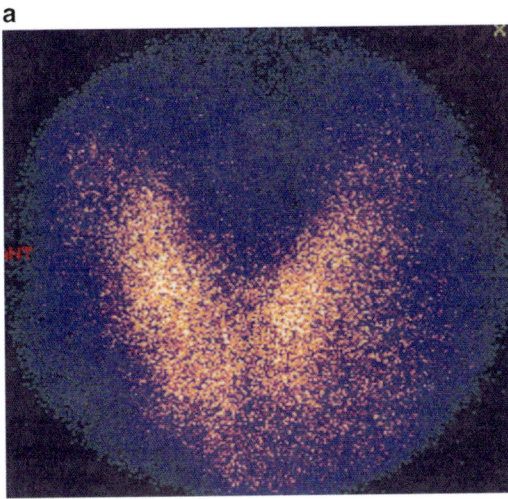

b

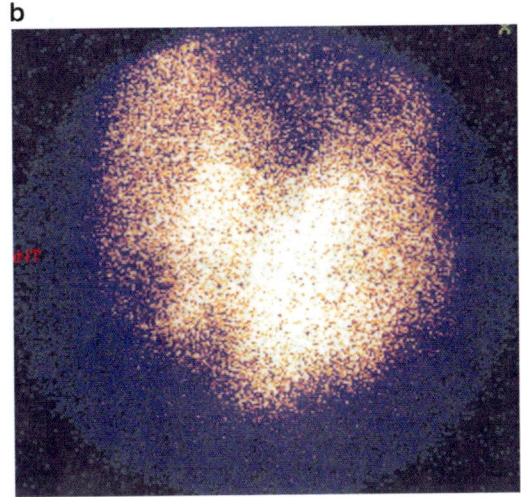

Fig. 17.9 Effect of low iodine diet on Tc-99m thyroid scan. (**a**) Uptake is moderately low in a patient with sub-clinical hyperthyroidism on thyroid scintigraphy performed as a part of pre-RAIT work-up. (**b**) The scan was repeated after a 14-day low iodine diet. Notable increase in the global thyroid uptake is seen on the repeat scan

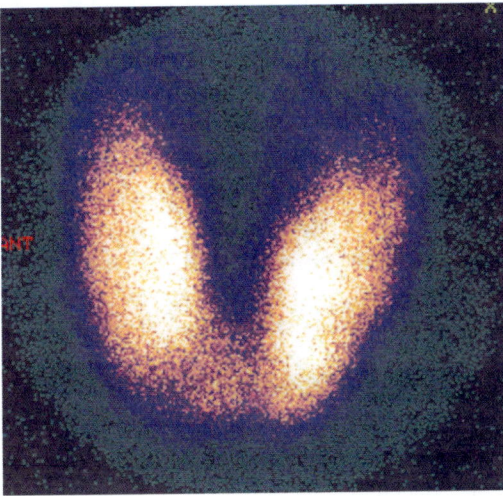

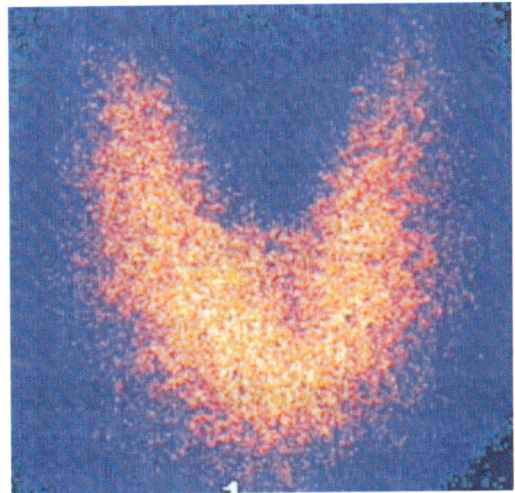

Fig. 17.10 Increased uptake in subclinical hypothyroidism. Thyroid scan of a 41-year-old woman with non-toxic goiter showing increased uptake mimicking Graves' disease

Fig. 17.11 Thyroid scan of a 33-year-old woman with non-toxic diffuse goiter. The uptake is not low, but notably heterogeneous. The serum thyroid stimulating hormone (TSH) level was 3.9 mIU/L

Preparation of Patients for RAIT

When a patient is diagnosed with hyperthyroidism, iodine intake should be restricted to augment the efficiency of anti-thyroid drugs and to reduce the severity of the hyperthyroid symptoms. This will also lead to increased radioiodine uptake in the thyroid allowing the administration of lower radionuclide activities if RAIT is chosen.

The success of RAIT regardless of indication lies in proper preparation of the patients. First rule is to reduce the iodine intake before RAIT regardless of the thyroid disease to be treated.

Measurement of urinary iodine excretion is a reliable tool to estimate the iodine intake of the patients, but due to high turnover of iodine within the thyroid and the body in hyperthyroid patients, the iodine excretion is lower in most of these patients, and thus may be misleading for the treating physician about the patient's iodine intake.

Although low iodine diet is a vital part of preparation for RAIT, it is not possible to completely isolate the patient from iodine. There are several protocols to reduce the iodine intake of the patients, but there is no standardization on this issue. Each department has its own protocol.

Low Iodine Diet
(Restricted food and medications)

- Iodinated salt
- Seafood
- Chinese, Japanese, and Far-East foods containing seaweed
- Pizza and other foods colored with red dye
- Food supplements containing kelp, seaweed, or iodine
- Radiologic contrast agents containing iodine
- Amiodarone, multivitamins, and medications containing iodine

---

Major source of iodine ingestion originates from the consumption of iodinated salt and seafood. A written instruction of preparation containing a list of "restricted" foods and drinks should be given to the patient after clearly explaining it verbally.

Also, there is no consensus on the time interval for low iodine diet before RAIT; we recommend that it should be initiated 14 days before RAIT although earlier initiation (i.e., at initial diagnosis) for hyperthyroid patient is recommended to relieve symptoms.

The written instruction for preparation should be written in plain, simple language. A detailed history of the patient should be taken about the recent administration (within the last 3 months) of iodinated contrast agents commonly used for diagnostic radiology procedures. Use of amiodarone, an anti-arrhythmic medication within 1

year before RAIT can also interfere with uptake of therapeutic iodine.

Anti-thyroid drugs, particularly propylthiouracil can increase radio-resistance and can interfere with the iodine uptake function of thyroid gland. If these drugs cannot be discontinued due to the risk of "thyroid storm," the dose should be reduced to a minimum.

If a combination of simultaneous use of antithyroid drugs and thyroid hormones is given to the patient (some practitioners prefer this combination in hyperthyroid patients), at least the thyroid hormones have to be discontinued before RAIT. The withdrawal of anti-thyroid drugs induces higher uptake, longer retention time, and higher radiosensitivity. There is no consensus on the time interval between the RAIT administration and the day of withdrawal of anti-thyroid drugs. While discontinuation of anti-thyroid drugs 3–5 days before the RAIT administration is found to be sufficient to obtain an optimal iodine uptake [32], we recommend to discontinue at least 7 days (2 weeks, if they have been taken for a long time) before the administration of radioiodine as these drugs can significantly interfere with the iodine uptake of thyrocytes [33–35]. Each patient should be handled individually and the decision should be based on the patient's age, presence, absence, and severity of hyperthyroidism, risk of coexistent diseases including cardiac diseases. If re-initiation of anti-thyroid drugs is needed after RAIT, it should be postponed 3–4 days after the administration of radioiodine.

If a patient receives thyroxin (a common treatment regimen in patients with non-toxic goiter and nodules) before RAIT, it would be useful to withdraw thyroxin medication at least 2–3 weeks before RAIT in order to increase TSH. Use of thyroxin also depresses iodine uptake function of thyroid gland and nodules. While high pretreatment serum TSH level is helpful to increase global thyroid uptake of radioiodine in patients with Graves' disease and non-toxic goiter or nodules, it should be avoided in patients with toxic nodules before RAIT. High serum TSH levels due to use of anti-thyroid drugs before RAIT in patients with solitary or multiple toxic nodules cause unnecessary irradiation of non-nodular thyroid tissue resulting in hypothyroidism.

Some experts propose to use iodine ingestion or thyroxin supplementation to suppress TSH before RAIT in patients with toxic nodules, but we suggest otherwise due to possible side-effects of these medications in these patients and propose to wait after discontinuation of anti-thyroid drugs until TSH is suppressed by secretion of thyroxin from these hyperfunctioning nodule(s), if hypothyroidism is a real concern.

Use of hydroclorothiazide before RAIT may increase the effect of iodine-deficient diet and thus induces higher radioiodine uptake. Currently, this method is not commonly employed in routine practice.

In Graves' disease, RAIT can be administered when the patient is hyperthyroid. Use of radioiodine when the patient is hyperthyroid is actually one of the benefits of RAIT over surgery. Due to the risk of thyrotoxicosis and thyroid storm, use of β receptor blockers with strong peripheral effects (i.e., propranolol) can protect against the effects of worsening of hyperthyroidism after RAIT administration. RAIT administration is therefore safe under β blocker protection even in hyperthyroid patients.

Fine needle aspiration biopsy should be performed before RAIT in all patients with thyroid nodules larger than 1 cm in size. Each and every nodule should be aspirated under ultrasonographic guidance to exclude malignancy if RAIT is chosen as the primary therapeutic modality.

A detailed history should be taken and local thyroid examination should be performed when the patient is referred for RAIT. The treating physician has the medico-legal responsibility to obtain a negative pregnancy test result (preferably a serum-based pregnancy test consisting of measuring β human chorionic gonadotropin-β-HCG) performed within the last 24 h before RAIT in each female patient within the reproductive age interval. Pregnant patients should not receive RAIT. In addition, the treating physician should assess the ability of the patient to follow the radiation protection instructions before making the final decision for RAIT. The presence of fecal and urinal incontinence should be definitely clarified.

Administration of RAIT

It is recommended by some (but not all) groups that the patient fasts at least 6 h in order to avoid interference with the gastrointestinal absorption of radioiodine. It is the Nuclear Medicine physician's responsibility to administer the therapeutic radioiodine to the patient under safe and optimal conditions. Universal radiation protection rules must be followed strictly during the administration. Radioiodine should be given to the patient by the treating Nuclear Medicine physician or under his/her responsibility and supervision by a well-trained technician or technologist. There should be a designated area with restricted access for the administration of radioiodine.

The patient should be given clear information about the procedure, expected therapeutic result, possible side-effects, and long-term follow-up. A written informed consent should be signed by the patient and the guardians, if the patient is of minor age or has medically documented mental incapacity.

Preference between an oral capsule and liquid form of I-131 depends on the choice of treating physician, departmental bias, availability of capsule form, and the cost concern. Liquid form is less expensive and more easily available, but the liquid form is associated with potentially higher radiation exposure to the treating medical staff. Some also argue against the use of liquid form based on concerns about higher radiation burden to the salivary glands and oral cavity as a result of direct exposure and also residual activity in the mouth. This view is not shared by all since the radioiodine is swallowed rapidly and eventually taken up and secreted by salivary glands after ingestion through blood circulation.

Water should be sipped after the ingestion of radioiodine of either liquid or capsule form of I-131. If the liquid form of radioiodine is used, a careful survey of the administration area where the treatment is administered should be carried out by the radiation physicist to identify any contamination. A record of the survey should be maintained. RAIT should be administered in a designated and licensed area in the Nuclear Medicine department.

Issues After RAIT

The patients should be given written and verbal instructions about the measures that should be taken in order to maintain an optimal therapeutic response, to prevent side-effects, and also to avoid unnecessary radiation exposure to the other members of the family and the public. The radiation protection measures for the close relatives who will live in the same dwelling with the treated patient should be addressed in these instructions. Presence of young children or pregnant woman in the house where the treated patient will stay creates significant concerns and thus taking appropriate, individualized radiation protection measures should become a priority for the therapy team.

Salivary stimulation by sipping lemon juice, chewing gum, or fruity candies is traditionally recommended for all patients to protect the salivary glands but some argue against these measures and claim that these can actually increase radiation burden to these glands, particularly if started in first hours of RAIT.

We recommend that the patient should keep fasting for at least 1 h after the ingestion of RAIT in order to maintain fast and maximum absorption. Patients should continue low iodine diet at least 3–4 days after RAIT.

The patient is allowed to go home if the activity of radioiodine and/or the radiation emitted by the patient does not exceed the locally allowable dose limits. If the activity is higher, then the patient should be hospitalized in accordance with the local and national regulations until the radiation emission from patient's body surface decreases to the locally allowable limits.

Outpatient administration of RAIT is encouraged, as the nursing services and the requirement of a shielded room for the hospitalized patient are logistically complicated. Staying in a hotel or in similar public accommodations after receiving RAIT is not recommended.

The allowed amount of activity of radioiodine and the radiation measured from patient's body surface after RAIT administration vary significantly in different parts of the world. Currently, the strictest country in relation to allowable radiation dose limit is Japan, followed by the countries that belong to European Union while currently most flexible country in this respect is Canada. The situation in the USA used to be as flexible as Canada, but due to the recently increased public concern and unsubstantiated movements against radioiodine treatment resulted in stricter rules in this country. According to current rules in the USA, any adult member of the public should not be exposed to a radiation level higher than 0.5 mSv (500 mrem), and the patient on discharge should not emit equal to or higher than 7 mrem/h at 1 m.

Patients who plan to travel soon after RAIT should be warned about the radiation detectors at the airports and the borders. If the patient plans to fly or cross the border of another country within a month after RAIT, a letter should be written explaining that the patient has received radioactive iodine for therapeutic purposes. Even very tiny amounts of radioactivity can trigger these detectors, which can even lead to detention of the patient.

Importance of Assessment of Radionuclide Thyroid Uptake Before RAIT

Radioiodine uptake is routinely used in most centers before RAIT in order to determine the therapeutic activity and predict the outcome of RAIT. If the uptake is high, the result of RAIT is favorable no matter what the iodine status of the patient and thyroid hormone levels are at the time of RAIT. The probability of hypothyroidism due to the use of high doses of anti-thyroid drugs before RAIT increases therapeutic radioiodine uptake of the thyroid following discontinuation of the anti-thyroid drugs. If the diagnosis of Graves' disease is based on clear evidence, but the uptake of thyroid gland is low, uptake measurement should be repeated after a 2-week strict low iodine diet.

Activity Versus Dose

Activity in Nuclear Medicine refers to the number of milliCuries (mCi) or MegaBequerels (MBq) of radioiodine ingested while the "dose" in therapeutic sense refers to the quantity of radiation absorbed in Grays (Gy) by the thyroid tissue. It is, however, not uncommon to see the amount of activity and radiation absorbed dose used interchangeably to mean the amount of radioiodine.

The Radioiodine Activity to Be Used for RAIT

Amount of activity to be used for RAIT is a controversial issue, and depends on several criteria including the type of benign thyroid disease to be treated. The amount of radioactivity used to treat patients is a function of radioiodine uptake of thyroid gland, efficient half-life of radioiodine in the gland, and the size of the thyroid tissue to be destructed.

The main question is whether to use a fixed (empiric) activity or an individually adjusted amount of activity based on absorbed dose calculation (calculated dosage). The thyroid radiation absorbed dose is determined by the amount administered, the thyroidal uptake and the volume of thyroid tissue to be treated as well as by the effective half-life of the I-131 in the thyroid. Dosimetric or non-dosimetric calculations are employed for determining individual activity for each patient. These calculations depend mainly on a predetermined target absorbed dose, thyroid volume/weight, and radioiodine uptake in 24 h. Dosimetric calculations are not yet universally standardized.

The aim of search for a precise method of dose calculation or estimate is to avoid unnecessary irradiation of the patient. There is no method of dose calculation or activity estimate for protecting patients from post-treatment hypothyroidism. The main difference between low activity RAIT and higher ablative activity of RAIT is that ingestion of lower activity is associated with more frequent relapse, but, if a permanent result (unavoidable hypothyroidism) is obtained, a lower dose of thyroxin replacement is still needed, and a lifelong dependency to thyroid tablets is still inevitable. Despite meticulous dosimetric methods, it is not yet possible to determine an amount of radioiodine for RAIT to render the patient permanently euthyroid [36–40].

In some patients with Graves' disease, a preliminary euthyroid status can be achieved in early months of RAIT, but in long-term follow-up inevitable hypothyroidism, at least subclinical hypothyroidism still requires the physician to prescribe thyroxin replacement. As a result, the current, increasingly accepted trend in Graves' disease is to use higher ablative activity of RAIT or to perform a near total thyroidectomy surgically. This trend guarantees a resultant hypothyroid status starting in earlier weeks but relapse and persistence of hyperthyroidism are almost completely avoided. Nevertheless, highly elaborative methods to induce euthyroidism are still studied and reported, which mainly consist of a combination treatment with low activity radioiodine and low-dose anti-thyroid drugs. Although a lower number of patients with resultant hypothyroidism were reported with this approach, there are still a significant number of patients with post-RAIT hypothyroidism and also there are no convincing long-term follow-up results yet [41].

> **Clinical Conditions Requiring Larger Amount of Activity**
>
> - Rapid radioiodine turnover/short effective half-life
> - Repeat therapies
> - Pediatric patients
> - Coexistent ophthalmopathy
> - Large multinodular goiter
> - Large diffuse toxic goiter

Generally, larger amount of activity is needed in patients with *nodular goiter, very large toxic diffuse goiter, rapid iodine turnover*, and for *repeat therapies* and *pediatric patients*.

Graves' Disease

Fixed (Empiric) Activity: Standard, fixed activity of radioiodine used for the treatment of Graves' disease varies between 5 and 30 mCi (185–1,110 MBq). A more precise approach is to calculate the amount of activity by glandular volume; activity per gram of thyroid tissue to be destructed. An amount of activity based on 50–200 µCi/g of thyroid tissue is sufficient to render a patient with Graves' disease hypothyroid, but the difference between 50 and 200 is so great that it requires the treating physician to use his/her experience and skills to find the optimal amount of activity in each patient individually taking into consideration the radioiodine uptake measurements, the amount of target volume in grams calculated by ultrasonography, duration of disease, use of previous anti-thyroid drugs, presence or absence of thyroid ophthalmopathy and patients' age.

A target radiation absorbed dose of 70 Gy for uncomplicated Graves' disease is preferred by some practitioners to achieve euthyroidism and avoid hypothyroidism. As a general rule, lower activities result in higher rate of treatment failure (persistence and relapse of hyperthyroidism, worsening of thyroid eye disease), delayed onset of hypothyroidism, less severe degree of hypothyroidism but still require lifelong thyroxin use. The choice of amount of activity mainly depends on patient's age, serum levels of thyroid hormones, levels of autoantibodies, duration of disease, presence or absence of previous RAIT treatment, relapse, previous use of anti-thyroid drugs, thyroid-related eye disease, and thyroid surgery.

Calculated Activity: A target absorbed radiation dose of 250 Gy is expected to be sufficient for ablative effect of hyperfunctioning thyroid gland in a middle-aged patient with moderately high level of thyroid hormones, antibodies, uptake value, short duration of disease, moderate volume of thyroid gland, and short-term use of anti-thyroid drugs. This is an estimate only in an ideal setting, and the activity and expected absorbed radiation dose should be calculated in each patient individually taking all relevant clinical parameters into consideration. As a general rule, higher activities (up to 300 Gy or higher) should be used in patients with ophthalmopathy to obtain a fast therapeutic result, cause extensive destruction of thyroid tissue, reduce the amount of antigenic tissue substances, render the patient hypothyroid in a short time, and to initiate thyroxin supplementation as early as possible, which results in further atrophy in antigenic thyroid tissue.

The amount of activity is generally accepted as an ablative dose for whole thyroid gland, and provides a quick destruction of thyrocytes and significant shrinkage of diseased thyroid parenchyma. This collateral therapeutic result (i.e., volume reducing effect) of RAIT can be termed as "*radiosurgical effect.*"

Toxic Multinodular Goiter and Toxic Adenoma

Fixed (Empiric) Activity: Radioiodine uptake in Plummer's disease is variable and is not as homogeneously high as Graves' disease. Thyroid glands with larger volumes require higher activity. Compared to Graves' disease, higher activities are needed to ablate toxic multinodular goiter.

For toxic multinodular goiter, 20–30 mCi for whole gland or 150–200 µCi I-131/g of thyroid tissue to be ablated corrected for 24 h radioiodine uptake is recommended to obtain an efficient therapeutic result, and to control hyperthyroidism in a reasonably short time [42]. This amount of activity is higher than that needed for the treatment of Graves' disease as discussed above. Pretreatment with thiamazole was found to be useful in increasing TSH, radioiodine uptake, and therapeutic efficacy but results in unnecessary irradiation of non-nodular thyroid tissue, and is thus controversial after RAIT [20]. Pretreatment with recombinant TSH may cause worsening of hyperthyroidism and thus is not recommended [42].

For solitary toxic adenoma, 15–25 mCi for the targeted hyperfunctioning nodule or 150–200 µCi I-131/g of thyroid tissue to be ablated corrected for 24 h radioiodine uptake is necessary, and usually it can be treated at one time [43]. Progressive hypothyroidism develops over time regardless of activity adjustment for nodule size [25]. Administering RAIT with suppressed TSH is recommended to protect the non-nodular thyroid tissue.

Calculated Activity: Estimates of radiation dose absorbed by the target tissue (hyperfunctioning nodule) is more useful in predicting response. A target dose of 300–400 Gy absorbed by the target tissue in a patient with single autonomic nodule is sufficient to obtain a response rate of higher than 95 % while the corresponding dose is

150–200 Gy for patients with multiple toxic nodules. An absorbed dose of 100–120 Gy for toxic multinodular goiter may result in less frequent hypothyroidism but more frequent treatment failure.

In the presence of smaller but multiple hyper-functioning nodules, absorbed doses as low as 80–250 Gy can be efficient and result in lower irradiation of the surrounding "normal," non-nodular thyroid tissue.

If high levels of doses cannot be delivered at one time due to radiation protection issues and patient discharge limitations, the aimed dose can be divided. For voluminous and highly hyper-functioning nodules, a lower dose should be pre-ferred on first application and the whole dose should be divided and given in multiple sessions.

Non-toxic Goiter and Nodules

Fixed (Empiric) Dose: Compared to Graves' dis-ease, the uptake is low and heterogeneous in patients with non-toxic goiter. The activity to be used is determined based on the volume to be ablated and the level of uptake.

Some recommend to use a simpler formula consisting of ingestion of 100 μCi/g of enlarged thyroid corrected for 24-h radioiodine uptake. If the thyroid volume to be ablated is so high that an activity higher than 1 GBq is needed, then the total activity should be administered in two ses-sions, which should be at least 3–4 months apart from each other. Longer period of time between two treatment sessions can be necessary for some patients in order to avoid the effects of "stunning."

These estimates should, however, be individu-ally modified for each patient considering multi-ple laboratory and clinical parameters. High serum TSH level before RAIT is helpful to obtain higher uptake in thyroid gland allowing to admin-ister lower activity of radioiodine. Obtaining high TSH levels by discontinuation of thyroxin sup-plementation and a strict iodine restricted diet is vital to have a satisfactory volume reduction and to administer lower doses. Pretreatment injection of recombinant TSH is an option to obtain high circulating TSH levels before RAIT for a higher therapeutic success rate [44–46].

Calculated Activity: Although published data are limited in RAIT of non-toxic goiter and nodules, a target absorbed dose of 100 Gy is recommended for a satisfactory volume reduction in most of the patients with non-toxic goiter.

In order to decrease the probability of post-treatment hypothyroidism, lower target absorbed doses are recommended by some practitioners: for adult patient 7,000 cGy for uncomplicated Graves' disease, 10,000–12,000 cGy re-treatment of Graves' disease, 10,000–12,000 cGy for toxic multinodular goiter, 15,000–20,000 cGy for toxic adenoma. These doses are lower than those rec-ommended above, and a higher probability of treatment failure, need for re-treatment, and relapse should be expected.

RAIT in Patients with Thyroid Eye Disease

Graves' ophthalmopathy, thyroid ophthalmopa-thy, and Graves' orbitopathy are also used in the same meaning. It is an inflammatory disease of the orbital structures seen in patients with current or past Graves' disease. Smoking is a risk factor and also a predictor of therapeutic response. In a significant number of patients, it can be the first sign of Graves' disease. It can be temporary and is expected to improve after the definitive treat-ment of Graves' disease, but it is not uncommon to see that the thyroid eye disease persists life-long or even deteriorates after the treatment of Graves' disease. The risk of developing Graves' ophthalmopathy after RAIT is between 15 and 30 % while the same risk for anti-thyroid drugs and surgery is 10 % and 16 %, respectively [47]. The risk is higher for smokers regardless of the modality of treatment [48].

It is a common judgment that thyroid ophthal-mopathy deteriorates after RAIT and thus these patients should be treated by surgery. The reason for worsening of eye disease just after RAIT is associated with post-treatment hypothyroidism and increasing serum level of autoantibodies [10, 32, 49, 50]. In nonsmokers, this worsening is thus reversible and temporary, and can be overcome to some extent by avoiding hypothyroidism through prompt initiation of thyroxin supplementation and corticoids. In smokers, the worsening of eye disease is more frequent and severe. It should be noted that Graves' ophthalmopathy may also develop anytime during or after anti-thyroid drug treatment and after surgery in Graves' disease.

If the patient has thyroid eye disease, a quicker and sharper therapeutic effect is needed in order to avoid rapidly increasing serum levels of autoantibodies due to slow destruction of thyrocytes [32]. Higher radioiodine activity is thus recommended. If lower activity of radioiodine is used, slow release of antigens from destructed thyrocytes can cause deterioration. Also, in these patients, earlier initiation of thyroxin replacement is recommended as hypothyroidism after RAIT can cause deterioration of eye disease.

Short-term and preferably low-dose corticoid use can be added to RAIT protocol starting day 1 after RAIT in nonsmokers or smokers with mild or inactive thyroid orbitopathy. In long-term follow-up, it is expected that the thyroid eye disease improves, probably due to decreased antigenic stimulus.

Although hypothyroidism and autoantibodies have definitive role, smoking is a stronger risk factor for developing Graves' ophthalmopathy and also worsening of the eye disease after RAIT [51, 52]. Corticoids should be given to smokers with active, severe ophthalmopathy if they are treated with radioiodine [32].

No form of Graves' ophthalmopathy is a contraindication for RAIT [32]. The activity of ophthalmopathy should be first determined before making any decision about RAIT. The American Thyroid Association recommends radioiodine therapy, surgery, or anti-thyroid drugs equally for the treatment of Graves' disease in patients with inactive and mildly active Graves' ophthalmopathy [32]. In active and severe cases of thyroid ophthalmopathy in patients with Graves' disease, surgery or anti-thyroid drugs (methimazole) is the first choice [32, 53], but RAIT can be administered with corticoids if RAIT is preferred.

As a general rule for RAIT in patients with Graves' ophthalmopathy, the amount of activity of radioiodine should be high and the supplementation of thyroxin should be initiated at an early stage before hypothyroidism becomes evident and severe.

RAIT in Subclinical Hyperthyroidism

Some experts propose low-dose anti-thyroid drug protocols for the treatment of subclinical hyperthyroidism, while others recommend β blocking agents and no anti-thyroid drugs. In recent years, however, RAIT is equally recommended for the treatment of subclinical hyperthyroidism. The most recent American Thyroid Association recommends to treat patients with subclinical hyperthyroidism like the patients with overt hyperthyroidism [32].

Changes in Serum Levels of Autoantibodies and Thyroglobulin After RAIT

Serum levels of thyroid autoantibodies can increase in early stages (in the first 1–6 months), but decrease gradually later due to decreased circulating antigens [47–50]. Thyroglobulin is high in almost all patients with Graves' disease despite high levels of anti-thyroglobulin antibody. It is our observation that the serum level of thyroglobulin increases in early stages after RAIT and decreases in long term, and may become undetectable in a significant number of patients in due course while the serum level of anti-thyroglobulin antibodies increases in early stages after RAIT and decreases in long term (unpublished data).

RAIT in Pediatric Patients

Pediatric Graves' Disease: American Thyroid Association recommends RAIT or thyroidectomy in pediatric patients if anti-thyroid drugs (methimazole) therapy fails to achieve a remission in 1–2 years. This medication should be discontinued 3–4 days before RAIT [32]. β blockers can be added to this protocol. Anti-thyroid drug use after RAIT can cause severe hypothyroidism as the decrease in serum thyroid hormone levels is expected as early as 1 week after RAIT without any anti-thyroid drug use. Hypothyroidism develops 2–3 months after RAIT in about 95 % of patients [11, 54–57].

Since the goal is the same as in adult patients (rendering the patient hypothyroid), sufficiently high amount of radioiodine should be given to ablate the thyroid tissue and control hyperthyroidism with a single dose [11]. Instead, lower amount of activities result in higher amount of partially irradiated residual thyroid tissue, which carries the risk of developing nodules and malignancy at a later stage.

The therapeutic activity should therefore be higher than 150 µCi/g of thyroid tissue [32]. If the gland is large (larger than 50 g), higher activities (200–300 µCi/g of thyroid tissue) are recommended for total ablation of pediatric thyroid. The volume of thyroid should be calculated ultrasonographically. Although the pediatric thyroid tissue is highly radiosensitive, it is not uncommon to see relapse of hyperthyroidism if suboptimal amount of activities is used. Calculated activity based on volume and radioiodine uptake allows the use of optimal amount of activities, although there is no study comparing the results of fixed and calculated activities.

Radiation protection measures should be followed more strictly both by the patients and by the families since saliva, urine, and stool are all contaminated by radioiodine for several days after RAIT. Proper diapering and bagging of urine and stool should be done in accordance with the local radiation safety regulations.

The risk of developing secondary malignancies including leukemia is theoretical only. There is no scientific proof showing any increased risk of thyroid cancer or secondary malignancies in pediatric children treated with radioiodine. The theoretical concerns about thyroid cancers and secondary malignancies after exposure to radioiodine result from the studies on the detrimental effects of radiation from nuclear fallout after Hiroshima atomic explosion and the Chernobyl nuclear accident [32]. It should be remembered that the children in those incidents were exposed to other radionuclides in addition to I-131 and the level of radiation absorbed from radioiodine was much lower than that used for therapeutic purposes. Exposure to lower amount of radioiodine activities is associated with greater risk of thyroid malignancy [57–61] as the thyroid tissue is irradiated but not destroyed. Also, iodine deficiency is a contributing factor for developing thyroid cancer when exposed to low level of radioiodine as seen in the comparison of Chernobyl (occurred in an iodine-deficient region) and Hanford nuclear accidents (occurred in iodine replete region).

Short-Term Interventions After RAIT

Short-term use of anti-thyroid drugs just after RAIT administration can be helpful in controlling the existing hyperthyroidism in patients with Graves' disease and to prevent thyroid storm due to release of excessive thyroid hormones from destructed follicles. Anti-thyroid drugs should be given to the patients only in whom the symptoms of hyperthyroidism cannot be controlled with β blockers. Patients should not take anti-thyroid medications in the following day after RAIT administration.

Low dose of "cold" iodine ingestion and administration of lithium were reported to prolong the half-life of radioiodine, but this approach is associated with serious side-effects [32]. Corticoids are recommended during the first 4 weeks after RAIT in patients with thyroid ophthalmopathy.

Corticoids can also be used to prevent thyroid storm in high-risk patients. Thyroxin supplementation just after RAIT is not recommended to prevent the detrimental effects of resultant hypothyroidism before the first follow-up visit as it can cause iatrogenic hyperthyroidism in the first weeks following RAIT. Instead, the first follow-up visit should be arranged for an earlier date to detect hypothyroidism at an early stage.

Although it is a rare clinical condition after RAIT, tracheal compression should be taken seriously, and thus patients should be advised to report immediately any signs and symptoms of compression including neck tightening, breathing difficulty, swelling, dysphagia, hoarseness, and stridor. Corticoids can alleviate major signs and symptoms, but if there is respiratory compromise, the patient should be handled and categorized as an acute case of tracheal compression.

Therapeutic Effect After RAIT

Graves' Disease: The expected therapeutic effect is the resolution of hyperthyroidism and reduction of thyroid volume. Resolution of hyperthyroidism can start as early as 2 weeks following the RAIT administration but the radiosensitivity of thyroid gland in each patient can differ, which determines the onset of therapeutic effect. In children and patients with young age, thyroid is highly radiosensitive while in older patients and those with a history of long-term use of anti-thyroid drugs before RAIT, a delayed therapeutic response should be expected. Larger glands and higher autoantibodies also can cause delayed therapeutic effect and even therapeutic failure. Generally, hypothyroidism is expected 4 weeks after RAIT but becomes evident 2–6 months after radioiodine ingestion. Decision about treatment failure should not therefore be made before 6 months.

It is important to detect subsequent hypothyroidism as early as possible. Thus, the first follow-up visit of the treated patient should not go beyond 1 month while patients with thyroid ophthalmopathy should be seen earlier (i.e., 2 weeks following RAIT) and the hypothyroidism in these patients should be more energetically treated by thyroid hormone replacement.

Toxic Multinodular Goiter and Toxic Adenomas: The therapeutic effect is the shrinkage of hyperfunctioning nodules, disappearance of hyperthyroidism, relief of compressive symptoms, and recovery of previously suppressed non-nodular thyroid tissue. If the non-nodular thyroid tissue has developed atrophy due to long-lasting hyperfunctioning nodules, the chance of the recovery of non-nodular tissue is slim even in long term.

Hyperfunctioning nodules, compared to Graves' disease, show a slower therapeutic effect. The control of hyperthyroidism is slow and can take months, and also the onset of hypothyroidism can take years. Volume reduction as

an indicator of therapeutic response is also slow and particularly in patients with large nodules, the expected shrinkage is limited to 30–50 % in the size of hyperfunctioning nodules. Volume reduction continues as long as 2 years after RAIT.

In some patients with mild hyperthyroidism (generally subclinical hyperthyroidism), worsening of thyrotoxicosis can be witnessed in the first follow-up results. If overt hyperthyroidism persists, the use of β blockers and anti-thyroid drugs is recommended. Although hypothyroidism should be expected in patients treated for their Plummer's disease, it is not as frequent, fast, and severe as seen in patients with Graves' disease.

If TSH is high before RAIT in patients with solitary hyperfunctioning nodules due to previous use of anti-thyroid drugs, the risk of the ablation of non-nodular thyroid tissue and the risk of hypothyroidism are high. Suppressed TSH before RAIT is therefore preferred in these patients in order to have a "pinpoint" ablation of hyperfunctioning nodule(s) and to save the non-nodular thyroid tissue and to avoid hypothyroidism.

Goiter: Net therapeutic effect is the global shrinkage of the thyroid gland and the nodules in it. Hypothyroidism is not uncommon but less severe and seen at a later stage than Graves' disease. Volume reduction continues as long as 2 years after RAIT.

Follow-Up

The time interval between RAIT and first follow-up visit differs greatly based on the primary indication for RAIT, patients' clinical status and associated cardiac risks and presence of comorbidities including diabetes mellitus. Also, the frequency of follow-up visits varies in different parts of the worlds. Generally, the first visit is planned for 1 month after RAIT to detect the early effects of radioablation and also signs of possible radiotoxic effects. Second visit should be no longer than 3 months. Hypothyroidism can be severe in most of the patients, and thus should be avoided to protect the patients from the serious detrimental effects of low thyroid hormones, particularly

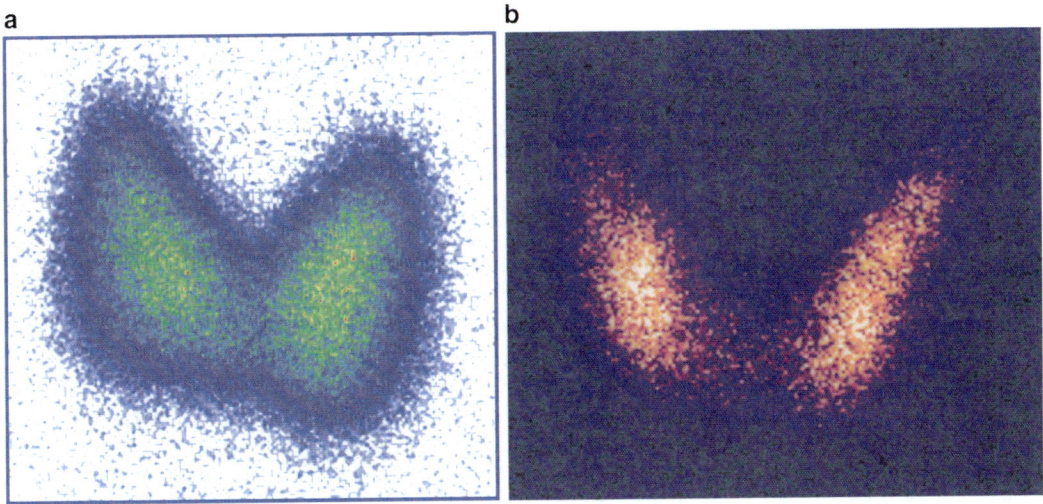

Fig. 17.12 Volume reducing effect of RAIT. (**a**) Enlarged thyroid gland on thyroid scan performed before RAIT in a patient with Graves' disease. (**b**) A smaller thyroid gland on the follow-up thyroid scan taken 28 months after RAIT

in patients with thyroid ophthalmopathy, hypertension or weight gaining. The evidence of hypothyroidism is the low serum levels of thyroid hormones and increased TSH, but particularly in patients with long-lasting hyperthyroidism and old age, TSH may remain suppressed for a longer time period despite low thyroid hormones.

Thyroxin Replacement

Once hypothyroidism is achieved within 1–2 months of RAIT, thyroxin replacement is initiated immediately to avoid serious hypothyroid symptoms and complaints including worsening of ophthalmopathy, gaining excessive weight, constipation, and bradycardia. The dose of thyroxin may be reduced later in follow-up probably due to the recovery and re-functioning of mildly damaged and "stunned" thyrocytes.

Thyroid Volume Changes

The two major effects of RAIT consist of reduction in serum levels of thyroid hormones and shrinkage in thyroid volume. Thyroid ultrasonography is the most reliable tool to document the volume reduction after RAIT [62, 63]. The volume change depends on the pre-RAIT thyroid volume, radioiodine uptake, and the radioiodine activity used for RAIT. The reduction of thyroid hormones is prompt and sharp but the decrease in volume starts at least 2 months after RAIT and continues for years (at least 2 years). The degree of volume change varies between mild reduction and complete atrophy (equivalent of total thyroidectomy). Volume reduction is dramatically prompt and evident in patients with Graves' disease (Fig. 17.12). The level of volume reduction in Plummer's disease and non-toxic goiter and nodules is moderate and slow. Also, thyroid scintigraphy performed 1–2 years after RAIT shows significant decrease in functional uptake and decrease in thyroid volume indicating its use as a tool for the assessment of long-term therapeutic response (Fig. 17.13).

Monitoring Changes in Thyroid Parenchyma and Volume

Ultrasonography, with its excellent spatial resolution and ability to detect submillimetric changes is the method of choice for measuring the thyroid volume and monitoring the early and the late effects in parenchyma including shrinkage of the nodules and the thyroid gland (Fig. 17.14).

a

b

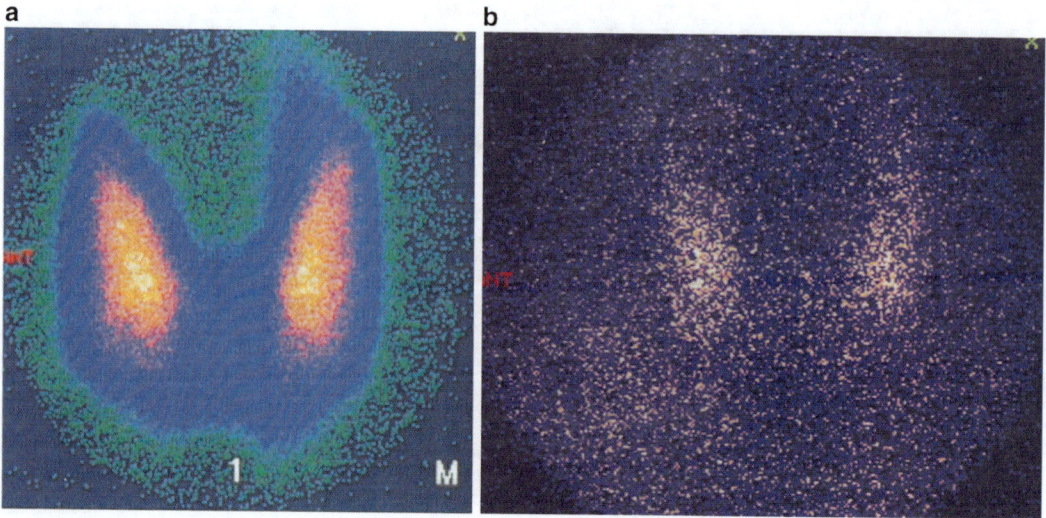

Fig. 17.13 Functional response assessed by thyroid scan in a 37-year-old man with Graves' disease. (**a**) Increased uptake in an enlarged gland on thyroid scintigraphy performed 7 days before RAIT. (**b**) Significantly decreased functional uptake in the thyroid gland on a follow-up thyroid scan taken 14 months after RAIT. Note the increased background activity and significant volume reduction in the thyroid gland

a

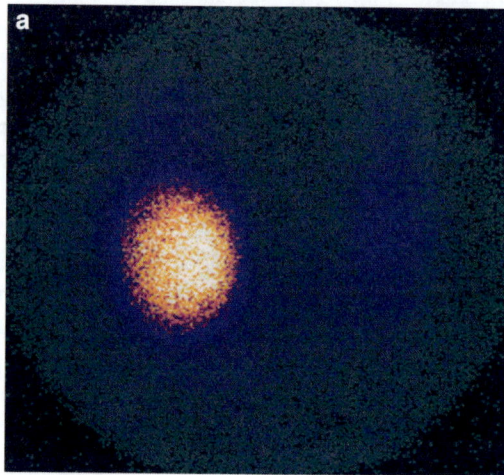

Fig. 17.14 Assessment of response to RAIT by ultrasonography in a patient with toxic adenoma (Below). (**a**) A hyperactive nodule in the lower pole of the right lobe and suppression of radionuclide uptake in the non-nodular thyroid tissue with lack of background activity. (**b–d**) Transaxial sections of thyroid ultrasonography taken on day 60 (18.6 × 18.1 mm), day 175 (10.8 × 9.7 mm) and day 372 (7.0 × 8.0 mm) after RAIT, respectively, showing gradual volume reduction of the nodule

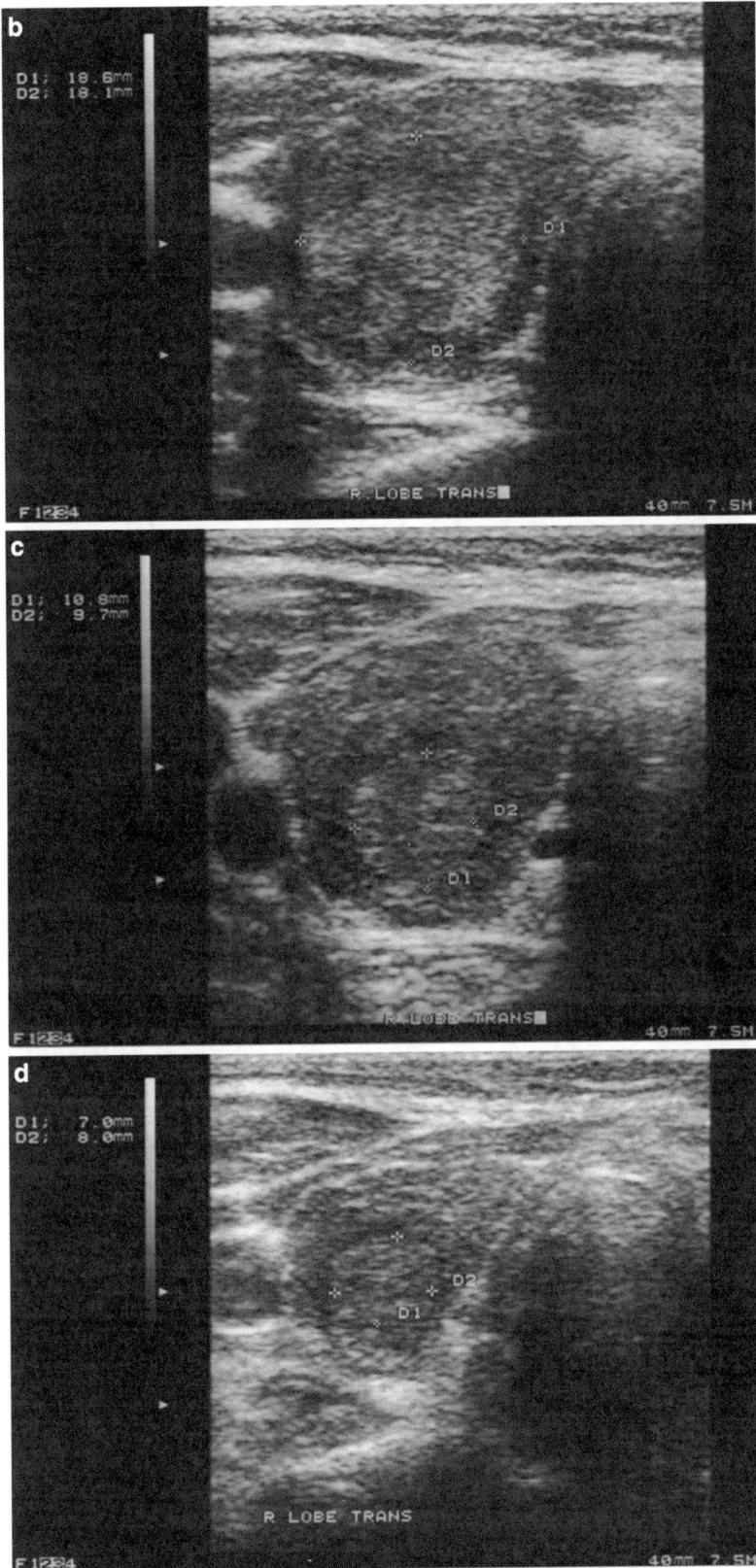

Fig. 17.14 (continued)

a

b

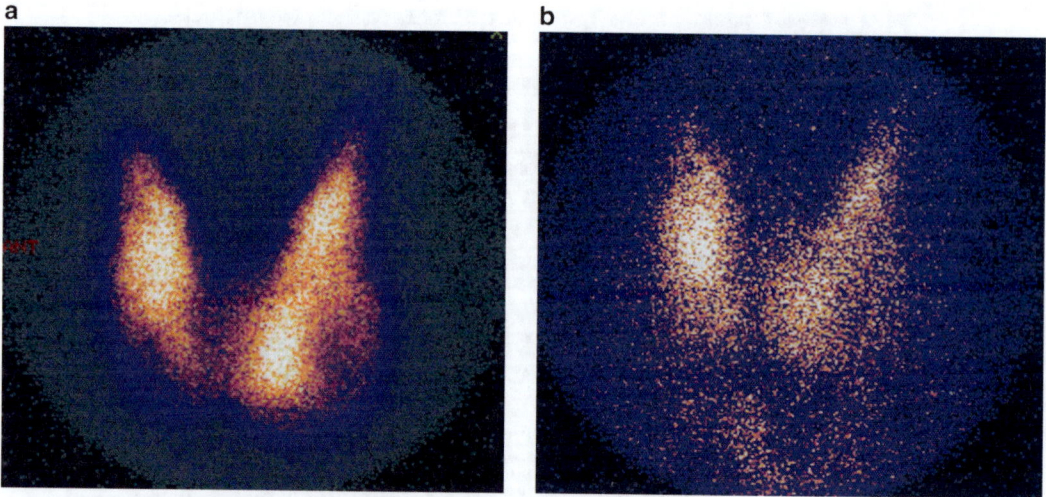

Fig. 17.15 Use of thyroid scan as a tool for the assessment of response to RAIT in a 59-year-old woman with Graves' disease and nodules: minimal volume reduction, significant functional response. (**a**) Asymmetrically been enlarged thyroid gland on scintigraphy taken before RAIT showing increased parenchymal uptake. (**b**) Significantly decreased radionuclide uptake in the thyroid parenchyma with almost no volume reduction on a follow-up thyroid scan performed 6 years after RAIT. The patient was clinically stable, hypothyroid, receiving thyroxin supplementation and had no symptoms of hyperthyroidism since RAIT

Radionuclide thyroid scan as a follow-up tool in the first 6 months of RAIT is not recommended and should be postponed to 6–12 months after RAIT as early scintigraphic changes can be subtle, and the effect of stunning and subsequent suppression are not uncommon before 1 year. Thyroid scan gives significant functional information, and can be used to assess the response to RAIT (Fig. 17.15). Ablated thyrocytes lose their function and thus do not take the up radionuclide used for scintigraphic imaging or radioiodine uptake study [64]. Hyperactive (hot) nodules before RAIT are seen as hypoactive (cold) or normoactive foci after successful RAIT on thyroid scan. Totally decreased global uptake is seen on 24-h radioiodine uptake studies and on thyroid scan after successful RAIT in patients with Graves' disease. Persistence of high uptake 6–12 months after RAIT in hyperfunctioning nodules in Plummer's disease or hyperfunctioning gland in Graves' disease after RAIT is an indication for treatment failure.

We studied the value of serial thyroglobulin measurements before and after RAIT in patients with Graves' disease and toxic multinodular goiter and toxic adenomas. We have found that serum thyroglobulin levels are usually high in patients with Graves' disease (despite high anti-thyroglobulin antibodies) and Plummer's disease, and gradually decrease after RAIT (unpublished data). Serial measurement of serum thyroglobulin after RAIT may be useful in the assessment of response to RAIT in patients with Graves' disease: after 3 months of RAIT, decreasing serum levels of thyroglobulin may be an indicator of therapeutic response (unpublished data).

Re-treatment with Radioiodine

Decision for re-treatment requires careful evaluation of response to therapy. For patients with Graves' disease, if hyperthyroidism does not resolve within 6 months of RAIT, re-treatment is indicated [32, 65]. It should be noted that the second administration of RAIT may be usually less effective, possibly due to stunning. Rarely, a third session may be needed to render the patient hypothyroid. If hyperthyroidism is still refractory to multiple RAIT, the patient should be referred to surgery [66].

For toxic nodules, the response criteria are the volume change and also the control of hyperthyroidism. If hyperthyroidism is not controlled within the first 6 months of RAIT, re-treatment is advised. The need for re-treatment is more frequent in patients with hyperfunctioning nodules than Graves' disease. It should be kept in mind that the therapeutic response is relatively slow, and thus the decision for re-treatment in Plummer's disease should be based on solid laboratory findings and persistence of hyperfunctioning nodules on radionuclide thyroid scan.

For patients with also large non-toxic nodules or goiter, re-treatment is possible. The criterion for response is the reduction in size of the thyroid and the nodule.

Effect of RAIT on Parathyroid Glands and Calcitonin

There is no evidence showing any detrimental effects of RAIT on parathyroid glands, and the serum levels of parathormone. Also, calcitonin, another thyroid hormone secreted from parafollicular (C-cells) cells of thyroid glands, is not affected from RAIT.

Therapeutic Action of Radioiodine in Thyroid

Once radioiodine is taken up by thyrocytes, the β particles of I-131 cause cellular damage and destruction through "*crossfire effect*" in a continuous fashion. Follicles are also destroyed and thus more thyroid hormones stored in these destructed follicles enter the circulation causing temporary (worsening of) hyperthyroidism. The treating physician should expect this change in thyroid hormone status and take the necessary measures including short-term use of β receptor blockers with prominent peripheral therapeutic effects after RAIT. The destruction (subsequent cell kill) is irreversible for most of the thyrocytes, but cells with mild damage can repair themselves and recover from the detrimental effects of radioiodine.

Table 17.6 Side-effects of RAIT in benign thyroid disease

Exacerbation of hyperthyroidism
Pain and swelling in thyroid gland (radiation thyroiditis)
Sialadenitis
Xerostomia
Xerophthalmia
Leukopenia
Thrombocytopenia
Hoarseness
Worsening of compressive symptoms
Laryngeal edema
Laryngeal nerve palsy
Dysgeusia
Precipitation of thyroid storm

Side-Effects

Treating physician should be aware of the exacerbation of symptoms within the first 2 weeks after RAIT, and necessary therapeutic interventions should be carried out using anti-thyroid drugs and β blocking agents. Sialadenitis and dry mouth (xerostomia) are the most frequent side-effects despite salivary stimulation after RAIT. The risk of sialadenitis and xerostomia is slightly higher when liquid form of I-131 is used for RAIT. Dry eye disease (xerophthalmia) is a rare condition that can be seen after RAIT. These side-effects may be temporary or permanent (Table 17.6). Temporary, mild leukopenia and thrombocytopenia can also be seen occasionally. No treatment is necessary for these hematological cytopenias, but if these conditions are severe and persistent, a consultation from hematology department should be arranged at an early stage.

Local swelling and pain in the thyroid gland due to radiation thyroiditis, a temporary condition causing local pain, requires medication to relieve the symptoms. Corticoids, acetaminophen or other non-narcotic analgesics or salicylate can be used for this purpose. The risk of bleeding and gastrointestinal side-effects of salicylate should be taken into consideration.

Laryngeal edema is a serious complication, which needs urgent medical intervention and collaboration with anesthesia and otolaryngology departments. Hoarseness is a mild and temporary condition that can be seen in patients with extremely high thyroid uptake of radioiodine or when the activity of ingested radioiodine is high.

Recurrent laryngeal nerve palsy and dysgeusia (distorted alteration of normal taste) are very rare side-effects of RAIT.

It should be kept in mind that possibility of tracheal compression just after RAIT is a reality in patients with very large goiter and nodules, particularly in patients with retrosternal extension. For patients with the risk of tracheal compression, RAIT should be avoided if close collaboration with otolaryngology department is not possible in case of compressive emergency. Compressive symptoms are more common in patients with large retrosternal goiter.

Serum testosterone levels can reversibly decrease but there is no clinical evidence about its clinical importance [67].

Contraindications

There are four absolute contraindications for RAIT: pregnancy, suspicion or presence of malignancy, breastfeeding/lactation, and the inability to comply with radiation safety precautions. Fecal or urinal incontinence is not an absolute contraindication, but meticulous diapering and bagging the contaminated material are necessary, and waste disposal must be done in accordance with local regulations.

The Conditions when RAIT is contraindicated

- Pregnancy
- Suspicion or presence of malignancy
- Breastfeeding/lactation
- Inability to comply with radiation safety precautions

RAIT should be postponed at least 6 weeks after lactation in order to protect the breast tissue from high amount of radioactivity. Fetuses accidentally exposed to I-131 after 10–11 weeks of pregnancy have a high risk of developmental abnormalities of thyroid gland. It is therefore mandatory for the treating physician to obtain a negative pregnancy test result performed in the last 24 h before RAIT in each female patient at reproductive age.

If the patient cannot follow radiation safety precautions, RAIT should not be administered.

RAIT in autonomic nodules and thyroid glands with large volume is not currently contraindicated but may require multiple, divided activities of radioiodine in more than one session.

Patients on dialysis, or having jejunostomy, colostomy or gastric feeding tube require special attention and detailed measures for radiation protection.

Malignancy Associated with RAIT

The "tool" (i.e., I-131) that is used for RAIT is "radioactive," and thus it was thought to be associated with the risk of development of malignancies. This issue has been debated extensively since the first use of I-131 in early 1940s, and tens of studies focusing on this "risk" have been reported in the literature. There is no convincing evidence in any of these reports that RAIT increases the risk of thyroid carcinoma or secondary malignancies [57–61]. Even the risk of secondary malignancies after much higher activities of I-131 used for the treatment of thyroid carcinoma is negligibly low. Hyperthyroidism itself, particularly Graves' disease, is associated with a high risk of malignancy [32].

Infertility

This issue has been investigated in many studies. The female patients are advised to postpone pregnancy 6 months after RAIT not due to the detrimental effects of radioiodine on ovaries but to maintain satisfactory and stable thyroxin replacement in the first 6 months after RAIT [32]. For men, a 3-month postponing of conception is sufficient to complete the sperm turnover. The key issue in this respect is to maintain euthyroidism by sufficient thyroxin replacement for both genders before conception and during pregnancy for female patients. While "accidental" pregnancies just after the ingestion of even much higher activities of I-131 for the treatment of thyroid carcinomas have been reported, even in these cases offspring were found to be healthy in long-term follow-up. It is therefore only an unsubstantiated speculation that RAIT could cause infertility, particularly with as low activities and doses as those used for benign thyroid disease. Also, there is no scientific evidence on the increased risk of congenital anomalies in the offspring of patients treated with radioiodine [68, 69].

Hypothyroidism After RAIT

Post-treatment hypothyroidism is shown in many texts as a "serious" side-effect. It is, however, an expected result indicating the "*success*" of RAIT. According to the recent guidelines of American Thyroid Association, the "aim" of RAIT in Graves' disease is to render the patient hypothyroid [32].

In some patients treated with radioiodine, early hypothyroidism is followed by a temporary period of euthyroidism and then comes permanent hypothyroidism. It should be made clear that even long-term high dose anti-thyroid drug use is also associated with subsequent hypothyroidism. Spontaneous subclinical hypothyroidism after months or years of anti-thyroid drug use is not an uncommon clinical condition causing lifelong thyroxin dependency.

Surgery is also associated with subsequent hypothyroidism. If the amount of tissue is large enough (i.e., subtotal, near total, or total thyroidectomy), post-surgical "overt" hypothyroidism occurs just after 1 week of surgical operation requiring immediate thyroxin replacement and resulting in life-long thyroxin dependency [32]. If the amount of thyroid tissue is small, despite current recommendations to do otherwise, the resultant hypothyroidism can be mild (subclinical hypothyroidism) and missed until it causes clinical symptoms and complaints later. Subclinical hypothyroidism also requires thyroxin supplementation.

In earlier years, it was expected that an activity of radioiodine, which could induce euthyroidism, was possible, and thus significant effort was spent to achieve this ultimate goal with limited success. Most of the criticisms about the subsequent hypothyroidism associated with RAIT date back to early days. Amount of activities as low as 2 mCi was recommended to render the patient euthyroid and to avoid the potential risk of malignancies. The approach was the same for surgery: removal of limited amount of thyroid tissue including total or partial lobectomy and subtotal thyroidectomy were the only recommended methods of surgery in those days. Relapse and persistence of hyperthyroidism were therefore frequent after both surgery and RAIT due to these concepts and expectations.

Today, particularly in North America, a concept consists of using a higher activity with ablative effect with RAIT in a single session or a surgical technique consisting of removing most of the gland tissue (near total thyroidectomy) is preferred and widely accepted. Resultant hypothyroidism is thus unavoidable in both choices associated with this concept, but the probability of relapse and persistence of the thyroid disease is much lower.

While in Europe and the rest of the world, subtotal thyroidectomy is still the most frequent technique despite the fact that even after single lobectomy or subtotal thyroidectomy, hypothyroidism (although subclinical) is still unavoidable and relapse is more frequent.

Hypothyroidism is thus not a side-effect of RAIT, but, an expected result and indicator of actual, definitive therapeutic response, particularly in hyperthyroid patients. It is easier to adjust the dose of the thyroxin replacement during follow-up after RAIT if the patient is permanently hypothyroid. As a general rule, hypothyroidism following RAIT is more common in patients with Graves' disease than those with Plummer's disease and non-toxic goiter and nodules.

In Plummer's disease, patients younger than 50 years have higher probability of hypothyroidism compared to older patients in long-term follow-up (61% vs. 36% in 16 years) [70]. Also, suppressed TSH level is a measure against hypothyroidism by protecting non-nodular thyroid tissue from high amount of radioiodine uptake in patients with Plummer's disease. The prevalence and severity of hypothyroidism in these patients are not related to the amount of activity used in RAIT [32]; the only difference between high and small amount of activity is earlier disappearance of hyperthyroidism and earlier appearance of hypothyroidism. Presence of anti-thyroid antibodies and non-suppressed TSH at the time of RAIT are important risk factors for developing post-treatment hypothyroidism in patients with solitary toxic adenomas [25, 71, 72].

Role of Nuclear Medicine Physician in RAIT

Nuclear Medicine physician should be involved in all stages of RAIT including decision of treatment (indication), patient preparation, timing of administration, administration of RAIT and follow-up (at least in early stages) to assess the therapeutic efficacy of RAIT, and possible radiation induced side-effects and toxicity. Close collaboration with endocrinologists is required in North America and in most of the other countries, but in some European countries, the patient who receives RAIT remains in the clinical responsibility of Nuclear Medicine physician even for long-term follow-up.

Conclusion

Radioiodine therapy of benign thyroid diseases is safe, cost-effective, and efficient. Patient reparations including low iodine diet before therapy is a vital part of RAIT. Malignancy should be excluded for each and every nodule existing in the thyroid gland. Meticulous activity calculation can be made using dosimetric techniques but administering fixed activities is also reliable. Hypothyroidism should be expected after RAIT, and early initia-

tion of thyroxin supplementation prevents the detrimental effects of hypothyroidism including worsening of ophthalmopathy. Nuclear Medicine physician should take part in the follow-up of the patient after RAIT, at least at early stages.

Appendix: Dosimetry

To avoid unnecessarily high irradiation of thyroid and the whole body by circulating radioiodine before being taken up by the thyroid gland, individualized calculation of activity necessary for optimal radiation dose to be absorbed by thyroid tissue to be ablated has always been an attractive approach [36, 73, 74]. This can be achieved through individualized dosimetric calculations, which mainly depend on target dose, 24-h radioiodine uptake (activity time interval), and amount of thyroid tissue to be ablated.

Amount of thyroid tissue and the volume to be ablated can be best calculated by ultrasonography. For thyroid glands with multiple autonomy (multiple toxic nodules), scintigraphic volume calculations can be used.

I-131 is the logistically ideal radionuclide for 24-h radioiodine uptake using a collimated probe (thyroid uptake device). I-123 can also be preferred if γ camera is used for counting. For Graves' disease, a 5-h uptake can be helpful for keeping to the fast kinetics of I-131, since iodine turnover is faster and time-to-reach peak is shorter in this disease than in any other thyroid diseases. Alternatively, 20-min Tc-99m uptake can be used on logistical grounds, but the information obtained from this method is not exactly the same with that obtained from a 24-h iodine uptake study. Anti-thyroid drugs should be withdrawn at least 1 day before the uptake studies.

Two main approaches are commonly used: the Marinelli formula (Marinelli–Quimby formula) and MIRD algorithm [36, 40, 73, 74], the latter differing from the former by about 10 %.

The Marinelli formula [75]:

$$ I\text{-}131\ activity\,(MBq) = \frac{Target\ dose\,(Gy) \times target\ weight\,(g) \times 24.67}{Maximal\ uptake\,(\%) \times effective\ half\text{-}life\,(days)}. $$

Modified Marinelli–Quimby–Hine formula:

$$I\text{-}131\ \text{activity(mCi)} = \frac{\text{Target dose(cGy)} \times \text{thyroid weight(g)} \times 6.67}{t_{1/2}\text{effective half-life(days)} \times 24\text{-h uptake(\%)}}.$$

Target dose is the desired radiation absorbed dose. Dosimetric calculations take into consideration the effective half-life of radioiodine in the gland and the time-integrated activity. Many physicians choose to calculate the target activity individually by performing multiple tracer dose activity measurements at various times. Some prefer to use four "target variables": time-integrated activity coefficient, time of maximum activity, effective half-life in the gland, and maximum activity. This approach increased accuracy only slightly [40].

Using a parameter k, thyroid absorbed dose and thyroid mass reduction as early as 1 month after RAIT month after therapy can be predicted before RAIT administration [76]. Dosimetric calculations were, however, found to be not useful in rendering the patient euthyroid and the performance of dosimetric calculations be low in this respect [77–79].

Dosimetry-based therapy of Graves' disease is still associated with significant controversies and challenges. Most of the formulas, models, and proposed modifications aim to calculate the individual activity in Graves' disease only. It is difficult to draw a reliable conclusion about the use of dosimetric calculations for Plummer's disease with the limited data published in the literature on this topic.

A simpler formula requires three variables: 24-h radioiodine uptake, gland weight, fixed activity in microgram per gram of thyroid tissue [32].

$$\text{Activity(mCi)} = \frac{\text{Gland weight(g)} \times \text{Microgram per each gram of thyroid tissue} \times 100}{24\text{-h uptake(percent)}}.$$

Currently, in clinical practice, most of the patients are eligible for a fixed activity-based treatment, but some patients still require elaborative dosimetric calculations. Although fixed activity method gives satisfactory results to achieve the targeted irradiation of thyroid gland in 80 % of the patients with Graves' disease, there is an obvious need to develop a reasonably fast, simple, and cost-effective method to measure the intra-thyroidal radioiodine kinetics for the routine calculation of optimal radioiodine activity.

Acknowledgement The authors would like to acknowledge the technical assistance of Arda Dora Aktolun in improving the quality of images and preparing them for publication using his excellent computer skills.

References

1. Trepacz PT, McCue M, Klein I, Levey GS, Greenhouse J. A psychiatric and neuropsychological study of patients with untreated Graves' disease. Gen Hosp Psychiatry. 1988;10:49–55.

2. Trepacz PT, Klein I, Roberts M, Greenhouse J, Levey GS. Graves' disease: an analysis of thyroid hormone levels and hyperthyroid signs and symptoms. Am J Med. 1989;87:558–61.

3. Bahn RS, Burch HS, Cooper DS, Garber JR, Greenlee CM, Klein IL, et al. The role of propylthiouracil in the management of Graves' disease in adults: report of a meeting jointly sponsored by the American Thyroid Association and Food and Drug Administration. Thyroid. 2009;19:673–4.

4. Sosa JA, Bowman HM, Tielsch JM, Powe NR, Gordon TA, Udelsman R. The importance of surgeon experience for clinical and economic outcomes from thyroidectomy. Ann Surg. 1998;228:320–30.

5. Röher HD, Goretzki PE, Hellman P, Witte J. Complications in thyroid surgery. Incidence and therapy. Chirurg. 1999;70:999–1000.

6. Sywak MS, Palazzo FF, Yeh M, Wilkinson M, Snook K, Sidhu SB, et al. Parathyroid hormone assay predicts hypocalcemia after total thyroidectomy. ANZ J Surg. 2007;77:667–70.

7. Abbas G, Dubner S, Heller KS. Re-operation for bleeding after total thyroidectomy and parathyroidectomy. Head Neck. 2001;23:544–6.

8. Jenkins K, Baker AB. Consent and anaesthetic risk. Anaesthesia. 2003;58:962–84.

9. Kraimps JL, Bouin-Pineau MH, Mathonnet M, De Calan L, Ronceray J, Visset J, et al. Multicenter study

of thyroid nodules in patients with Graves' disease. Br J Surg. 2000;87:1111–3.

10. Gorman CA. Radioiodine therapy does not aggravate Graves' ophthalmopathy. J Clin Endocrinol Metab. 1995;80:340–2.

11. Rivkees SA, Dinauer C. An optimal treatment for pediatric Graves' disease is radioiodine. J Clin Endocrinol Metab. 2007;92:797–800.

12. Vitti P, Ragio T, Chiovato L, Pallini S, Santini F, Fiore E, et al. Clinical features of patients with Graves' disease undergoing remission after antithyroid drug treatment. Thyroid. 1997;7:369–75.

13. Erickson D, Gharib H, Li H, van Heerden JA. Treatment of patients with toxic multinodular goiter. Thyroid. 1998;8:277–82.

14. Nygaard B, Hegedüs L, Ulriksen P, Nielsen KG, Hansen JM. Radioiodine therapy for multinodular toxic goiter. Arch Intern Med. 1999;159:1364–8.

15. Kang AS, Grant CS, Thompson GB, van Heerden JA. Current treatment of nodular goiter with hyperthyroidism (Plummer's disease): surgery versus radioiodine. Surgery. 2002;132:916–23.

16. Vidal-Trecan GM, Stahl JE, Eckman MH. Radioiodine or surgery for toxic thyroid adenoma: dissecting an important decision. A cost-effective analysis. Thyroid. 2004;14:933–45.

17. Pappalardo G, Guadalaxara A, Frattaroli FM, Illomei G, Falaschi P. Total compared with subtotal thyroidectomy in benign nodular disease: personal series and review of published reports. Eur J Surg. 1998; 164:501–6.

18. Thomusch O, Machens A, Sekula C, Ukkat J, Lippert H, Gastinger I, et al. Multivariate analysis of risk factors for postoperative complications in benign goiter surgery: prospective multicenter study in Germany. World J Surg. 2000;24:1335–41.

19. Hisham AN, Azlina AF, Aina EN, Sarojah A. Total thyroidectomy: the procedure of choice for multinodular goiter. Eur J Surg. 2001;167:403–5.

20. Albino CC, Graf H, Sampaio AP, Vigario A, Paz-Filho GJ. Thiamazole as an adjuvant to radioiodine for volume reduction of multinodular goiter. Expert Opin Investig Drugs. 2008;17:1781–6.

21. Regalbuto C, Salamone S, Scollo C, Vigneri R, Pezzino V. Appearance of anti-TSH receptor antibodies and clinical Graves' disease after radioiodine therapy for hyperfunctioning thyroid adenoma. J Endocrinol Invest. 1999;22:147–50.

22. Kendall-Taylor P, Keir M, Ross WM. Ablative radioiodine therapy for hyperthyroidism: long term follow-up study. Br Med J. 1984;289:361–3.

23. Reiners C. Functional autonomy of the thyroid: volume reduction after radioiodine treatment. Exp Clin Endocrinol. 1993;101:136–8.

24. Kinser JA, Roesler H, Furrer T, Grütter D, Zimmerman H. Nonimmunogenic hyperthyroidism: cumulative hypothyroidism incidence after radioiodine and surgical treatment. J Nucl Med. 1989;30:1960–5.

25. Ceccarelli C, Bencivelli W, Vitti P, Grasso L, Pinchera A. Outcome of radioiodine-131 therapy in hyperfunctioning thyroid nodules: a 20-years' retrospective study. Clin Endocrinol (Oxf). 2005;62:331–5.

26. Kahraman D, Keller C, Schneider C, Eschner W, Sudbrock F, Schbrsmidt M, et al. Development of hypothyroidism during long term follow-up of patients with toxic nodular goiter after radioiodine therapy. Clin Endocrinol (Oxf). 2012;76:297–303.

27. Manders JMB, Corstens FHM. Radioiodine therapy of euthyroid multinodular goiters. Eur J Nucl Med. 2002;29:466–70.

28. Kaniuka S, Lass P, Sworczak K. Radioiodine-an attractive alternative to surgery in large non-toxic multinodular goiters. Nucl Med Rev Cent East Eur. 2009;12:23–9.

29. Ceccarelli C, Brozzi F, Bianchi F, Santini P. Role of recombinant human TSH in the management of large euthyroid multinodular goiter: a new therapeutic option? Pros and cons. Minerva Endocrinol. 2010;35:161–71.

30. Braverman L, Kloos RT, Law Jr B, Kipnes M, Dionne M, Magner J. Evaluation of various doses of recombinant human thyrotropin in patients with multinodular goiters. Endocr Pract. 2008;14:832–9.

31. Baczyk M, Pisarek M, Czepczyński R, Ziemnicka K, Gryczyńska M, Pietz L, et al. Therapy of large multinodular goiter using repeated doses of radioiodine. Nucl Med Commun. 2009;30:226–31.

32. Bahn RS, Burch HB, Cooper DS, Garber JR, Greenlee MC, Klein I, et al. Hyperthyroidism and other causes of thyrotoxicosis: management guidelines of American Thyroid Association and American Association of Clinical Endocrinologists. Thyroid. 2011;21:593–646.

33. Sabri O, Zimny M, Schulz G, Schreckenberger M, Reinartz P, Willmes K, et al. Success rate of radioiodine therapy in Graves' disease: influence of thyrostatic medication. J Clin Endocrinol Metab. 1999; 84:1229–33.

34. Andrade VA, Gross JL, Maia AL. The effect of methimazole pretreatment on the efficacy of radioactive iodine therapy in Graves' hyperthyroidism: one-year follow-up of a prospective, randomized study. J Clin Endocrinol Metab. 2001;86:3488–93.

35. Walter MA, Briel M, Christ-Crain M, Bonnema SJ, Connel J, Cooper DS, et al. Effects of antithyroid drugs on radioiodine treatment: systematic review and meta-analysis of randomized controlled trials. BMJ. 2007;334:514.

36. Bockish A, Jamitzky T, Derwenz R, Biersack HJ. Optimized dose planning of radioiodine therapy of benign thyroidal diseases. J Nucl Med. 1993;34: 1632–8.

37. Peters H, Fischer C, Bogner U, Rainers C, Schleusener H. Radioiodine therapy of Graves' hyperthyroidism: standard versus calculated 131-iodine activity. Results from a prospective, randomized, multicentric study. Eur J Clin Invest. 1995;25:186–93.

38. de Rooij A, Vandenbroucke JP, Smit JW, Stokkel MP, Dekkers OM. Clinical outcomes after estimated versus calculated activity of radioiodine for the treatment of hyperthyroidism: systematic review and meta-analysis. Eur J Endocrinol. 2009;161:771–7.

39. Salvatori M, Luster M. Radioiodine dosimetry in benign thyroid disease and differentiated thyroid carcinoma. Eur J Nucl Med Mol Imaging. 2010;37:821–8.

40. Merrill S, Horowitz J, Traino AC, Chipkin SR, Hollot CV, Chait Y. Accuracy and optimal timing of activity measurements in estimating the absorbed dose of radioiodine in the treatment of Graves' disease. Phys Med Biol. 2011;56:557–71.

41. Liu CJ, Dong YY, Wang YW, Wang KH, Zeng QY. Efficiency analysis of using tailored individual doses of radioiodine and fine tuning using a low-dose anti-thyroid drugs in the treatment of Graves' disease. Nucl Med Commun. 2011;32:227–32.

42. Magner J. Problems associated with the use of thyrogen in patients with a thyroid gland. N Engl J Med. 2008;359:1738–9.

43. Zakavi SR, Mousavi Z, Davachi B. Comparison of four different protocols of I-131 therapy for treating single toxic thyroid nodule. Nucl Med Commun. 2009;30:169–75.

44. Bonnema SJ, Nielsen VE, Hegedüs L. Radioiodine therapy in non-toxic multinodular goiter. The possibility of effect-amplification with recombinant human TSH (rhTSH). Acta Oncol. 2006;45:1051–8.

45. Fast S, Nielsen VE, Bonnema SJ, Hegedüs L. Time to re-consider non-surgical therapy of benign non-toxic multinodular goiter: focus on recombinant TSH augmented radioiodine therapy. Eur J Endocrinol. 2009; 160:517–28.

46. Fast S, Bonnema SJ, Hegedüs L. Radioiodine therapy in non-toxic multinodular goiter. Potential role of recombinant human TSH. Ann Endocrinol (Paris). 2011;72:129–35.

47. Tallstedt L, Lundell G, Torring O, Wallin G, Ljunggren JG, Blomgren H, et al. Occurrence of ophthalmopathy after treatment for Graves' hyperthyroidism. The Thyroid Study Group. N Eng J Med. 1992;326:1733–8.

48. Bartalena L, Marcocci C, Bogazzi F, Manetti L, Tanda ML, Dell'Unto E, et al. Relation between therapy for hyperthyroidism and the course of Graves' ophthalmopathy. N Eng J Med. 1998;338:73–8.

49. Laurberg P, Walling G, Tallstedt L, Abraham-Nording M, Lundell G, Torring O. TSH-receptor autoimmunity in Graves' disease after therapy with anti-thyroid drugs, surgery, or radioiodine: a 5-year prospective randomized study. Eur J Endocrinol. 2008;158:69–75.

50. Bahn RS. Graves' ophthalmopathy. N Eng J Med. 2010;362:726–38.

51. Pfeilschifter J, Ziegler R. Smoking and endocrine ophthalmopathy: impact of smoking severity and current vs lifetime cigarette consumption. Clin Endocrinol (Oxf). 1996;45:477–81.

52. Regensburg NI, Wiersinga WM, Berendschot TT, Saeed P, Mourits MP. Effect of smoking on orbital fat and muscle volume in Graves' orbitopathy. Thyroid. 2011;21:177–81.

53. De Bellis A, Conzo G, Cennamo G, Pane E, Bellastella G, Colella C, et al. Time course of Graves' ophthalmopathy after total thyroidectomy alone or followed by radioiodine therapy: a 2-year longitudinal study. Endocrine. 2012;41(2):320–6.

54. Nebesio TD, Siddiqui AR, Pescovitz OH, Eugster EA. Time course to hypothyroidism after fixed dose radioablation therapy of Graves' disease in children. J Pediatr. 2002;141:99–103.

55. Rivkees SA, Cernelius EA. Influence of iodine-131 dose on the outcome of hyperthyroidism in children. Pediatrics. 2003;111:745–9.

56. Bonnema SJ, Bennedbaek FN, Gram J, Veje A, Marving J, Hegedus L. Resumption of methimazole after I-131 therapy of hyperthyroid diseases: effect on thyroid function and volume evaluated by a randomized clinical trial. Eur J Endocrinol. 2003;149: 485–92.

57. Dolphin GW. The risk of thyroid cancers following irradiation. Health Phys. 1968;15:219–28.

58. Ron E, Lubin JH, Shore RE, Mabuchi K, Modan B, Pottern LM, et al. Thyroid cancer after exposure to external radiation: a pooled analysis of seven studies. Radiat Res. 1995;141:259–77.

59. Boice Jr JD. Radiation and thyroid cancer: what more can be learned? Acta Oncol. 1998;37:321–4.

60. Sigurdson AJ, Ronckers CM, Mertens AC, Stovall M, Smith SA, Liu Y, et al. Primary thyroid cancer after a first tumour in childhood (the Childhood Cancer Survivor Study): a nested case-control study. Lancet. 2005;365:2014–23.

61. Boice Jr JD. Radiation-induced thyroid cancer — what's new? J Natl Cancer Inst. 2005;97:703–5.

62. Gómez-Arnaiz N, Andía E, Gumà A, Abós R, Soler J, Gómez JM. Ultrasonographic thyroid volume as a reliable prognostic index of radioiodine-131 treatment outcome in Graves' disease hyperthyroidism. Horm Metab Res. 2003;35:492–7.

63. Nakatake N, Fukata S, Tajiri J. Prediction of post-treatment hypothyroidism using changes in thyroid volume after radioactive iodine therapy in adolescent patients with Graves' disease. Int J Pediatr Endocrinol. 2011;2011:14.

64. Carpentier WR, Gilliland PF, Piziak VK, Petty FC, McConnell BG, Verdonk CA, et al. Radioiodine uptake following iodine-131 therapy for Graves' disease: an early indicator of need for retreatment. Clin Nucl Med. 1989;14:15–8.

65. Leslie WD, Peterdy AE, Dupont JO. Radioiodine treatment outcomes in thyroid glands previously irradiated for Graves' hyperthyroidism. J Nucl Med. 1998;39:712–6.

66. Alexander EK, Larsen PR. High dose of 131-I therapy for the treatment of hyperthyroidism caused by Graves' disease. J Clin Endocrinol Metab. 2002;87:1073–7.

67. Ceccarelli C, Canale D, Battisti P, Caglieresi C, Moschini C, Fiore E, et al. Testicular function after I-131 therapy for hyperthyroidism. Clin Endocrinol (Oxf). 2006;65:446–52.

68. Baxter MA, Stewart PM, Daykin J, Sheppard MC, Franklyn JA. Radioiodine therapy for hyperthyroid-

ism in young patients-perception of risk and use. Q J Med. 1993;86:495–9.

69. Rosário PW, Barroso AL, Rezende LL, Padrão EL, Borges MA, Guimarães VC, et al. Testicular function after radioiodine therapy in patients with thyroid cancer. Thyroid. 2006;16:667–70.

70. Holm LE, Lundell G, Israelson A, Dahlqvist I. Incidence of hypothyroidism occurring long after iodine-131 therapy for hyperthyroidism. J Nucl Med. 1982;23:103–7.

71. Goldstein R, Hart IR. Follow-up of solitary autonomous thyroid nodules treated with I-131. N Engl J Med. 1983;309:1473–6.

72. Nygaard B, Hegedüs L, Nielsen KG, Ulriksen P, Hansen JM. Long-term effect of radioactive iodine on thyroid function and size in patients with solitary autonomously functioning toxic thyroid nodules. Clin Endocrinol (Oxf). 1999;50:197–202.

73. Peters H, Fischer C, Bogner U, Rieners C, Schleusener H. Radioiodine therapy of Graves' hyperthyroidism: standard vs. calculated 131-iodine activity. Results from a prospective, randomized, multicentric study. Eur J Clin Invest. 1995;25:186–93.

74. Haase A, Bähre M, Lauer I, Meller B, Richter E. Radioiodine therapy in Graves' hyperthyroidism: determination of individual optimum target dose. Exp Clin Endocrinol Diabetes. 2000;108:133–7.

75. Marinelli LD, Quinby EH, Hine GJ. Dosage determination with radioactive isotopes; practical considerations in therapy and protection. Am J Roentgenol Radium Ther. 1948;59:260–81.

76. Traino AC, Di Martino F, Lazzeri M. A dosimetric approach to patient-specific radioiodine treatment of Graves' disease with incorporation of treatment-induced changes in thyroid mass. Med Phys. 2004;31: 2121–7.

77. Catargi B, Leprat F, Guyot M, Valli N, Ducassou D, Tabarin A. Optimized radioiodine therapy of Graves' disease: analysis of delivered dose and of other possible factors affecting outcome. Eur J Endocrinol. 1999;141:117–21.

78. Traino AC, Di Martino F, Lazzeri M, Stabin MG. Study of the correlation between administered activity and radiation committed dose to the thyroid in 131-I therapy of Graves' disease. Radiat Prot Dosimetry. 2001;95:117–24.

79. Traino AC, Xhafa B. Accuracy of two simple methods for estimation of thyroidal 131-I kinetics of for dosimetry-based treatment of Graves' disease. Med Phys. 2009;36:1212–8.

Radiosynoviorthesis

18

Gynter Mödder and Renate Mödder-Reese

Abbreviations

AC	Acromioclavicular joint
RA	Rheumatoid arthritis
RSO	Radiosynoviorthesis = radiation synovectomy
OA	Osteoarthritis = activated arthrosis
MCP	Metacarpophalangeal joint
PIP	Proximal interphalangeal joint
DIP	Distal interphalangeal joint
MTP	Metatarsophalangeal joint

Introduction

Radiosynoviorthesis (RSO), also called radiation synovectomy and radiosynovectomy, is a therapeutic modality for the local treatment of chronic inflammatory joints. RSO, first used in 1968, means rebuilding (*orthesis*) of the synovium by means of radionuclides [1]. It is a procedure attempting to modify the synovial proliferative process by intra-articular application of radiopharmaceuticals as an alternative to surgical synovectomy and avoiding escalation of antirheumatic drug treatment. In Anglo-American literature, the term "radiosynovectomy" or "radiation

G. Mödder (✉) • R. Mödder-Reese
NURAMED, German Centre for Radiosynoviorthesis,
Max-Planck-Str. 27 a, 50858 Köln, Germany
e-mail: Gynter.moedder@t-online.de

synovectomy" is commonly used. It may be argued that these synonyms may be incorrect because this method is actually not an "-ectomy" (excision of the synovium). The procedure was first described in 1923 in animals, and in 1953 in human beings [2, 3].

The radionuclides (mainly beta emitters) used for RSO penetrate only a few millimeters in tissue and are not absorbed or excreted. It is usually performed on outpatient basis. Currently, RSO is performed in about 70,000 joints per year in Germany, almost equal to the number of radioiodine therapy for thyroid diseases. Close collaboration with orthopedists and rheumatologists is vital to ensure optimal medical care and increase the number of referrals (Fig. 18.1).

Indications

Basically, RSO is indicated for the local treatment of almost all kinds of chronic synovitis [4–8]. The main indications for RSO as stated in German [9] and European guidelines [10] are as below:
- Rheumatoid arthritis (RA)
- Seronegative spondarthropathy (i.e., reactive arthritis, psoriatic arthritis)
- Hemarthrosis in hemophilia
- Recurrent joint effusions (i.e., after arthroscopy)
- Pigmented villonodular synovitis (PVNS)
- Osteoarthritis (activated arthrosis)
- Persistent effusions

C. Aktolun and S.J. Goldsmith (eds.), *Nuclear Medicine Therapy: Principles and Clinical Applications*,
DOI 10.1007/978-1-4614-4021-5_18, © Springer Science+Business Media New York 2013

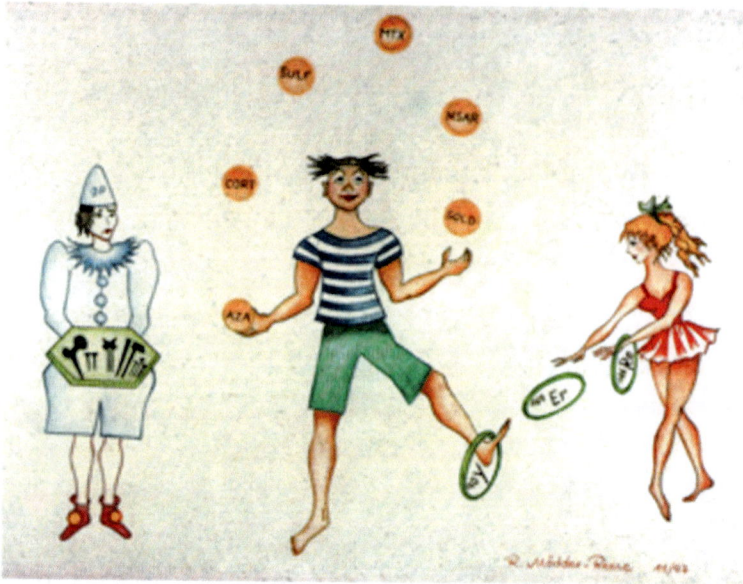

Fig. 18.1 At the centre is the rheumatologist. It is often an artistic work to juggle with anti-rheumatoid drugs. Sometimes a drug fails or the whole show ends up as a complete flop. If he recognizes the attractive help by RSO throwing Yttrium-90, Rhenium-186 or Erbium-169 to him he is able to enhance the quality of his art-work. For the sake of non-invasive treatment the orthopedic surgeon stands aside

- Polyethylene disease after joint prosthesis
- Undifferentiated arthritis (where the arthritis is characterized by synovitis, synovial thickening, or effusion)

Rheumatoid Arthritis

"Rheumatism" includes a number of diseases presenting with degenerative or inflammatory symptoms involving either the bony joint (local/intra-articular) or the connective tissue (systemic/extra-articular). Rheumatoid arthritis (RA) is a chronic disease manifested primarily in the synovium including joints, tendon sheaths, and bursas. Involvement of larger joints with painful dysfunction can be seen, although joints of the fingers and toes are usually involved at the onset. Various manifestations of inflammation, such as effusion, are common in the acute phase. In later stages, destruction may result in fibrous ankylosis. In addition to progressive joint involvement (mono-, oligo- or polyarticular), generalized manifestations may be seen.

Synovitis, inflammation of the synovial membrane (synovium), and vascularization that lead to hyperplastic synovial tissue (pannus), which may erode cartilage, subchondral bone, articular capsule, and ligaments is characteristic for RA. The final stage of synovitis is characterized with loss of function after progressive joint destruction resulting in ulnar deviation of the hands, swan neck, Baker's cysts, subluxation of the atlanto-axial joint, caput-ulnae-syndrome, deformation, axial malposition and instability of the knee joints, secondary arthrosis, disabling mutilating joint destructions, fibrous or bony ankylosis and extra-articular manifestations as well as a reactive depressive syndrome.

Treatment Options for Rheumatoid Arthritis

The aim of therapy is to improve the quality of life by reducing the pain, improving the mobility, and preserving the function. Treatment options include medication, surgical therapy, RSO, and physical therapy rehabilitation.

Systemic treatment such as non-steroidal anti-inflammatory drugs (NSAIDs) is employed to slow the inflammatory process (down-regulation). These "disease-modifying anti-rheumatoid drugs" (DMARDs) act by suppression, stimulation, or modulation of immunity. Immunosuppressive drugs include methotrexate (MTX), azathioprine, cyclophosphamide, and systemic corticosteroids. Recently, new biologic agents including anti-TNFα have made an impact on the quality of life.

Local treatment options include intra-articular corticosteroid injection, chemosynoviorthesis (rarely preferred), surgical intervention, and RSO. Local joint therapeutic methods become increasingly attractive due to the potential toxicities associated with systemic treatment options [11]. Surgical methods rank low due to unfavorable expense-to-benefit ratio. In this respect, intra-articular steroid injection is undoubtedly the most preferred procedure; however, it is associated with septic complications that are difficult to foresee. Systemic treatment fails to control some of the highly aggressive local inflammatory courses. Among these options, RSO as an outpatient procedure is most favorable because of its low cost-to-benefit ratio, high efficiency, and fewer side-effects.

RSO can be applied to all joints, especially small peripheral joints, while a few joints are only technically eligible for surgical synovectomy. In general, RSO performed at an early stage is more efficient in rheumatoid joint involvement. The most favorable results are obtained in patients with Steinbrocker stages I and II. RSO makes a positive impact on joint function and quality of life even in advanced stages of RA.

Osteoarthrosis and osteoarthritis

Differential diagnosis between osteoarthrosis and osteoarthritis is important since RSO is used in osteoarthritis only, and not recommended for osteoarthrosis, which is basically a degenerative joint disease. The prevalence of osteoarthrosis increases with age and the etiology is still unknown [4, 12].

Osteoarthritis (OA) is usually classified as primary (idiopathic) or secondary to metabolic conditions, anatomic abnormalities, trauma, or inflammatory arthritis. The changes in bone and synovium are the sources of pain [13]. In osteoarthritic synovial tissues, low-grade inflammation contributes to disease pathogenesis. Clinical symptoms and signs in joints (e.g., joint swelling, effusion, stiffness, and occasional redness) reflect synovial inflammation clearly [14]. Arthroscopy demonstrates localized synovial proliferative and inflammatory changes in the knee joints in up to 50% of patients with OA. Proteases and cytokines secreted by activated synovium accelerate deterioration of contiguous cartilage lesions [14–16].

Mediators of inflammation (lysosomal enzymes) released from cartilage degradation, detritus, and phagocytosis as well as mechanical stimulation lead to irritation of the synovium. This reactive synovitis (proliferative, frequently villous, pannus-like new connective tissue formation) frequently turns the clinically "silent" arthrosis into "activated arthrosis" or "osteoarthritis" with painful limitation of motion associated with joint effusion. Recurrent episodes may lead to fibrosis and retraction of the capsule with increasing stiffness and contraction of the joint. This additional damage in capsule, ligament, and muscle (apparatus) is called "decompensated arthrosis."

Cartilage should not be the source of pain as it has no nerve endings inside. This is the basis for the poor relationship between the extent of morphological changes (radiologic or pathologic) and clinical problems including pain [17]. The pain confined to the joints is correlated with findings on *soft tissue scintigraphy* [4].

Osteoarthritis of Finger Joints

Involvement of the distal interphalangial (DIP) and proximal interphalangial (PIP) joints is known as Heberden and Bouchard finger polyarthrosis, respectively. The disease is traditionally regarded as a degenerative disease but there is some contradicting evidence. RA should be suspected when metacarpophalangial (MCP) joints are inflamed first. Right-handed individuals often have more symptoms compared to their left hand. There is no well-defined difference between OA and RA in *soft tissue scintigraphy* [18].

Osteoarthritis of the Knee Joint

Osteoarthritis of the knee joint is the most common form of arthritis among the synovial joints. It is characterized by progressive loss of cartilage with peri-articular bone remodeling (osteophytes) leading to pain, disability, and handicap in aging populations. Subchondral membrane destruction by osteoarthritic progression or arthroscopy with wash-out or joint debridement may happen resulting in bone marrow edema and increased pressure in subchondral bone, the most serious source of pain in severe osteoarthritis, which is best seen with MRI.

Sometimes sources of pain generated in osteoarthritis are muscle pain, stretching of the capsule, strain of ligament, and tendon insertion and elevation of periosteum. RSO in osteoarthritis (i.e., knee joint) would not be beneficial if mechanical problems including severe instability or axis deviation persist. Synovial membrane inflammation and low-grade synovitis that are frequently present in patients with symptomatic osteoarthritis play a critical role in disease process, which is best seen by soft tissue scintigraphy.

The management of knee osteoarthritis includes administration of intra-articular corticosteroids to reduce synovitis. This procedure is also a prognostic test for RSO: if intra-articular steroid brings pain relief for days or weeks, then RSO will usually be effectively significant for longer periods.

The synovitis in OA has a major role in the disease pathogenesis, and some forms of OA are as much an inflammatory as a degenerative form of arthritis [17]. Varus and valgus deformity usually occurs when the medial or lateral compartments are involved, respectively. Retropatellar arthrosis may be seen after involvement of the patello-femoral joint.

Pigmented Villonodular Synovitis

The histological diagnosis is usually established after arthroscopic examination or other surgical procedures. The abundant synovitis should be removed and arthroscopic synovectomy will be sufficient as surgical procedure for this purpose. RSO should be performed 6 weeks later when the extensive iatrogenic wounds are healed and leakage is unlikely. In a meta-analysis, therapeutic outcome was favorable in $77.3\pm25.3\%$ of patients [19].

Contraindications

Absolute Contraindications

- Pregnancy
- Breast feeding
- Local skin infection
- Actual rupture of popliteal cyst (Baker's cyst)

Relative Contraindications

- RSO should only be used in children and young patients (<20 years) if the benefits of treatment are likely to outweigh the potential hazards. RSO is routinely applied in hemophilic children.
- Extensive joint instability with bone destruction

Side-Effects

Side-effects are not common, and are well tolerated by the patients. A temporary worsening of synovitis may be relieved by local cooling. A nationwide survey in Germany has shown that RSO is associated with complications in about 1:1,000 cases [20]. Local radionecrosis may be seen if the administered colloid refluxes through the needle track or due to incorrect injection technique. Such necrosis heals slowly (in several months) and usually leaves only a small depigmented area in the skin.

Thrombosis due to immobilization may occur in the treated limb. This can be avoided by administration of heparin for a few days. Joint infection is very rare (1: 35,000 joint punctures) and can be avoided by employing a strict sterile technique [21].

Side-Effects

- Worsening of synovitis
- Local radionecrosis
- Thrombosis

Risk of Malignancy

There is no reported evidence of radiation-induced malignancy. Determination of the frequency of dicentric chromosomes in peripheral lymphocytes is the most sensitive method available today to detect radiation effects. In a recent study, the number of dicentric chromosomes was determined immediately before and 4 weeks after RSO with ^{90}Y colloid. After RSO, 41 dicentric chromosomes were found in 10,000 cells (0.41%), whereas 25 were found in 10,000 cells (incidence rate 0.25%) before RSO. The difference was not statistically significant [22].

In a meta-analysis of 9,300 patients who underwent yttrium-90 RSO, only two cases of leukemia were detected (chronic myelocytic leukemia after 4 years and lymphatic leukemia after 6 months). The short time interval between RSO and the diagnosis of leukemia suggests that RSO unlikely causes leukemia in these patients [23].

In another study, no case of treatment-related malignancy has been reported within 25 years of ^{90}Y-RSO [24]. In a 7-year study including 1,228 patients, it was found that those treated with RSO had a lower rate of malignancies than those who were not [25]. Our experience with RSO since 1972 (6,000 RSO cases per year in the last decade) showed no increase in prevalence of RSO-induced malignancy.

Radiopharmaceuticals

The most common radiopharmaceuticals used for RSO (Fig. 18.2):

- ^{90}Y-yttrium colloid (knee joints)
- ^{186}Re-rhenium colloid (middle-sized joints)
- ^{169}Er-erbium colloid (small joints)

The physical characteristics of these radionuclides are described in Fig. 18.2, and recommended dosages are listed in Table 18.1. These radiopharmaceuticals are β-emitters in colloidal suspensions. Other radiocolloids including dysprosium-165-ferric-hydroxide, holmium-166-hydroxy apatite, and sammarium-153-hydroxy apatite are used less frequently for RSO.

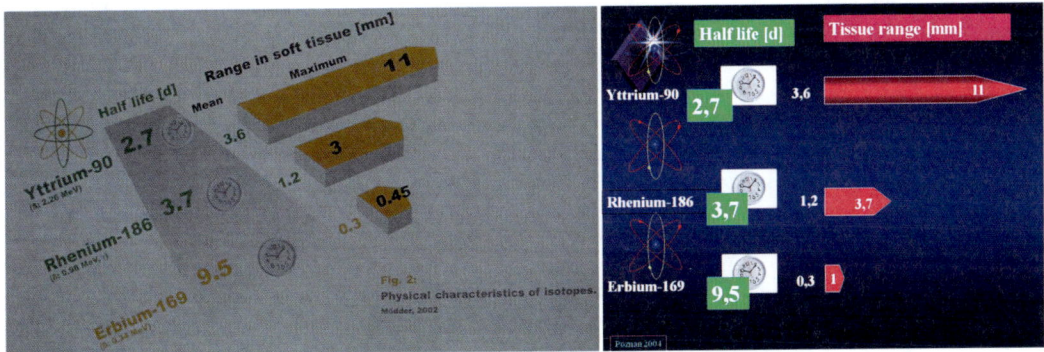

Fig. 18.2 Radioisotopes for radiosynoviorthesis

Table 18.1 Amount of activity for radionuclides used in RSO of various joints (MBq)

Joint	Yttrium-90	Rhenium-186	Erbium-169
Knee joint	185–222		
Glenohumeral joint		74	
Elbow joint		74	
Wrist joint		55–74	
Hip joint		111–185	
Ankle joint		74	
Talonavicular/Subtalar joint		55	
Thumb base joint			30
Metacarpophalangeal (MCP) joint			22
Proximal interphalangeal (PIP) joint			18
Distal interphalangeal (DIP) joint			15
Cuneonavicular joint			37
Tarsometatarsal joint			22
Metatarsophalangeal (MTP) joint I			30
MTP joint II–V			22

A study for absorbed dose calculation was performed for ^{90}Y-yttrium colloid, ^{186}Re-rhenium colloid, and [^{169}Er]-erbium colloid radionuclides. Radiation absorbed by the synovium was found to be about 130 Gy [26].

Ideal radiopharmaceuticals for RSO should emit β-radiation sufficient to penetrate and ablate the synovial tissue, avoid damaging the underlying articular cartilage or overlying skin and provide the smallest minimal lymphatic clearance. The particles attached to beta emitting radionuclides should be small enough to be phagocytozed and large enough to remain with uniform distribution within the joint cavity and should be biodegradable. The ideal particle size should be about 10 nm [27].

Mechanism of Action

After intra-articular administration, the radioactive particles in colloidal form are phagocytozed by synovial macrophages lining the synovial cavity [28]. A particle size of about 10±5 nm is essential to avoid leakage and provide homogenous distribution on the surface of synovium. β-radiation leads to coagulation necrosis, sclerosis,

and fibrosis of the synovial tissue including vessels and pain receptors, thus results in reducing effusion, swelling, and pain of the joint. The cartilage is not a target for the radiation effects and has no ability for phagocytosis [2].

The remark "synovitis is the villain of the drama" is valid not only for rheumatic diseases but also for osteoarthritis (activated arthrosis). Arthrosis with typical joint space narrowing as a result of cartilage defects is not associated with pain because cartilage has no nerve endings and vessels, as mentioned before. Activated arthrosis (osteoarthritis) results from inflammation and causes pain, swelling, and effusions only after synovitis by detritus [4, 18, 29]. The healing effects of RSO in osteoarthritis (i.e., knee joint) will not be fully obtained if mechanical problems such as severe instability and axis deviation are predominating factors.

Simultaneous intra-articular injection of corticosteroids (i.e., triamcinolone hexacetonide or triamcinolone acetonide) is recommended to reduce local inflammation and prolong residence time of the radiopharmaceutical agent in the joint [30]. Moreover, steroids reduce synovial edema allowing penetration of the radiocolloid more effectively, thus reaching to the deteriorating pannus, and eventually improving the efficacy of RSO.

Patient Selection

Patients with rheumatoid arthritis are treated with systemic anti-rheumatoid drugs as it is a systemic disease. Joints with no adequate improvement after at least 6 months of systemic therapy even after corticosteroid injections are selected for RSO, and thus escalation of systemic therapy with its possible side-effects is avoided. In mono- or oligo-arthritis, RSO can be the first-choice-therapy if locally administered corticosteroids fail [7, 31].

The guidelines of the German Society of Rheumatology require at least one failure of intra-articular corticosteroid administration before the joint is regarded suitable for RSO. Orthopedic patients should be referred after failure of local corticoid injection and/or ineffective conservative treatment. Efficacy of RSO has been demonstrated after total knee replacement and in patients with effusions after arthroscopy [32–34]. The time interval between arthroscopy or joint surgery (i.e., PVNS) and RSO should be 4–6 weeks.

Diagnostic Studies Prior to RSO

Diagnostic studies prior to RSO basically include:
- Medical history and clinical examination of the joint
- Ultrasonography
- Scintigraphy
- X-ray images
- Laboratory tests

Ultrasonography (Arthrosonography)

Examination with ultrasound is useful to evaluate synovial structure and thickness, extent of effusion, possible tenosynovitis or rotator cuff tears (shoulder), osteophytes, and capsule swelling (in the knee joint). Ultrasound is obligatory prior to performing RSO of the knee joint to rule out problems including Baker's cyst puncture.

Bone and Joint Scintigraphy

Multiphase scintigraphy (3-phase scintigraphy) using ^{99m}Tc-MDP (or similar radiopharmaceuticals) is the best diagnostic tool to detect synovial inflammation and to select joints for RSO. Three-phase bone scintigraphy provides detailed information in each phase of the study.

First phase (radionuclide angiography): Initial blood flow is demonstrated by imaging the arrival of the radiopharmaceutical.

Second phase (10 min p.i.) (*soft tissue scintigraphy*) visualizes the blood pool and detects active inflammation of the synovium. Multiple views should be obtained if necessary (e.g., medial, lateral, and plantar views) (Fig. 18.3)

Third phase (3 h p.i.) (*bone scintigraphy*) assesses bone involvement.

Second phase is useful to evaluate activated arthrosis (osteoarthritis) while focal accumulation in the third phase not demonstrated in the second phase suggests inactive arthrosis, in which RSO is not indicated. Focal accumulation in both phases suggests activated arthrosis (osteoarthritis), in which RSO can be successfully used.

Whole-body bone scan provides an overview to assess multiple joint involvement in polyarthritis, both rheumatoid and seronegative arthritis [4]. Single photon emission computed tomography (SPECT) and magnetic resonance imaging (MRI) are useful in selected cases for detailed local assessment (i.e., bone edema, femoral head necrosis).

X-Ray Fluoroscopy and Arthroscopy

Most procedures are completed by arthrography but all joints except the knee should be punctured under fluoroscopy during RSO procedure. Dye distribution that is injected immediately afterwards predicts the distribution of radionuclide and the control for perfect needle position in the cavity of the joint is ensured (Fig. 18.4). Otherwise, intra-articular injection of radiopharmaceuticals is not guaranteed. It is best to use a surgical picture intensifier ("C-arm"), for this

Fig. 18.3 Bone scan (second phase, soft tissue): Psoriatic arthritis with typical "stream-like" pattern. Hand is the "visiting card" of the rheumatic patient

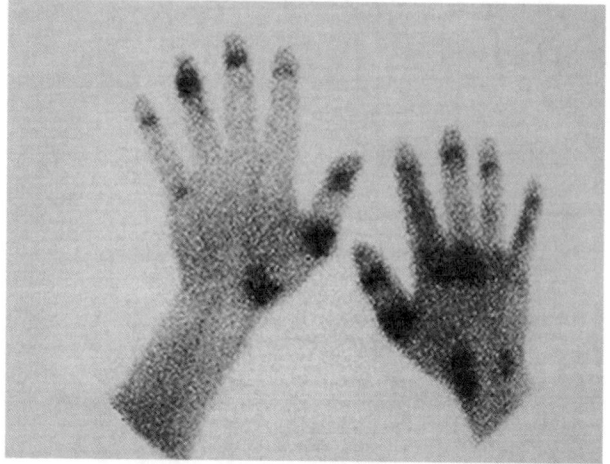

Fig. 18.4 (a) Arthrogram of MTP I. The joint cavity with its synovium is target for RSO. (b) Arthrogram of a PIP joint. Intraarticular position of the needle, but *not in the cavity*. The contrast medium is injected into a villous. If it happened with Erbium-169, serious side effects should have been seen

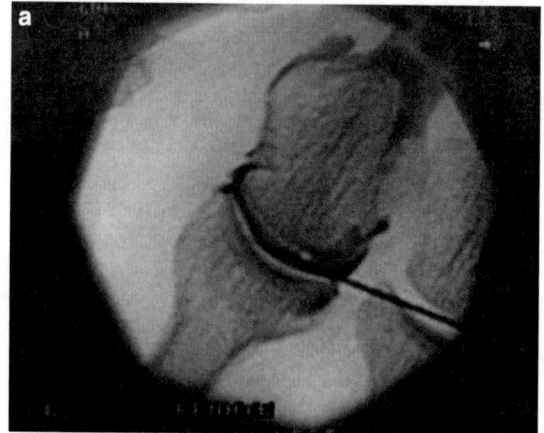

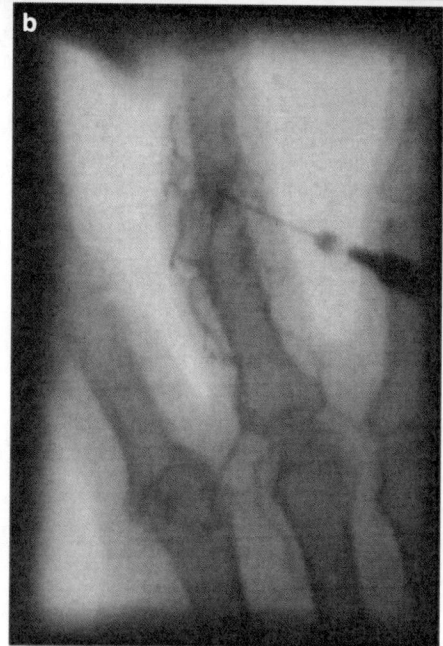

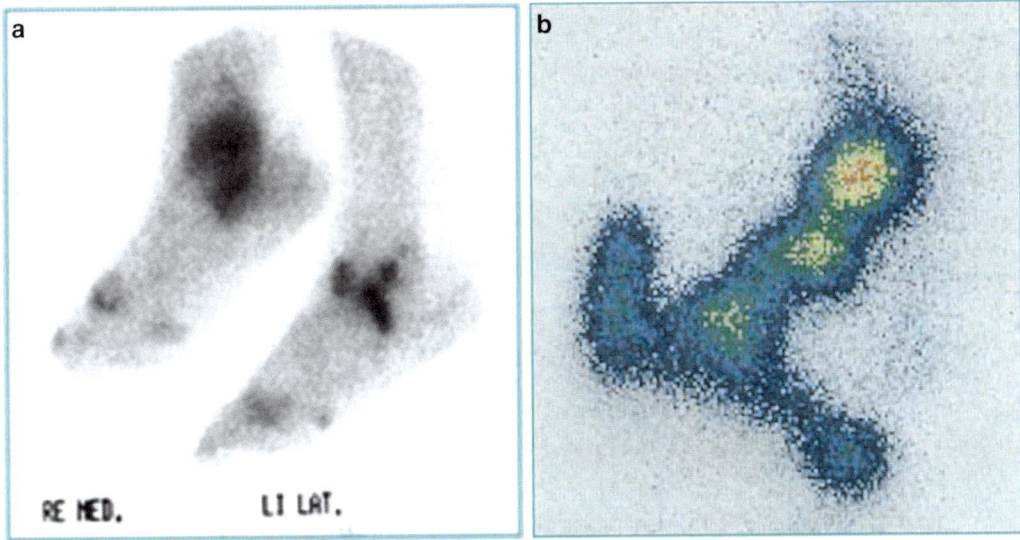

Fig. 18.5 The patient with rheumatoid arthritis should undergo a triple arthrodesis of the left foot. Is that a case for RSO? (**a**) *Soft tissue scintigraphy* detects inflammatory involvement in the talonavicular, subtalar and calcaneo- cuboid joints. (**b**) *Distribution scintigram* in the same position demonstrating distribution in the identical joints marked in the diagnostic scintigram

purpose, to allow a complete free access to all joints and the closest contact of the joint to the X-ray tube for optimal picture quality.

Distribution Scintigraphy

A distribution scintigraphy is performed after RSO with yttrium-90 and Rhenium-186 after immobilizing the joint.

- The joint is immobilized for 48 h to prevent leakage and necrosis in the injection channel or skin caused by reflux and to avoid transporting radioactive particles through the lymphatic vessels (leakage).
- Distribution scintigram confirms the appropriate intra-articular distribution of the radiopharmaceutical (Fig. 18.5). Scintigraphy is performed acquiring Bremsstrahlung emission of yttrium-90 and 140 keV gamma photon of rhenium-186.
- Scintigraphy is not possible with [^{169}Er] erbium because of short range (1 mm) of its beta particles.

RSO Procedure

The patient should be given written and verbal instruction about the procedure. An informed consent should be signed by the patient before the procedure.

Principles of Joint Puncture Technique

- Nuclear Medicine physician is responsible for the whole procedure including the puncture of the joint.
- Joint punctures should be performed providing strict asepsis in a designated room complying with the local radiation safety regulations. Joint puncture is needed for intra-articular instillation of radiopharmaceuticals, aspirating joint effusion during follow-up, puncturing Baker's cyst, and intra-articular corticoid injection.
- Attention should be paid to a convenient position of the patient and the physician. The skin at the injection site is shaved and disinfected. Disposable instruments should be used and

the area surrounding the joint should be covered with a sterile hole sheet.

- Knowledge of joint anatomy and skill for the puncture technique are essential for the success of RSO [4, 31]. Instillation of radionuclide out of the joint capsule could have disastrous consequences (extended necrosis).
- The joint should be first punctured with a syringe containing local anesthetic, and the syringe should be then replaced with another syringe containing the therapeutic radionuclide without displacing the needle in the joint.
- Most of the existing synovial fluid should be aspirated; but a small amount of fluid should remain to allow better distribution of the radionuclide throughout the joint.
- The injection needle and the puncture channel have to be flushed afterwards (e.g., with the rest of local anesthetic), so that a radiation necrosis along the puncture channel can be avoided.

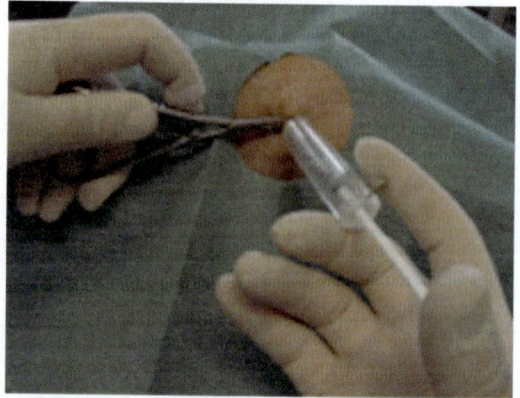

Fig. 18.6 Radioprotection during RSO of a knee joint. Forceps lengthens the distance from the conus of the syringe when the syringe is replaced for corticosteroid after injection of yttrium-90. A beta radiation finger ring dosimeter measures the dose

Radiation Safety Considerations

Necessary radiation safety measures should be taken to protect both the patient and the medical staff performing the procedure. No radiation-induced stochastic side-effects were observed in long-term follow-up [35]. The effective dose to the whole body is estimated to be 30 times lower than in Iodine-131-therapy of benign thyroid diseases [35]. Acrylic syringe protectors, nitril or vinyl gloves, β-finger-dosimeters or forceps (Fig. 18.6), and other relevant measures are used to reduce radiation exposure to the fingers [6].

Joints and Clinical Applications

Sternoclavicular joint: The sternoclavicular joint may be involved in cases of psoriatic arthritis, especially in Sappho syndrome, and OA. Normally, this joint is either completely or incompletely divided by a longitudinal disc.

Glenohumeral joint: Apart from RA or OA, special cases such as "omarthritis of the elderly woman" or "Milwaukee shoulder" with very painful osseous destruction and bloody effusions may be seen. Ventral vertical and horizontal ultrasonographic sections in the intertubercular sulcus show the long bicipital tendon and its recess that may also be filled with effusion. A partial or complete rotator cuff tears, usually with leakage of the effusion into the bursae (subacromial or subdeltoideal) should always be investigated. However, rotator cuff tears are not contraindicated for RSO because the radiopharmaceutical distributed intra-articularly will not leave the glenohumeral cavity by leaking into periarticular tissues. It may enter the bursa subacromialis and remain in a closed cavity. AP and lateral views are best for scintigraphic imaging. Necessary items for puncture include puncture needle 20G × 2 3/4 in., 0.9 × 70 (long No.1 needle), and a connecting tube for dye. Recommended activity for RSO is 74–111 MBq (2–3 mCi) [186Re] rhenium sulfide.

Elbow joint: On ultrasonography, a cubital arthritis is most easily verified with a dorsal longitudinal plane above the olecranonal fossa (effusion: echo-free to poor interior structure). Attention must be paid to osteodestructive changes (erosions at the osseous surface, e.g., of the olecranon), furthermore to cysts, olecranonal bursitis. On arthrography, there are no synovial tendon sheaths at the elbow joint and a striped distribution pattern of the dye shows an

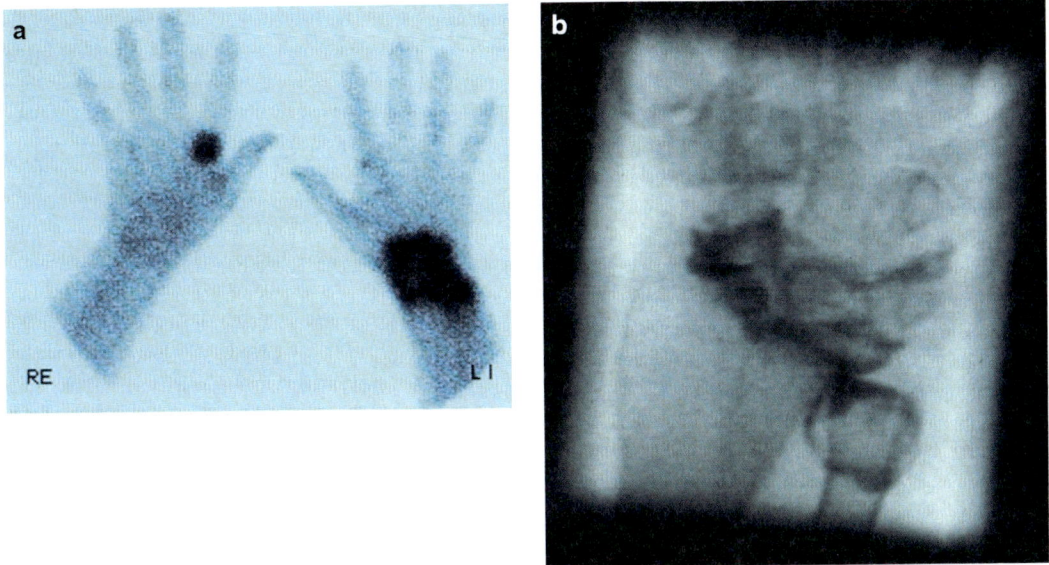

Fig. 18.7 (a) "Soft tissue scintigram" of hands of a patient with rheumatoid arthritis involving the (proximal) wrist joint, whole carpus and the distal radioulnar joint are involved. The ligamentum triangulare is destroyed. (b) Arthrogram during RSO demonstrates good distribution of the contrast agent even into the distal radioulnar joint

extra-articular injection. Rarely, the joint cavity communicates with the large olecranon bursa. Recommended activity for RSO is 55.5–74 MBq (1.5–2 mCi) [^{186}Re] rhenium [36]. The most convenient position for the patient is the sitting position; the upper arm elevated laterally and horizontally; the elbow fixed at 90°, lies horizontal on the fluorescent tube.

Joints of the Hand (MCP, PIP, and DIP): There are characteristic patterns of distribution for every disease best recognized on soft tissue scintigraphy (phase 2) (Fig. 18.7). In *rheumatoid arthritis*, MCP and PIP joints are often affected while involvement of DIP joints is rare. Involvement is mostly symmetrical. Asymmetric ipsilateral involvement of the finger joints and the "stream-like" affection (*sausage fingers*) or a transverse involvement of the DIP joints is typical in *psoriatic arthritis* (Fig. 18.3). In finger polyarthrosis, DIP joints (Heberden) and/or PIP joints (Bouchard) and/or the first metacarpophalangeal joint (rhizarthrosis) are affected.

The injection of corticosteroids is the easiest intervention for *local therapeutic management*. However, its effect does not last long and becomes even shorter with repetition, apart from the unfavorable side-effects in long term (e.g., pseudo-Charcot-joint). The results of surgical interventions including early or late synovectomy, tenosynovectomy, tendon reconstructions (tears), nerve decompressions, resection (interposition) arthroplasties, arthrodesis, and alloarthroplasty are often disappointing.

On the contrary, the RSO with [^{169}Er] erbium has longlasting success rates. A repetition (Re-RSO) may strengthen and stabilize the result for many years. RSO is simple and not less effective than some surgical efforts especially in the finger joints. In advanced Heberden's arthrosis, the only useful surgical procedure available is often surgical fusion (e.g., arthrodesis with Kirschner wires), whereas a single injection with [^{169}Er] erbium is sufficient for substantial relief of pain in the majority of cases.

Wrist joints: Ultrasonography often gives valuable additional information with equivocal clinical findings. It is most useful in distinguishing the carpal arthritis from a tenosynovitis (maybe also additional). The tenosynovitis appears in the longitudinal section as an echo-rich structure (tendon) in an echo-poor tubular structure. A synovitis of the wrist is best documented in volar and dorsal longitudinal sections. The caput-ulnae syndrome becomes apparent through erosions of the ulnar head with surrounding effusion. In rheumatoid arthritis, the destructive synovitis may devastate normal anatomy in various ways. Therefore, arthrography is often successful to demonstrate all compartments including the intercarpal joints and the distal radioulnar joint with a single injection. On scintigraphy, the intensity of pathologically increased accumulation on the second phase images (soft tissue scintigraphy) correlates with the pain, swelling, and motion limitation. The radiopharmaceutical spreads to all diseased regions corresponding with the arthrographic distribution (Fig. 18.7).

RSO is not contraindicated in an existing tenosynovitis; in fact, it is often very effective. By common joint puncture of the wrist, it is possible to demonstrate the diseased tendon sheath and the reach of the instilled [186]Re arthrographically. Recommended activity for RSO is 55.5 MBq (1.5 mCi) [[186]Re] rhenium. It is usually not necessary to develop a sophisticated puncture technique for different joint spaces, as the destruction of structures in arthritis will frequently lead to obliteration of the physiologic separations between spaces. A puncture of the proximal wrist joint is almost sufficient while the usual puncture site should be situated between the middle third of the scaphoid and the distal articular facet of the radius.

Joints of the fingers: Ultrasonography offers little advantage (except for the first carpometaphalangeal joint) over inspection, palpation, and radiographic findings. In activated rhizarthrosis, a narrowing distinct joint space and the swelling capsule can be demonstrated. Scintigraphy of the finger joints provides important information. The hands show typical patterns of involvement in rheumatoid arthritis, psoriatic arthritis, activated rhizarthrosis, and finger polyarthrosis.

First carpometacarpal joint (thumb base): Rhizarthrosis is detected radiographically in many asymptomatic patients. There may be a focal intense tracer uptake on skeletal scintigraphy (late phase). The findings of painful symptomatic problems in activated rhizarthrosis (rhizarthritis)

correlate with the findings of soft tissue scintigraphy (second phase). The trapezscaphoid joint is involved additionally in 25% of the cases.

Recommended activity for RSO of metacarpophalangeal Joints (MCP) is 22–37 MBq (0.6–1 mCi) [[169]Er] erbium. Lower power in fluoroscopy should be used for PIP and DIP joints to reduce the radiation load for the therapist. We recommend using a finger-grasp-forceps with a long handle which can bend the joint slightly. The DIP joints, affected in polyarthritis or Heberden's polyarthrosis, may often be swollen and/or changed after osteodestruction. In these cases, making a puncture can become difficult. For these small joints, the skill of the therapist is vital as these are highly sensitive joints ("fingertip instinct"). The patient should be closely followed up during the RSO procedure as she/he may faint during the puncture. It is thus better to treat the patient on supine position. The finger should be held with a forceps at the distal phalanx.

Hip joint: On ultrasonography, the leading finding in hip arthritis is joint effusion with elevation of the joint capsule from the femoral neck. A two-phase scintigraphy of the hip is recommended, as the proportion of the arthritic component (activated coxarthrosis) and the arthrosis can be differentiated by this technique. Images should be taken in AP and PA views and additionally in a "perineal view" (patient sitting on the gamma-camera).

A 20G × 2 3/4 in. 0.9 × 70 long No.1 needle is recommended for puncture. The ventral approach with a negligible risk is the best. The needle tip is directed to the midline of the femoral neck just distal to the femoral head. The distance to the medially located vessels is usually far enough to spare them. The injection into the joint space is dangerous due to the risk of damaging the ligamentum capitis femoris containing blood vessels, and thus possibly inducing a femoral head necrosis (Fig. 18.8). If no effusion is aspirated, saline can be injected to unfold the joint space locally. In coxitis, pain will be typically felt by the patient in the groin. If the patient describes the pain in lateral of the hip—often with spreading to the lateral thigh downward to the knee—then think of bursitis trochanterica.

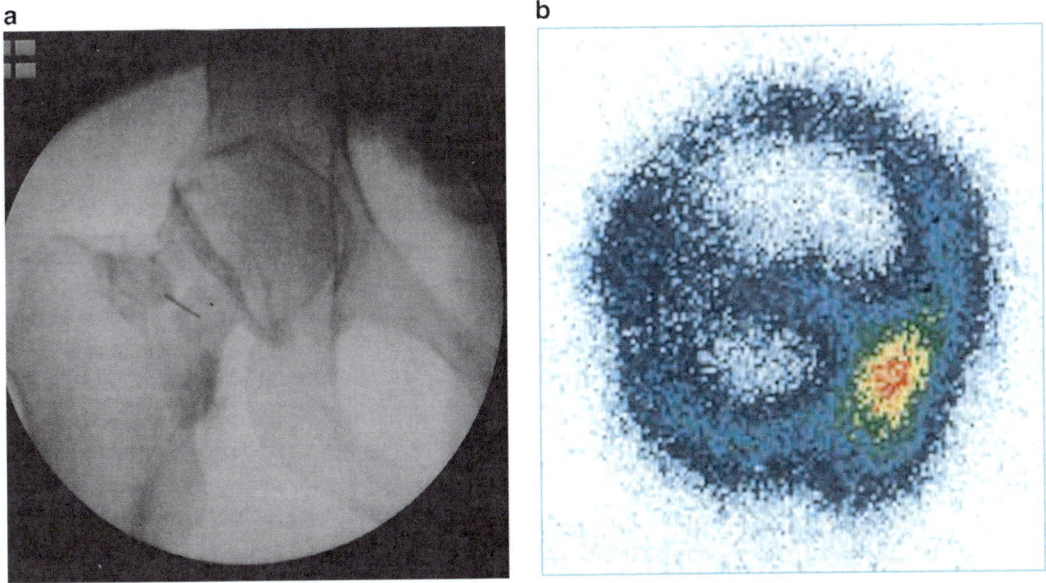

Fig. 18.8 (**a**) Arthrogram of a hip joint. The image shows perfect and safe needle position. Beware of injecting into the joint space as usually recommended! You would risk destroying the ligamentum capitis femoris and thus cause femur head necrosis. (**b**) Perfect distribution scintigram after injection of Rhenium-186—colloid in the hip joint

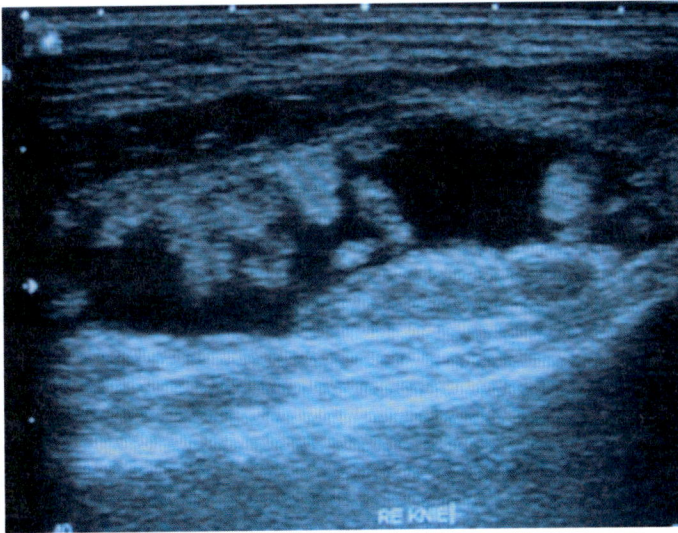

Fig. 18.9 Ultrasonography of the knee joint

Knee joint

Ultrasound is an obligatory examination before RSO of knee joints. With the patient in supine position, a medially or laterally obtained suprapatellar longitudinal section gives information about involvement of the medial or lateral compartment and demonstrates existence and quality of an effusion (no echo: liquid; multiple oval interior echos: gelatinous) and quality of the synovium (synovial thickness, smooth or villous-like ("coral-reef") surface, adhesions) (Fig. 18.9). The suprapatellar transverse plane of the knee with flexed position allows assessment of the

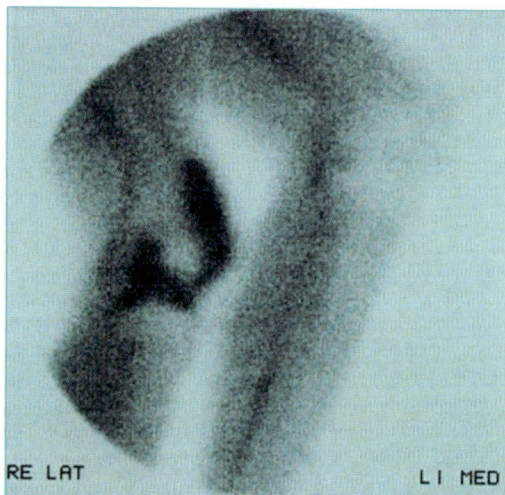

Fig. 18.10 *Soft tissue scintigram* with 99m-Tc MDP, 10 min after intravenous injection. Increased accumulation in the synovitis above the arthrotic right knee joint. The tracer distribution reflects the cavity of the knee joint including the recessus suprapatellaris. The left knee is free of complaints and is scintigraphically intact

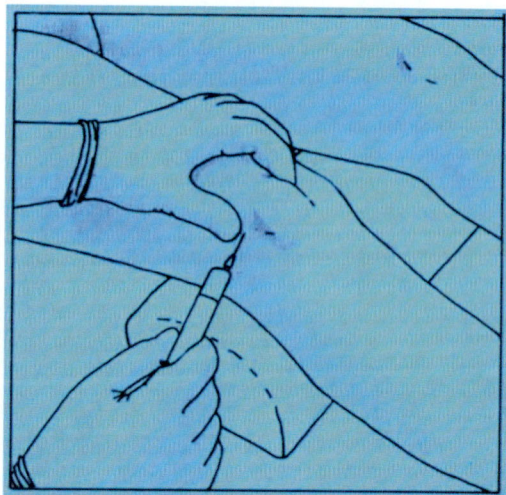

Fig. 18.11 Injection technique for the knee joint. Avoid injecting beside the ligamentum patellae with the patient in sitting position, otherwise there is a risk of injecting yttrium-90 into the crucial ligaments or in Hoffa's fat body

femoropatellar space. Ultrasonography is essential in the diagnosis of Baker's cyst [4, 36]. The soft tissue scintigraphy (10 min p.i.) detects the degree of active inflammation of synovium (Fig. 18.10). The bone scintigraphy (3 h p.i.) assesses the bone involvement in the painful process. If there is increased accumulation in knee arthrosis suggesting associated synovitis, a good therapeutic outcome for RSO is expected.

Puncture

The best puncture technique for the knee joint is shown in Fig. 18.11. The list of items necessary for knee joint puncture includes:

- Sterile gloves and drape, mouth guard
- 5 mL syringe with local anesthetic, puncture needle No.1
- 10 mL syringe (for aspiration of synovial fluid)
- 1 mL syringe with yttrium-90 colloid suspension
- 2 mL syringe filled with corticosteroid
- Small basin for collection of synovial fluid
- Swabs, bandage, splint

Recommended activity for knee joint *RSO* is 185–222 MBq (5–6 mCi) yttrium-90 colloid suspension. Smaller amount of activity (111–148 MBq, 3–4 mCi) is recommended for joints without effusion. Most convenient position for the patient is the supine position; knee gently flexed on an underlying cushion.

Technique: The patella is pushed slightly lateral with the fingers of the left hand, so that the left thumb can easily palpate the place between the lateral upper border of the patella and the insertion of the tendon of m. rectus femoris. The needle is inserted slightly dorsal to the patella. The local anesthetic is first injected subcutaneously, so that the tiny skin-punch-cylinders are not carried into the joint. Then the needle is quickly pushed into the joint cavity. Injection through or medial or lateral to the ligamentum patellae (with the patient sitting) could deposit the radiopharmaceutical into the swollen Hoffa's fat body leading to fat necrosis. This could also destroy the anterior crucial ligament.

Arthrography is not necessary and not recommended when yttrium-90 colloid is preferred for RSO. It was reported that yttrium-90 and colloid are dissolved due to contrast medium possibly EDTA [37] while this effect is not seen when erbium-169 or rhenium-186 is used for RSO. If there is effusion, complete aspiration is not recommended which provide a sufficient distribution volume.

If there is no effusion, instillation of about 10–20 mL saline is necessary to provide a sufficient distribution volume. Aspiration of fluid confirms the right positioning of the needle tip. Eventually additional instillation of air is preferred by some practitioners to be certain about the intra-articular position. After instillation, of yttrium-90, a corticosteroid agent (e.g., 20–40 mg triamcinolonehexacetonide) is injected to flush the injection channel. It is also useful

1. To avoid an iatrogenic effusion resulting from irritation.
2. To reduce the thickness of the edematous superficial layer of synovium for yttrium-90 beta radiation with its limited penetration to become more effective.

After, instillation of radionuclide, firm pressure is gently applied to the puncture site, and the knee joint is then wrapped with an elastic bandage and a splint. A distribution scintigram under the gamma camera is done using the Bremsstrahlung radiation of yttrium-90 to verify homogeneous distribution of the radiopharmaceutical within the joint cavity. Alternatively, distribution scintigram can be performed with yttrium-90 and 20 MBq of technetium-99m pertechnetate instilled simultaneously.

Baker's cyst: Baker's cyst is ultrasonographically diagnosed in about 25% of our patients who underwent RSO in our institution. The Baker's cyst is usually located in the region of the medial gastrocnemic head. Persisting inflammatory activity of the main joint, enhanced by flexion movements in the knee joint results in more effusion to be pumped into the Baker's cyst. This effusion cannot flow back due to a functionally one-way valve mechanism that can eventually lead to spontaneous rupture of the Baker's cyst [4].

The existence of a Baker's cyst is stated in numerous publications as a "contraindication" for RSO, but the reason is nowhere mentioned. It seems to be a question of unchecked quoting of quotes. Occasionally, a rupture occurs spontaneously mimicking lower leg thrombosis. If RSO

procedure and subsequent effusion cause a rupture in the Baker's cyst, the radionuclide spreads into the calf muscles resulting in serious consequences. In case of a valve mechanism, the Baker's cyst as a "divisioned joint" may be over- or under-accessed by the radionuclide.

The Baker's cyst has also some problems for the surgeon: As the synovitis is located in the knee joint, it has to be rehabilitated at least by arthroscopy. The Baker's cyst is usually removed surgically from a dorsal approach. Recurrence of the Baker's cyst after surgery is not uncommon.

On ultrasonography, which is performed with patient in prone position, the Baker's cysts can vary considerably in position, size, form, interior lining, and echo pattern of the contents. The cyst is usually filled with clear liquid without considerable wall thickening, may show an extended villous-like synovial hypertrophy, adhesions, real septations, and pseudo-septations. The connecting duct is identified in the popliteal transverse section. The cyst gets smaller in size and the duct dilates by pressing slightly with the transducer in the absence of valve mechanism (Fig. 18.12).

If the duct cannot be identified (obliterated) and/or the firm cyst not be compressed, a valve mechanism is assumed to exist. The Baker's cyst should be punctured under ultrasonographic guidance, which also allows drainage. Infusion of 20 mg triamcinolone is advisable. The ultrasound of the Baker's cyst is decisive if the Baker's cyst reaches to the distal third of the calf, surgery is the procedure of choice. Usually, no drainage is required prior to RSO if the cyst is hardly palpable. For RSO, the main joint should be punctured, not the Baker's cyst. If a reactive inflammation with effusion after RSO is foreseen, the amount of activity is fractionated (a smaller initial activity is followed by a second fraction given 3 months later).

The patient always should be informed in detail before the RSO about the complications regarding the Baker's cyst. The importance of immobilization after RSO and the possibility of complications due to joint movement and subsequent effusion should be emphasized. In a personal prospective study of 150 joints with a Baker's cyst, no side-effect or complication was

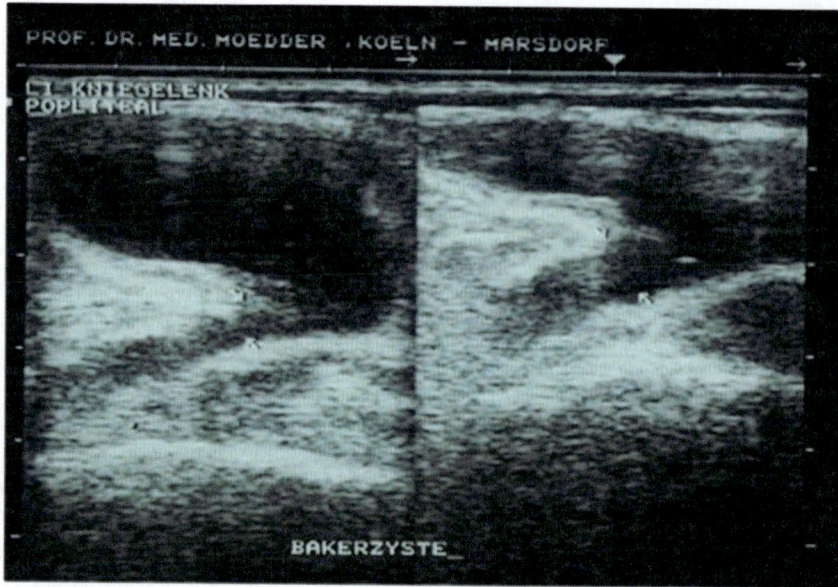

Fig. 18.12 Ultrasonographic appearance of a Baker's cyst (transverse section). Check for valve mechanism. *Left*: the connecting duct between knee joint (*below*) and Baker's cyst is seen. *Right*: by the pressure of transducer, the cyst decreased in size and the duct dilates. No valve mechanism

experienced. The Baker's cyst disappeared in 87 patients after the first RSO and in 54 patients after the second application [4].

RSO after total knee replacement: In contrast to the relatively unproblematic total hip replacement, the total knee replacement is not always successful. The complaints become sometimes worse, even after revision of the knee replacement. Clinically, relapsing effusions with a painful joint movement is common. Polyethylene disease after surgery poses a problem for RSO.

No thickened synovium is detectable in most of the patients, but sometimes villous- and cushionlike synovial hypertrophy is seen on ultrasonography. In patients with moderate effusion, a wide echo-poor zone is seen, which may extend beyond the synovium into the surrounding soft tissue. On scintigraphy, the knee implant contrasts with the surrounding tissue as a photopenic area. Intensely increased accumulation around the implant, frequently affecting the tibial component is often suggestive of aseptic implant loosening.

RSO procedure: Experience is vital to avoid complications. The post-surgical scar tissue can cause difficulty in puncture. The synovial fluid aspirated during RSO should be sent for culture and antibiogram. If the effusion is hemorrhagic, flushing with saline should be repeated until the fluid gets clear. For fractionated therapy, the first radioactivity of yttrium-90 should be 185 MBq (5 mCi), and the corresponding amount for the second session after 3 months should be 222 MBq (6 mCi).

In the first report in 1994 describing the results of 18 patients treated with RSO, the effusions disappeared in all patients [38]. Pain relief was reported in 15 patients and persistence of pain in three (one patient had an extreme instability, one patient axial malposition, and one patient had a unicompartmental slide implant with erosion of the tibial plateau). Recent reports confirmed these findings in larger number of patients [32]. In 107 patients who underwent RSO after total knee replacement, effusion up to 780 mL disappeared in 93 cases and decreased in 8 cases. Symptom improvement was reported in 89% patients.

The main reason for soft tissue problems and aseptic loosening after total knee replacement is the polyethylene wear which may cause severe granulomatosis. Additionally, staphylococcus epidermidis adheres and grows on polymer surfaces producing extracellular slime. Clinical findings include warmth and swelling of the joint, limitation of mobility, and

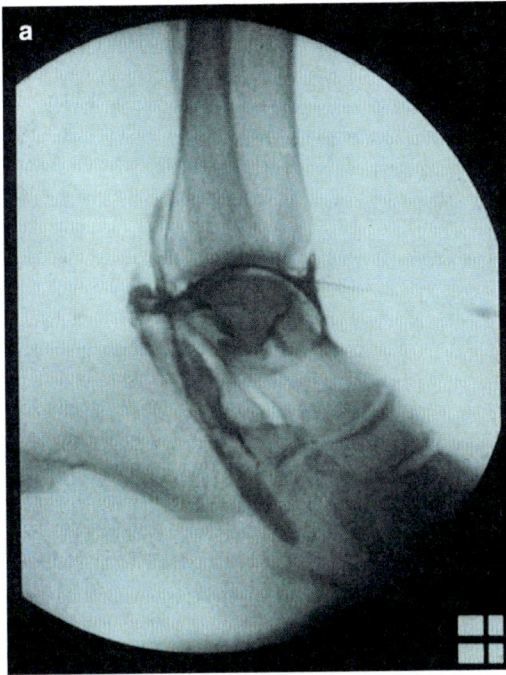

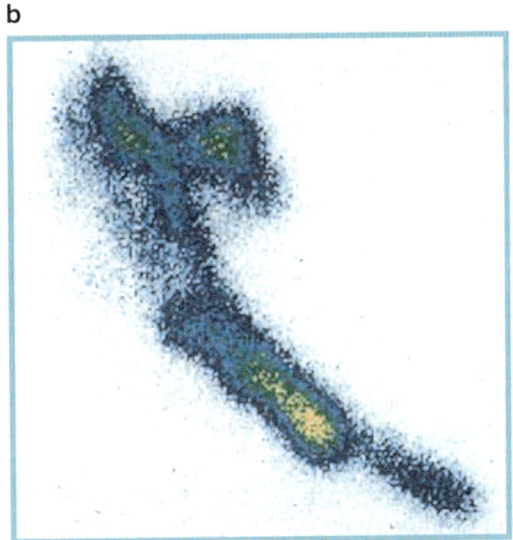

Fig. 18.13 Ankle joint. (**a**) Arthrogram of a patient with Rheumatoid arthritis. (Note the co-representation of the common peroneal tendon sheath). (**b**) The distribution scintigram after RSO demonstrates the distribution of ^{186}Re within the ankle joint and the peroneal tendon sheath

recurrent effusions. Ultrasound of the knee joint and soft tissue scintigraphy are the best methods to document the pathological process. RSO is an adequate therapy to remove the effects of polyethylene wear: β-emission stops the growth of the foreign body granulomas.

Joints of the Foot

Tarsal joints and midfoot: Ultrasonographic examinations on longitudinal and transverse sections, ventrally and dorsally, reveal valuable information. Arthritis of the superior or inferior tarsal joints is best recognized on the plane above the dorsum pedis. Ultrasound is very helpful especially in patients with rheumatoid arthritis, psoriatic arthritis, or seronegative spondyloarthritis who cannot localize the pain exactly. The joint to be treated with RSO must be determined precisely before intra-articular delivery of the radiopharmaceutical. A peroneal or tibialis posterior tenosynovitis that often co-exists in tarsal joint arthritis is detected on ultrasonographic examination as a broad, light longitu-dinal lane (tendon), which lies in a long dark field (effusion border). Soft tissue scintigraphy (second phase) may occasionally be helpful in revealing an enthesitis or localizing pathology when the patient complains about "pain in the whole foot."

Superior tarsal joint (ankle joint): During puncture, patient should be in a comfortable lateral position (for right superior tarsal joint: right lateral position; for left superior tarsal joint: left lateral position). Puncture should be guided by fluoroscopy. For anterior approach: the extensor hallucis longus tendon is palpated with the joint slightly plantar flexed. The needle should be inserted just lateral to the tendon (height and insertion angle are easily to ascertain by fluoroscopy). It is important to have the foot in a lateral position. Contrary to the common belief, tenosynovitis is effectively treated by RSO. On arthrogram, the peroneal tendon sheath is visualized by the instilled ^{186}Re (Fig. 18.13).

Inferior tarsal joint: The inferior tarsal joint is anatomically composed of three joints (talocalca-neonavicular, subtalar, and posterior compartment).

Fig. 18.14 Ultrasono-
graphy of foot. Effusion in
ankle joint (*left*) and
talonavicular joint (*right*).
RSO using [169]Re has been
performed separately to
both joints

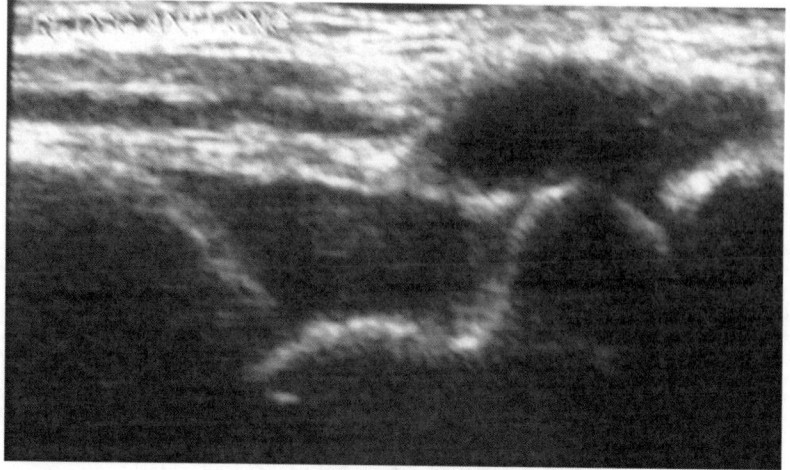

They lose their anatomical separation during the
course of arthritis. Currently, RSO is usually performed for talocalcaneonavicular joint.
Ultrasonographic and scintigraphic examinations
are essential prior to RSO. Two joints can be
treated in the same session (Fig. 18.14).
Differentiation between arthritis of the inferior
tarsal joint and neuropathic arthropathy in diabetes should be made before proceeding to RSO.

Other joints of the tarsus: The cuneonavicular
joint and the tarsometatarsal joints are injected
in the same position as the talonavicular joint.
Tarsometatarsal joints 4 and 5 have a common cavity. In RA or OA, the joints may lose normal separations of the cavities. The whole inflamed synovium
of this area is reached with a single injection.

Toe joints: Rheumatoid arthritis, psoriatic arthritis, also activated arthrosis of the first metatar-
sophalangeal (MTP) joint can be treated with
RSO. Sonography has limited use in the assessment of joints distal of MTP joints. It sometimes
reveals that the toe joints are not directly affected,
but the toe complaints are due to the disease of a
more proximal joint including the tarsometatarsal
area. Scintigraphy, especially in plantar view is
useful in the foot area, particularly in patients
who cannot precisely localize the pain. As in
other small joints, [169Er] erbium is the radionuclide of choice for RSO. Recommended dose for
MTP joint I (MTP I) is 26 MBq (0.7 mCi), for

interphalangeal joint I (IP I) 18 MBq (0.5 mCi)
and for other MTP 15 MBq (0.4 mCi). The needle
should be inserted in oblique dorsal aspect when
the patient is in supine position with the knee
bent and the plantar surface of the foot lies flat on
the table. It may be difficult to insert the needle to
MTP joints II to V with subluxation and osteodestructive changes.

Follow-Up

The first follow-up visit is recommended about 6
months after RSO. An earlier visit is arranged when
reactive inflammation, suspect of infection, relapsing effusions, tear of the rotator cuff, or swelling of
Baker's cyst is expected or occurs. Clinical evaluation and ultrasonography are essential for the first
visit 6 months after RSO, but scintigraphy is performed generally 12 months after RSO.

Repeated Radiosynoviorthesis

RSO should be performed at the early stage of
the disease when the cartilage damage is minimal.
Reasons for unsuccessful RSO include recurring
effusions, development of thick synovial villous,
enlargement of the joint cavity by additional cavities (Baker's cyst, bursa subdeltoidea), unfavorable Larsen stage. The decision for a repeat-RSO
(Re-RSO) should be made no earlier than 6

months following RSO [4]. Re-RSO of the wrist i.e., will not only treat the proximal wrist joint but additionally reach the intercarpal compartments. After total knee replacement, the deeper layers of polyethylene disease can be reached by Re-RSO, which is usually more effective than the first RSO [35].

Reported Clinical Studies

The success rates reported in the literature range between 60 and 80% for all joints, often with greater success rate for rheumatoid diseases than for osteoarthritis [39–46].

In non-rheumatoid diseases with chronic inflammatory synovium including OA, the response rate of RSO is between 40 and 80% [8, 39, 41, 46, 47]. The success rate in 97 patients covering 174 joints was 55% for rheumatoid arthritis, 23% for OA, and 22% for other chronic joint diseases associated with synovitis. Pain relief was reported in 78% of the patients 6 months after RSO depending on the age of the patient and the duration of illness [46].

In another study in 136 patients covering 424 joints (RA in 313 and OA in 111), subjective success rate was 79–89% for RA and OA, respectively, while the corresponding figures for scintigraphy-based success rate was 69–81%

[43]. In a well-designed multicentre study, the success rate was 78% for both RA and OA without significant difference between these two clinical entities [40]. In a comparative study in patients with RA, RSO was superior to triamcinolone with significant improvement in pain and swelling and also radiological regression in destruction was found [48].

Two recent multicentre trials have confirmed the superiority of RSO using Er-169 and Re-186 against placebo and high-dose corticosteroid in pain relief, improvement in swelling, and joint movements [49, 50]. The results of RSO using yttrium-90 colloid were similarly favorable [51]. In a double-blind three-arm study ^{90}Y colloid, three different protocols were compared: ^{90}Y colloid alone, ^{90}Y colloid plus intra-articular triamcinolone, and triamcinolone alone [52]. "Y-90 alone protocol" was recommended based on efficacy criteria. Y-90 RSO was found to be an effective treatment option in patients with osteoarthritic knee pain and scintigraphically established synovial inflammation, which are inadequately controlled by pharmacotherapy [53]. The success rate was 75 and 76% in psoriatic arthritis and ankylosing spondylitis, respectively [54–57]. The success rate in an individual joint is best assessed subjectively by the patient and objectively by the comparison of soft tissue scintigrams taken before and after RSO (Fig. 18.15).

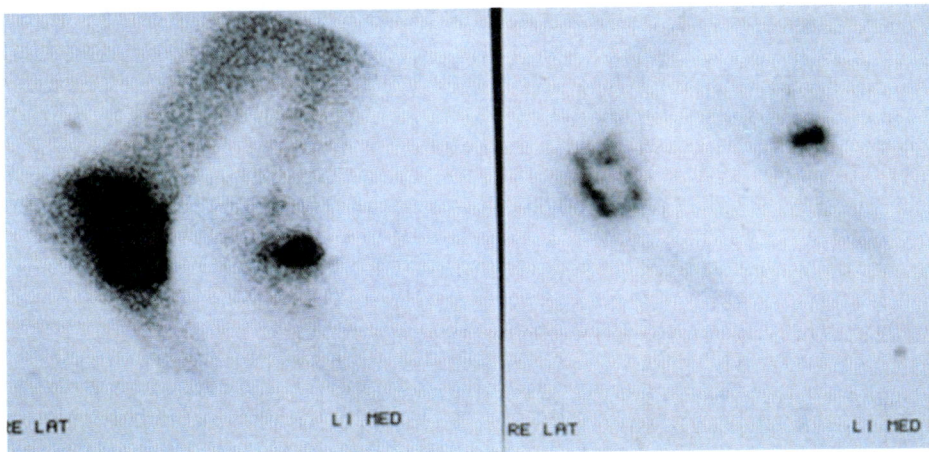

Fig. 18.15 *Left: Soft tissue scintigram* prior to RSO (*lateral view*). Severe arthritic-secondary arthrotic process in the right foot (inoperable). *Right:* Images after RSO to ankle joint, talonavicular and subtalar joints. Significant scintigraphic improvement

Conclusion

RSO is a safe and effective tool in patients with RA and OA. It provides significant improvement in joint movements and pain relief, especially in small joints. RSO offers slightly better results in rheumatoid arthritis than in osteoarthritis. Minimal or moderate changes according to Steinbrocker stages I and II respond better to RSO than do stages III and IV. Application of RSO at an earlier stage is recommended. Treatment failure is more frequent in deformed or unstable joints and thus surgery should be preferred in these patients. Close collaboration with orthopedists and rheumatologists is necessary.

References

1. Delbarre F, Cayla J, Menkes CJ, Aignan J, Roucayrol JC, Ingrand J. La synoviorthèse par les radioisotopes. Presse Med. 1968;76:1045–50.
2. Ishido C. Über die Wirkung des Radiothoriums auf die Gelenke. Strahlentherapie. 1923;15:537–44.
3. Fellinger K, Schmid J. Die lokale Behandlung der rheumatischen Erkrankungen. Wiener Z Inn Med. 1952;33:351–63.
4. Mödder G. Radiosynoviorthesis. Involvement of nuclear medicine in rheumatology and orthopaedics. Meckenheim: Warlich Druck; 2001. p. 1–119.
5. Kampen WU, Brenner W, Kroeger S, Sawula JA, Bohuslavizki KH, Henze E. Long-term results of radiation synovectomy: a clinical follow-up study. Nucl Med Commun. 2001;22:239–46.
6. Brenner W. Grundlagen und Technik der Radiosynoviorthese. Der Nuklearmediziner. 2006;29:5–14.
7. Fischer M, Mödder G. Radionuclide therapy of inflammatory diseases. Nucl Med Commun. 2002; 23:829–31.
8. Hoefnagel CA, Clarke SEM, Fischer M, Chatal J-F, et al. Radionuclide therapy practice and facilities in Europe. Eur J Nucl Med. 1999;26:277–82.
9. Farahati J, Chr R, Fischer M, Mödder G, Franke C, Mahlstedt J, Sörensen H. Leitlinie für die Radiosynoviorthese. Nuklearmedizin. 1999;38:254–5.
10. EANM. Procedure guidelines for radiosynovectomy. Eur J Nucl Med. 2003;30:BP12–6.
11. Karger TH. Stellungnahme des Berufsverbandes Deutscher Rheumatologene. V. zur Radiosynoviorthese. In: Mödder G, editor. Die Radiosynoviorthese. Nuklearmedizinische Gelenktherapie (und diagnostik) in Rheumatologie und Orthopädie. Meckenheim: Warlich Druck; 1994. p. 16–7.
12. Sharma L, Kapoor D. Epidemiology of Osteoarthritis. In: Moskowitz RW, Altman RD, Hochberg MC, Buckwalter JA, Goldberg VM, editors. Osteoarthritis: diagnosis and medical/surgical management. 4th ed. Philadelphia: Lippincott Williams & Wilkins; 2007. p. 3–26.
13. Hill CL, Gale DG, Chaisson CE, et al. Knee effusions, popliteal cysts, and synovial thickening: association with knee pain in osteoarthritis. J Rheumatol. 2001;28:1330–7.
14. Poole AR, Guilak F, Abramson SB. Etiopathogenesis of Osteoarthritis. In: Moskowitz RW, Altman RD, Hochberg MC, Buckwalter JA, Goldberg VM, editors. Osteoarthritis. Diagnosis and Medical/Surgical Management. 4th ed. Philadelphia: Lippincott Williams & Wilkins; 2001. p. 27–49.
15. Lindblatt S, Hedfors E. Arthroscopic and immunohistologic characterization of knee joint synovitis in osteoarthritis. Arthritis Rheum. 1987;30:1081–8.
16. Ayral X, Pickering EH, Woodworth TG, et al. Synovitis: a potential predictive factor of structural progression of medial tibiofemoral knee osteoarthritis—results of a 1 year longitudinal arthroscopic study in 422 patients. Osteoarthritis Cartilage. 2005;13:361–7.
17. Dieppe P. Osteoarthritis. In: Klippel JH, Dieppe PA, editors. Rheumatology. London: Mosby; 1994.
18. Mödder G. Radiosynoviorthese bei aktivierter Fingerpolyarthrose. Der Nuklearmediziner. 2006;29: 21–7.
19. Kresnik E, Mikosch P, Gallowitsch HJ, Jesenko R, Just H, Kogler D, Gasser J, Heinisch M, Unterweger O, Kumnig G, Gomez I, Lind P. Clinical outcome of radiosynoviorthesis: a meta-analysis including 2190 treated joints. Nucl Med Commun. 2002;23(N7):683–8.
20. Kampen WU, Matis E, Czech N, Massoudi S, Brenner W, Henze E. Komplikationen nach Radiosynoviorthese: erste Ergebnisse einer Umfrage zu Häufigkeit und therapeutischen Optionen. Nuklearmedizin. 2004; 43(Suppl):A21.
21. Kaiser H, Kley HK. Corticoide in Klinik und Praxis. Stuttgart: Georg Thieme; 1992.
22. Voth M, Klett R, Lengsfeld P, Stephan G, Schmid E. Biological dosimetry after Y-90 citrate radiosynviorthesis (RSO). Nuklearmedizin. 2005;44(Suppl):A134.
23. Kos-Golja M, et al. Long term follow-up after radiosynovectomy with Yttrium-90 in patients with different rheumatic diseases. Radiol Oncol. 1997;31:353–7.
24. Deckart H, Reuter U, Hüge W et al. Radiosynovectomy—radiosynoviorthesis. 25 Years experience. Treatment of rheumatoid arthritis. In: Lanthanoids in clinical therapy. Wien: Facultas-Universitäts; 1996.
25. Vuorela J, Sokka T, Pukkala E, Hannonen P. Does yttrium radiosynovectomy increase the risk of cancer in patients with rheumatoid arthritis? Ann Rheum Dis. 2003;62:251–3.
26. Johnson LS, Yanch JC, et al. Beta particle dosimetry in radiation synovectomy. Eur J Nucl Med. 1995; 22(9):977–88.

27. Ingrand J. Characteristics of radioisotopes for intra-articular therapy. Ann Rheum Dis. 1973;Suppl (3):32–5.

28. Isomäki AM, Inoue H, Oka M. Uptake of 90Y resin colloid by synovial fluid cells and synovial membrane in rheumatoid arthritis. Scand J Rheumatol. 1972;1:53–60.

29. Otte P. Der Arthrose-Prozeß. Gelenkerhaltung—Gefährdung—Destruktion. Teil 1: Osteochondrale Strukturen. Rheumatologie Orthopädie 11. Novartis Pharma, Nürnberg; 2000.

30. Bridgman JF, Bruckner FE, Blehen NM. Radioactive Yttrium (90 Y) in the treatment of rheumatoid knee effusions. Ann Rheum Dis. 1971;30:180.

31. Mödder G. Radiosynoviorthese, 224Radiumtherapie und Röntgenstrahlentherapie. In: Zeidler H, Zacher J, Hiepe F, editors. Interdisziplinäre klinische Rheumatologie. Berlin: Springer; 2001. p. 361–77.

32. Mödder G, Mödder-Reese R. Radiosynoviorthese nach Knieendoprothesen: Effektive Therapie bei „Polyethylene disease". Der Nuklearmediziner. 2001; 2(24):97–103.

33. Kerschbaumer F, Herresthal J. Arthroskopische Synovektomie und Radiosynoviorthese. Z Rheumatol. 1996;55:388–93.

34. Thabe H. Operative Behandlungskonzepte, Kapitel 5.3. In: Thabe H, editor. Praktische Rheumatherapie. Chapman & Hall: Weinheim; 1997. p. 117–34.

35. Manil L, Voisin P, Aubert B, Guerreau D, Verrier P, Lebegue L, Wargnies JP, Di Paola M, Barbier Y, Chossat F, Menkes CJ, Tebib J, Devaux JY, Kahan A. Physical and biological dosimetry in patients undergoing radiosynoviorthesis with erbium-169 and rhenium-186. Nucl Med Commun. 2001;22:405–16.

36. Kampen WU, Voth M, Pinkert J, Krause A. Therapeutic status of radiosynoviorthesis of the knee with yttrium [90Y] colloid in rheumatoid arthritis and related indications. Rheumatology. 2007;46:16–24.

37. Schomäcker K, Dietlein M, Mödder G, Boddenberg-Pätzold B, Zimmermanns B, Fischer T, Schicha H. Stability of radioactive colloids for radiation synovectomy: influence of X-ray contrast agents, anaesthetics and glucocorticoids in vitro. Nucl Med Commun. 2005;26:1027–935.

38. Mödder G. Radiosynoviorthese bei Z.n. Knie-Totalendoprothese. Nucl Med. 1994;33:A39.

39. Farahati J, Schulz G, Wendler J. Multivariate analysis of factors influencing the effect of radiosynovectomy. Nuklearmedizin. 2002;41:114–9.

40. Farahati J, Kenn W, Körber C, et al. Zeit bis zur Remission nach Radiosynovektomie (RSV). Nuklearmedizin. 1999;38:254–5.

41. Gumpel JM, Matthews SA, Fisher M. Synoviorthesis with erbium-169; a double-blind controlled comparison of erbium-169 with corticosteroid. Ann Rheum Dis. 1979;38:341–3.

42. Kröger S, Sawula JA, Klutmann S, et al. Wirksamkeit der Radiosynoviorthese bei degenerativ-entzündlichen und chronisch-entzündlichen Gelenkerkrankungen. Nucl Med. 1999;38:279–84.

43. Zuderman L, Liepe K, Zöphel K, et al. Radiosynoviorthesis (RSO): influencing factors and therapy monitoring. Ann Nucl Med. 2008;22:735–41.

44. Deutsch E, Brodack JW, Deutsch KF. Radiation synovectomy revisited. Eur J Nucl Med. 1993;20: 1113–27.

45. Savaser AN, Hoffmann K-T, Sörensen H, Banzer DH. Die Radiosynoviorthese im Behandlungsplan chronisch-entzündlicher Gelenkerkrankungen. Z Rheumatol. 1999;58:71–8.

46. Schneider P, Farahati J, Chr R. Radiosynovectomy in rheumatology and orthopedics. J Nucl Med. 2005;46: 48S–54.

47. Jones G. Yttrium synovectomy: a meta-analysis of the literature. Aust N Z J Med. 1993;23:272–5.

48. Göbel D, Gratz S, von Rothkirch T, Becker W. Chronische Polyarthritis und Radiosynoviorthese: Eine prospektive, kontrollierte Studie der Injektionstherapie mit Erbium-169 und Rhenium-186. Z Rheumatol. 1997;56:207–13.

49. Kahan A, Mödder G, Menkes CJ, et al. 169-Erbium-citrate synoviorthesis after failure of local corticosteroid injection to treat rheumatoid arthritis-affected finger joints. Clin Exp Rheumatol. 2004;22:722–6.

50. Tebib JG, Manil LM, Mödder G, Verrier P, et al. Better results with rhenium-186 radiosynoviorthesis than with cortivazol in rheumatoid arthritis (RA): a two-year follow-up randomized controlled multicenter study. Clin Exp Rheumatol. 2004;22:609–16.

51. Mödder G, Langer H-E. Evidence for the efficacy of radiation synovectomy with yttrium-90: Comment on the article by Jahangier et al. (Letter to the editor). Arthritis Rheum. 2007;56:386.

52. Urbanová Z, Gatterová J, Olejárová M, Pavelka K. Radiosynoviorthesis with 90Y—results of a clinical study. Ées Revmatol. 1997;5:140–2.

53. Chatzopoulos D, Moralidis E, Markoud P, Makris V. Yttrium-90 radiation synovectomy in knee osteoarthritis: a prospective assessment at 6 and 12 months. Nucl Med Commun. 2009;30:472–9.

54. Jahangier ZN, Moolenburgh JD, Jacobs JW, et al. The effect of radiation synovectomy in patients with persistent arthritis: a prospective study. Clin Exp Rheumatol. 2001;19:417–24.

55. Jahangier ZN, Jacobs JW, van Isselt JW, Bijlsma JW. Persistent synovitis treated with radiation synovectomy using yttrium-90: a retrospective evaluation of 83 procedures for 45 patients. Br J Rheumatol. 1997;36:861–9.

56. Jahangier ZN, Jacobs JWG, Lafeber FPJG, Moolenburgh JD, Swen WAA, Bruyn GAW, Griep EN, ter Borg E-J, Bijlsma JWJ. Is radiation synovectomy for arthritis of the knee more effective than intraarticular treatment with glucocorticoids? Arthritis Rheum. 2005;52:3391–402.

57. Van der Zant FM, Jahangier ZN, Moolenburgh JD, Swen WAA, Boer RO, Jacobs JWG. Clinical effect of radiation synovectomy of the upper extremity joints: a randomised, double-blind, placebo-controlled study. Eur J Nucl Med Mol Imaging. 2007;34:212–8.

Part III

Special Topics in Radionuclide Therapy

The Chemistry of Therapeutic Radiopharmaceuticals

19

Shankar Vallabhajosula

Introduction

Radiation therapy or radiotherapy is the medical use of ionizing radiation, generally as part of cancer treatments to control malignant cells. Historically, the three main divisions of radiation therapy are (1) external beam radiation therapy (EBRT or XRT) or teletherapy, (2) brachytherapy or sealed source radiation therapy, and (3) systemic radioisotope therapy or unsealed source radiotherapy.

Conventional radiotherapy plays a major role in the treatment of cancer in a specific region in the body, but it is not useful for the treatment of wide spread metastases. Since 1936, when Dougherty and Lawrence first introduced ^{32}P for the treatment of leukemia, the use of radiopharmaceuticals to deliver therapeutic doses of ionizing radiation has been extensively investigated. The term *unconjugated* radiopharmaceutical has been generally defined as referring to those radionuclides that target specific disease sites by virtue of chemical, biologic, or physical affinity of

radioisotope itself, rather than by virtue of carrier agents to which they are tagged. Because of the untagged nature of their use, *unconjugated* radiopharmaceuticals are also referred as *naked* radiopharmaceuticals.

During the last couple of decades, there has been significant increase in the application of *conjugated* radiopharmaceuticals for targeted radionuclide therapy (TRT), mainly due to the development of a range of new carrier molecules, which can transport the radionuclide to a molecular target at the disease site. The most important factors that influence tumor localization of *conjugated* radiopharmaceuticals include the chemical and biochemical nature of the carrier molecule transporting the radionuclide of choice to the targeted area. A century ago, Paul Ehrlich postulated the notion that a *magic bullet* could be developed to selectively target disease. He envisioned that antibodies could act as magic bullets. The first demonstration of TRT was the use of ^{131}I labeled polyclonal antibodies for the treatment of patients with melanoma. A number of radiopharmaceuticals are now available for the treatment of different benign diseases and malignancies, and the current forms of TRT using *unconjugated* or *conjugated* radiopharmaceuticals with specific examples are described in Table 19.1 and Fig. 19.1. Several review articles and book chapters have extensively discussed the development of radiopharmaceuticals for therapy [1–9].

S. Vallabhajosula, Ph.D. (✉)
Division of Nuclear Medicine and Molecular Imaging, New York-Presbyterian Hospital-Weill Cornell Medical Centre, Weill Cornell Medical College, 525 E 68th Street, STARR 2-21, New York, NY, USA
e-mail: svallabh@med.cornell.edu

C. Aktolun and S.J. Goldsmith (eds.), *Nuclear Medicine Therapy: Principles and Clinical Applications*,
DOI 10.1007/978-1-4614-4021-5_19, © Springer Science+Business Media New York 2013

Table 19.1 Radiopharmaceuticals for targeted radionuclide therapy (TRT)

Therapy	Radiopharmaceutical	Target	Clinical application	
Oral therapy	^{131}I sodium iodide	Active transport via Na-I symporter	Hyperthyroidism, thyroid cancer (local and metastatic)	
Systemic therapy	^{32}P sodium orthophosphate		Polycythemia vera	
			Chronic myelogenous leukemia	
	^{89}Sr chloride (Metastron)	Hydroxyapatite	Palliative therapy of pain due to bone metastasis	
	^{153}Sm-EDTMP (Quadramet)			
	^{223}Ra chloride			
	^{188}Re- or ^{186}Re-HEDP			
	^{131}I-Tositumomab (Bexxar)	CD20	Non-Hodgkin lymphoma	RIT
	^{90}Y-Ibritumomab Tiuxetan (Zevalin)			
	^{131}I-cTNT mAb	Intracellular DNA in necrotic tissue	Advanced lung cancer	RIT
	^{90}Y-DOTATOC or DOTATATE	SSTR	Neuroendocrine tumors	PRRT
	^{177}Lu-DOTATOC or DOTATATE			
	^{131}I-MIBG (Iobenguane I 131)	NET Adrenergic tissue		
Local/Regional therapies	^{90}Y-Labeled glass microspheres (TheraSphere)		Primary and secondary malignancies of liver	Radioembolization
	^{90}Y-Labeled resin microspheres (SIR-Spheres)			
	^{32}P, ^{90}Y, ^{86}Re, and ^{198}Au colloids		Therapy of malignant effusions and or ascites	Intracavitary (peritoneum or pleura) therapy
	^{90}Y, ^{186}Re, and ^{169}Er colloids		Therapy of rheumatoid arthritis	Radiation synovectomy

RIT radioimmunotherapy; *PRRT* peptide receptor radiation therapy

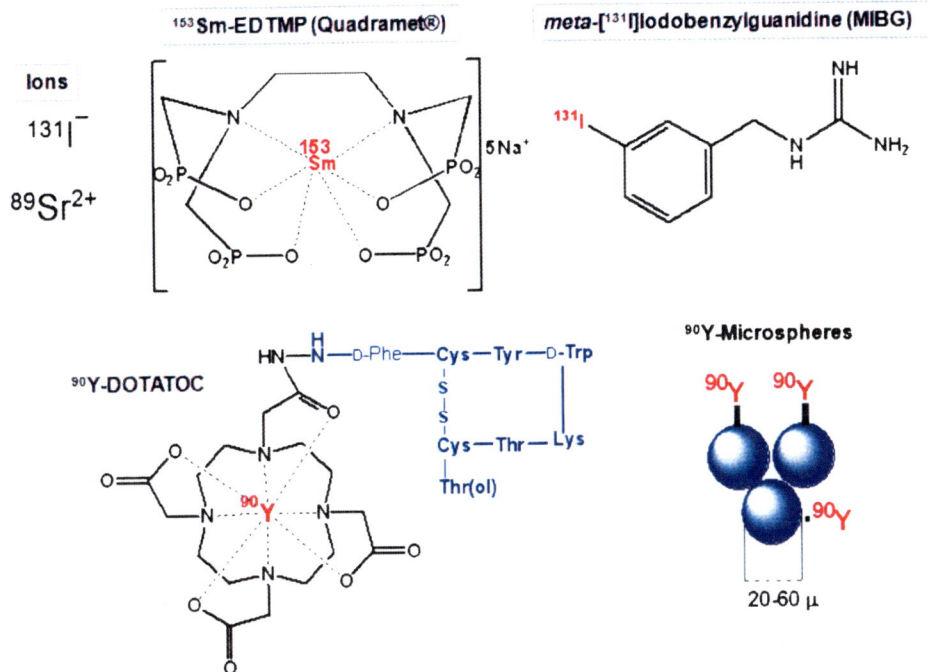

Fig. 19.1 Diverse chemistry of radiopharmaceuticals used in radionuclide therapy (TRT). These drugs may be structurally simple ions (^{131}I sodium iodide), small molecules (^{131}I-MIBG and ^{153}Sm-EDTMP), biomolecules (^{131}I, ^{90}Y or ^{177}Lu labeled mAbs or peptides) or even particles (^{90}Y labeled microspheres)

Therapeutic Radionuclides

Various radionuclides used for therapy are listed in Table 19.2. The ideal radionuclides for therapy are those with an abundance of non-penetrating radiations such as charged particles (α^{2+} and β^-) and lack of penetrating radiations (γ or X-rays). The energy of the charged particle determines the amount of energy deposited in a given volume of the tissue, expressed as the linear energy transfer (LET). The higher the LET of a specific radionuclide, the greater is the relative biological effectiveness (RBE). While penetrating radiation is not essential for TRT, a small amount or abundance with an appropriate energy (100–400 KeV) may be useful for imaging studies to demonstrate tumor localization or altered biodistribution.

Most of the radionuclides in routine clinical use are β^- emitters (^{131}I, ^{90}Y, ^{153}Sm, and ^{177}Lu) with a wide range of half-lives ranging from 0.7 to 8 days. Among the α-emitting radionuclides,

^{211}At with a relatively longer half-life (7.21 h) has generally been considered as a more useful and versatile α-emitter to prepare radiopharmaceuticals for TRT, compared to ^{212}Bi or ^{213}Bi radionuclides. The physical half-life ($T_{\frac{1}{2}p}$) of the therapeutic radionuclide is very important since the time course of irradiation of a target is related to both the physical half-life and biological turnover or biological half-life ($T_{\frac{1}{2}b}$) of the radiopharmaceutical. One must select an appropriate radionuclide depending on the carrier molecule used to develop the therapeutic agent. For example, with an intact antibody molecule, radioisotopes with medium $T_{\frac{1}{2}p}$ (3–8 days) are preferable, while with small molecules and peptides, radioisotopes with shorter $T_{\frac{1}{2}p}$ may be acceptable.

The β particles have low LET values (0.2 keV/μ) and their RBE is unity. The path length (range) is quite variable, ranging from 1 to 12 mm. When a radiopharmaceutical has a non-uniform distribution within the tumor (>1 mm), radionuclides with high energy β^- particles

Table 19.2 Radionuclides for the preparation of therapeutic radiopharmaceuticals

RN	$T_{1/2}$ (d)	Decay	Energy (MeV)		Range (mm)		γ emission	
			Max	Mean	Max	Mean	MeV	%
^{90}Y	2.67 d	β$^-$	2.28	0.935	12.0	2.76	None	
^{188}Re	0.71 d	β$^-$, γ	2.12	0.779	10.8	2.43	155	15
^{166}Ho	1.12 d	β$^-$, γ	1.854		9.0			
^{32}P	14.3 d	β$^-$	1.71	0.695	8.7	1.85	None	
^{89}Sr	50.5 d	β$^-$	1.463	0.583	8.0	1.78	None	
^{186}Re	3.77 d	β$^-$, γ	1.07	0.336	5.0	0.92	137	9
^{153}Sm	1.95 d	β$^-$, γ	0.81	0.225	3.0	0.53	103	29
^{131}I	8.04 d	β$^-$, γ	0.61	0.20	2.4	0.40	364	81
^{67}Cu	2.58 d	β$^-$, γ	0.577		2.2	0.27	92, 185	24 and 49
^{177}Lu	6.70 d	β$^-$, γ	0.497	0.133	1.8		113, 208	6.4 and 11
^{117m}Sn	13.6 d	β$^-$, γ	0.16				159	97
^{213}Bi	45.6 m	α	8.0 (98 %)		<0.10		440	17
^{212}Bi	60.6 m	α	6.0 (36 %) 9.0 (64 %)		90 μ		727	7
^{211}At	0.30 d	α	6.0 (42 %) 7.5 (58 %)		65 μ		670	0.3
^{223}Ra	11.4 d	α	6.0					
^{125}I	60.3 d	EC	0.40 KeV (Auger e^-)		10 nm		25–35 KeV	

deposit energy in cells that do not take up the radioisotope, by the cross-fire effect. In contrast, for the treatment of microscopic disease (<1.0 mm in diameter), α particles are ideal since they deposit their energy (5–9 Mev) over short distances (40–80 μ) and are of high LET(80 keV/μ) and RBE. Radionuclides with Auger electrons or other low energy electrons have a very short range (<50 nm) and, if the radionuclide is localized in the nucleus, most of the energy will be deposited locally and, thus, damage cellular DNA.

Production of Therapeutic Radionuclides

All the β$^-$ emitting radionuclides used for therapy are man-made, and produced either using nuclear reactors or radionuclide generators [2, 10–12]. The nuclear reactions involved in the production of beta and α-emitting nuclides are summarized in Table 19.3. Radionuclides decaying by β$^-$ emission are generally produced in a reactor either by fission of ^{235}U or by neutron capture

reactions (n,γ or n,p) involving absorption of a thermal neutron by a stable isotope of an element. Radionuclide generators are designed to separate shorter $T_{1/2p}$ daughter radionuclide from a parent radionuclide with a longer $T_{1/2}$ that was originally produced in a reactor or cyclotron. The radionuclides produced directly by the fission of ^{235}U or obtained using a radionuclide generator, generally have very high specific activities and are preferable for the preparation of radiopharmaceuticals for TRT.

Among the α-emitters, ^{211}At is produced in a medium energy cyclotron on a natural bismuth target using a beam of α particles (22–28.5 MeV) based on the nuclear reaction ^{209}Bi(α, 2n)^{211}At. Subsequently, ^{211}At can be isolated from the cyclotron target using a dry distillation procedure. It is important to appreciate that most of the cyclotrons used to prepare PET drugs are relatively low energy cyclotrons (<20 MeV) and do not have the capability to accelerate α particles. Not many institutions in the world have appropriate facilities for producing this radionuclide.

Table 19.3 Production of therapeutic radionuclides

Source	Radionuclide	Nuclear reaction	
Reactor	^{131}I	^{235}U(n, fission)^{131}I or ^{130}Te(n, γ)^{131}Te $\xrightarrow{\beta-}$ ^{131}I	
	^{32}P	^{31}P(n,γ)^{32}P or ^{32}S(n, p)^{32}P	
	^{67}Cu	^{67}Zn(n,p)^{67}Cu	
	^{177}Lu	^{176}Lu(n,γ)^{177}Lu	
	^{89}Sr	^{88}Sr(n,γ)^{89}Sr	
	^{186}Re	^{185}Re(n,γ)^{186}Re	
	^{153}Sm	^{152}Sm(n,γ)^{153}Sm	
	^{117m}Sn	^{117}Sn(n,n'γ)^{117m}Sn	
Cyclotron	^{211}At	^{209}Bi(α, 2n)^{211}At	
Generator	^{90}Y	^{235}U(n, fission)^{90}Sr $\xrightarrow[28.8 \text{ yr}]{\beta-}$ ^{90}Y	^{90}Sr→^{90}Y generator
	^{188}Re	^{187}W(n,γ)^{188}W $\xrightarrow[69.4 \text{ d}]{\beta-}$ ^{188}Re	^{188}W→^{188}Re generator
	^{212}Bi	^{228}Th$\xrightarrow[\text{decay chain}]{}$^{224}Ra→^{212}Pb $\xrightarrow[10.64 \text{ h}]{\beta-}$ ^{212}Bi	^{224}Ra generator
	^{213}Bi	^{229}Th$\xrightarrow[\text{decay chain}]{}$^{225}Ac $\xrightarrow[10 \text{ d}]{\alpha}$ ^{221}Fr $\xrightarrow{\alpha}$^{217}At $\xrightarrow{\alpha}$^{213}Bi	^{225}Ac generator

Therapeutic Radiopharmaceuticals

Characteristics

Therapeutic radiopharmaceuticals may be structurally simple ions (^{131}I$^-$ and ^{89}Sr^{2+}), small molecules (^{131}I-MIBG and ^{153}Sm-EDTMP), complex molecules (^{131}I, ^{90}Y, or ^{177}Lu labeled intact antibodies or antibody fragments), colloids (^{32}P chromic phosphate), or even particles (^{90}Y labeled microspheres). The tumor localization properties of a specific therapeutic radiopharmaceutical and the clinical application will depend on the route of administration, such as intravenous, intra-arterial, intracavitary, and intra-articular approaches. The ideal physical and biological properties of a radiopharmaceutical intended for therapy should be such that a large absorbed radiation is deposited in the tumor, or diseased tissue, with minimal dose to normal tissues. This requires the use of an appropriate radionuclide, administered in a suitable chemical form with optimal specific activity (mCi or MBq/μmole), and by an appropriate route of administration, which will allow selective uptake in the target tissue in sufficient concentration to elicit a therapeutic response. Different mechanisms, however, are involved in the delivery and accumulation of the therapeutic agent within the tumor cells (Fig. 19.2).

Radiopharmaceuticals used for bone pain palliation (Metaston®, Quadramet®) do not accumulate in the tumor cells, but are deposited in the bone cells in response to the osteoblastic activity of the metastatic lesions in the bone marrow. The ^{90}Y labeled particles (Theraspheres® and Sirspheres®) are deposited in the tumor tissue due to capillary blockade. In contrast, in TRT, the choice of a chemical carrier (*ligand* or *vector*) is very important since the tumor localization of a particular radiopharmaceutical depends on the specific mechanism of the ligand interaction with specific binding sites (ligand-receptor or antigen-antibody binding) on the tumor cells, or within the tumor cells. The specific tumor cell uptake of the radiopharmaceutical depends on the chemical and biological properties of the ligand. Specifically, the selection of a suitable ligand depends on the following factors:

- Biologic specificity and in vivo stability
- The *affinity* of ligand (K_d) to the binding site (antigen, receptor, or an enzyme)
- The stability of ligand-binding complex
- The ligand's ability to bind to complex radionuclide without losing biologic specificity and affinity

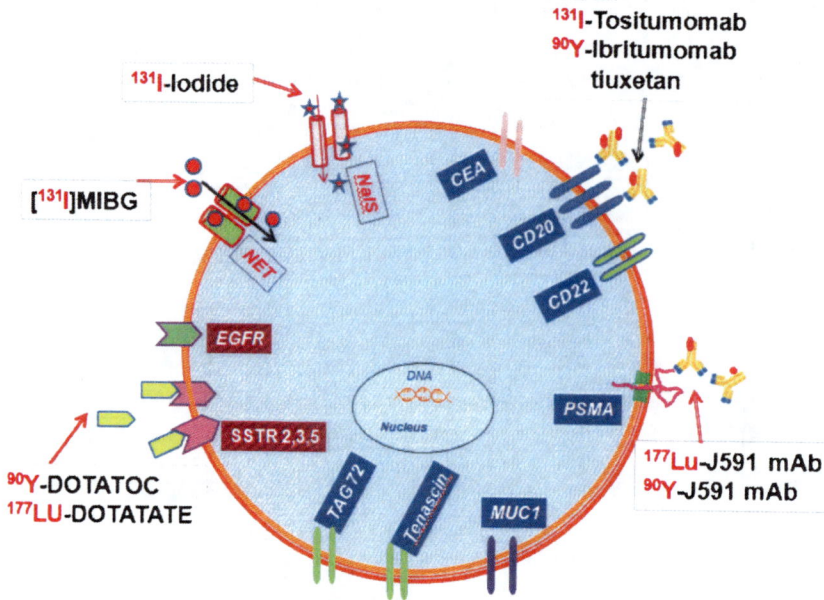

Fig. 19.2 Mechanisms of tumor localization of radiopharmaceuticals for TRT

A Suitable Ligand Depends on the Following Factors

- Biologic specificity and in vivo stability
- *Affinity* to the binding site
- Stability of ligand-binding complex
- Ability to bind to complex radionuclide without losing biologic specificity and affinity

In the design of a target (binding site) specific radiopharmaceutical, the choice of a specific target in the tumor tissue depends on the following important factors:

- The accessibility of the target for the ligand is a very important consideration. In this context, the microscopic environment of the target, including tumor vascularity, permeability, and oxygenation would all contribute to the net uptake of the radiopharmaceutical by the tumor.
- The number of binding sites (B_{max}) per tumor cell and the relative distribution and the expression of target molecules within the tumor tissue during each phase of the cell cycle.

- The expression of binding sites in the non-target sites, such as blood and soft tissues (liver, kidney, spleen, and muscle).

In summary, an ideal radiopharmaceutical for TRT, under ideal conditions must have the following characteristics:

- High specificity and affinity for tumor cells
- In vivo stability in blood and within the tumor tissue with minimal metabolite formation
- Rapid blood clearance (to minimize bone marrow dose)
- Rapid targeting and significant retention of the therapeutic radionuclide (3–4 half-lives of the radionuclide)
- Rapid excretion from the body with minimal uptake and retention by normal tissues and cells
- Minimal hematologic toxicity in order to increase the maximum tolerated dose (MTD) to preserve dose-rate effect
- Acceptable toxicity to liver, spleen, and kidney
- No radiation-induced biologic effects such as mutation, transformations leading to secondary cancers

- High specificity and affinity for tumor cells
- In vivo stability with minimal metabolite formation
- Rapid blood clearance
- Rapid targeting and significant retention of the therapeutic radionuclide
- Minimal uptake and retention by normal tissues and cells
- Minimal hematologic toxicity
- Acceptable toxicity to liver, spleen, and kidney
- No radiation-induced biologic effects such as mutation and transformations

In order to meet all the requirements described above, the design and development of a successful therapeutic radiopharmaceutical for TRT requires careful multistep matching of (a) the target and the ligand molecule, (b) the ligand and the radionuclide, (c) the tumor and radionuclide, and, finally, (d) the radiopharmaceutical (ligand-linker-BFC-radionuclide combination).

Design Strategies

A classic example of TRT is the use of ^{131}I as sodium iodide (I^-) for the post-surgery treatment of thyroid cancer. The radioiodide selectively accumulates in thyroid cancer cells by active transport via an ion pump known as sodium iodide symporter (SIS). In this mechanism (Fig. 19.2), the radionuclide as iodide ion is the active ingredient of the radiopharmaceutical and no specific ligand or carrier is required. Similarly, with ^{89}Sr chloride, $^{89}Sr^{2+}$ localizes in the hydroxyapatite ($Ca_{10}(PO_4)_6(OH)_2$), the mineral content of bone as strontium ion and no specific carrier is required. In contrast, with ^{153}Sm, the radionuclide is complexed by a metal chelating agent, EDTMP and ^{153}Sm-EDTMP complex, similar to ^{99m}Tc-MDP, and is taken up by the bone hydroxyapatite

due to transchelation of radiometal complex. Finally, in order to prepare ^{90}Y labeled microspheres (20–60 μ) for radioembolization, the radiometal ^{90}Y is bound to glass or resin microspheres, which localize in the liver tumors following radioembolization and capillary blockade. In these two examples, the therapeutic radionuclide is transported to the tumor site by a carrier agent, either by a bone seeking phosphone chelator, or simply by glass or resin particles. While ^{153}Sm-EDTMP and ^{90}Y labeled microspheres can be regarded as therapeutic radiopharmaceuticals for TRT, these agents have not been designed specifically to target tumor cells. These agents do not bind to the tumor cells in vivo.

For TRT to be truly effective and specific, the carrier molecule (ligand or vector), ideally, seeks the tumor cells and delivers the radionuclide to the tumor cells by specific binding to a target site, either on the cell surface, or within the tumor cell. For example, ^{131}I-MIBG, a norepinephrine analog, is actively transported into the tumor cell by the norephrine transporter (NET) although some passive diffusion may occur[13]. The concept of a magic a bullet in TRT was demonstrated successfully with radiolabeled monoclonal antibodies (mAb) against tumor-specific antigens. The two Food and Drug Administration (FDA) approved drugs for radioimmunotherapy (RIT) of Non-Hodgkin's lymphoma (NHL), Zevalin and Bexxar target the CD20 surface antigen on B-cells using anti-CD20 intact mAbs and deliver either ^{90}Y or ^{131}I radionuclides to the primary and metastatic tumor sites. In addition, a number of different carriers are under preclinical and clinical investigation for the selective delivery of radionuclides for TRT. These carrier molecules include small organic molecules, peptides, affibody molecules, aptamers, and nanostructures (e.g., liposomes, microparticles, nanoparticles, spheres, nanoshells, and minicells).

Monoclonal Antibodies and Antibody Fragments

To date, the U.S. FDA has approved *five* mAbs for diagnosis: *four* for the detection of cancer and only *two* radiolabeled mAbs for RIT (Table 19.4).

Table 19.4 Food and Drug Administration (FDA) approved monoclonal antibodies for diagnosis and therapy in oncology

Year	Generic (trade) name	Target	Type	FDA approved Indication
1992	^{111}In-satumomab pendetide (OncoScint™)	Tumor associated glycoprotein-72	Murine IgG	Ovarian and colorectal cancer
1996	^{99m}Tc-acritumomab (CEA-Scan™)	Carcinoembryonic antigen (CEA)	Murine F(ab')	Colorectal cancer
1996	^{99m}Tc-Nofetumomabmerpentan (Verluma™)	Epithelial cell adhesion molecule (EGP-1)	Murine Fab	Small cell lung cancer
1996	^{111}In-capromab pendetide (ProstaScint™)	Prostate specific membrane antigen (PSMA)	Murine IgG$_1$	Prostate cancer
1997	Rituximab (Rituxan®)	CD20	Chimeric IgG$_1$	CD20(+) low-grade lymphoma, diffuse large B-cell lymphoma, follicular lymphoma
1998	Trastuzumab (Herceptin®)	Human epidermal growth factor receptor (HER-2 neu)	Humanized IgG$_1$	Her2/neu(+) breast cancer
2000	Gemtuzumab ozogamicin (Myelotarg®)	CD33	Humanized gG$_4$ conjugated to calicheamicin	Acute myelogenous leukemia
2001	Alemtuzumab (Campath®)	CD52	Humanized IgG$_1$	Chronic lymphatic leukemia
2002	^{90}Y-ibritumomab tiuxetan (Zevalin®)	CD20	Murine IgG$_1$	CD20(+) low-grade lymphoma
2003	^{131}I-Tositumomab (Bexxar®)	CD20	Murine IgG$_{2A}$	CD20(+) low-grade lymphoma
2004	Bevacizumab (Avastin®)	VEGF	Humanized IgG$_1$	Colorectal cancer
2006				Non-small cell lung cancer
				Metastatic breast cancer
2004	Cetuximab (Erbitux®)	Epidermal growth factor receptor (EGFR)	Chimeric IgG$_1$	EGFR(+) metastatic colorectal cancer
2006				Head and neck cancer
2006	Panitumumab (Vectibix®)	EGFR	Human IgG$_1$	Colorectal cancer

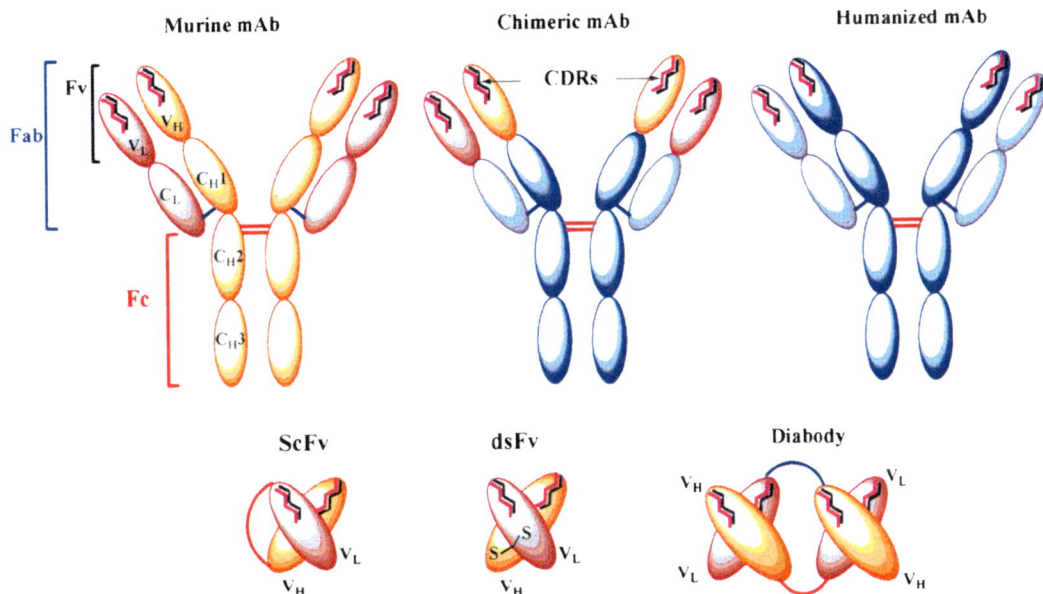

Fig. 19.3 The classification of monoclonal antibodies (mAbs): The fundamental structure of an intact, single immunoglobulin G (IgG) molecule has a pair of light chains and a pair of heavy chains. Light chains are composed of two separate regions (one variable region (V_L) and one constant region (C_L)), whereas heavy chains are composed of four regions (V_H, $C_H 1$, $C_H 2$ and $C_H 3$). The complementarity-determining regions (CDRs) are found in the variable fragment (Fv) portion of the antigen-binding fragment (Fab). In a chimeric antibody, the mouse heavy- and light-chain variable region sequences are joined onto human heavy-chain and light-chain constant regions. In a humanized antibody, the mouse CDRs are grafted onto human V-region FRs and expressed with human C-regions. Monovalent and multivalent antibody fragments are shown at the *bottom* of the figure; Single chain Fv fragments *scFv*, Disulfide-stabilized Fv fragments *dsFv*, Noncovalent scFv dimer *diabody*

Hundreds of new mAbs are under development worldwide [13–15]. Also, a variety of promising antigens/targets are currently being evaluated in clinical trials at various stages [14, 16]. Tumor-associated antigens and receptors present on the tumor cell surface include CD20, CD22, PSMA, mucin 1 (MUC1), Carcinoembryonic antigen, pancarcinoma antigen (TAG-72), sialyl Lewis antigen, HER2/neu receptor, tumor-necrosis-factor-related apoptosis-inducing ligand receptor, and epidermal growth factor receptor (EGFR). In contrast, VEGF and integrins are more abundant on vascular endothelial cells within newly sprouting blood vessels that nourish the nearby tumor during angiogenesis.

The introduction of hybridoma technology for mAb development turned this magic bullet concept into a realistic option [17]. The first generations of mAbs were of murine origin and had limitations for clinical use, but developments in recombinant DNA technology resulted in the production of chimeric (c-mAb), humanized (h-mAb), and complete human mAbs (Fig. 19.3). Chimeric mAbs are constructed with variable regions (V_L and V_H) derived from a murine source and constant regions derived from a human source. Humanized therapeutic mAbs are predominantly derived from a human source, except for the CDRs, which are murine. There is a significant difference between the IgG subclasses in terms of their half-lives in the blood (IgG$_1$, IgG$_2$, and IgG$_4$ approximately 21 days; IgG$_3$ approximately 7 days) and in terms of their capability to activate the classical complement pathway and to bind Fc receptors. The choice of an IgG subclass is a key factor in determining the efficacy of therapeutic mAbs. Most of the FDA approved mAbs belong to the IgG$_1$ subclass, which has a long half-life and triggers potent immune-effector functions, such as complement-dependent

Table 19.5 Comparison of targeting properties of representative forms of antibody and chemically prepared or engineered fragments

Antibody/ fragment	Size (kDa)	Relative $T_{1/2}$ rank[a]	Target Organ	Tumor binding properties		
				Relative uptake[b]	Relative duration[c]	Time to optimum accretion time
IgG	150	1 d	Liver	1	1	Day(s)
F(ab')$_2$	100	2 d	Liver	2	2	Day
Fab'	50	3 h	Kidneys	3	3	Hours
Daibody	40	3 h	Kidneys	3	3	Hours
ScFv	20	4 h	Kidneys	4	4	Hour

The above table from Sharky and Goldenberg [77]
[a]Relative biologic half-life from blood (grading: slowest (1) and fastest (4))
[b]Based on intravenous infusion. Numbers represent grading from highest (1) to lowest (4)
[c]Numbers represent grading from longest (1) to shortest (4)

cytotoxicity (CDC), complement-dependent cell-mediated cytotoxicity (CDCC), and antibody-dependent cellular cytotoxicity (ADCC).

In addition to intact mAb molecules, mAb fragments like F(ab')$_2$, F(ab'), Fab, engineered variants such as single chain Fv (scFv), the covalent dimers scFv$_2$ diabodies, and minibodies (molecular weights ranging from 25 to 100 kDa) have all been developed to improve pharmacokinetics, tumor localization, and antigen binding [6, 15, 18]. More recently, it has also become possible to produce totally human recombinant antibodies derived either from antibody libraries, single immune B cells, or from transgenic mice bearing human immunoglobulin loci. Single chains are formed by linking the variable light (V$_L$) and variable heavy (V$_H$) chains with amino acid (AA) linker. Diabodies, triabodies, and even tetrabodies are formed spontaneously when smaller length AA chains are used to hold the V$_H$ and V$_L$ units together. Recombinant bispecific diabodies and other bispecific constructs can be prepared by pairing V$_H$ and V$_L$ of two antibodies with different specificities [6].

Size, Penetration, and Clearance rate of Antibodies and Fragments: Intact mAbs have a long residence time in humans, ranging from a few days to weeks, which results in optimal tumor-to-non-tumor ratios at 2–4 days post injection. In contrast, mAb fragments have a much faster blood clearance and as a result optimal tumor-to-nontumor ratios can be obtained at earlier time points, but the absolute tumor uptake may be much lower compared to intact mAbs is often lower. The targeting properties of antibody molecules of different sizes are compared in Table 19.5. In general, intact mAbs are preferable for therapy, while the optimal format for immunoimaging is still under discussion.

Size is one factor that impacts the circulation time of Abs [14]. A full IgG mAb is a large 150-kDa protein that can remain in circulation for 3–4 weeks while being metabolized slowly by the reticuloendothelial system (RES). In contrast, a 25-kDa monovalent fragment (scFv) has a blood clearance time of <10 h with primarily renal excretion in 2–4 h. The Fv fragment consisting only of the V$_H$ and V$_L$ domains is the smallest immunoglobulin fragment available that carries the whole antigen-binding site, but scFvs have never fared well in the clinic, despite their small size (25 kDa) because of their poor tumor retention. Molecules with molecular weights above >70 kDa (the glomerular filtration threshold) remain in circulation much longer than smaller more rapidly eliminated molecules. Recent protein engineering has been used to produce designer bispecific antibody that are based on antibody Fv or scFv fragments as building blocks rather than whole antibodies. One such fragment is the diabody, a dimer, and each chain comprising two domains. Each chain consists of a V$_H$ domain connected to a V$_L$ domain using a linker too short to allow pairing between domains on the same chain [19]. Diabodies (55 kDa) are the smallest engineered fragments that are bivalent, retaining the chief advantage of whole antibodies, namely,

Table 19.6 Peptide receptors as targets for developing therapeutic radiopharmaceuticals in oncology

Peptide	Receptor/subtype	Tumor expression	Peptide labeled with ^{99m}Tc, ^{111}In, or ^{123}I
Somatostatin	SSTR I–V	Neuroendocrine, small-cell lung, breast, monocytes and lymphocytes	Octreotide analogs
Bombesin	GRP-bombesin	Prostate, breast, small cell lung cancer (SCLC), gastric, ovarian, colon and pancreatic caners	Bombesin
Substance P	NK1	Glial tumors, astrocytomas, medullary thyroid cancer (MTC), and breast cancer	Substance-P
VIP	VPAC1	GI and other epithelial tumors	VIP, TP3654
RGD analogs	$A_v\beta_3$ integrin	Insulinomas	
CCK/gastrin	CCK2	MTC, insulinoma, SCLC, GISTs	Minigastrin
Glucagon-like peptide 1 (GLP-1)	GLP-1-R	Insulinoma, gastrinoma	GLP-1
Neuropeptide-Y	NPY-R	Breast, ovarian, and adrenal tumors	Neuropeptide-Y
Neurotensin	NT-R1	Exocrine pancreatic cancer, meningioma, Ewing sarcoma, and prostate cancer	Neurotensin

avidity. Increased tumor uptake has been observed for intermediate-sized bivalent Ab formats, such as 75-kDa triabodies and 80-kDa minibodies (scFv-CH$_3$); however, slower blood clearance was evident. Larger bivalent antibody fragments, such as F(ab')$_2$ fragments, have slower blood clearance than diabodies, resulting in optimal tumor-to-normal tissue ratios only at prolonged times (18–24 h) relative to those of diabodies (3–5 h).

Receptor Binding Peptides

Peptides are formed when two or more amino acids are condensed together with the formation of a secondary amide bond, the so-called peptide bond or peptide unit. Peptides of natural or synthetic origin are compounds involved in a variety of biologic interactions. Peptides are hormones, protein substrates and inhibitors, opioids, regulators of biologic functions, antibiotics, and so on. They bind to specific binding sites or receptors on the cell membrane or within the cell in order to initiate specific actions. Various peptides, peptide receptors, and the corresponding eligible target-related tumors are summarized in Table 19.6. The over-expression of peptide receptors on tumor cells lead to the development of radiolabeled peptides for diagnosis and therapy. It has been demonstrated that only tumors

expressing a high density of receptors can be selected for targeted therapy. Since peptide agonists are quickly metabolized (or inactivated) by amino peptidases, following binding to receptors, peptide radiopharmaceuticals are generally developed using chemically modified peptide analogs that may have greater affinity for the receptor, but block the receptor function. Following intravenous administration, peptides are generally cleared from the circulation rapidly and excreted through the liver and kidneys.

Somatostatin Receptors: Because the majority of NETs express somatostatin (SS) receptors, they have been successfully targeted with radiolabeled SS analogs in vivo. Somatostatin, a 14-amino acid cyclic peptide is secreted throughout the body and has multiple physiological functions, including inhibition of secretion of growth hormone, glucagon, insulin, gastrin, and other hormones secreted by the pituitary and gastrointestinal tract. The diverse biological effects of SST are mediated through a family of G protein coupled receptors of which five subtypes have been identified. Human SST receptors (SSTR1-SSTR5) have been identified on most of the neuroendocrine tumors, small cell lung cancers, and medullary thyroid carcinoma, express high densities of SSTRs [20–22]. The expression of SSTR subtypes in human tumor tissues, however, seems

Ala – Gly – Cys – Lys – Asn – Phe – Phe – Trp – Lys – Thr – Phe – Thr – Ser – Cys   **Somatostatin**

DTPA - D-Phe – Cys – Phe – D-Trp – Lys – Thr – Cys – Thr(ol)   **DTPA-Octreotide**

DOTA- D-Phe – Cys – Tyr – D-Trp – Lys – Thr – Cys – Thr(ol)   **DOTATOC**

DOTA- D-Phe – Cys – Tyr – D-Trp – Lys – Thr – Cys – Thr(OH)   **DOTATATE**

DOTA- D-Phe – Cys – Nal – D-Trp – Lys – Thr – Cys – Thr(ol)   **DOTANOC**

(Nal = 3- (1-naphtalenyl)-L-alanyl)

Fig. 19.4 Amino acid sequence of Somatostatin and DTPA or DOTA conjugated octreotide analogs

to vary among different tumor types. Although various SS receptor subtypes are expressed in tumors, SSTR2 is the predominant receptor subtype expressed in NETs. The clinically used SS analogs bind predominantly to SSTR2. It is the presence of SSTR2 as well as its density which provides the molecular basis for a number of radiolabeled SS analogs (Fig. 19.4) that were developed for diagnosis and peptide receptor therapy (PRT).

Other Peptide Receptors: Many other peptide receptors have been identified in the last two decades and are known to be over-expressed in several different cancers (Table 19.6). A number of radiolabeled peptides are being developed to target specific receptors for Vasoactive intestinal peptide (VIP), glucagon-like peptide 1 (GLP-1), neurotensin (NT), substance-P, gastrin, cholecystokinin, and neuropeptide-Y. While several preclinical studies have shown some potential for imaging studies, no major therapeutic analogs are under clinical investigation, at this time.

Adrenergic Presynaptic Transporters

Tumors arising from the neural crest share the characteristic of amine precursor uptake and decarboxylation (APUD) and contain large amounts of adrenaline, dopamine, and serotonin within the secretary granules in cytoplasm. Tumors of the adrenergic system include pheochromocytoma (arise in adrenal medulla), or paragangliomas (extra-adrenal tissue). Meta-iodobenzylguanidine (MIBG) is an analog of

noradrenaline, originally developed by linking the benzyl portion of bretylium with the guanidine group of guanethidine [23]. It was observed that [131I]MIBG accumulated in the chromaffin cells of adrenal medulla. Since MIBG is structurally similar to noradrenaline, MIBG is believed to be transported into the cell by the re-uptake pathways of the adrenergic presynaptic neurons. Within the cells, MIBG is transported into the catecholamine-storing granules by means of ATPase-dependent proton pump. The major difference between MIBG and noradrenaline is that MIBG does not bind to post-synaptic adrenergic receptors. [131I]MIBG was initially used to image pheochromocytoma. MIBG, also known as Iobenguane I 131 intravenous, received FDA approval in 1994 as an imaging agent. Recently in 2008, 123I-MIBG (AdreView™, GE Healthcare) was also approved by the FDA as a tumor imaging agent. [131I]MIBG as an experimental treatment for metastasized pheochromocytoma was first reported in 1984. Since that time, [131I]MIBG has been used as a therapeutic agent for the treatment of neuroendocrine tumors. A therapeutic indication utilizing [131I]MIBG for TRT, however, has not been approved in the United States.

Chemistry of Therapeutic Radiopharmaceuticals

The periodic table (Fig. 19.5) shows the position of different chemical elements used to develop therapeutic radiopharmaceuticals. Among the halogens (Group 17), the radioisotopes of iodine (131I) and astatine (211At) are the most important

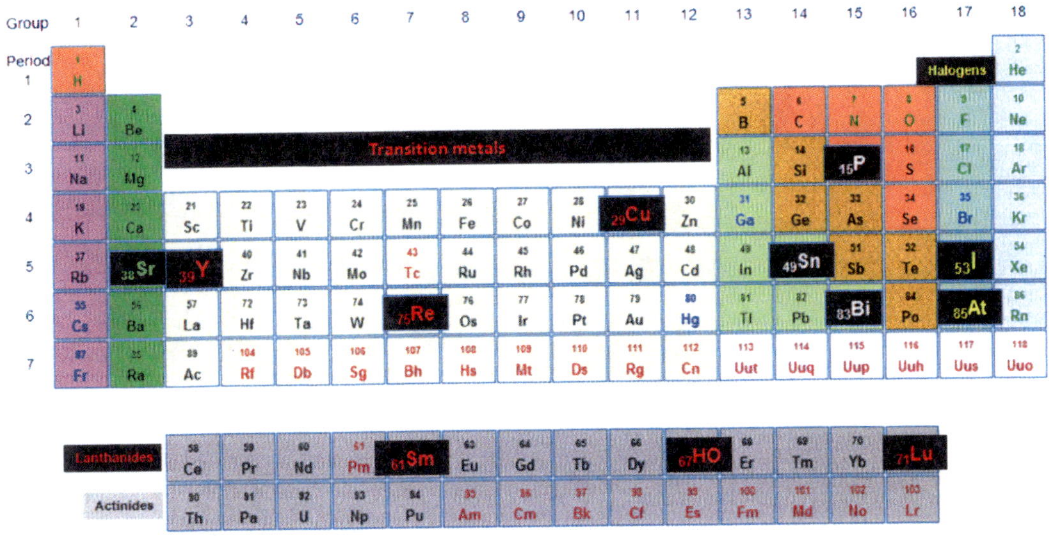

Fig. 19.5 The periodic table

radionuclides used to develop therapeutic agents. The majority of other radionuclides used in TRT belong to a category of elements known as transition metals (Groups 3–12), such as copper (^{67}Cu), yttrium (^{90}Y), rhenium (^{188}Re, ^{186}Re), samarium (^{153}Sm), holmium (^{166}Ho), and lutetium (^{177}Lu). The post-transition metals, gallium (^{67}Ga, ^{68}Ga, ^{66}Ga) and indium (^{111}In), are mainly useful to develop radiopharmaceuticals for imaging studies. Among the alkaline earth metals, strontium (^{89}Sr) and radium (^{223}Ra) are also important, but are used less frequently in TRT. Since halogens and metals (especially transition metals) are of particular interest in developing therapeutic radiopharmaceuticals, the radiochemistry of halogens and transition metals is presented here in greater detail.

Chemistry of Halogens

All halogens are characterized by the presence of two s electrons and five p electrons in the outer most valence shell (ns^2, np^5). The electronegativity values reveal that among halogens, fluorine has the greatest attraction for electrons and astatine the least. This means that the F$^-$ ion is more stable than the I$^-$ or At$^-$ ion. Since fluorine is the most electronegative element, it has only one

oxidation state (-1). In contrast, the other halogens may attain positive oxidation states when interacting with more electronegative element, oxygen. The higher ionization potentials of halogens suggest that it is difficult to remove an electron from halogen atoms. Also among halogens, fluorine is the most powerful oxidizing agent, while iodine is the most powerful reducing agent. In general, halogens can react as *electrophiles*, electron-deficient positively charged species or *nucleophiles*, electron-rich negatively charged species. *Electrophiles* (X$^+$) seek electron-rich reactants such as carbon atoms with high local electron densities, while *nucleophiles* (X$^-$) seek electron-deficient reactants. Astatine is the heaviest halogen with some of its chemical properties similar to those of iodine. In certain circumstances, however, astatine also has significant metallic characteristics. An important consideration is that the carbon-halogen bond strength for astatine is lower than that for iodine.

Radioiodination

The free molecular iodine (I$_2$) has the structure of I$^+$–I$^-$ in aqueous solution. However, the electrophilic species (I$^+$) does not exist as a free species, but forms complexes with nucleophilic entities,

Electrophilic Radioiodination

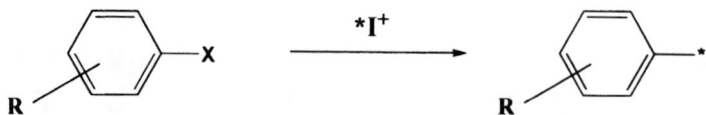

where X = H, HgCl, Tl(OCOCF$_3$)$_2$, Sn(CH$_3$)$_3$, Si(CH$_3$)$_3$

Nucleophilic Radioiodination

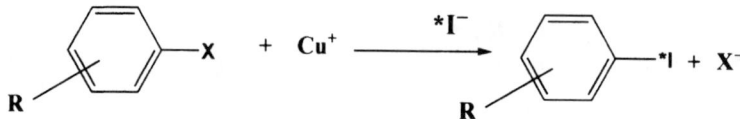

where X = I, Br

Fig. 19.6 Iodination based on electrophilic and nucleophilic aromatic substitution (or halogen-halogen exchange reaction) catalyzed by copper

such as water or pyridine. The reactions with water can be written as follows:

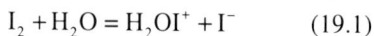

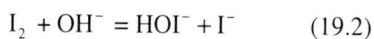

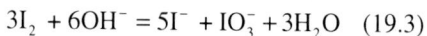

$$I_2 + H_2O = H_2OI^+ + I^- \qquad (19.1)$$

$$I_2 + OH^- = HOI^- + I^- \qquad (19.2)$$

$$3I_2 + 6OH^- = 5I^- + IO_3^- + 3H_2O \qquad (19.3)$$

The hydrated iodonium ion, H$_2$OI$^+$, and the hypoiodous acid, HOI, are believed to be highly reactive electrophilic species. In an iodination reaction, iodination occurs by (a) electrophilic substitution of a hydrogen ion by an iodonium ion in a molecule of interest or (b) nucleophilic substitution (isotope exchange) where a radioactive iodine atom is exchanged with a stable iodine atom that is already present in the molecule. Other cationic species such as I$_2$Cl$^+$, ICl$_2^+$, I$_2$Br$^+$ may exist under special conditions and may also behave as powerful electrophiles.

The advantages and disadvantages of different radioiodination techniques were recently reviewed [24, 25]. In general, the aliphatic carbon–iodine bond is relatively weak and as a result, in vivo deiodination occurs either by nucleophilic substitution or by β-elimination. In the preparation of radioiodinated compounds, the radioiodine is preferentially attached to a carbon atom, in a vinylic or aromatic moiety, in which the carbon–iodine bond strength is higher.

Therefore, the radioiodination is often implemented by electrophilic or nucleophilic aromatic substitution (Fig. 19.6).

Electrophilic labeling reactions can often be performed fast and under mild reaction conditions. The electrophilic species (HO*I, H$_2$O*I) generated from radioiodide and the oxidant react directly with the aromatic moiety of the compound to be labeled. The most frequently used oxidizing agents are peracetic acid and the N-chloro compounds, such as chloramine-T, iodogen, and succinimides. The N-chloro compounds are by far the most popular oxidants, however, their relatively strong oxidizing properties often induce by-products. In order to limit these oxidative side reactions, chloramine-T is immobilized on spherical polystyrene particles (iodobeads), while iodogen, which contains four functional chlorine atoms, is coated as a thin layer on the walls of a reaction vessel. In order to label small organic molecules, peracetic acid is often preferred due to its mild oxidizing properties. The aromatic amino acids, tyrosine, and histidine are the sites of iodination in protein molecules [26, 27]. With tyrosine, substitution of a hydrogen ion with the reactive iodonium ion occurs ortho- to the phenolic hydroxyl group. With histidine, substitution occurs at the second position of the imidazole ring. Electrophilic substitutions can often be carried out on a non-derivatized substrate. However, in case of low reactivity or lack of

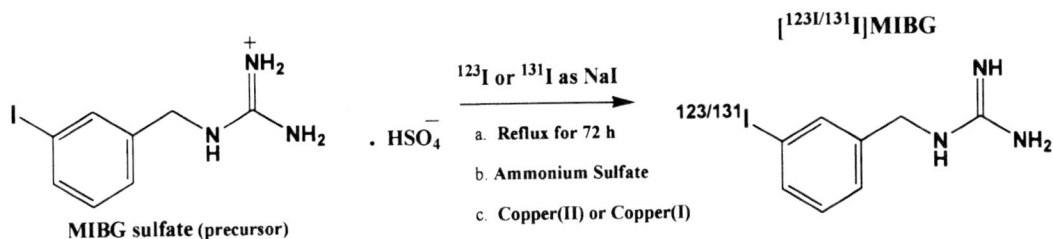

Fig. 19.7 Synthesis of [$^{123/131}$I] meta-iodobenzylguanidine (MIBG) based on nucleophilic radioiodination or radioiodide exchange reaction. MIBG can be synthesized by reflexing cold MIBG sulfate for 72 h at RT. The synthesis can be improved by using catalysts such as ammonium sulfate or copper ions at higher temperature

regioselectivity, radioiodo destannylation has become more and more the method of choice.

The method of choice in nucleophilic radioiodination is the well-established Cu(I)-catalysed halogen–halogen exchange reaction in an acidic, aqueous medium (Fig. 19.4). The exchange reactions can be either isotopic exchange (*I/I) or non-isotopic exchange (*I/Br), which specifically enables the synthesis of a high SA radiopharmaceutical [28]. A nucleophilic exchange can be successfully applied on activated (presence of electron-deficient substituents, e.g., carbonyl group) or non-activated (e.g., alkyl group) aromatic compounds. However, in organic media, electron-donating substituents are also well tolerated. The purity, the labeling yield, and the SA can be controlled by carefully optimizing the concentration of copper and the precursor. The synthesis of radioiodinated MIBG is used as an example to describe several radioiodination techniques routinely used in the preparation of 1^{23}I or ^{131}I labeled small organic molecules.

Synthesis of [^{131}I]MIBG

Commercial formulations of [^{131}I]MIBG are based on isotope exchange reaction, and contain large mass amounts of unlabeled MIBG, or "cold carrier" molecules[13]. Studies have reported that more than 99 % of the MIBG molecules in commercial formulations are not radiolabeled. Since the cold MIBG molecules, competitively inhibit the uptake of radiolabeled MIBG molecules by tumor cells expressing NET, no carrier added (n.c.a), high specific activity (SA) radioiodinated

MIBG preparations have been developed in the last decade for both diagnostic and therapeutic studies based on MIBG [29].

Nucleophilic Radioiodination: Radioiodide Exchange Reaction: In the original liquid-phase exchange method [23], the precursor, MIBG sulfate (5 mg in 2 mL of water) was added to 5 mCi of carrier-free ^{131}I sodium iodide solution and was refluxed for 72 h. Radiolabeled MIBG was purified using anion exchange cellulose column to remove the unreacted radioiodide and iodate. The radiochemical yield (labeling efficiency) was 60–80 %, resulting in a SA of 0.6–0.8 mCi/mg. In order to increase both radiochemical yield and radiochemical purity (RCP), a solid-phase exchange facilitated by ammonium sulfate was developed [30, 31]. Subsequently, a liquid-phase copper (Cu^{2+} or Cu^{1+} ion) catalyzed exchange radioiodination (Fig. 19.7) turned out to be an attractive alternative to ammonium sulfate facilitated method [32] and the current commercial methods to produce [^{131}I]MIBG utilize the copper catalyzed isotope exchange reaction. Therapeutic doses of MIBG can also be prepared by copper(I) assisted nucleophilic isotope exchange reaction [33]. In a typical procedure, 2–4 mg of cold MIBG, 5–6 mg sodium metabisulphite, 68 mg CuSO$_4$.5H$_2$O, and 50 mL of glacial acetic acid are taken in a 10-mL vial to which 1–1.5 Ci [^{131}I] NaI activity is added and crimped with a silicone rubber and heated at 160 °C for 35–40 min. Upon completion of the reaction, the pH is adjusted to 5.0 using 2 mL of 0.76 M sodium acetate solution. The purification of the reaction mixture is carried, using a small ion exchange syringe

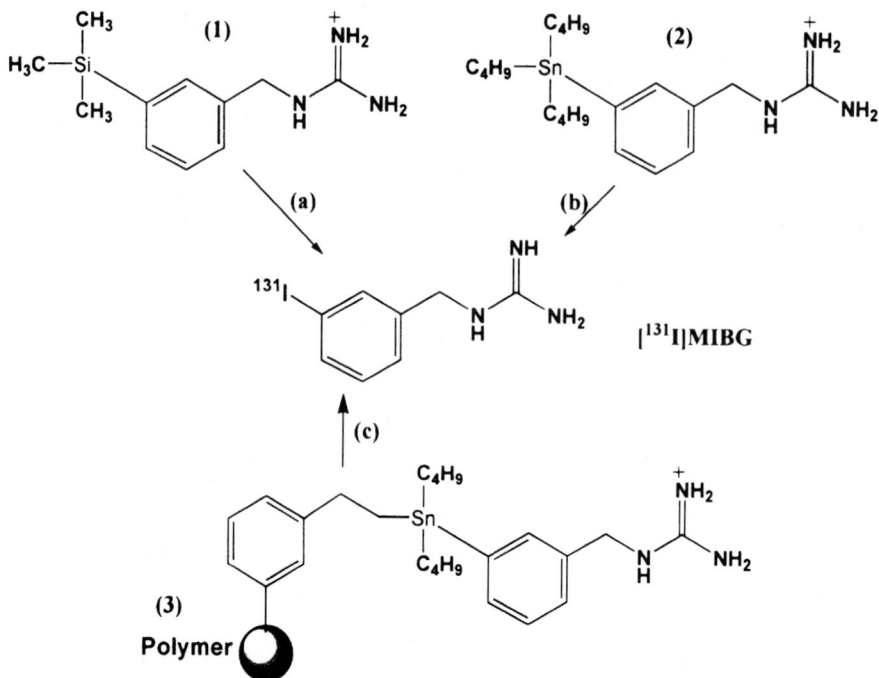

Fig. 19.8 Electrophilic iodination reactions to synthesize no carrier added (N.C.A) radioiodinated MIBG based on a tri-methylsilicon precursor (1), tri-butyltin precursor (2), or di-butyltin precursor attached to a polymer.

Incubation of radioiodide in the presence of an oxidizing agent (H$_2$O$_2$.HOAc) promotes the electrophilic reaction. MIBG synthesis based on polymer-linked di-butyltin precursor does not require HPLC purification

Dowex column. The purified [^{131}I]MIBG is diluted with saline containing 1 % benzyl alcohol to have a final concentration of 15 mCi/mL. The final drug product is then prepared by aseptic filtration through 0.22 μ membrane filter.

Electrophilic Radioiodination: Preparation of N.C.A Radioiodinated MIBG: In order to produce very high specific activity MIBG, no-carrier added (n.c.a) methods based on electrophilic iodination reaction were developed. The original method, based on a silicon precursor [34], requires HPLC purification to prepare the final drug product. Since then, several methods based on different precursors (Fig. 19.8) were developed to improve the radiochemical yields.

A more practical method based on polymer-linked precursor requiring no HPLC purification was developed [35], where the benzylguanidine precursor is bound to a polystyrene-based resin through a di-butyltin. Radiolabeling is performed simply by heating radioiodide with an oxidizing

agent (H$_2$O$_2$.HOAc) and filtering the mixture through a C18 solid-phase cartridge in order to purify radiolabeled MIBG preparation. Radiochemical yields can be increased to about 85 %, when 10 mg of polymer-linked precursor is reacted with radioiodide at 85 °C using H$_2$O$_2$.HOAc as an oxidant and phosphate buffer/ethanol mixture as the solvent. The intrinsic implication of this technique is that very high SA radioiodinated MIBG can be rapidly produced with no other components in the solution, except the aqueous vehicle. This process offers a true carrier-free or n.c.a radioiodinated MIBG.

High SA [^{131}I]MIBG for therapy was produced by Molecular Insight Pharmaceuticals using the Ultratrace solid-phase method [36]. The Ultratrace process uses a solid polystyrene resin containing the covalently bound stannylbenzylguanidine precursor, which undergoes a 1:1 displacement reaction with radioiodine. Briefly, the solid-phase precursor is suspended in a dilute mixture of radioactive ^{131}I-sodium iodide, H$_2$O$_2$/HOAc at

25 °C for 60 min. The oxidized ^{131}I-iodine reacts to disrupt the covalent bond between the tin and benzylguanidine precursor with radioiodine insertion at the *meta* position of the phenyl ring to form [^{131}I]MIBG, which simultaneously cleaves from the resin and dissolves in to the liquid phase. The labeled [^{131}I]MIBG is then purified by using cation exchange cartridge. The formulated final product solution is membrane filtered and aseptically filled into 30-mL glass vials, which are then aseptically capped, sealed, and frozen. The RCP of the drug product is >97 % and the minimum SA is about 1,650 mCi/mg or 460 mCi/μmol.

Radioiodination of Peptides and Proteins: In order to preserve the functional integrity of peptides and proteins, various methods were developed for the radioiodination under mild reaction conditions. Some of these methods include direct nucleophilic labeling of proteins through radioiodination of tyrosine residues with electropositive iodine, as discussed earlier. Chloramine T, iodogen®, and various oxidative enzymes (such as *lactoperoxidase*) are useful for the in situ oxidation of radioiodide for direct protein labeling. Since 1980s, a number of antibodies and antibody fragments were labeled based on direct halogenations methods.

BEXXAR® Formulation: The radioiodination of the mouse IgG$_{2a}$ anti-B1 (anti-CD20) mAb was performed according to the iodogen method [37, 38]. Following purification through an ion-exchange resin column, >90 % of ^{131}I was protein bound with a maximum specific activity of 8.8 mCi/mg. The BEXXAR therapeutic regimen is supplied commercially as a sterile, clear, preservative-free liquid for intravenous administration. The dosimetric dosage form is supplied at nominal protein and activity concentrations of 0.1 mg/mL and 0.61 mCi/mL (at the time of calibration), respectively. The therapeutic dosage form is supplied at 1.1 mg/mL and 5.6 mCi/mL, respectively. Even though the SA of the therapeutic preparation is 5.1 mCi/mg, the SA is not a major issue for the therapeutic dose since 450 mg of cold antibody is administered 1 h prior to the radiolabeled preparation.

In order to perform indirect labeling of proteins, various prosthetic groups have been developed such as Bolton-Hunter reagent, N-succinimidyl 3-(4-hydroxy-5-[^{131}I]iodophenyl) propionate ([^{131}I]I-SHPP). The Boton-Hunter reagent reacts with the lysine residues of peptides or proteins and is more stable towards radio-deiodination. The reagent SHPP is first iodinated using iodogen and subsequently the [^{131}I]I-SHPP is reacted with protein at pH 8.5 to generate ^{131}I labeled protein, as shown in Fig. 19.9a.

211At Labeled Radiopharmaceuticals

The potential applications of α-emitters in TRT is in the treatment of micrometastases, tumors of circulation (leukemias and lymphoma), and compartmental tumors (cystic, ovarian, and neoplastic meningitis). In the last two decades, a number of small aromatic molecules, peptides, intact mAbs, and antibody fragments have been radiolabeled with [211]At. The fact that there are no stable isotopes of astatine (the naturally occurring astatine is radioactive) complicates the synthetic and analytical chemistry of [211]At-labeled radiotracers. For example, 0.1 mCi (3.7 MBq) of [211]At is equivalent to 2×10^{-13} moles of astatine mass, which is far below the mass needed for conventional analytical techniques based on UV, NMR, and IR spectroscopy.

Since astatine is a halogen and directly below iodine in the periodic table, methods used for radioiodination based on electrophilic halogenation of tyrosine residues were used to prepare [211]At labeled proteins and small peptides. However, it was shown that the carbon-astatine bond in the presence of oxidants is not very stable. Just as in the preparation of MIBG, reactions involving astatodestannylation are also useful in the electrophilic labeling of [211]At to proteins and small molecules. This procedure involves the production of N-succinimidyl 3-[211]At-astatobenzoate (SAB) by destannylation of N-succinimidyl 3-(tri-n-butylstannyl)benzoate (BuSTB) or N-succinimidyl 3-(trimethylstannyl)benzoate (MeSTB) [39, 40]. Subsequently, SAB is coupled to the protein as shown in Fig. 19.9b.

a

b

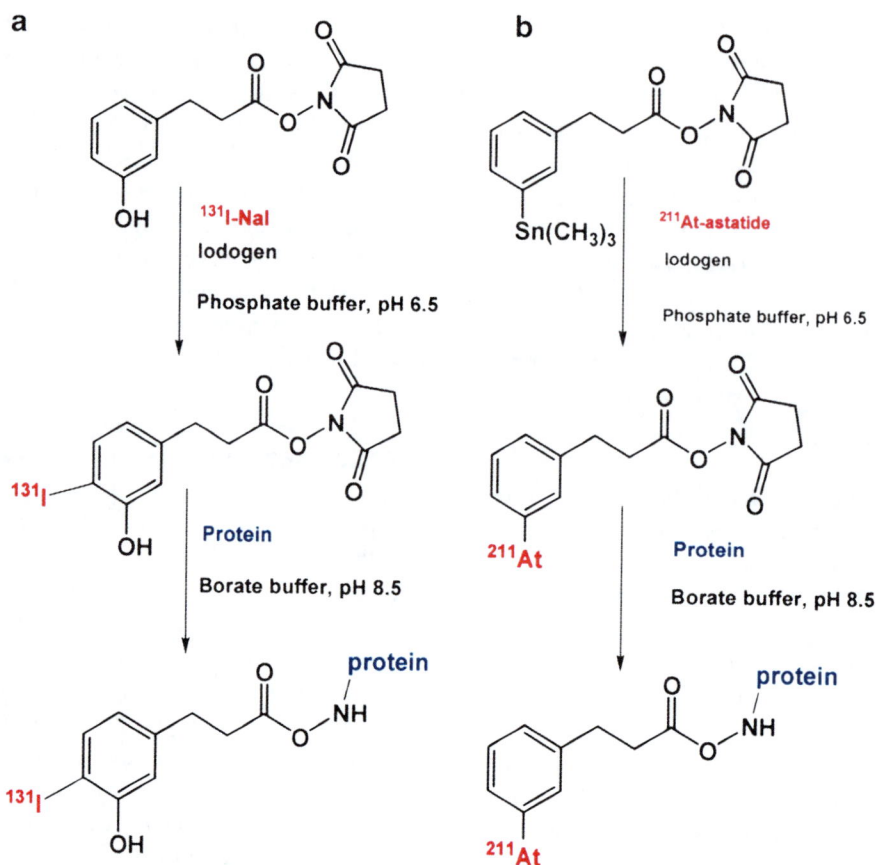

Fig. 19.9 Indirect radioiodination technique: (**a**) The Bolton-Hunter reagent, *N*-succinimidyl 3-(4-hydroxy-5-[[131I]iodophenyl) propionate ([131I]I-SHPP) is first prepared by labeling the reagent SHPP using the iodogen method. Subsequently [131I]I-SHPP reacts with the lysine residues of peptides or proteins to generate 131I labeled protein. (**b**) In a similar manner, *N*-succinimidyl 3-211 At-astatobenzoate ([211At]At-SAB) by destannylation of *N*-succinimidyl 3-(trimethylstannyl)benzoate (MeSTB). Subsequently, ([211At]At-SAB) is coupled to the protein

Astatine-211 labeled radiopharmaceuticals that have been investigated for TRT include astatide, naphthoquinone derivatives, methylene blue, DNA precursors, *meta*-astatobenzylguanidine (MABG), biotin conjugates, bisphosphonates, monoclonal antibodies and antibody fragments, and, finally, particles [41].

Labeling of Biomolecules with Radiometals

Three different strategies are used in the design of therapeutic radiopharmaceuticals for TRT: the integrated approach, bifunctional approach, and the hybrid approach [4]. The integrated approach involves replacement of part of a known high affinity biomolecule (BM) or ligand with an "unnatural" radiometal-chelate complex. Through metal chelation, all parts are arranged in such a way that the whole metal complex becomes a high affinity radiopharmaceutical. This approach is very complicated and difficult to meet all the necessary criteria necessary for an optimal therapeutic agent.

The bifunctional approach as shown in Fig. 19.10 uses a high affinity ligand, a bifunctional chelate (BFC) for conjugation of the biomolecule on one side, a chelation of the radiometal on the other side, and a linker for pharmacokinetic

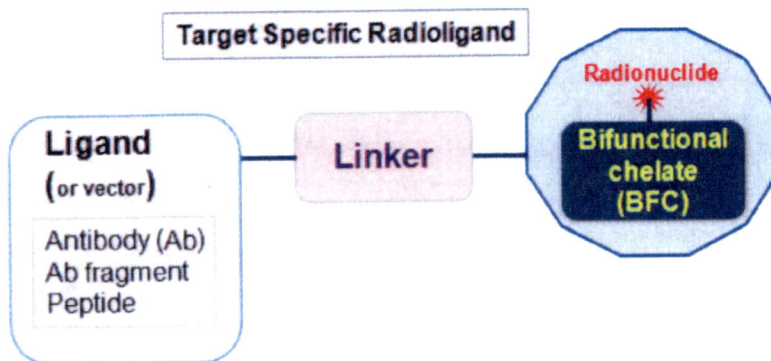

Fig. 19.10 Preparation of a target specific radioligand: The bifunctional chelate (BFC) is first conjugated to a ligand or a biomolecule (BM) via a linker molecule. The BFA-BM complex is then labeled with a radiometal by chelation of the metal with the electron donating atoms (such as nitrogen and oxygen) in the BFA to form coordinate covalent bonds

modification. The choice of BFC is largely determined by the nature and oxidation state of the radiometal. The radiometal chelate is often kept at a distance away from the ligand binding motif to minimize possible interference with the binding site. Linker molecules may be necessary to join the biomolecule to BFC. In addition, pharmacokinetic modifiers within linkers can also impart desirable distribution characteristics. This is a more popular approach for the development of target-specific radiopharmaceuticals for TRT. The two most clinically used radiopharmaceuticals, OctreoScan® and Zevalin®, were developed based on this approach.

In the hybrid approach, the radiometal (^{188}Re or ^{99m}Tc) is chelated by a peptide sequence containing an N_4, N_3S, or N_2S_2 donor set. The radiometal can also be incorporated as part of a macrocyclic peptide framework. The "unchelated" linear peptide has a relatively low binding affinity for the intended receptor and the chelation of radiometal results in a constrained macrocyclic metallopeptide with increased receptor binding affinity. A major advantage of this approach is that the bonding of radiometal may increase the receptor binding affinity of the polypeptide. Since this approach was successful in the development of several ^{99m}Tc radiopharmaceuticals (such as MAG3), the methodology could be adopted to develop ^{188}Re labeled therapeutic radiopharmaceuticals.

Chelating Agents

In 1970s, ligands known as *bifunctional chelating agents* (BFC) were introduced to complex radiometals such as ^{111}In and ^{67}Ga. Various BFCs (Table 19.8) have been designed and synthesized over the years to develop a wide variety of radiopharmaceuticals based on radiometals [42, 43]. A *ligand* is a neutral molecule or an ion having a lone pair of electrons that can be donated to form a bond with a metal ion. A chelating agent (or a chelate) is a molecule containing more than one ligand or an atom (such as N, O, and S) that can donate a lone pair of electrons. All the chelating agents listed in Table 19.7 contain N and O atoms that can form coordinate covalent bonds with the central metal ion.

The chelates such as EDTA and DTPA are open chain polyaminopolycarboxylic acids, while NOTA, DOTA, and TETA are cyclic polyaminoploycarboxylates (or macrocyclics) consisting of triaza or tetraaza macrocycle ranging from 9 to 14 membered ring size. BFCs based on bis(thiosemicarbozone) or BTS containing N and S atoms have been developed specifically to bind to Cu metal. Similarly, BFCs such as PnAOs, DADTs, and MAG3 containing N and S atoms were designed to develop ^{99m}Tc radiopharmaceuticals. A wide variety of derivatives of the BFCs have been designed to improve the in vivo stability and optimize the kinetics of

Table 19.7 Bifunctional chelating agents

Polyaminocaboxylic acids	Diethylenetriamenepentaacetic acid	DTPA
	Ethylenediaminetetraacetic acid	EDTA
Macrocyclics	1,4,7,10-tetraazacyclododecane-N,N'',N''',N''''-tetraacetic acid	DOTA
	1,4,8,11-tetraazacyclotetradecane-N,N'',N''',N''''-tetraacetic acid	TETA
	1,4,7,-triazacyclododecane-N,N'',N''',N''''-tetraacetic acid	NOTA
Others	Bis(thiosemicarbazone)	BTS
	Propyleneamine oxime	PnAO
	Diaminedithiol	DADT
	Mercaptoacetylglycylglycylglycine	MAG_3
	Desferrioxamine	DFO

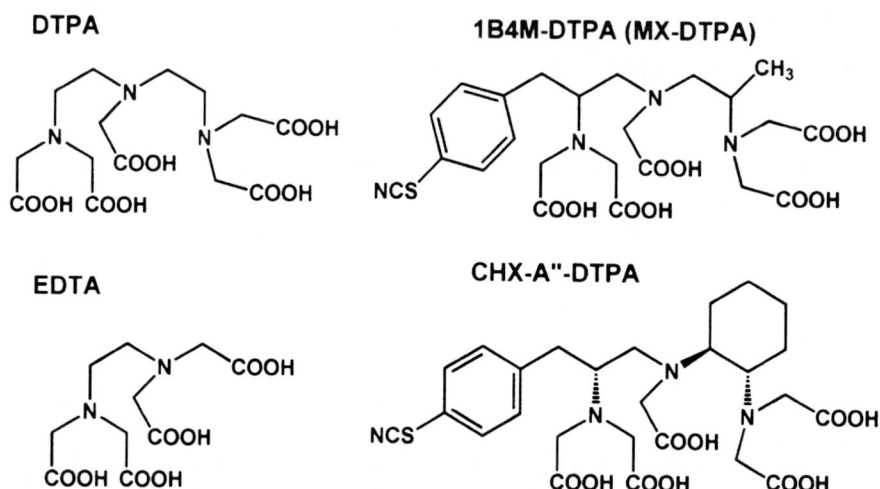

Fig. 19.11 Polyaminocaboxylic acids, EDTA and DTPA as bifunctional chelating agents; Radiometal complexes of the derivatives of DTPA (MX-DTPA and CHX-DTPA) provide greater in vivo stability of radiometal complex compared to DTPA alone

a specific metal-chelate complex. The structures of various BFCs are shown in Figs. 19.11, 19.12, 19.13, and 19.14.

The BFCs contain a side chain for conjugation to a peptide or protein. The side chain can be attached to the carbon backbone of the chelate (c-functionalized chelate) or by substitution to one of the nitrogen atoms in the molecule. C-functionalized chelating agents are preferable and provide greater stability to metal-chelate complex since all the nitrogen and oxygen atoms will be available for coordination with the metal ion. It is also preferable to conjugate the chelating agent to the peptide or protein of interest first, before complexation with the radiometal.

In coordination compounds, the metal ions have two types of valence: the *primary valence* (also known as oxidation state) refers to the ability of metal ion to form ionic bonds with oppositely charged ions, while the *secondary valence* (also known as coordination number) refers to the ability of a metal ion to bind to Lewis bases (ligands) to form complex ions. Therefore, the coordination number is the number of bonds formed by the metal ion with the atoms (that can donate a pair of electrons) in a chelating agent. This number varies from 2 to 9, depending on the size, charge, and electron configuration of the metal ion. The ligand geometric arrangements of coordination compounds can be linear, square

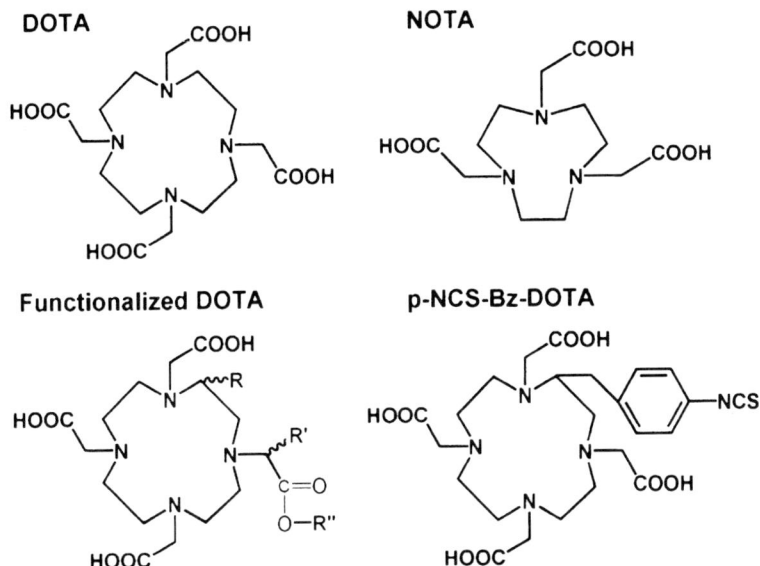

Fig. 19.12 Macrocyclic bifunctional chelating agents useful to prepare therapeutic radiopharmaceuticals with trivalent radiometals (such as ^{111}In, ^{90}Y and ^{177}Lu)

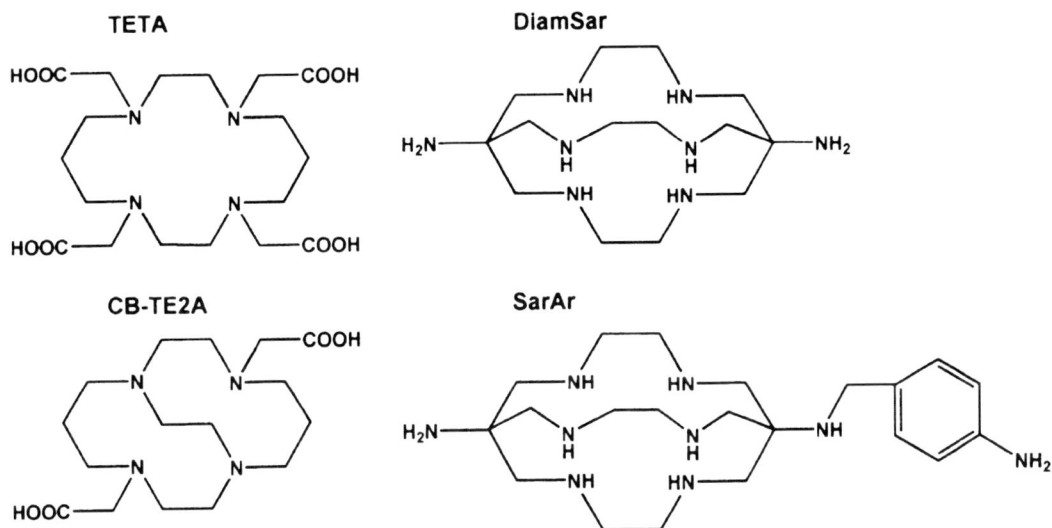

Fig. 19.13 Macrocyclic bifunctional chelating agents useful to prepare therapeutic radiopharmaceuticals with radio-isotopes of copper (^{64}Cu and ^{67}Cu)

planar, tetrahedral, or octahedral depending on the coordination number.

Stability of Metal-Ligand Complex: As shown in Table 19.8, except for Ga and In, all other metals used in radiation therapy are transition metals. The electronegativity and the oxidation state play a major role in the formation of metal-ligand complexes. Since the metal ions form insoluble hydroxides in water at physiological pH, direct labeling of peptides and proteins with metallic radionuclides is relatively difficult. Chelating agents can complex and stabilize the metal. Therefore, it is necessary to first attach a chelating agent, by covalent

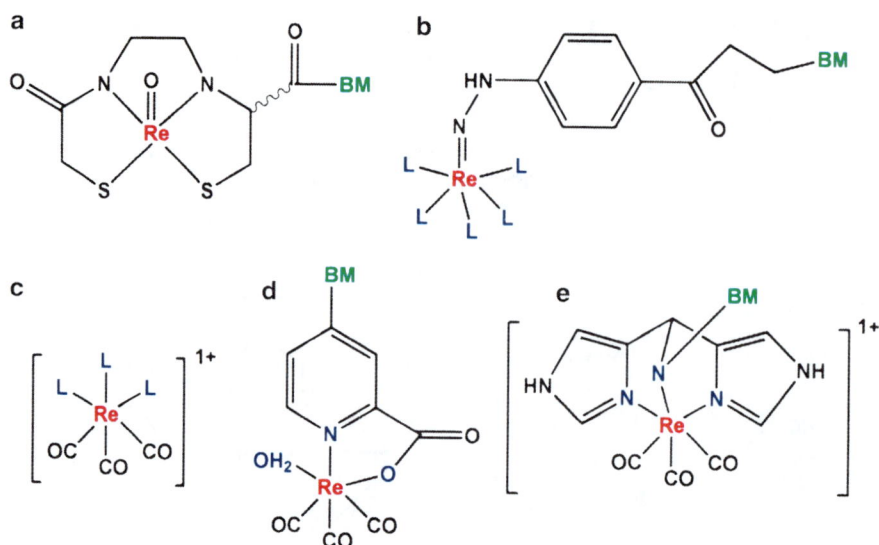

Fig. 19.14 Examples of bidentate and tridentate bifunctional chelating agents to label biomolecules (BM) with $^{186/188}$Re: (**a**) Re-N$_3$S ligand, (**b**) Re-HYNIC complex, (**c–e**) Re-tricarbnyl complexes where nitrogen and oxygen atoms in ligand molecules form complexes with Re. The biomolecules (BM) is attached to the carbon atoms in the backbone of the chelating agent

Table 19.8 Physical properties and electron configuration of metals

Physical property	Element							
	Cu	Ga	Y	In	Lu	Re	Tc	Zr
Atomic number	29	31	39	49	71	75	43	40
Atomic radius (pm)	128	122	181	163	174	137	136	160
Ionic radius (pm)	2$^+$, 71–87	3$^+$, 61–76	3$^+$, 90–108	3$^+$, 92	3+, 86–103	5$^+$, 58	5$^+$, 60	4$^+$, 59–89
Electron structure	[Ar]	[Ar]	[Kr]	[Kr]	[Xe]	[Xe]	[Kr]	[Kr]
	3d^{10}	3d^{10}	4d^1	4d^{10}	4f^{14}	4f^{14}	4d^5	4d^2
	4s^1	4s^2	5s^2	5s^2	5d^1	5d^5	5s^2	5s^2
		4p^1		5p^1	6s^2	6s^2		
Electronegativity	1.90	1.81	1.22	1.78	1.27	1	1.9	1.33
Oxidation state	+1, +2	+3	+3	+3	+3	−1 to +7	−1 to +7	+4, +2
Coordination number	4–6	4–6	6–9	4–6	6–9	6	6	4–9

bonds, to a peptide or protein, and then label the chelate-biomolecule complex with the radiometal. The metal ions dissolved in water are complexed to form aqua ions. However, in the presence of a chelating agent or the ligand (L) with greater affinity for the metal than the affinity of OH$^-$ ion for the metal, formation of metal-chelate complex is preferred, as shown below.

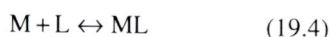

$$M + L \leftrightarrow ML \qquad (19.4)$$

$$K_s = \frac{[ML]}{[M][L]} \qquad (19.5)$$

In the above equation, [ML] represents the concentration of metal-ligand complex, while [M] and [L] represent the concentrations of free metal and the free ligand. The stability of the metal-ligand complex is defined by the stability constant (K_s) when the system reaches equilibrium between the interacting chemical species [44]. The higher the value of K_s, the greater is the thermodynamic stability of the metal-ligand complex. The values of K_s (such as 10^4 or 10^{30}) are normally represented as log K_s values (such as 4 and 30). It is important to appreciate that the stability constant can reveal only the direction of reaction (formation or dissociation), but not the rate of reaction. For example, when a purified metal-ligand complex is injected into the circulation, the rate of dissociation of the complex may be significantly increased, due to the extreme dilution of the complex. Therefore, the *kinetic stability* of the metal-ligand complex is very important under in vivo conditions where competing ions and ligands may augment the transchelation of radiometal [44]. The K_s values are usually determined for reaction in ideal conditions of buffer, pH, temperature, etc., and do not necessarily reflect the stability of metal-ligand complex in vivo. A quantity known as *conditional stability constant* can be measured or estimated as a function of pH and in the presence of different amounts of other competing ligands.

Chemistry of Metals

As discussed earlier, among various transition metals, ^{67}Cu, ^{90}Y, and $^{186/188}Re$ have been used extensively for developing radiopharmaceuticals for TRT. There are several lanthanides, such as ^{177}Lu, ^{153}Sm, and ^{166}Ho that are also of special interest. Yttrium and lanthanide metals share similar coordination chemistry. In addition, the tracer chemistry of these transition metals is similar to the chemistry of post-transition radiometals ^{67}Ga and ^{111}In, which have a filled d shell and three electrons in the outermost shell (Table 19.6). In contrast, yttrium has an incomplete d shell with one electron and two electrons in the outermost $(5S^2)$ shell. Lutetium also lies in the d-block of the periodic table with one electron and two electrons in the outermost $(6S^2)$ shell. However, for all these metals (M), the most important oxidation state is M^{III}. Their coordination chemistry is somewhat similar; however, due to small differences in their ionic radii and electronegativities, minor, but significant differences do exist in their chemistries. These four trivalent metals also share chemical characteristics with the ferric ion (Fe^{3+}). This similarity with ferric ion is important in the development of radiopharmaceuticals with

these three metals since iron is an essential element in the human body and a number of iron binding proteins such as transferrin (in blood) do exist to transport and store iron in vivo. As a result, the atoms of iron always compete with these radiometals in vivo for specific binding with proteins such as transferrin, lactoferrin, and ferritin [45].

Zirconium-89 is a β^+ emitting radionuclide that is becoming increasingly popular as an ideal radionuclide to develop radiolabeled antibodies for immunoPET. Like other transition metals, zirconium forms a wide range of inorganic compounds and coordination complexes. In contrast to the more familiar coordination chemistry of trivalent radionuclides discussed above, ^{89}Zr displays a number of distinct differences. In particular, the 4+ oxidation state imparts a strong preference for $^{89}Zr^{4+}$ ions to bind to highly electronegative (class a) hard donor atoms including oxygen, nitrogen, and fluoride. Zirconium complexes have a high propensity towards hydrolysis in aqueous solution. In addition, the relatively large ionic radius of $^{89}Zr^{4+}$ allows the first coordination sphere to accommodate up to eight donor atoms. In this respect, the ionic nature of most Zr^{4+} complexes and the higher coordination numbers means that the chemistry more closely resembles that of radio-lanthanides and radio-actinides such as Lu and Ac [46].

The chemistry of copper is dominated by two oxidation states, I and II [47]. Copper salts form the aqua ion $[Cu(OH)_6]^{2+}$ and the compounds of Cu (I) oxidation state are unstable in aqueous solution and readily oxidize to Cu(II) which can form 4, 5, or 6 coordination bonds with ligands. In Cu (II) oxidation state, the metal binds strongly with N and S containing molecules forming coordination complexes. Complex formation with chelating agents occurs at pH <7 since formation of insoluble $Cu(OH)_2$ is not a major concern. The ability to fully exploit Cu radionuclides for TRT is limited, at least in part, by the high lability of Cu(II) complexes (i.e., high k_d). In circulation, Cu binds to human serum albumin (HSA), which typically exists at a concentration of 5×10^{-4} M. Since the concentration of HSA is relatively high compared to the mass of Cu, the amount of Cu that is transferred from the chelate complex to the endogenous proteins is of major concern. Therefore, the choice of BFC used for labeling copper radionuclides to peptides and proteins is very important.

Rhenium is a third row transition metal directly under technetium in Group 7 of the periodic table (Fig. 19.7). For both these metals, the chemistry is diverse with compounds in oxidation states ranging from −1 through +7. The most important oxidation states for the development of radiopharmaceuticals, however, are +5, +3, and +1. The radioisotopes of both Tc and Re are available as the permetallate (MO_4^-), which means that the metal must be reduced from +7 oxidation state to lower oxidation states in order to complex the metal by a chelating agent [4].

The aqueous chemistry of trivalent metals is dominated by their ability to form strong complexes (both soluble and insoluble) with the hydroxyl ion. The fully hydrated (hexaaquo) M^{3+} ions are only stable under acidic conditions. As the pH is raised above 3, these metals form insoluble hydroxides ($M(OH)_3$). A variety of OH intermediates are formed as a function of pH and the mass of the metal. Ga is more amphoteric at physiological pH, and it exists predominantly as a soluble species, $[Ga(OH)_4]^-$ (gallate) [48]. With indium, the soluble $[In(OH)_4]^-$ starts forming only at pH values higher than 7.0. Since the ionic radius of Y or Lu is relatively larger than Ga, they bind to a larger number of water molecules or ligands. The total solubility of these metals at physiological pH is very limited. Very high SAs of radiometals are needed to keep them soluble in water. However, it is a common practice to add weak chelating agents, such as citrate, acetate, or tartrate ion, to complex the metal and prevent precipitation at neutral pH.

BFCs for Trivalent Metals: The coordination chemistry of the metallic radionuclide will determine the geometry and stability of "metal-chelate complex." Different metallic radionuclides have different coordination chemistries and require BFC with different donor atoms and chelator frameworks. Both Ga and In are classified as hard acids and prefer hard bases [45]. It has been shown that in +3 oxidation state, both Ga and In

form thermodynamically stable complexes with either 4, 5, or 6 coordinate ligands, with 6-coordiante being the most stable, while Y and Lu prefer octadentate coordinating ligands. The advantage of using the acyclic chelators (DTPA and EDTA) is their extremely fast and high radiolabeling efficiency under mild conditions and greater thermodynamic stability; however, their kinetic lability often results in dissociation of the radiometal. The macrocyclic chelates (NOTA and DOTA), however, provide greater thermodynamic stability as well as kinetic stability. While Ga and In radionuclides form greater thermodynamically stable complexes with NOTA, DTPA, or EDTA, the Y and Lu radionuclides prefer the macrocyclic chelator, DOTA to form stable complexes [43, 49–51]. In order to improve in vivo stability, a number of derivatives of DTPA were prepared in which the DTPA carbon backbone has been methylated or which used a "built-in" cyclohexyl group (Fig. 19.10). Due to the presence of a carbon stereocenter in the DTPA backbone, the chelate preparation contains a mixture of stereo and constitutional isomers, referred to as "MX-DTPA." Another series of DTPA derivatives, referred to as CHX-DTPA, contain a cyclohexyl group. It has been reported that one of the isomers, known as "CHX-A" DTPA (Fig. 19.10) is an effective chelators for ^{111}In, ^{90}Y, and [177]Lu. This DTPA analog has been used to develop therapeutic radiopharmaceuticals based on the α-emitter, [212/213]Bi.

DOTA is a 12-membered tetraaza macrocycle with four carboxylate arms (Figure 12). While several DOTA derivatives have been reported, the most common agent used extensively in the preparation of radiolabeled antibodies and peptides is the original DOTA chelate. A number of ^{90}Y and ^{177}Lu labeled antibodies and peptides are based on DOTA. The labeling kinetics of DOTA-based BFCs is usually slow, and much more dependent on the radiolabeling conditions, including the DOTA-conjugate concentration, pH, reaction temperature, heating time, buffer agent and concentration, and presence of other metallic impurities, such as Fe^{3+} and Zn^{2+} [49, 50]. High SA of the radiometal is also very important, especially in the synthesis of therapeutic radiopharmaceuticals based on peptides.

153Sm-EDTMP: In the preparation of ^{153}Sm-EDTMP (Quadramet®), ^{153}Sm forms the thermodynamically stable complex with the linear acyclic ligand, ethylenediamine tetramethylenephosphonic acid (EDTMP). To prevent dissociation, however, it is necessary to have ligand-^{153}Sm ratio to be 250–300:1 [8]. Since the half-life of ^{177}Lu is much longer than that of ^{153}Sm, ^{177}Lu-EDTMP has been prepared recently and is under clinical evaluation for bone pain palliation.

Radiolabeled mAbs

A number of reviews have been published describing the techniques of labeling mAbs with trivalent radiometals [4, 8, 43, 52]. One of the earliest reports of a BFA conjugated to an antibody made use of a natural product, desferrioxamine (DFO), for radiolabeling with ^{111}In [53]. Subsequently, the derivatives of EDTA were used to prepare ^{111}In and ^{90}Y labeled antibodies. However, due to their limited stability, DTPA derivatives were developed to provide a more appropriate coordination number and stability [54]. The cyclic anhydride of DTPA (ca-DTPA) and the isobutylcarbonic anhydride (carb-DTPA) were also introduced to label macromolecules such as albumin and mAb [55]. Antibodies labeled with ^{111}In and ^{90}Y using ca-DTPA, however, showed suboptimal in vivo stability and potential toxicity [52]. The full octadentate bifunctional DTPA derivatives such as MX-DTPA and CHX-DTPA provided greater in vivo stability [56]. One of these MX-DTPA isomers, specifically 1B4M-DTPA, has been used in the preparation of chelate tiuxetan [51, 57]. Zevalin, the ^{90}Y or ^{111}In labeled Ibritumomab tiuxetan mAb, is the only FDA approved radiopharmaceutical based on straight chain polyaminopolycarboxylate.

111In or 90Y-Zevalin: In the commercial kit for the preparation of Radiolabeled Zevalin, 3.2 mg of Ibritumomab Tiuxetan in 2 mL of saline is supplied. However, to prepare ^{111}In-Zevalin, ^{111}In chloride (5.5 mCi/0.5 mL) is first mixed with 50 mM sodium acetate buffer (0.6 mL) and the mixture is then added to only 1 mL of antibody (1.6 mg) solution. To prepare ^{90}Y-Zevalin, ^{90}Y-chloride (40 mCi/0.5 mL) is first mixed with 50 mM sodium acetate buffer and then mixed with 1.3 mg of antibody (2.1 mg). At the end of 30 min incubation period, a formulation buffer (containing albumin, pentetic acid in phosphate buffer) is added to the incubation mixture to make the final volume of 10 mL. The specific activity of ^{90}Y-Zevalin is around 20 mCi/mg of antibody.

In the last two decades, most of the mAbs have been labeled with ^{111}In, ^{90}Y, and ^{177}Lu using DOTA or DOTA derivatives. Several studies have demonstrated that conjugation of 2–6 DOTAs per mAb molecule would provide optimal labeling yield with higher specific activity (10–20 mCi/mg) and immunoreactivity [58, 59]. In addition, DOTA-mAb binds ^{90}Y with extraordinary stability, minimizing the toxicity of ^{90}Y-DOTA immunoconjugates arising from loss of ^{90}Y to bone. Typical radiolabeling procedure involves first mixing the radiometal (in HCl) with ammonium acetate buffer (0.5–1.0 M, pH 7.0) and subsequently incubating the radiometal-acetate complex with DOTA-mAb. Raising the reaction temperature from 25 °C to 37–45 °C markedly increases the labeling efficiency.

Radiolabeled Octreotide Analogs: The most successful somatostatin (SS) analog or derivative is the cyclic octapeptide, Octreotide (developed by Sandoz, now Novartis), which binds to SSTR with very high affinity. ^{111}In-DTPA-octreotide (OctreoScan®) has become the main imaging technique for NETs and is used routinely in clinical practice. Starting from the Octreotide (OC) sequence, many other analogs (Fig. 19.4, Table 19.9) were developed to optimize SSTR binding affinity in order to develop radiopharmaceuticals for both imaging and therapy. Since the peptide structure is not affected when conjugated, molecules are covalently bound to the N-terminus, DTPA and DOTA were conjugated to D-Phe^1 [60, 61]. While preserving the critical sequence D-Trp^4-Lys^5 for receptor binding, modifications have been performed on the side-chain amino acids, Phe^3 and Thr^6 [62]. It has been shown that when Phe^3 is replaced by Tyr^3 in order to increase hydrophilicity, the resulting Octreotide analog (DOTA-TOC) exhibited improved SSTR2 affinity and a lower affinity for the SSTR3 subtype [20]. Also, converting

Table 19.9 Somatostatin analogs: affinity profiles (IC50a) for the somatostatin receptor (SSTR) subtypes

Peptide	SSTR1	SSTR2	SSTR3	SSTR4	SSTR5
Somatostatin	5.2	2.7	7.7	5.6	4.0
DTPA-Octreotide	>10,000	22	182	>1,000	237
In-DOTA-TOC	>10,000	4.6	120	230	130
Ga-DOTA-TOC	>10,000	2.5	613	>1,000	73
DOTA-TATE	>10,000	1.5	>1,000	453	547
In-DOTA-NOC	>10,000	2.9	8.0	227	11.2
Ga-DOTANOC	>1,000	1.9	40	–	7.2
In-DOTA-BOC-ATE	>1,000	1.4	5.5	135	3.9

The values in the above table are from Rufini et al. [61]
[a]IC_{50} values expressed in nanomoles

Table 19.10 177Lu-DOTA-TATE (200 mCi dose) preparation using 177Lu with different specific activity (SA)

SA of [177]Lu (Ci/mg)/in0.2 mL	Required DOTA-TATE (µg)	AA Buffer (mL)	Required Gentic acid (mg)	Final volume (mL)	SA of ^{177}Lu-DOTA-TATE (mCi/µmol)
20	324	1.57	63	2.10	885
25	259	1.38	55	1.84	1,504
30	216	1.25	50	1.66	1,325
35	185	1.16	46	1.54	1,550
40	162	1.09	43	1.45	1,770

Modified from Das et al. [66]

octreotide to octreotate (DOTA-TATE), by replacing C-terminal Thr(ol) with a natural amino acid, Thr[8] results in a peptide with increased receptor binding, high tumor uptake, and improved internalization. Finally, replacing Phe[3] with a more lipophilic residue, β-naphtyl alanine (NaI), the resulting peptide (DOTA-NOC), showed high affinity for SSTR2, SSTR3, and SSTR5 [63]. The affinity profiles for human SSTR subtypes of several octreotide analogs [20, 61] are summarized in Table 19.9. While the clinical utility of ^{90}Y-DOTA-TOC and ^{177}Lu-DOTATATE for therapy of NETs has been well documented, the advantage of PET studies using ^{68}Ga-DOTATOC or DOTA-NOC is still under clinical evaluation.

^{177}Lu-DOTA-TATE: In peptide receptor radionuclide therapy (PRRT), ^{177}Lu-DOTA-TATE has emerged as the most promising agent for the treatment of patients suffering from inoperable neuroendocrine-originated tumors [12, 64]. One of the challenges involved in carrying out PRRT with this radiopharmaceutical, however, is to prepare the radiolabeled conjugate with adequately high specific activity in order that sufficient activity can be deposited in the cancerous

lesions without saturating the limited number of receptors present in the cancerous site. The source of ^{177}Lu, the production method, and specific activity are all very important considerations. While optimizing conditions with ^{177}Lu have been reported previously [65], a recent publication evaluated the role of specific activity of ^{177}Lu in the preparation of patient-specific doses [66]. ^{177}Lu-DOTA-TATE was prepared using a precalculated amount of DOTA-TATE based on the available specific activity of ^{177}Lu at the time of preparation, keeping a minimum molar ratio of DOTATATE/Lu is about 4:1, so that the final specific activity was in the range of 32.74–65.49 GBq/µmol (885–1770 mCi/µmol). DOTA-TATE solution was prepared by dissolving the peptide in high-purity water (1 mg/mL) in the necessary volume of 0.1 M ammonium acetate buffer, pH 5 containing 40 mg/mL gentisic acid. The pH of the resultant solution was adjusted to 5, if required, after the addition of required volume of [177]LuCl$_3$. Subsequently, the reaction mixture was incubated at 85–90 °C for 45 min. Table 19.10 shows the composition of ^{177}Lu-DOTA-TATE (200 mCi dose) prepared with different ^{177}Lu specific activities. After the quality control studies, the preparation was subjected to Millipore filtration prior to the administration to the patients.

BFCs for Copper: In order to bind radionuclides of copper to biomolecules, macrocyclic chelators, such as TETA, have been developed [67, 68]. However, Cu (II)-TETA complexes were not optimal as imaging agents since they are not stable in vivo [69]. Recently, a new class of bicyclic tetraazamacrocycles (Fig. 18.13), the ethylene "crossbridged" cyclam derivatives (CB-2ETA) were developed which form highly kinetically stable complexes with Cu(II) and are less susceptible to transchelation in vivo [70, 71]. Similarly, another series of TETA analogs, known as hexaaza-cryptand ligands, SarAr and SarArNCS, were also reported to form strong and stable Cu (II) complexes by wrapping the Cu atom more tightly [72, 73]. This approach does not, however, take into account other factors that may affect complex stability in vivo, such as chelate ring size, chelate flexibility, and ring substitution. While several ^{64}Cu labeled peptides are under clinical evaluation as molecular probes for PET, radiopharmaceuticals based on ^{67}Cu labeled mAbs are not being considered as appropriate or ideal for RIT.

BFCs for Rhenium: BFCs with N_3S and N_2S_2 configuration (Fig. 19.14) are tetradentate basal plane chelates that were originally developed to prepare stable complexes with Tc and Re radionuclides. These chelates can be covalently linked to the biomolecule through functional groups on their carbon backbone as well as internal and terminal amine/amides [4]. Tc and Re have similar chemistries, however, labeling with radioisotopes of Re often requires a low pH, higher temperatures, and long reaction times when compared with the conditions needed for Tc-99m labeling [51].

Since Abrams and coworkers first reported the use of [Tc]HYNIC core for ^{99m}Tc-labeling of polyclonal IgG, the pyridyl azide ligand, 6-hydrazinopyridine-3-carboxylic acid (HYNIC) has been used as a BFC for labeling of proteins and small biomolecules with Tc(V) and Re(V) radionuclides [4, 8]. The +5 oxidation state of the metal is generated simply by reduction using reducing agents such as stannous chloride. The HYNIC chelate takes up only one coordination site on the metal complexes leaving five coordination sites to be filled by coligands, such as glucoheptonate and tricine. The overall charge of the complex is dependent on the coligands and protonation state of the HYNIC ligand.

A major advancement in Tc and Re chemistry occurred when it was discovered that a highly adaptable tricabonyl Tc core makes it possible to prepare organometallic complexes in aqueous solution [74, 75]. In an effort to develop new organometallic precursors for the preparation of ^{99m}Tc-complexes, the investigators showed that by treating pertechnetate (TcO_4^-) with sodium borohydride ($NaBH_4$) in the presence of carbon monoxide (CO) gas, they could produce the reactive Tc(I) species, $[Tc(CO)_3(OH_2)_3]^+$ [74, 76]. The Tc(I) and Re(I) tricarbonyl cores have three open, facially oriented coordination sites. The geometry of the core allows for the use of many different BFCs. Several different ligand backbones for $Re(CO)_3$ are shown in Fig. 19.14. In this complex, the three facially oriented water molecules are sufficiently labile so that they can be readily displaced by a variety of mono-, bi-, and tridentate ligands. Since it is difficult to work with CO gas, the technology is based on the use of a solid reagent, potassium boranocarbonate ($K_2H_3BCO_2$), which acts as both a reducing agent and a source of CO gas [75]. The kit is available from Mallinckrodt (Tyco) Medical under the trade name *Isolink*. It has been shown that both bidentate and tridentate chelates bind rapidly to the $[Tc(CO)_3]^+$ core on a macroscopic scale and at the tracer level.

Summary

During the last couple of decades, there has been significant increase in the application of radiopharmaceuticals for TRT, mainly due to the development of a range of new carrier molecules, which can transport a therapeutic radionuclide to a molecular target at the disease site. Most of the radionuclides in routine clinical use are β⁻ emitters (^{131}I, ^{90}Y, ^{153}Sm, and ^{177}Lu) with a wide range of half-lives ranging from 0.7 to 8 days. Among the α-emitting radionuclides, [211]At with a relatively longer half-life (7.21 h) has generally been considered as a more useful and versatile nuclide for TRT. For TRT to be truly effective and specific, the carrier molecule (ligand or vector), ideally, seeks the tumor cells and delivers the radionuclide to the tumor cells by specific binding to a target site, either on the cell surface, or within the tumor cell. The tumor localization properties of a specific therapeutic radiopharmaceutical and the clinical application will depend on the route of administration, such as intravenous, intra-arterial, intracavitary, and intra-articular approaches. Therapeutic radiopharmaceuticals may be structurally simple ions ([131]I[-] and [89]Sr[2+]), small molecules (^{131}I-MIBG and [153]Sm-EDTMP), complex molecules (^{131}I, ^{90}Y or ^{177}Lu labeled intact antibodies or antibody fragments), colloids (^{32}P chromic phosphate), or even particles (^{90}Y labeled microspheres). Among ^{131}I labeled radiopharmaceuticals, ^{131}I labeled Bexxar® is the only mAb approved by FDA for therapy. While ^{123}I-MIBG (AdreView™, GE Healthcare) was approved as a tumor imaging agent, the therapeutic indication utilizing [^{131}I]MIBG for TRT, however, has not been approved in the United States. Among the radiometal labeled biomolecules, ^{90}Y-Zevalin is the only FDA approved drug for RIT. However, hundreds of mAbs labeled with ^{131}I, ^{90}Y, or ^{177}Lu are under extensive clinical evaluation. In PRRT, while ^{90}Y-DOTA-TOC has demonstrated significant clinical utility in treating patients with neuroendocrine tumors, ^{177}Lu-DOTA-TATE has also emerged as the most promising agent for the treatment of patients suffering from inoperable neuroendocrine-originated tumors.

References

1. Volkert WA, Hoffman TJ. Therapeutic radiopharmaceuticals. Chem Rev. 1999;99:2269–92.
2. IAEA-TECDOC-1228. Therapeutic applications of radiopharmaceuticals. Vienna, 2001.
3. IAEA-TECDOC-1359. Labeling techniques of biomolecules for targeted radiotherapy. Vienna, 2003.
4. Liu S. The role of coordination chemistry in the development of target specific radiopharmaceuticals. Chem Soc Rev. 2004;33:445–61.
5. Pandit-Taskar N, Batraki M, Divgi CR. Radiopharmaceutical therapy for palliation of bone pain from osseous metastases. J Nucl Med. 2004;45:1358–65.
6. Sharkey RM, Goldenberg DM. Targeted therapy of cancer: new prospects for antibodies and immunoconjugates. CA Cancer J Clin. 2006;56:226–43.
7. IAEA-TRS No. 458. Comparative evaluation of therapeutic radiopharmaceuticals. Vienna, 2007.
8. Jurisson S, Cutler C, Smith SV. Radiometal complexes: characterization and relevant in vitro studies. Q J Nucl Med Mol Imaging. 2008;52:222–34.
9. Correia JDG, Paulo A, Raposinho PD, et al. Radiometallated peptides for molecular imaging and targeted therapy. Dalton Trans. 2011;40:6144–67.
10. Zalutsky MR, Zhao X-G, Alston KL, et al. High-level production of α-particle-emitting [211]At and preparation of [211]At-labeled antibodies for clinical use. J Nucl Med. 2001;42:1508–15.
11. Neves M, Kling A, Lambrecht RM. Radionuclide production for therapeutic radiopharmaceuticals. Appl Radiat Isotop. 2002;57:657–64.
12. IAEA-TRS No. 470. Therapeutic radionuclide generators: [90]Sr/^{90}Y AND [188]W/[188]Re generators. Vienna, 2009.
13. Van Dongen GAMS, Visser GWM, Lub-De Hoodge MN, et al. Immuno-PET: a navigator in monoclonal antibody development and applications. Oncologist. 2007;12:1379–89.
14. Boswell CA, Brechbiel MW. Development of radioimmunotherapeutic and diagnostic antibodies: an inside-out view. Nucl Med Biol. 2007;34:757–78.
15. Olafsen T, Wu AM. Antibody vectors for imaging. Semin Nucl Med. 2010;40:167–81.
16. Oyen WJG, Bodei L, Giammarile F, et al. Targeted therapy in nuclear medicine—current status and future prospects. Ann Oncol. 2007;18:782–92.
17. Köhler G, Milstein C. Continuous cultures of fused cells secreting antibody of predefined specificity. Nature. 1975;256:495–7.
18. Holliger P, Hudson PJ. Engineered antibody fragments and the rise of single domains. Nat Biotechnol. 2005;23:1126–36.
19. Holliger P, Winter G. Diabodies: small bispecific antibody fragments. Cancer Immunol Immunother. 1997;45:128–30.
20. Reubi JC, Schar JC, Waser B, et al. Affinity profiles for human somatostatin receptor subtypes SST1-SST5 of somatostatin radiotracers selected for scintigraphic and radiotherapeutic use. Eur J Nucl Med. 2000; 27:273–82.
21. Reubi JC. Peptide receptors as molecular targets for cancer diagnosis and therapy. Endocr Rev. 2000;24:389–427.
22. Reubi JC, Mäcke HR, Krenning EP. Candidates for peptide receptor radiotherapy today and in the future. J Nucl Med. 2005;46:67S–75.
23. Wieland DM, Wu J, Brown LE, et al. Radiolabeled adrenergic neuron-blocking agents: adrenomedullary imaging with [^{131}I]iodobenzylguanidine. J Nucl Med. 1980;21:349–53.

24. Kabalka GW, Mereddy AR. A facile no-carrier-added radioiodination procedure suitable for radiolabeling kits. Nucl Med Biol. 2004;31:935–8.
25. Eersels JLH, Travis MJ, Herscheid JDM. Manufacturing I-123-labelled radiopharmaceuticals: pitfalls and solutions. J Label Compd Radiopharm. 2005;48:241–57.
26. Greenwood FC, Hunter WM, Glover JS. The preparation of ^{131}I-labelled human growth hormone of high specific radioactivity. Biochem J. 1963;89:114–23.
27. Bolton AE, Hunter WM. The labeling of proteins to high specific radioactivities by conjugation to a ^{125}I containing acylating agent. Biochem J. 1973;133:529–38.
28. Mertens JJR, et al. Cu(I) supported isotopic exchange of arylbound iodide, new future for fast high yield labelling. In: Cox PH editor. Progress in radiopharmacy. The Hague, Nijhoff M. Publisher, Dordrecht, p. 101–9.
29. Vallabhajosula S, Nikolopoulou A. Radioiodinated metaiodobenzylguanidine (MIBG): radiochemistry, biology, and pharmacology. Semin Nucl Med. 2011;41:323–88.
30. Mangner JT, Wu J-L, Wieland DM. Solid-phase exchange radioiodination of aryl iodides: facilitation by ammonium sulfate. J Org Chem. 1982;47:1484–8.
31. Mangner JT, Anderson-Davis H, Wieland DM, et al. Synthesis of I-131 and I-123 metaiodobenzylguanidine for diagnosis and treatment of pheochromocytoma. J Nucl Med. 1983;24:p118.
32. Verbruggen RF. Fast high-yield labeling and quality control of [123I]- and [131I]MIBG. Appl Radiat Isot. 1987;38:303–4.
33. Prabhakar G, Mathur A, Shunmugam G, et al. Efficient production of therapeutic doses of ^{131}I-MIBG for clinical use. Appl Radiat Isot. 2011;69:63–7.
34. Vaidyanathan G, Zalutsky MR. No-carrier-added synthesis of meta-[131I]iodobenzylguanidine. Appl Radiat Isot. 1993;44:621–8.
35. Hunter GH, Zhu X. Polymer supported radiopharmaceuticals: ^{131}I-MIBG and ^{123}I-MIBG. J Label Compd Radiopharm. 1999;42:653–61.
36. Barrett JA, Joyal JL, Hillier SM, et al. Comparison of high-specific-activity Ultratrace[123/131]I-MIBG and carrier added [123/131]I-MIBG on efficacy, pharmacokinetics, and tissue distribution. Cancer Biother Radiopharm. 2010;25:299–308.
37. Press OW, Eary JF, Applebaum FR, et al. Radiolabeled-antibody therapy of B-cell lymphoma with autologous bone marrow transport. N Engl J Med. 1993;329:1219–24.
38. Kaminsky MS, Zasadny KR, Francis IR, et al. Radioimmunotherapy of B-cell lymphoma with [131I] anti- B1 anti (CD20) antibody. N Engl J Med. 1993;329:459–65.
39. Pozzi OR, Zalutsky MR. Radiopharmaceutical chemistry of targeted radiotherapeutics, part 2: radiolytic effects of 211At α-particles influence N-Succinimidyl 3-211At-Astatobenzoate synthesis. J Nucl Med. 2005;46:1393–400.
40. Pozzi OR, Zalutsky MR. Radiopharmaceutical chemistry of targeted radiotherapeutics, part 3: α-particle–induced radiolytic effects on the chemical behavior of 211At. J Nucl Med. 2007;48:1190–6.
41. Zalutsky MR, Vaidyanathan G. Astatine-211-labeled radiotherapeutics: an emerging approach to targeted alpha-particle radiotherapy. Curr Pharm Des. 2000;6:1433–55.
42. Meares CF, McCall MJ, Reardan DT, et al. Conjugation of antibodies with bifunctional chelating agents: isothiocyanate and bromoacetamido reagents, methods of analysis, and subsequent addition of metal ions. Anal Biochem. 1984;142:68–78.
43. Meares CF, Moi MK, Diril H, et al. Macrocyclic chelates of radiometals for diagnosis and therapy. Br J Cancer Suppl. 1990;10:21–6.
44. Brunner UK, Renn O. Radiometals and their chelates. In: Ki M, Wagner Jr HN, Szabo Z, Buchanan JW, et al., editors. Principles of nuclear medicine. Philadelphia: WB Saunders Company; 1995.
45. Weiner RE, Thakur ML. Chemistry of gallium and indium radiopharmaceuticals. In: Welch MJ, Redvanly CS, editors. Handbook of radiopharmaceuticals. West Sussex, England: Wiley; 2003.
46. Holland JP, Sheh Y, Lewis JS. Standardized methods for the production of high specific-activity zirconium-89. Nucl Med Biol. 2009;36:729–39.
47. Anderson CJ, Green MA, Fujibayashi Y. Chemistry of copper radionuclides and radiopharmaceutical products. In: Welch MJ, Redvanly CS, editors. Handbook of radiopharmaceuticals. West Sussex, England: Wiley; 2003.
48. Green MS, Welch MJ. Gallium radiopharmaceutical chemistry. Int J Rad Appl Instrum B. 1989;16:435–48.
49. Kukis DL, DeNardo SJ, DeNardo GL, et al. Optimized conditions for chelation of yttrium-90-DOTA immunoconjugates. J Nucl Med. 1998;39:2105–10.
50. Lewis MR, Kao JY, Anderson AL, et al. An improved method for conjugating monoclonal antibodies with N-hydroxysulfosuccinidyl DOTA. Bioconjug Chem. 2001;12:320–4.
51. Wilson AD, Brechbiel MW. Chelation chemistry. In: Speer TW, editor. Targeted radionuclide therapy. Philadelphia: Lippincott Williams & Wilkins; 2011. p. 88–107.
52. Brechbiel MW. Bifunctional chelates for metal nuclides. Q J Nucl Med Mol Imaging. 2008;52:166–73.
53. Pritchard JH, Ackerman M, Tubis M, et al. Indium-III-labeled antibody heavy metal chelate conjugates: a potential alternative to radioiodination. Proc Soc Exp Biol Med. 1976;151:297–302.
54. Krejcarek GE, Tucker KL. Covalent attachment of chelating groups to macromolecules. Biochem Biophys Res Commun. 1977;77:581–5.
55. Hnatowich DJ, Layne WW, Childs RL, et al. Radioactive labeling of antibody: a simple and efficient method. Science. 1983;220:613–5.

56. Nemoto H, Cai J, Yamamoto Y. A new synthetic method of all carboxylate-free DTPA derivatives and its application to the synthesis of Gd-carborane complex. Tetrahedron Lett. 1996;37:539–42.

57. ZEVALIN®, package insert. Irvine, CA: Spectrum Pharmaceuticals, Inc.; 2009.

58. Smith-Jones PM, Vallabhajosula S, Goldsmith SJ, et al. In vitro characterization of radiolabeled monoclonal antibodies specific for the extracellular domain of prostate-specific membrane antigen. Cancer Res. 2000;60:5237–43.

59. Vallabhajosula S, Kuji I, Hamacher KA, et al. Pharmacokinetics and biodistribution of ^{111}In- and ^{177}Lu-labeled J591 antibody specific for prostate-specific membrane antigen: prediction of ^{90}Y-J591 radiation dosimetry based on ^{111}In or ^{177}Lu? J Nucl Med. 2005;46:634–41.

60. Alberto R, Smith-Jones P, Soltz B, et al. Direct synthesis of [DOTA-DPhe^1]-octreotide and [DOTA-DPhe^1, Tyr^3]-octreotide (SMT487): two conjugates for systemic delivery of radiotherapeutical nuclides to somatostatin receptor positive tumors in man. J Pless Bioorg Med Chem Lett. 1998;8:1207–10.

61. Rufini V, Calcagni ML, Baum RP. Imaging of neuroendocrine tumors. Semin Nucl Med. 2006;36:228–47.

62. Reuter JK, Mattern R, Zhang L, et al. Synthesis and biological activities of sandostatin analogs containing stereochemical changes in positions 6 or 8. Biopolymers. 2000;53:497–505.

63. Ginj M, Schmitt JS, Chen J, et al. Design, synthesis and biological evaluation of somatostatin-based radiopeptides. Chem Biol. 2006;13:1081–90.

64. Kwekkeboom DJ, de Herder WW, Kam BL, et al. Treatment with the radiolabeled somatostatin analog [^{177}Lu-DOTA0,-Tyr^3]octreotate: toxicity, efficacy, and survival. J Clin Oncol. 2008;26:2124.

65. Breeman WAP, de Jong M, Visser TJ, et al. Optimising conditions for radiolabeling of DOTA-peptides with ^{90}Y, ^{111}In and ^{177}Lu at high specific activities. Eur J Nucl Med Mol Imaging. 2003;30:917–20.

66. Das T, Chakraborty S, Kallur KG, et al. Preparation of patient doses of ^{177}Lu-DOTA-TATE using indigenously produced ^{177}Lu: the Indian experience. Cancer Biother Radiopharm. 2011;26:395–400.

67. Blower PJ, Lewis JS, Zweit J. Copper radionuclides and radiopharmaceuticals in nuclear medicine. Nucl Med Biol. 1996;23:957–80.

68. Anderson CJ, Dehdashti F, Cutler PD, et al. Copper-64-TETA-octreotide as a PET imaging agent for patients with neuroendocrine tumors. J Nucl Med. 2001;42:213–21.

69. Bass LA, Wang M, Welch MJ, et al. In vivo transchelation of Copper-64 from TETA-octreotide to superoxide dismutase in rat liver. Bioconjugate Chem. 2000;11:527–32.

70. Boswell CA, Sun X, Niu W, et al. Comparative in vivo stability of copper-64 labeled cross-bridged and conventional tetraazamacrocyclic complexes. J Med Chem. 2004;47:1465–74.

71. Anderson CJ, Wadas TJ, Wong EH, et al. Cross-bridged macrocyclic chelators for stable complexation of copper radionuclides for PET imaging. Q J Nucl Med Mol Imaging. 2008;52:185–92.

72. Di Bartolo NM, Sargeson AM, Donlevy TM, et al. Synthesis of a new cage ligand, SarAr, and its complexation with selected transition metal ions for potential use in radioimaging. J Chem Soc Dalton Trans. 2001;15:2303–9.

73. Smith SV. Sarar technology for the application of copper-64 in biology and materials science. Q J Nucl Med Mol Imaging. 2007;51:1–10.

74. Alberto R, Schlibi R, Schubiger AP. First application of fac-[^{99m}Tc(OH$_2$)$_3$(CO)$_3$]$^+$ in bioorganometallic chemistry: design, structure, and in vitro affinity of a 5-HT$_{1A}$ receptor ligand labeled with ^{99m}Tc. J Am Chem Soc. 1999;121:6076–7.

75. Alberto R, Ortner K, Wheatley N, et al. Synthesis and properties of boranocarbonate: a convenient in situ CO source for the aqueous preparation of [^{99m}Tc(OH$_2$)$_3$(CO)$_3$]$^+$. J Am Chem Soc. 2001;123:3135–6.

76. Waibei R, Alberto R, Willude J, et al. Stable one-step technetium-99m labeling of His-tagged recombinant proteins with a novel Tc(I)-carbonyl complex. Nat Biotechnol. 1999;17:897–901.

77. Sharkey RM, Goldenberg DM. Perspectives on cancer therapy with radiolabeled monoclonal antibodies. J Nucl Med. 2005;46:115S–27.

Pretargeting: Advancing the Delivery of Radionuclides

20

Robert M. Sharkey and David M. Goldenberg

Introduction

The use of radiolabeled antibodies started in the late 1940s, when investigators radioiodinated ammonium-sulfate precipitated antiserum from animals immunized with different normal rodent tissues to determine if the immunoglobulins would localize selectively in these tissues in vivo [1–5]. They subsequently developed antisera to rodent tumors and showed the immunoglobulin fraction would localize selectively in the syngeneic tumor [6, 7]. In these first studies, they found immunoglobulins from tumor-immunized animals also bound to other normal tissues, suggesting that tumors shared cross-reactive antigen with other organs and that purifying the immunoglobulin fraction by immune absorption with normal tissues enhanced tumor binding [6]. They also developed the technique widely used today, paired radioiodine labels; e.g., tagging the specific immunoglobulin fraction with ^{131}I and an irrelevant immunoglobulin fraction with ^{125}I to show differential targeting specificity in vivo [8].

With radioiodine being used to treat thyroid cancer, it was clear that if a suitably specific immunoglobulin fraction to a human cancer could be developed, antibodies could carry the radionuclide to sites of tumor for therapeutic use [9]. By the mid-1960s, procedures for radioiodinating an immunoglobulin fraction for human use had been developed [10–12], and ^{131}I-labeled antibodies to human fibrin/fibrinogen would be examined in 50 patients with various tumors [13]. The scans were considered unremarkable, but tumors were said to be localized in 29 patients (58 %), with data showing slow, but improving tumor-to-heart ratios over 10 days. Uptake measured by scanning or by surgery was highly variable, averaging ~0.01 %.

Problems and Solutions

Looking back, this technology was investigated well before its time, using crudely prepared antibody fractions that were not sufficiently specific for cancer, immature imaging instrumentation, and questionable radionuclide purity. Better markers for human tumors, such as carcinoembryonic antigen (CEA), were just beginning to be identified in the mid-1960s [14], but it would take nearly 10 more years before affinity-purified polyclonal anti-CEA IgG labeled with ^{131}I would be tested in animals bearing human colon cancer xenografts and then later in humans [15–18]. Even in this maiden clinical study, investigators had to use computer-

R.M. Sharkey, Ph.D. (✉)
Center for Molecular Medicine and Immunology,
The Garden State Cancer Center, 300 The American
Road, Morris Plains, NJ 07950, USA
e-mail: rmsharkey@gscancer.org; dmg.gscancer@att.net

D.M. Goldenberg, Sc.D., M.D.
IBC Pharmaceuticals, Inc. and Immunomedics, Inc.,
Morris Plains, NJ, USA

Garden State Cancer Center, Center for Molecular
Medicine and Immunology, 300 The American Road,
Morris Plains, NJ, USA

C. Aktolun and S.J. Goldsmith (eds.), *Nuclear Medicine Therapy: Principles and Clinical Applications*,
DOI 10.1007/978-1-4614-4021-5_20, © Springer Science+Business Media New York 2013

ized-subtraction procedures to account for activity in the blood pool and interstitium to disclose selective uptake in sites of tumor. The difficulty in detecting tumors was not related to the antibody binding to normal tissues, but because IgG does what it is designed to do: it stays in the blood, giving it ample time to circulate, find, and bind to the target antigen. The problem with the slow clearance of the IgG was soon solved by enzymatically removing the Fc-portion of the IgG, with F(ab')$_2$ and monovalent Fab' fragments improving tumor/nontumor ratios more quickly [19–22]. With the advent of monoclonal antibodies, molecular engineering allowed investigators to dissect the antibody into its smallest binding fragment, the single chain Fv (scFv). Although reasonably good for imaging because of its rapid blood clearance and quick tumor localization, the monovalent binding of the scFv often resulted in low signal at the tumor that diminished within day. However, it was not long before a multitude of multivalent constructs were prepared and evaluated. Over the same period of time when different antibody structures were being developed, new discoveries in chelation chemistry greatly expanded the ability to bind isotopes of many different elements stably to proteins. No longer were investigators limited to radioiodine (almost exclusively ^{131}I), but a new age of coupling radionuclides with improved imaging and therapeutic properties had finally come, nearly 30 years from the first radiolabeled antibody targeting studies. While this new age brought fresh possibilities for antibody-targeted radionuclides, a new reality also set in; these other radionuclides (radiometals) faithfully remained associated with the antibody and became entrapped in the tissues where they were catabolized. Thus, high liver or kidney retention became a major problem for directly radiolabeled antibodies and their fragments.

It is ironic that the main difficulty with directly radiolabeled antibodies for therapy is derived from the fact that the radionuclide is tightly bound to protein. Because of this, the blood-rich, radiation-sensitive bone marrow is exposed for a protracted period, resulting in dose-limiting hematologic toxicity. As illustrated in Fig. 20.1a, directly radiolabeled IgG clears slowly from the blood and can take 1–3 days before reaching peak concentrations. During this time, the radionuclide attached to the antibody is undergoing decay, but most of this decay is occurring outside the tumor. The marrow is so sensitive that a directly radiolabeled IgG, which has the highest tumor uptake of all antibody forms, is unable to reach sufficient concentration (total dose) quickly enough (dose rate) to produce the desired therapeutic outcome, at least in solid tumors. Hematopoietic cancers are more radiosensitive, and therefore they do respond well in most instances to the targeted radiation.

In an effort to reduce red marrow exposure, various enzymatic or engineered modifications of the parent IgG that accelerate blood clearance have been examined. Unfortunately, a shorter residence time in the blood means they have less time to accrue in tumors as the native IgG. Thus, progres-

---

Fig. 20.1 Comparison of radionuclide targeting using a directly conjugated IgG or a bispecific antibody pretargeting procedure using a radiolabeled hapten-peptide. (**a**) With direct targeting, the radiolabeled IgG injected intravenously flows through the bloodstream, being slowly eliminated primarily in the liver. Tumor uptake also takes several days to reach peak levels, and often by this time tumor/blood ratios are just beginning to favor the tumor. The radiolabeled antibody stays in the tumor for a sustained period, while the levels in the blood gradual decrease. Antibodies are eventually eliminated from the tumors, and apart from physical decay, radioactivity from radiometal-labeled IgG's will accumulate over time, but radioiodinated antibodies, particularly if internalized, will expel the radioiodine, with decreasing concentrations of radioactivity over time. (**b**) With bsMAb pretargeting, the radionuclide dose is withheld until the unlabeled bsMAb has time to localize in the tumor and clear from the blood and tissues. With the DNL Tri-Fab bsMAb, at least 95 % is cleared from the blood within 1 day, allowing the radiolabeled hapten-peptide to be given without appreciable interaction with the bsMAb in the blood. The hapten-peptide is designed to have two haptens that increase binding avidity (AES, affinity enhancement system), as well as potentially cross-linking bsMAb bound to surface antigen. The hapten-peptide distributes very rapidly in the extravascular space, reaching maximum levels of binding to the pretargeting bsMAb in the tumor within 1 h. The remaining hapten-peptide clears from the blood and tissues just as quickly by urinary elimination. Thus, pretargeting rapidly deposits the radiation in the tumor and creates very high tumor/nontumor ratios much more quickly than a radiolabeled IgG

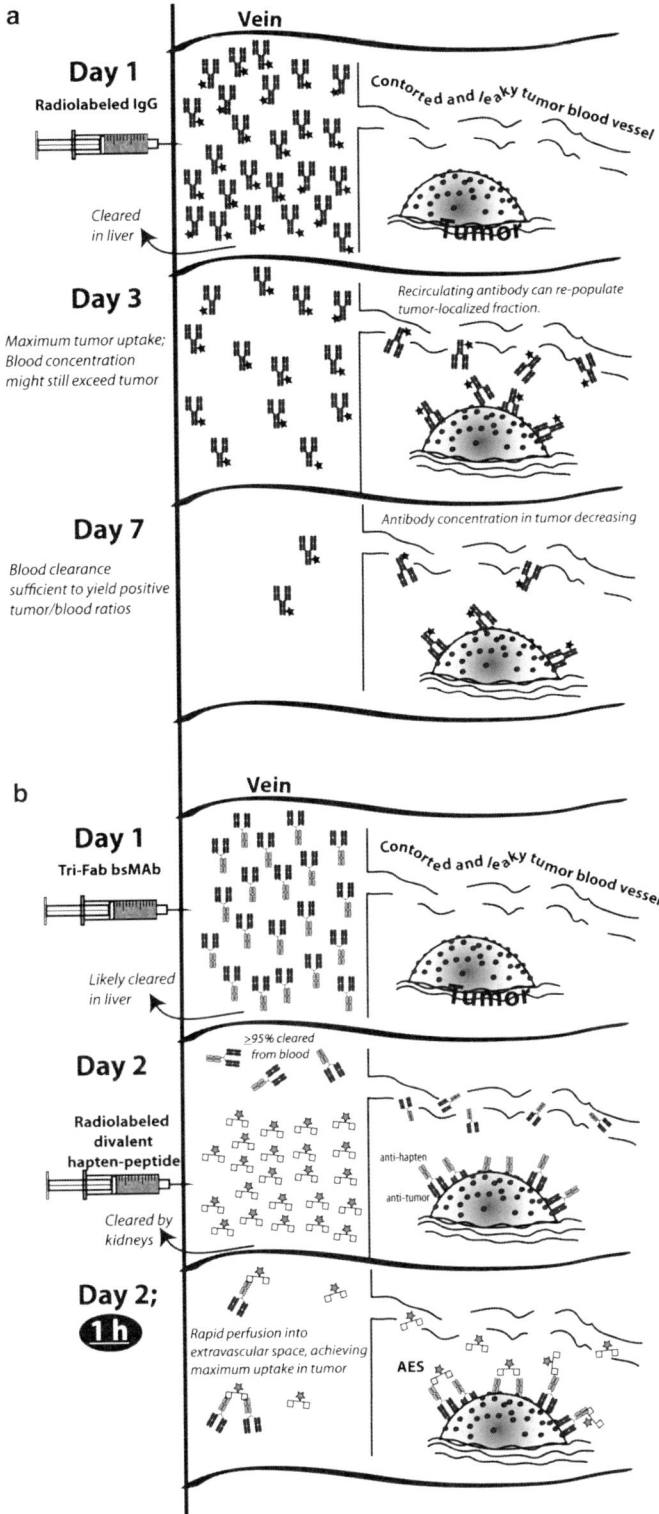

a

Vein

Day 1
Radiolabeled IgG

Contorted and leaky tumor blood vessel

Tumor

Cleared in liver

Day 3

Maximum tumor uptake;
Blood concentration
might still exceed tumor

Recirculating antibody can re-populate
tumor-localized fraction.

Day 7

Blood clearance
sufficient to yield positive
tumor/blood ratios

Antibody concentration in tumor decreasing

b

Vein

Day 1
Tri-Fab bsMAb

Contorted and leaky tumor blood vessel

Tumor

Likely cleared
in liver

Day 2

**Radiolabeled
divalent
hapten-peptide**

>95% cleared
from blood

anti-hapten

anti-tumor

Cleared by
kidneys

Day 2;
1 h

Rapid perfusion into
extravascular space, achieving
maximum uptake in tumor

AES

sively smaller and faster clearing fragments have lower tumor uptake, and monovalent fragments have shorter retention times than multivalent forms. However, smaller fragments have the advantage of localizing more quickly, thereby increasing the rate at which the radiation is delivered to the tumor, and are potentially more uniformly distributed than an IgG. From this perspective, it is not surprising that antibody fragments occasionally have been found in some preclinical studies to improve therapeutic responses compared to whole IgG [23–27]. Nevertheless, because the radionuclide is tightly bound to an antibody fragment, if the fragment is small enough to be cleared renally, the radioactivity from a radiometal-labeled fragment will be retained in the kidneys for extended periods, while the radioactivity from a radioiodinated form will be released over a short period of time (over several hours to 1 day). Renal uptake for these smaller, radiometal-labeled fragments is often very much higher than the uptake achieved in the tumor. While renal uptake can be tempered to some degree with the addition of various blocking agents, most of these procedures will reduce renal uptake by no more than twofold, which still puts the tumor at a disadvantage compared to the kidney [28, 29].

Thus, the tight bond between the radionuclide and the antibody causes high red marrow exposure and elevated uptake in the liver or the kidneys, depending on the size of the construct. Therefore, what is needed is a procedure that can minimize radiation exposure to normal tissue by rapidly clearing the IgG from the blood and body, but it would also need to provide reasonably high uptake and retention in the tumor. This just does not happen with a directly radiolabeled antibody, regardless of the form. However, one group of investigators took a different perspective, noting that chelated radiometals were cleared rapidly and efficiently from the body with minimal tissue retention. So how can these nontargeted agents be engineered to localize in tumors?

Pretargeting

They introduced a novel concept of developing a specialized antibody that had the ability to bind to the tumor as well as to the chelated

radiometal [30]. They had prepared antibodies to derivatives of the chelating agent EDTA (ethylenediaminetetraacetic acid), and over time, a procedure known as *pretargeting* was developed.

The premise of the pretargeting procedure in its simplest form was that a nonradiolabeled *bispecific antibody* (bsMAb) would be administered and given time to localize in the tumor and clear from the blood with no radiation exposure. Then, the chelated radiometal would be given. Figure 20.1b illustrates the bsMAb pretargeting procedure as compared to targeting with a directly radiolabeled IgG (Fig. 20.1a). Its small size allowed it to escape the vasculature quickly, whereupon entering the tumor's extravascular space, it would encounter the pretargeted bsMAb on the tumor cells and be captured by the antichelate binding arm. There it would be retained while the remaining chelated radiometal would clear rapidly from the body. Since the chelated radiometal had minimal retention in the kidneys, even renal uptake would be drastically reduced as compared to a radiometal-labeled antibody fragment.

Steps of the Pretargeting Procedure

- Administer a nonradiolabeled *bispecific antibody.*
- Wait for it to localize in the tumor and clear from the blood.
- Give the chelated radiometal.

Indeed, experiences with this and other types of pretargeting procedures have shown that most of the radiolabeled pretargeting agent, whether it is a hapten-peptide, biotin, or an oligomer, is cleared from the blood within a few hours, with very low whole-body retention [31, 32]. However, peak concentrations in the tumor are achieved within 1 h, and therefore most of the radionuclide's decay will occur in the tumor.

Hapten and Affinity Enhancement System

In addition to ensuring rapid clearance from the blood and body, a pretargeting system also must efficiently capture the radionuclide in the specific locations where the primary targeting agent is deposited. The original bsMAb pretargeting system used a chemically cross-linked anti-CEA Fab′ × antichelate Fab′ to bind the chelate-radiometal complex (the hapten), showing successful targeting of hepatic metastases in patients [33, 34]. This was a significant advance, since at this time, directly radiolabeled ^{111}In-anti-CEA antibodies showed similar lesions as photopenic areas, because more activity was deposited in the normal liver than in the tumor. However, in this first model system, antibody binding to the tumor and to the chelate (i.e., hapten) was monovalent. A group of French investigators improved the bsMAb pretargeting system, using two chelating groups tethered together with a short amino acid linker. This divalent hapten model became known as the *affinity enhancement system* (AES) (Fig. 20.1b), which enhanced uptake and retention of the radiolabeled hapten-peptide by increasing the avidity of the hapten-peptide [35, 36]. Indeed, the divalent hapten-peptide could potentially cross-link two bsMAb on the cell surface, creating a structure that was divalently bound to the tumor antigen. Using a bsMAb with a divalent hapten-peptide, tumor uptake was found to rival a directly radiolabeled F(ab′)$_2$ [37]. Hnatowich et al. [38] introduced another pretargeting system based on the ultra-high binding affinity of avidin/streptavidin for biotin. Two procedures based on this system were successfully developed for clinical use [31]. One of these reported that tumor uptake of radiolabeled biotin pretargeted with an antibody (NR-LU-10)-streptavidin conjugate was equal to that of the directly radiolabeled IgG [39, 40]. Thus, pretargeting systems minimized radiation exposure to normal tissues, while enjoying the benefit of high tumor uptake that could equal that of a directly radiolabeled F(ab′)$_2$ or even IgG.

Streptavidin-Biotin System

The NR-LU-10-streptavidin/^{90}Y-biotin pretargeting system was examined extensively, optimizing the amount of conjugate and labeled biotin as well as the use of a clearing agent to achieve excellent tumor localization in patients [41]. These studies revealed mild-to-moderate hematologic toxicity

at doses of up to 140 mCi/m^2 of ^{90}Y-biotin, but severe GI toxicity was encountered at doses higher than 100 mCi/m^2 [42]. As it turned out, the GI toxicity was not a secondary toxicity related to the pretargeting procedure in general, but instead was directly related to the binding of the NR-LU-10 antibody to the colon that then bound the ^{90}Y-biotin. NR-LU-10 eventually was shown to be specific for EpCam, also known as the 17.1a antigen. Fortunately, some of these advanced cancer patients enrolled in the Phase I studies survived long enough, and evidence for elevated serum creatinine levels was found, indicating that renal toxicity also was a dose-limiting concern. A Phase II trial was performed in advanced CRC patients, testing a fixed dose of 110 mCi of the ^{90}Y-biotin/m^2 [43]. Unfortunately, only two partial and four stable disease cases were found in the 25 patients treated. In the two patients where tumor dosimetry was determined, the procedure also did not appear to deliver substantially higher doses than that reported in many of the directly radiolabeled IgG trials. A newly engineered fusion protein composed of four scFv fragments of the CC49 humanized anti-TAG-72 antibody with streptavidin showed more promising results in a Phase I therapy setting in CRC [44]. Dosimetry data predicted that some lesions would have received ≥5,000 cGy if the administered ^{90}Y-biotin dose was adjusted so that the kidneys received 2,000 cGy (~200 mCi ^{90}Y-biotin), but patients were given only 10 mCi/m^2 of the ^{90}Y-biotin. This new construct was not fully evaluated, possibly because the streptavidin portion of the fusion protein was immunogenic.

Hapten-Peptide

Another pretargeting procedure using a chemically conjugated anti-CEA Fab′ × anti-DTPA Fab′ also was evaluated in patients with CEA-producing tumors, first examining biodistribution and tumor localization in CRC patients with an ^{111}In(In)-diDTPA-tyrosine-lysine hapten-peptide [45, 46], and then later with an ^{131}I-(In)DTPA-peptide for therapy. While this group performed a number of important preclinical studies in models of CRC [37, 47, 48], their preclinical and clinical efforts focused on the use of this pretargeting method for the treatment of medullary thyroid cancer (MTC) [49–56]. Initial studies in MTC found that CEA was highly expressed, providing an excellent target, and there was also a highly reliable and sensitive tumor marker, calcitonin [49, 56, 57]. While investigating the pretargeting procedure in patients with MTC and other CEA-producing cancers, they found MTC patients had a lower tolerance for the ^{131}I-hapten-peptide [58, 59]. Later studies offered a possible explanation; many patients with advanced MTC had bone and bone marrow involvement [60]. A retrospective analysis of their complete clinical experience in treating MTC with the pretargeting procedure revealed a subset of patients who had a more rapid doubling time of their serum calcitonin levels had a significantly improved survival [50]. They speculated that this group of patients likely deteriorated more quickly because of more active disease in the bone and bone marrow, and that the pretargeted therapy may have had a positive effect on the metastatic disease, leading to their improved survival.

bsMAb and Anti-HSG Hapten Antibody

Our group initially took an interest in pretargeting by examining a streptavidin conjugate of the hMN-14 anti-CEACAM5 (labetuzumab) antibody and ^{90}Y-biotin [61]. While the pretargeting procedure was successful [62], we were concerned that the immunogenicity of streptavidin would compromise its utility. We then collaborated with the French investigators who had been working with the anti-CEA bsMAb pretargeting procedure and found that it too could achieve rapid tumor localization, with evidence that it may have some therapeutic utility as well [63]. However, this initial evaluation focused on the prospects for using ^{188}Re, since the anti-DTPA bsMAb pretargeting could not be used with ^{90}Y. Indeed, this was a potential limitation for bsMAb pretargeting systems that relied on antichelate antibodies as the anti-hapten binding arm; the antibodies were too specific for the chelate-metal complex, and chelates also were often best used

with a restricted number of radiometals. We subsequently evaluated a second pretargeting system, first mentioned by LeDoussal et al. [35] and later examined by Janevik-Ivanovska et al. [64], that utilized an antibody to the hapten histamine-succinyl-glycine (HSG) [65]. Since this anti-HSG hapten antibody did not bind to the radionuclide or a radionuclide carrier, it opened the possibility to synthesize peptides containing two HSG moieties to maintain the principle of AES, but with any radionuclide-binding group. The lead hapten-peptide compound attached DOTA to a short peptide backbone, which was then used successfully with ^{111}In, ^{90}Y, and ^{177}Lu, as well as another compound with a group for binding ^{99m}Tc/^{188}Re [65]. A subsequent compound was synthesized to include a tyrosine residue as part of the peptide backbone, allowing it to be radioiodinated, but it also contained a DOTA moiety, allowing it to be radiolabeled with ^{111}In [66], and it was later used with ^{90}Y and ^{177}Lu for therapy, as well as ^{68}Ga for PET imaging [67–71]. The diversity of this pretargeting system also was expanded recently to include a novel way of radiolabeling peptides with an aluminum-^{18}fluoride complex [72–75]. Imaging studies using anti-CEA×anti-HSG bsMAbs in xenograft models have found pretargeting enhances detection sensitivity over directly radiolabeled Fab' [76] (Fig. 20.2) and even ^{18}F-FDG [77], but it is also more specific than ^{18}F-FDG because the targeting is dependent on the bsMAb that localizes to a tumor-expressed antigen rather than an enhanced metabolism [66, 74].

Bispecific antibodies can be humanized to reduce immunogenicity and engineered to have desirable pharmacokinetic or therapeutic properties [78–80]. For pretargeting, our early work with chemically conjugated bsMAb found an antitumor F(ab')$_2$×anti-hapten Fab' to be a preferred configuration, in part because its divalent binding to the tumor antigen provided higher tumor uptake than a Fab'×Fab' conjugate, but it cleared more quickly than an IgG×Fab' conjugate [81]. This led to the development of engineered bsMAbs that bound to the tumor antigen divalently, with monovalent binding to the hapten [82, 83]. Monovalent binding to the hapten

^{99m}Tc-anti-CEACAM5 Fab'

Anti-CEA bispecific antibody pretargeted ^{99m}Tc-hapten-peptide

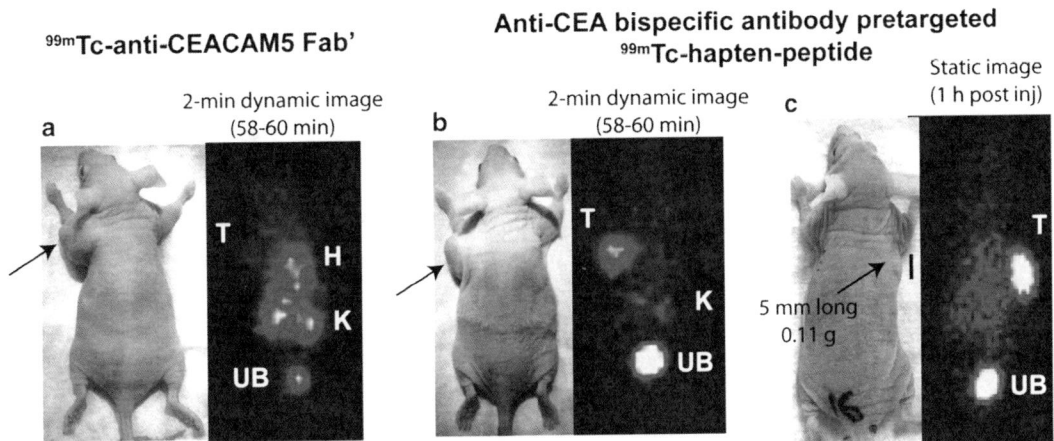

Fig. 20.2 Pretargeting improves tumor targeting even when compared to a rapidly clearing directly radiolabeled Fab' fragment. Nude mice bearing ~1.5 g human colon cancer xenografts were injected with ^{99m}Tc-Fab' (**a**) or an anti-CEA bsMAb followed 1 day later with a ^{99m}Tc-hapten-peptide (**b**). Immediately following the injection of the radiolabeled compound, dynamic imaging, using 2-min intervals over 60 min, was initiated to tract the kinetics of tumor localization for each procedure. The images shown in (**a**) and (**b**) were acquired in the last 2 min of the session.

Heart and kidney localization in the primary tissues showing localization with the ^{99m}Tc-anti-CEA Fab'; the tumor is barely seen. With pretargeting, majority of the background activity is cleared from the body into the urinary bladder, with faint uptake seen in the kidneys, but clear, intense uptake in the tumor. (**c**) A static image (20-min acquisition time) of a mouse pretargeted with the same anti-CEA bsMAb followed 1 day later with a ^{99m}Tc-hapten-peptide shows intense localization of a 0.11 g tumor, illustrating the sensitivity of tumor targeting with this method

minimizes the possibility for the formation of more stable complexes in the blood when the bsMAb comes in contact with a divalent hapten-peptide. However, as mentioned above, in the tumor microenvironment, where the bsMAb will be in higher concentration than the blood, the divalency of the hapten-peptide will encourage retention.

Our first generation hBS14 construct that targeted CEA provided excellent imaging qualities, as well as improved therapeutic results when compared to a ^{90}Y-labeled anti-CEA IgG [66, 84]. However, we then turned to another engineering platform called Dock-and-Lock (DNL) that tethered Fab fragments of antibodies in a manner that allowed divalent binding to the tumor antigen and monovalent binding to the hapten [85] (Fig. 20.3). Although these constructs were larger than the hBS14 (156 kDa vs. 80 kDa), they still cleared quickly from the blood, probably because they lack the Fc-portion of the immunoglobulin responsible for extended circulation half-lives. Thus, the DNL constructs provide rapid pretargeting

capabilities, and this modular format allows bsMAbs to a number of different tumor antigens to be prepared easily [67–69, 77, 86–88].

An anti-CEA bsMAb, TF2, prepared by the DNL method is currently being evaluated in combination with a ^{177}Lu-labeled hapten-peptide in advanced CRC [87]. This trial's first objective is to assess a series of different pretargeting conditions, varying the bsMAb dose, interval, and even the amount of hapten-peptide given. The treatment plan is designed for the patient to undergo an imaging study using a preplanned set of pretargeting conditions with the ^{111}In-labeled hapten-peptide. From this study, dosimetry predictions are made with respect to the amount of ^{177}Lu-hapten-peptide that could be administered, based on prescribed limits to the red marrow and kidneys. The estimated total ^{177}Lu-activity is divided into four equal fractions that would be given at 2–3-month intervals (preclinical studies have indicated that repeated injections of ^{177}Lu would be required for maximum therapeutic benefit [71, 89]). The first treatment is given ~1

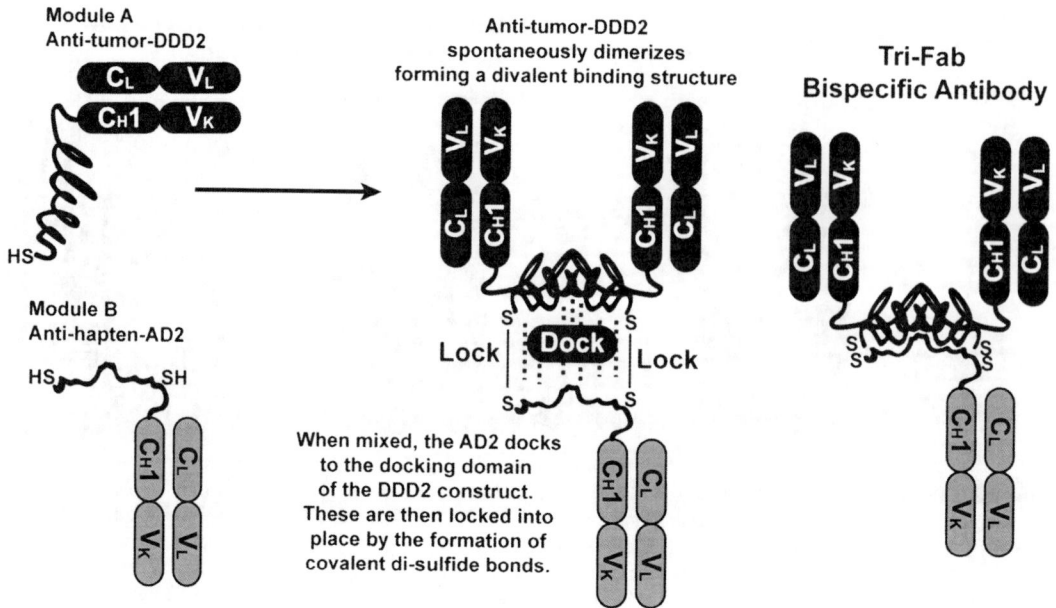

Fig. 20.3 Tri-Fab bsMAb prepared using the Dock-and-Lock (DNL) procedure. The DNL procedure as described by Rossi et al. [85] starts with two modules. The (A) module is a fusion protein between the antitumor Fd fragment and 44-amino acid sequence taken from the human regulatory II-alpha protein. The (B) module is the Fd fragment of the anti-hapten antibody fused to a 17-amino acid sequence taken from the anchoring domains of the A-kinase anchoring protein. Both of the amino acid sequences were modified by strategically placing cysteines in their sequence, so they

will be able to interact when the two modules are brought together. The antitumor-DDD2 module naturally forms homodimers as a consequence of the interaction between the regulatory II-alpha sequences. This then forms a docking domain that the A-kinase anchoring portion of the anti-hapten-AD2 module will bind. Once bound noncovalently, the interaction between the cysteine residues will covalently lock the two modules in place, forming the Tri-Fab bsMAb with divalent binding to the tumor antigen and monovalent binding to the hapten

week after completing the ^{111}In-hapten-peptide imaging study, with the patient receiving the same amount of bsMAb and hapten-peptide at the same interval as in the imaging study, but replacing the ^{111}In-hapten-peptide with the ^{177}Lu-hapten-peptide. The early results show promising targeting capability, but further adjustments to the pretargeting methods are still being evaluated. A second clinical trial in advanced CRC is also planned, which will evaluate the same pretargeting agents, but having the hapten-peptide radiolabeled with ^{90}Y. This trial will build on the experience of the first to select more optimal pretargeting conditions and will pursue a more traditional Phase I dose escalation plan examining the MTD for a single treatment.

Conclusion

Molecular engineering and other technologies allow antibody-based constructs to be designed in a number of configurations that will optimize their use in imaging or therapeutic applications. Rarely will one form be optimized for the both imaging *and* therapy. In therapeutic applications, some of these constructs limit the choice of radionuclide to ^{131}I.

Pretargeting procedures have the unique capacity of being ideally suited for imaging and therapeutic applications. By separating the radionuclide-targeting step, the radiolabeled agent is bound to a compound that rapidly leaves the vascular system, being able to equilibrate quickly in the extravascular volume, where it can bind to the pretargeted antibody-based agent, and then just as quickly be removed from the body. The rapid throughput of the radioactivity in the body, with selective retention in the tumor and minimal uptake in normal tissues, certainly seems to be an ideal way of delivering radionuclides. Using the HSG hapten-peptide system, any number of different ligands can be incorporated into a short peptide bearing two HSG haptens to ensure optimal binding and retention at the tumor site, while ensuring the ligand has optimal binding affinity for the radionuclide. The peptide core can also be modified if necessary to minimize tissue binding of the radiolabeled complex. Indeed, even with receptor-binding peptides, modifications to the peptide structure that might improve clearance could alter receptor binding, but with pretargeting, a bsMAb to the receptor paired with radiolabeled hapten-peptide could provide less background without sacrificing tumor binding. The HSG hapten-peptides can be radiolabeled at high specific activities, even with heating at 100 °C, and peptides are usually more amenable to purification than antibodies should the need arise.

Pretargeting is a multistep process, and therefore additional testing needs to be performed before suitable localization conditions are determined. The amount of bsMAb required to optimize the capture of the hapten-peptide and the interval between the bsMAb and hapten-peptide injections are the main issues for this mode of pretargeting. Preclinical studies have indicated that amount of bsMAb given does not have to saturate the antigen present in the tumor, but it should be enough to ensure efficient capture of the amount of hapten-peptide given [90]. Thus, the specific activity of the hapten-peptide will influence bsMAb dose selection. For therapy, considerably higher amounts of radioactivity will be tolerated than with an agent that clears more slowly, which raises special issues for dosimetry, similar to those found for targeted peptides [29, 91–93].

There is no question that pretargeting offers an exceptional imaging experience. If, as preclinical studies suggest, pretargeting can deliver the same amount of radioactivity to tumors as a directly radiolabeled IgG with significantly lower uptake in normal tissue, pretargeting may be poised to provide more than just an incremental improvement in radionuclide deliver that most of the newly designed direct conjugates appear to provide. Pretargeting also appears to be very amenable to combinations with other therapeutics, which may further enhance therapeutic prospects. Therefore, pretargeting technologies have the potential to open new opportunities in a wide number of applications.

References

1. Pressman D, Keighley G. The zone of activity of antibodies as determined by the use of radioactive tracers; the zone of activity of nephritoxic antikidney serum. J Immunol. 1948;59:141–6.
2. Pressman D. The zone of localization of antibodies; the specific localization of antibodies to rat kidney. Cancer. 1949;2:697–700.
3. Pressman D, Hill RF, Foote FW. The zone of localization of anti-mouse-kidney serum as determined by radioautographs. Science. 1949;109:65–6.
4. Pressman D. The zone of localization of antibodies; the in vivo disposition of anti-mouse-kidney serum and anti-mouse-plasma serum as determined by radioactive tracers. J Immunol. 1949;63:375–88.
5. Pressman D. The zone of localization of antitissue antibodies as determined by the use of radioactive tracers. J Allergy. 1951;22:387–96.
6. Pressman D, Korngold L. The in vivo localization of anti-Wagner-osteogenic-sarcoma antibodies. Cancer. 1953;6:619–23.
7. Day ED, Korngold L, Planinsek J, Pressman D. Tumor-localizing antibodies purified from antisera against Murphy rat lymphosarcoma. J Natl Cancer Inst. 1956;17:517–32.
8. Pressman D, Day ED, Blau M. The use of paired labeling in the determination of tumor-localizing antibodies. Cancer Res. 1957;17:845–50.
9. Bale WF, Spar IL. Studies directed toward the use of antibodies as carriers of radioactivity for therapy. Adv Biol Med Phys. 1957;5:285–356.
10. Spar IL, Bale WF, Goodland RL, Izzo MJ. Preparation of purified I-131-labeled antibody which reacts with human fibrin. Preliminary tracer studies on tumor patients. Cancer Res. 1964;24:286–93.
11. Balewf SIL. Fibrinogen and antibodies to fibrin as carrier of 131-I for cancer therapy. Nucl Med (Stuttg). 1965;2:323–35.
12. Bale WF, Helmkamp RW, Davis TP, Izzo MJ, Goodland RL, Contreras MA, et al. High specific activity labeling of protein with I-131 by the iodine

monochloride method. Proc Soc Exp Biol Med. 1966;122:407–14.

13. McCardle RJ, Harper PV, Spar IL, Bale WF, Andros G, Jiminez F. Studies with iodine-131-labeled antibody to human fibrinogen for diagnosis and therapy of tumors. J Nucl Med. 1966;7:837–47.

14. Gold P, Freedman SO. Specific carcinoembryonic antigens of the human digestive system. J Exp Med. 1965;122:467–81.

15. Primus FJ, Wang RH, Goldenberg DM, Hansen HJ. Localization of human GW-39 tumors in hamsters by radiolabeled heterospecific antibody to carcinoembryonic antigen. Cancer Res. 1973;33:2977–82.

16. Goldenberg DM, Preston DF, Primus FJ, Hansen HJ. Photoscan localization of GW-39 tumors in hamsters using radiolabeled anticarcinoembryonic antigen immunoglobulin G. Cancer Res. 1974;34:1–9.

17. Primus FJ, Macdonald R, Goldenberg DM, Hansen HJ. Localization of GW-39 human tumors in hamsters by affinity-purified antibody to carcinoembryonic antigen. Cancer Res. 1977;37:1544–7.

18. Goldenberg DM, DeLand F, Kim E, Bennett S, Primus FJ, van Nagell Jr JR, et al. Use of radiolabeled antibodies to carcinoembryonic antigen for the detection and localization of diverse cancers by external photoscanning. N Engl J Med. 1978;298:1384–6.

19. Mach JP, Forni M, Ritschard J, Buchegger F, Carrel S, Widgren S, et al. Use of limitations of radiolabeled anti-CEA antibodies and their fragments for photoscanning detection of human colorectal carcinomas. Oncodev Biol Med. 1980;1:49–69.

20. Wahl RL, Parker CW, Philpott GW. Improved radioimaging and tumor localization with monoclonal F(ab')$_2$. J Nucl Med. 1983;24:316–25.

21. Larson SM, Carrasquillo JA, McGuffin RW, Krohn KA, Ferens JM, Hill LD, et al. Use of I-131 labeled, murine Fab against a high molecular weight antigen of human melanoma: preliminary experience. Radiology. 1985;155:487–92.

22. Herlyn D, Powe J, Munz DL, Alavi A, Herlyn M, Meinken GE, et al. Radioimmunodetection of human tumor xenografts by monoclonal antibody F(ab')2 fragments. Int J Rad Appl Instrum B. 1986;13:401–5.

23. Blumenthal RD, Sharkey RM, Kashi R, Goldenberg DM. Comparison of therapeutic efficacy and host toxicity of two different ^{131}I-labelled antibodies and their fragments in the GW-39 colonic cancer xenograft model. Int J Cancer. 1989;44:292–300.

24. Buchegger F, Pfister C, Fournier K, Prevel F, Schreyer M, Carrel S, et al. Ablation of human colon carcinoma in nude mice by ^{131}I-labeled monoclonal anti-carcinoembryonic antigen antibody F(ab')$_2$ fragments. J Clin Invest. 1989;83:1449–56.

25. Buchegger F, Pelegrin A, Delaloye B, Bischof-Delaloye A, Mach JP. Iodine-131-labeled MAb F(ab')$_2$ fragments are more efficient and less toxic than intact anti-CEA antibodies in radioimmunotherapy of large human colon carcinoma grafted in nude mice. J Nucl Med. 1990;31:1035–44.

26. Behr TM, Memtsoudis S, Sharkey RM, Blumenthal RD, Dunn RM, Gratz S, et al. Experimental studies on the role of antibody fragments in cancer radio-immunotherapy: influence of radiation dose and dose rate on toxicity and anti-tumor efficacy. Int J Cancer. 1998;77:787–95.

27. Behr TM, Blumenthal RD, Memtsoudis S, Sharkey RM, Gratz S, Becker W, et al. Cure of metastatic human colonic cancer in mice with radiolabeled monoclonal antibody fragments. Clin Cancer Res. 2000;6:4900–7.

28. Behr TM, Goldenberg DM, Becker W. Reducing the renal uptake of radiolabeled antibody fragments and peptides for diagnosis and therapy: present status, future prospects and limitations. Eur J Nucl Med. 1998;25:201–12.

29. Vegt E, de Jong M, Wetzels JF, Masereeuw R, Melis M, Oyen WJ, et al. Renal toxicity of radiolabeled peptides and antibody fragments: mechanisms, impact on radionuclide therapy, and strategies for prevention. J Nucl Med. 2010;51:1049–58.

30. Reardan DT, Meares CF, Goodwin DA, McTigue M, David GS, Stone MR, et al. Antibodies against metal chelates. Nature. 1985;316:265–8.

31. Goldenberg DM, Sharkey RM, Paganelli G, Barbet J, Chatal JF. Antibody pretargeting advances cancer radioimmunodetection and radioimmunotherapy. J Clin Oncol. 2006;24:823–34.

32. Meredith RF, Buchsbaum DJ. Pretargeted radioimmunotherapy. Int J Radiat Oncol Biol Phys. 2006;66:S57–9.

33. Stickney DR, Slater JB, Kirk GA, Ahlem CN, Chang CH, Frincke JM. Bifunctional antibody: ZCE/CHA [111]indium-BLEDTA-IV clinical imaging in colorectal carcinoma. Antibody Immunoconjug Radiopharm. 1989;2:1–13.

34. Stickney DR, Anderson LD, Slater JB, Ahlem CN, Kirk GA, Schweighardt SA, et al. Bifunctional antibody: a binary radiopharmaceutical delivery system for imaging colorectal carcinoma. Cancer Res. 1991;51:6650–5.

35. Le Doussal JM, Martin M, Gautherot E, Delaage M, Barbet J. In vitro and in vivo targeting of radiolabeled monovalent and divalent haptens with dual specificity monoclonal antibody conjugates: enhanced divalent hapten affinity for cell-bound antibody conjugate. J Nucl Med. 1989;30:1358–66.

36. Boerman OC, Kranenborg MH, Oosterwijk E, Griffiths GL, McBride WJ, Oyen WJ, et al. Pretargeting of renal cell carcinoma: improved tumor targeting with a bivalent chelate. Cancer Res. 1999;59:4400–5.

37. Gautherot E, Rouvier E, Daniel L, Loucif E, Bouhou J, Manetti C, et al. Pretargeted radioimmunotherapy of human colorectal xenografts with bispecific antibody and ^{131}I-labeled bivalent hapten. J Nucl Med. 2000;41:480–7.

38. Hnatowich DJ, Virzi F, Rusckowski M. Investigations of avidin and biotin for imaging applications. J Nucl Med. 1987;28:1294–302.

39. Axworthy DB, Fritzberg AR, Hylarides MD, Mallet RW, Theodore LJ, Gustavson LM, et al. Preclinical

evaulation of an anti-tumor monoclonal antibody/streptavidin conjugate for pretargeted ^{90}Y radioimmunotherapy in a mouse xenograft model. J Immunother. 1994;16:158.

40. Axworthy DB, Reno JM, Hylarides MD, Mallett RW, Theodore LJ, Gustavson LM, et al. Cure of human carcinoma xenografts by a single dose of pretargeted yttrium-90 with negligible toxicity. Proc Natl Acad Sci U S A. 2000;97:1802–7.

41. Breitz HB, Weiden PL, Beaumier PL, Axworthy DB, Seiler C, Su FM, et al. Clinical optimization of pretargeted radioimmunotherapy with antibody-streptavidin conjugate and ^{90}Y-DOTA-biotin. J Nucl Med. 2000;41:131–40.

42. Breitz HB, Fisher DR, Goris ML, Knox SJ, Ratliff B, Murtha AD, et al. Radiation absorbed dose estimation for ^{90}Y-DOTA-biotin with pretargeted NR-LU-10/streptavidin. Cancer Biother Radiopharm. 1999;14: 381–95.

43. Knox SJ, Goris ML, Tempero M, Weiden PL, Gentner L, Breitz H, et al. Phase II trial of yttrium-90-DOTA-biotin pretargeted by NR-LU-10 antibody/streptavidin in patients with metastatic colon cancer. Clin Cancer Res. 2000;6:406–14.

44. Shen S, Forero A, LoBuglio AF, Breitz H, Khazaeli MB, Fisher DR, et al. Patient-specific dosimetry of pretargeted radioimmunotherapy using CC49 fusion protein in patients with gastrointestinal malignancies. J Nucl Med. 2005;46:642–51.

45. Le Doussal JM, Chetanneau A, Gruaz-Guyon A, Martin M, Gautherot E, Lehur PA, et al. Bispecific monoclonal antibody-mediated targeting of an indium-111-labeled DTPA dimer to primary colorectal tumors: pharmacokinetics, biodistribution, scintigraphy and immune response. J Nucl Med. 1993;34: 1662–71.

46. Chetanneau A, Barbet J, Peltier P, Le Doussal JM, Gruaz-Guyon A, Bernard AM, et al. Pretargetted imaging of colorectal cancer recurrences using an ^{111}In-labelled bivalent hapten and a bispecific antibody conjugate. Nucl Med Commun. 1994;15: 972–80.

47. Gautherot E, Bouhou J, Le Doussal JM, Manetti C, Martin M, Rouvier E, et al. Therapy for colon carcinoma xenografts with bispecific antibody-targeted, iodine-131-labeled bivalent hapten. Cancer. 1997;80:2618–23.

48. Gautherot E, Le Doussal JM, Bouhou J, Manetti C, Martin M, Rouvier E, et al. Delivery of therapeutic doses of radioiodine using bispecific antibody-targeted bivalent haptens. J Nucl Med. 1998;39: 1937–43.

49. Barbet J, Peltier P, Bardet S, Vuillez JP, Bachelot I, Denet S, et al. Radioimmunodetection of medullary thyroid carcinoma using indium-111 bivalent hapten and anti-CEA x anti-DTPA-indium bispecific antibody. J Nucl Med. 1998;39:1172–8.

50. Chatal JF, Campion L, Kraeber-Bodere F, Bardet S, Vuillez JP, Charbonnel B, et al. Survival improvement

in patients with medullary thyroid carcinoma who undergo pretargeted anti-carcinoembryonic-antigen radioimmunotherapy: a collaborative study with the French Endocrine Tumor Group. J Clin Oncol. 2006;24:1705–11.

51. Hosono M, Hosono MN, Kraeber-Bodere F, Devys A, Thedrez P, Fiche M, et al. Biodistribution and dosimetric study in medullary thyroid cancer xenograft using bispecific antibody and iodine-125-labeled bivalent hapten. J Nucl Med. 1998;39:1608–13.

52. Kraeber-Bodere F, Bardet S, Hoefnagel CA, Vieira MR, Vuillez JP, Murat A, et al. Radioimmunotherapy in medullary thyroid cancer using bispecific antibody and iodine 131-labeled bivalent hapten: preliminary results of a phase I/II clinical trial. Clin Cancer Res. 1999;5:3190s–8.

53. Kraeber-Bodere F, Faibre-Chauvet A, Sai-Maurel C, Gautherot E, Fiche M, Campion L, et al. Bispecific antibody and bivalent hapten radioimmunotherapy in CEA-producing medullary thyroid cancer xenograft. J Nucl Med. 1999;40:198–204.

54. Kraeber-Bodere F, Sai-Maurel C, Campion L, Faivre-Chauvet A, Mirallie E, Cherel M, et al. Enhanced antitumor activity of combined pretargeted radioimmunotherapy and paclitaxel in medullary thyroid cancer xenograft. Mol Cancer Ther. 2002;1:267–14.

55. Kraeber-Bodere F, Salaun PY, Oudoux A, Goldenberg DM, Chatal JF, Barbet J. Pretargeted radioimmunotherapy in rapidly progressing, metastatic, medullary thyroid cancer. Cancer. 2010;116:1118–25.

56. Rouvier E, Gautherot E, Meyer P, Barbet J. Targeting medullary thyroid carcinomas with bispecific antibodies and bivalent haptens. Results and clinical perspectives. Hormone Res. 1997;47:163–7.

57. Barbet J, Campion L, Kraeber-Bodere F, Chatal JF. Prognostic impact of serum calcitonin and carcinoembryonic antigen doubling-times in patients with medullary thyroid carcinoma. J Clin Endocrinol Metab. 2005;90:6077–84.

58. Kraeber-Bodere F, Rousseau C, Bodet-Milin C, Ferrer L, Faivre-Chauvet A, Campion L, et al. Targeting, toxicity, and efficacy of 2-step, pretargeted radioimmunotherapy using a chimeric bispecific antibody and ^{131}I-labeled bivalent hapten in a phase I optimization clinical trial. J Nucl Med. 2006;47:247–55.

59. Kraeber-Bodere F, Faivre-Chauvet A, Ferrer L, Vuillez JP, Brard PY, Rousseau C, et al. Pharmacokinetics and dosimetry studies for optimization of anti-carcinoembryonic antigen x anti-hapten bispecific antibody-mediated pretargeting of Iodine-131-labeled hapten in a phase I radioimmunotherapy trial. Clin Cancer Res. 2003;9:3973S–81.

60. Mirallie E, Vuillez JP, Bardet S, Frampas E, Dupas B, Ferrer L, et al. High frequency of bone/bone marrow involvement in advanced medullary thyroid cancer. J Clin Endocrinol Metab. 2005;90:779–88.

61. Karacay H, Sharkey RM, Govindan SV, McBride WJ, Goldenberg DM, Hansen HJ, et al. Development of a streptavidin-anti-carcinoembryonic antigen antibody,

radiolabeled biotin pretargeting method for radioim-munotherapy of colorectal cancer. Reagent develop-ment. Bioconjug Chem. 1997;8:585–94.

62. Sharkey RM, Karacay H, Griffiths GL, Behr TM, Blumenthal RD, Mattes MJ, et al. Development of a streptavidin-anti-carcinoembryonic antigen antibody, radiolabeled biotin pretargeting method for radioim-munotherapy of colorectal cancer. Studies in a human colon cancer xenograft model. Bioconjug Chem. 1997;8:595–604.

63. Karacay H, McBride WJ, Griffiths GL, Sharkey RM, Barbet J, Hansen HJ, et al. Experimental pretargeting studies of cancer with a humanized anti-CEA x murine anti-[In-DTPA] bispecific antibody construct and a ^{99m}Tc-/^{188}Re-labeled peptide. Bioconjug Chem. 2000; 11:842–54.

64. Janevik-Ivanovska E, Gautherot E, Hillairet de Boisferon M, Cohen M, Milhaud G, Tartar A, et al. Bivalent hapten-bearing peptides designed for iodine-131 pretargeted radioimmunotherapy. Bioconjug Chem. 1997;8:526–33.

65. Sharkey RM, McBride WJ, Karacay H, Chang K, Griffiths GL, Hansen HJ, et al. A universal pretarget-ing system for cancer detection and therapy using bispecific antibody. Cancer Res. 2003;63:354–63.

66. McBride WJ, Zanzonico P, Sharkey RM, Noren C, Karacay H, Rossi EA, et al. Bispecific antibody pre-targeting PET (immunoPET) with an ^{124}I-labeled hapten-peptide. J Nucl Med. 2006;47:1678–88.

67. Sharkey RM, Karacay H, Litwin S, Rossi EA, McBride WJ, Chang CH, et al. Improved therapeutic results by pretargeted radioimmunotherapy of non-Hodgkin's lymphoma with a new recombinant, triva-lent, anti-CD20, bispecific antibody. Cancer Res. 2008;68:5282–90.

68. Sharkey RM, Karacay H, Johnson CR, Litwin S, Rossi EA, McBride WJ, et al. Pretargeted versus directly targeted radioimmunotherapy combined with anti-CD20 antibody consolidation therapy of non-Hodgkin lymphoma. J Nucl Med. 2009;50:444–53.

69. Karacay H, Sharkey RM, Gold DV, Ragland DR, McBride WJ, Rossi EA, et al. Pretargeted radioimmu-notherapy of pancreatic cancer xenografts: TF10-^{90}Y-IMP-288 alone and combined with gemcitabine. J Nucl Med. 2009;50:2008–16.

70. Karacay H, Sharkey RM, McBride WJ, Rossi EA, Chang CH, Goldenberg DM. Optimization of hapten-peptide labeling for pretargeted immunoPET of bispecific antibody using generator-produced 68Ga. J Nucl Med. 2011;52:555–9.

71. Schoffelen R, van der Graaf WT, Franssen G, Sharkey RM, Goldenberg DM, McBride WJ, et al. Pretargeted ^{177}Lu radioimmunotherapy of carcinoembryonic anti-gen-expressing human colonic tumors in mice. J Nucl Med. 2010;51:1780–7.

72. McBride WJ, Sharkey RM, Karacay H, D'Souza CA, Rossi EA, Laverman P, et al. A novel method of ^{18}F radiolabeling for PET. J Nucl Med. 2009;50:991–8.

73. McBride WJ, D'Souza CA, Sharkey RM, Karacay H, Rossi EA, Chang CH, et al. Improved ^{18}F labeling of peptides with a fluoride-aluminum-chelate complex. Bioconjug Chem. 2010;21:1331–40.

74. Schoffelen R, Sharkey RM, Goldenberg DM, Franssen G, McBride WJ, Rossi EA, et al. Pretargeted immuno-positron emission tomography imaging of carcinoem-bryonic antigen-expressing tumors with a bispecific antibody and a ^{68}Ga- and ^{18}F-labeled hapten peptide in mice with human tumor xenografts. Mol Cancer Ther. 2010;9:1019–27.

75. D'Souza CA, McBride WJ, Sharkey RM, Todaro LJ, Goldenberg DM. High-yielding aqueous ^{18}F-labeling of peptides via Al18F chelation. Bioconjug Chem. 2011;22:1793–803.

76. Sharkey RM, Cardillo TM, Rossi EA, Chang CH, Karacay H, McBride WJ, et al. Signal amplification in molecular imaging by pretargeting a multivalent, bispecific antibody. Nat Med. 2005;11:1250–5.

77. Sharkey RM, Karacay H, Vallabhajosula S, McBride WJ, Rossi EA, Chang CH, et al. Metastatic human colonic carcinoma: molecular imaging with pretar-geted SPECT and PET in a mouse model. Radiology. 2008;246:497–507.

78. Chames P, Baty D. Bispecific antibodies for cancer therapy: the light at the end of the tunnel? MAbs. 2009;1:539–47.

79. Muller D, Kontermann RE. Bispecific antibodies for cancer immunotherapy: current perspectives. BioDrugs. 2010;24:89–98.

80. Thakur A, Lum LG. Cancer therapy with bispecific antibodies: clinical experience. Curr Opin Mol Ther. 2010;12:340–9.

81. Karacay H, Sharkey RM, McBride WJ, Griffiths GL, Qu Z, Chang K, et al. Pretargeting for cancer radioim-munotherapy with bispecific antibodies: role of the bispecific antibody's valency for the tumor target anti-gen. Bioconjug Chem. 2002;13:1054–70.

82. Rossi EA, Chang CH, Losman MJ, Sharkey RM, Karacay H, McBride W, et al. Pretargeting of carcino-embryonic antigen-expressing cancers with a trivalent bispecific fusion protein produced in myeloma cells. Clin Cancer Res. 2005;11:7122s–9.

83. Rossi EA, Sharkey RM, McBride W, Karacay H, Zeng L, Hansen HJ, et al. Development of new multivalent-bispecific agents for pretargeting tumor localization and therapy. Clin Cancer Res. 2003;9: 3886S–96.

84. Karacay H, Brard PY, Sharkey RM, Chang CH, Rossi EA, McBride WJ, et al. Therapeutic advantage of pre-targeted radioimmunotherapy using a recombinant bispecific antibody in a human colon cancer xeno-graft. Clin Cancer Res. 2005;11:7879–85.

85. Rossi EA, Goldenberg DM, Cardillo TM, McBride WJ, Sharkey RM, Chang CH. Stably tethered multi-functional structures of defined composition made by the dock and lock method for use in cancer targeting. Proc Natl Acad Sci U S A. 2006;103:6841–6.

86. Gold DV, Goldenberg DM, Karacay H, Rossi EA, Chang CH, Cardillo TM, et al. A novel bispecific, trivalent antibody construct for targeting pancreatic carcinoma. Cancer Res. 2008;68:4819–26.

87. Sharkey RM, Rossi EA, McBride WJ, Chang CH, Goldenberg DM. Recombinant bispecific monoclonal antibodies prepared by the dock-and-lock strategy for pretargeted radioimmunotherapy. Semin Nucl Med. 2010;40:190–203.

88. Karacay H, Sharkey R, Rossi E, McBride B, Chang C-H, Goldenberg D. A new tri-Fab recombinant bispecific antibody (bsMAb) for pretargeting epithelial cancers: studies with TF12 and ^{111}In-labeled hapten-peptide (IMP 288) in ovarian cancer. J Nucl Med. 2010;51:Abst 1148.

89. Frampas E, Maurel C, Remaud-Le Saec P, Mauxion T, Faivre-Chauvet A, Davodeau F, et al. Pretargeted radioimmunotherapy of colorectal cancer metastases: models and pharmacokinetics predict influence of the physical and radiochemical properties of the radionuclide. Eur J Nucl Med Mol Imaging. 2011;38(12):2153–64.

90. Sharkey RM, Karacay H, Richel H, McBride WJ, Rossi EA, Chang K, et al. Optimizing bispecific antibody pretargeting for use in radioimmunotherapy. Clin Cancer Res. 2003;9:3897S–913.

91. Barone R, Borson-Chazot F, Valkema R, Walrand S, Chauvin F, Gogou L, et al. Patient-specific dosimetry in predicting renal toxicity with (90)Y-DOTATOC: relevance of kidney volume and dose rate in finding a dose-effect relationship. J Nucl Med. 2005;46 Suppl 1:99S–106.

92. Cremonesi M, Ferrari M, Bodei L, Tosi G, Paganelli G. Dosimetry in peptide radionuclide receptor therapy: a review. J Nucl Med. 2006;47:1467–75.

93. Siegel JA, Stabin MG, Sharkey RM. Renal dosimetry in peptide radionuclide receptor therapy. Cancer Biother Radiopharm. 2010;25:581–8.

Radiobiology as Applied to Radionuclide Therapy with an Emphasis on Low Dose Rate Radiation Effects

David Murray, Razmik Mirzayans, and Alexander J. McEwan

Introduction

The last 20 years has seen an explosive growth in our understanding of the molecular underpinnings of the response of human cells and tissues to ionizing radiation (IR) and the application of this information to the treatment of cancer. For reasons such as ease of data interpretation and relevance to conventional external-beam radiotherapy (XRT) for cancer, much of this understanding has been derived from studies of single or fractionated doses of X-rays or γ-rays in the 1–10 Gy dose range, typically delivered at a relatively high dose rate (HDR) on the order of 1 Gy/min. How realistically do such studies inform us of the biological basis of systemic radionuclide therapy (SRT) when the dose is delivered via the decay of a radiopharmaceutical at a low dose rate (LDR) over a protracted period of time? The sense that there may be some issues in extrapolating these earlier radiobiological principles to SRT derives in part from a number of recent observations that are not easily explained by conventional thinking. First are the unexpectedly good tumor responses to SRT that have sometimes been reported in the clinical literature. Second are a number of new questions that are raised by laboratory studies using LDR exposures, including whether phenomena such as bystander effects and inverse dose-rate effects contribute to the efficacy of SRT.

D. Murray (✉)
Department of Oncology, Division of Experimental Oncology, Cross Cancer Institute, School of Cancer, Engineering and Imaging Sciences, University of Alberta, 11560 University Avenue, Edmonton, ABT6G 1Z2, Canada
e-mail: David.Murray5@albertahealthservices.ca

R. Mirzayans
Department of Oncology, Division of Experimental Oncology, School of Cancer, Engineering and Imaging Sciences, University of Alberta, 11560 University Avenue, Edmonton, ABT6G 1Z2, Canada
e-mail: Razmik.Mirzayans@albertahealthservices.ca

A.J. McEwan
Division of Oncologic Imaging, Department of Oncology, School of Cancer, Engineering and Imaging Sciences, University of Alberta, 11560, University Avenue, Edmonton, ABT6G 1Z2, Canada
e-mail: mcewan@ualberta.ca

External Beam Versus Systemic Radiation Therapy

There are important similarities and yet major differences in the scientific and clinical features of SRT and XRT. Modern XRT techniques involve the image-guided localized delivery of IR from a sophisticated computer-controlled external device such as a linear accelerator. The intent is usually to deliver a relatively homogeneous high dose to the tumor while minimizing the dose to critical normal structures in the radiation field. This is achieved by precise physical control of the direction and intensity of the radiation beam which in turn depends on accurate imaging of the tumor. The dose is delivered at HDR, in the

C. Aktolun and S.J. Goldsmith (eds.), *Nuclear Medicine Therapy: Principles and Clinical Applications*,
DOI 10.1007/978-1-4614-4021-5_21, © Springer Science+Business Media New York 2013

general range of 1–5 Gy/min, and typically involves giving daily fractions of ~2 Gy five times a week for 6–8 weeks, such that the total dose to the tumor will be in the range of 60–70 Gy. The classical radiobiological principles that influence cell and tissue responses to fractionated IR exposures and that guide clinical practice in XRT are embodied in the "4 Rs of Radiotherapy": these are Repair, Redistribution, Regeneration (or Repopulation), and Reoxygenation [1]. The same principles are important in SRT, although not always to the same degree, as will become apparent.

In contrast to XRT, SRT involves the systemic delivery of different types of radioactive isotopes to the tumor utilizing unsealed source/radionuclides or targeted approaches such as the use of metabolic precursors, ligands, and peptides. An example of a radiopharmaceutical used to treat solid tumors is ^{131}I-meta-iodobenzylguanidine (^{131}I-mIBG); it is a physiological analog of noradrenaline which is taken up by cells of neuroectodermal origin via the noradrenaline transporter (NAT) and is widely used in the treatment of neuroendocrine tumors [2]. An alternative is to use monoclonal antibodies for "radioimmunotherapy," as illustrated by the use of anti-CD20 antibodies such as Bexxar® and Zevalin® for the treatment of B-cell lymphomas [3, 4]. The most common radionuclides used to label SRT agents emit β-particles which have a typical range in tissue of several millimeters; the most widely used of these is ^{131}I although, as will be discussed later, other β-emitters as well as α-particle and Auger-electron emitters are under active investigation.

The expectation of therapeutic efficacy in SRT is based on the preferential accumulation of the radiopharmaceutical in the tumor by virtue of it being directed to a specific cancer-associated target, with little uptake by (and thus sparing of) normal tissue [5]. Another feature that distinguishes SRT from XRT is that the former delivers radiation to the tumor continuously at an exponentially decreasing LDR; the actual dose rate depends on factors such as the extent of uptake of the radiopharmaceutical and the half-life of the radionuclide [6]. The typical average dose rate in SRT is between ~10 and 40 cGy/h, with the

integrated dose to tumor being up to 50 Gy over a period of days [7]. As for any cancer therapy, it is important in SRT to have an optimized therapeutic index such that tumor responses are achieved without unacceptable risk of normal tissue toxicity. In general, if patients are appropriately selected, the normal tissue toxicity and morbidity associated with SRT/LDR therapies can be modest [8, 9].

High Dose Rate Versus Low Dose Rate Radiation

- The dose delivered at HDR (external beam) XRT: 1–5 Gy/min, the total dose to the tumor: 60–70 Gy.
- The typical average dose rate in SRT: 10–40 cGy/h, with the integrated dose to the tumor: 50 Gy over a period of days.

Clinical Observations on SRT

Although considerable effort has gone into studying novel or experimental strategies for SRT, translation of this knowledge into the clinic has been slow. This is partly because of issues involving optimum dosing and scheduling as well as inadequate understanding of the mechanistic basis of SRT [6, 10]. As this understanding has improved, clinical responses to SRT have been found to not always be consistent with predictions based on classical radiobiological modeling. Indeed, SRT is sometimes effective for palliation and tumor control even when the estimated doses to tumor are significantly lower than those delivered by conventional XRT regimens [6, 9, 11–15]. A similar scenario has been described in some animal models (e.g., [16]).

Despite such caveats, the basic radiobiological principles that are assumed to apply to SRT have been mainly derived by extrapolation of data obtained following homogeneous acute exposures to single or fractionated doses of IR and have assumed that the doses delivered by XRT and SRT are biologically equivalent [17, 18]. However, both experimental and clinical evidence suggest that LDR therapeutic radiopharmaceuticals may in fact have radiobiological features that are mechanistically distinct from HDR therapies [6, 19].

Linear-Quadratic Model of Cell Killing and Dose-Rate Effects

Survival curves for single HDR exposures. Early models for mammalian-cell survival curves after single HDR exposures were developed primarily using data obtained with the clonogenic survival assay. Implicit in these early models were the concepts that a cell could only be "killed" if it was physically traversed by an IR track and that the chromosomal DNA was the principal cellular "target" for radiation injury, with DNA double-strand breaks (DSBs) being the key events underlying cell death.

Survival curves for cells exposed to low-LET beams such as X-rays and γ-rays are typically curvilinear, with an initial "shoulder" region below ~1.5 Gy, indicative of relatively inefficient cell killing, followed by a steeper component between ~3 and 10 Gy. Several models were developed to describe the shape of this curve. Early among these was "Target Theory," which embodied the concept that each cell must accumulate a number of sublethal "hits" in critical subcellular targets for it to be killed [20]. Later the linear-quadratic (LQ) model (Fig. 21.1) became widely used, mostly because it was useful for clinical purposes rather than any inherently superior mechanistic or curve-fitting characteristics. The LQ model describes IR-induced cell killing by a combination of two components: the first is a 1-hit/linear component (αD) that is proportional to dose; the second is a 2-hit/quadratic component (βD^2) in which a lethal event requires an interaction between two sub-lesions, each sub-lesion being produced in proportion to dose. Whereas the contribution of linear/α-type events to cell death is independent of exposure time, and thus of dose rate, the contribution of quadratic/β-type events is reduced by decreasing the dose rate. From this point on, we will consider only the LQ model; it is preferred by many because of its simplicity, having only the two parameters, α and β, and because

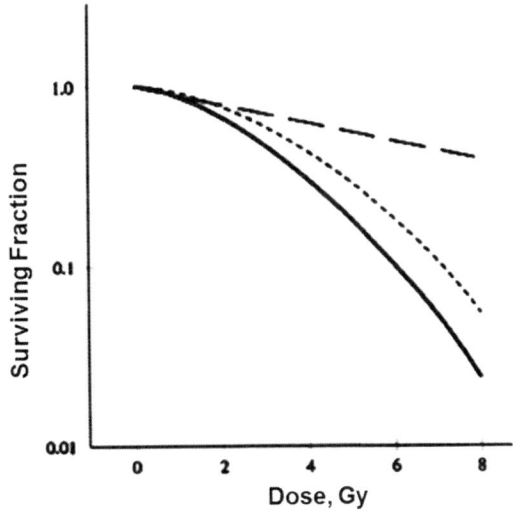

Fig. 21.1 Clonogenic survival curve for a typical human tumor cell line exposed to low-LET radiation beams such as γ- or X-rays. The *solid line* is the fit to the linear-quadratic (LQ) model: $-\ln[SF] = \alpha D + \beta D^2$, where SF is the surviving fraction at dose D. The *dashed curves* represent the α/single-hit (*dashed lines*) and β/two-hit (*dotted lines*) components of the LQ equation

the ratio of the two parameters, the α/β ratio, is useful to assess the biological and clinical impact of changes in dose fractionation or dose rate on biological effect in cells and tissues/tumors.

Survival curves for differing dose rates: the "conventional" dose-rate effect. For the HDR exposures typically used in XRT and radiobiological studies (~1–5 Gy/min), it takes only a minute or so to deliver a dose of 2 Gy, during which time biological processes such as the DNA damage response (DDR) (see below) are only just beginning to engage. However, for lower dose rates in the range of ~100 cGy/min down to ~1 cGy/min (when it would take more than 3 h to deliver a dose of 2 Gy), the individual β-type sub-lesions can be repaired during the protracted exposure rather than interacting to generate potentially cytotoxic lesions, so radiosensitivity should progressively decrease with decreasing dose rate over this range [21]. The LQ model predicts that the survival curve will become shallower and straighter as the dose rate decreases, ultimately approaching the initial slope (α) of the HDR curve when the β-type sub-lesions can be

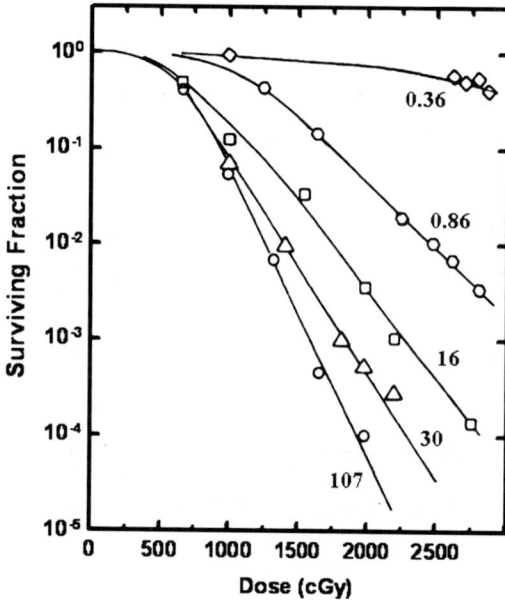

Fig. 21.2 Dose rate dependency of the killing of asynchronous log-phase Chinese hamster lung fibroblast CHL-F cells by γ-rays. The slope of the survival curve becomes progressively shallower as the dose rate decreases from 107 to 0.36 cGy/min. Adapted from Bedford and Mitchell [22], with permission

optimally repaired. Such behavior is illustrated in Fig. 21.2, which covers a range of dose rates from 107 cGy/min down to 0.36 cGy/min [22]; similar behavior has been observed for other biological endpoints such as division delay, chromosomal aberrations, and animal survival [23]. The half-time $(t_{1/2})$ for the repair of β-type sub-lesions in human cells is on the order of an hour, and for normal tissues ranges from ~0.5 to ~1.5 h. At very LDRs (below ~1 cGy/min), the cells can proliferate during the radiation exposure and repopulate the pool of clonogens, leading to a further (albeit non-radiobiological) increase in radioresistance [21].

The clinical implication of this behavior is that a given dose of IR delivered in the SRT context (i.e., as a protracted LDR exposure) should be less effective against the tumor clonogens/repopulating cells than the same dose of XRT (i.e., an acute HDR exposure). As noted above, this expectation is not always borne out by clinical findings. This is one of the important points that suggests that there might be unanticipated

radiobiological differences in the cellular response to LDR vs. HDR exposures.

LQ modeling of normal tissue complications. The major rationale for fractionation in XRT is to reduce the incidence of severe late normal tissue complications that could otherwise be life threatening. This would be of little value if the tumor response was not spared to a lesser extent, which both laboratory and clinical experience tell us to (mostly) be the case (a notable exception being prostate cancer). In general, the changes in normal tissue complication probability with altered fractionation or dose rate are consistent with the LQ model and depend predictably on the α/β ratio for the single-dose HDR survival curve. Late normal tissue complications such as lung-related death have a small α/β ratio and display large fractionation and dose-rate sparing effects; early complications such as death from bone marrow failure have a large α/β ratio and show minimal sparing with fractionation or decreasing dose rate. This is illustrated for mice in Fig. 21.3 [23]. The anticipated lack of bone marrow sparing with LDR therapies [24] is unfortunate given that myelosuppression is the major dose-limiting side effect for most radiopharmaceuticals. This is seen in the use of ^{131}I-mIBG to treat neuroblastoma: many centers use relatively low cumulative administered doses of the radiopharmaceutical that do not usually result in severe hematological toxicity; however, the use of higher doses does result in significant hematological toxicity that requires either bone marrow or stem cell transplantation [25].

The DNA Damage Response Network

The last two decades have heralded remarkable advances in our knowledge of the chemical nature of IR-induced DNA damage and of the biological pathways that cells and tissues use to circumvent the deleterious effects of such damage. Damage to the genetic material activates a complex molecular network collectively termed the "DNA damage response" (DDR) that integrates downstream processes such as DNA repair, cell-cycle checkpoint activation, and cell death, via a cascade of

Fig. 21.3 Effect of dose rate on the killing of mice by X-rays. As the dose rate was reduced from 1.8 to 0.025 Gy/min there was a significant sparing of late lung injury (end-point: lethality at 9 months after irradiation of the thorax) but little sparing of early bone marrow injury (end-point: lethality at 30 days after total-body exposure). This differential sparing is presumed to reflect differences in shape of the survival curves of the putative target cells that underlie these two tissue responses. Reproduced from Travis [23], with permission

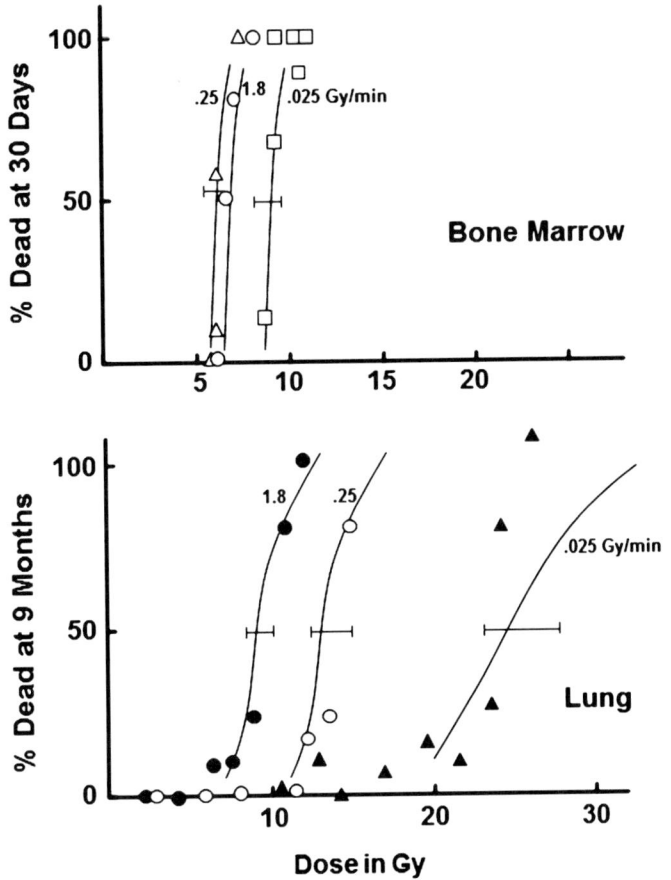

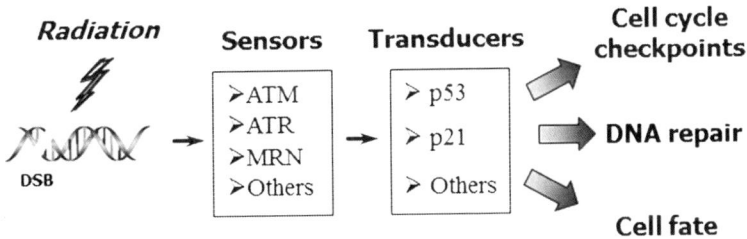

Fig. 21.4 Simplified cartoon of the cellular DNA damage response (DDR) networks activated by IR. The DDR involves four classes of proteins: sensors, mediators, transducers, and effectors. Sensors are DNA damage-binding proteins that bind to the various types of DNA damage, illustrated here for a DSB induced by IR, and activate

signaling events that alter the activity of specific DDR proteins [26–28]. The holistic function of the DDR is to promote genetic stability and the survival of cells that have processed these DNA lesions appropriately, as well as invoking the

transducers such as the ATM (mutated in ataxia telangiectasia) serine/threonine kinases that amplify and transmit these signals to the effector proteins, such as p53, which execute the various functional outcomes of the damage-response network, such as the activation of cell-cycle checkpoints, DNA repair, apoptosis, and premature senescence

death of cells that fail to achieve this objective. A general outline of the DDR is shown in Fig. 21.4.

DNA lesions induced by IR. Exposing cells to IR generates a number of types of simple DNA lesions such as base and sugar damage and single-strand breaks which involve only one strand of the DNA helix. Such lesions are fairly easy for the cell to process because the undamaged strand can serve as a template for their repair. What is distinctive about IR is that it also generates complex clustered lesions involving both strands of the DNA helix that arise because of the microheterogeneity of energy deposition along the track of the ionizing particle [29]. These clustered lesions, which include DSBs, are generally regarded as the main initiators of IR-induced cell killing [30] and are much more difficult for the DDR to process.

DDR components. For an irradiated cell to remain genetically stable and survive, it needs to rapidly detect and repair DNA lesions such as DSBs. Sensor proteins bind to the DSBs and recruit/activate additional DDR proteins such as mediators (which are critical for the assembly of damage-signaling and chromatin-remodeling protein complexes) and signal-transducing proteins. The major transducers are serine/threonine kinases (i.e., enzymes that transfer a phosphate group to a serine or threonine residue of a substrate protein) belonging to the phosphatidylinositol 3-kinase-related kinase or "PIKK" family [27]. Additional protein kinases amplify and transmit these signals to downstream effectors such as p53 that implement the functional consequences of the DDR network. An effective DDR requires that the chromatin (the combination of DNA and proteins located in the nucleus of the cell) is rapidly remodeled to facilitate access by DNA repair and checkpoint-activator proteins; this is carried out by various chromatin-remodeling complexes; these events may be particularly important to understand in the context of LDR IR exposures when chromatin remodeling will be occurring simultaneously with ongoing damage induction.

The DDR proteins mediate both pro-survival (e.g., DNA repair and cell-cycle checkpoint activation) and pro-death (e.g., apoptosis; see below) responses. The ATM (mutated in ataxia telangiectasia, AT) protein, a member of the PIKK family, is the major sensor/signaling kinase for IR-induced DSBs [31]. Activation of the kinase activity of ATM in response to a DSB requires its autophosphorylation, as well as its relocation to the DSB site, which requires additional DDR proteins such as the "MRN" (MRE11/RAD50/NBS1) complex and MDC1 (mediator of DNA damage checkpoint protein 1) [32–34]. ATM is subject to a variety of posttranslational modifications, such as phosphorylation and acetylation, that modulate its various functions [35]. The ATM kinase activity, either directly or indirectly through one of its substrates, the CHK2 checkpoint kinase protein, can phosphorylate a broad range of substrates including sensors, mediators, DNA repair and cell-cycle checkpoint proteins as well as wild-type p53, resulting in p53 stabilization and cellular accumulation as well as its functional activation [27, 31, 36–38]. DSBs can also be processed by other PIKKs such as DNA-PK (DNA-dependent protein kinase) and ATR (ATM and RAD3 related) under some circumstances (Fig. 21.4).

DSB-repair foci. Another substrate of ATM is the H2AX variant histone, a chromatin protein whose rapid (within minutes) phosphorylation in the chromatin surrounding the DSB appears to recruit other DSB-repair factors to the site of the DSB, generating discrete entities known as "IR-induced foci" or "IRIFs" [39, 40]. IRIFs involving the phosphorylated form of H2AX (γ-H2AX) can be visualized using a microscope after staining the cells with an antibody that recognizes γ-H2AX [41]. This provides the basis for a sensitive method to indirectly detect DSBs in cells and tissues that has proven valuable for studying low-dose exposures. For example, γ-H2AX IRIFs were clearly detectable in skin fibroblasts from prostate cancer patients who had received XRT [42], in skin biopsies from prostate cancer patients who had received XRT and for whom the absorbed dose to skin was in the range of 0.05–1.1 Gy [43], in blood lymphocytes from cancer patients who had received a low dose diagnostic CT scan to the chest and/or abdomen [44, 45], and in lymphocytes from patients after angiography who received doses as low as 2 mGy [46]. This assay has enormous potential for application to SRT studies.

DNA repair pathways. Human cells mainly repair DSBs by non-homologous end joining (NHEJ) or

Table 21.1 Key components of the DNA damage-response network

Component	Characteristics and key players
NHEJ pathway for DSB repair	"Classical" NHEJ is believed to be the preferred mechanism for DSB repair in human cells, especially in G_1/G_0-phase [48]
	Catalyzes the direct rejoining of incompatible DNA ends [48–50], so it often results in deletion of nucleotides
	Key factors include the MRN complex and the DNA-PK complex that is composed of a catalytic subunit (DNA-PK$_{cs}$) as well as KU70 and KU80 [51]
	Recently an "alternative" NHEJ pathway was described, the importance of which is only now being uncovered [48]
HRR pathway for DSB repair	Requires extensive homology and can thus repair a DSB with high fidelity [52]
	Most efficient in S- and G_2-phase where recombination can occur between the sister chromatids
	Key factors include RAD51 and the BRCA1/BRCA2 tumor-suppressor proteins [51, 53, 54]
Chromatin remodeling complexes	NuRD (nucleosome remodeling and histone deacetylation)
	NuA4 (nucleosome acetyltransferase of histone H4)
	Ino80 (inositol auxotroph 80)
	SMARCA1 (SWI/SNF related, matrix associated, actin-dependent regulator of chromatin, subfamily a, member 1)
Cell-cycle checkpoints	Key checkpoints are in G_1, S, and G_2 phase
	Wild-type p53 is a major regulator of the G_1 checkpoint
	The S-phase checkpoint is triggered by parallel pathways in which ATM phosphorylates a number of substrates including CHK2 and the MRN constituent NBS1 (the protein mutated in the radiosensitivity-associated condition "Nijmegen breakage syndrome") [60]
	The "conventional" G_2 checkpoint has both p53-dependent and -independent components [61]
	A second checkpoint early-G_2 phase [62] is activated through ATM, but the involvement of p53 therein is uncertain

homologous recombination repair (HRR) (Table 21.1 [47–54]). The two pathways share some elements, such as the MRN complex [47], but other proteins are pathway-specific. The repair of simple non-DSB lesions such as oxidized or missing bases is carried out by another pathway, base excision repair (BER) [55, 56]. An important BER enzyme, poly(ADP-ribose)polymerase 1 (PARP-1), has been the focus of intense interest because of its potential exploitation in cancer therapy involving "synthetic-lethal" interactions with HRR factors such as BRCA1 that are defective in many human cancers; specifically, BRCA1-deficient cancer cells are highly susceptible to killing by PARP-1 inhibitors [57]. There is some evidence that PARP-1 inhibitors may be particularly effective sensitizers of LDR IR exposures [58].

Cell-cycle checkpoints. The activation of checkpoints in the G_1, S, and G_2 phases that temporarily delay progression through the cell cycle is a key feature of the DDR (Table 21.1 [59–62]).

Checkpoint activation is presumed to promote cell survival by providing time for the various DNA repair pathways to operate on the damaged genome without the complication of ongoing DNA synthesis or mitosis [59]. The early-G_2 checkpoint [62] may be particularly relevant to LDR IR exposures, as will be discussed below.

p53. Wild-type p53 regulates several key steps in the DDR network, including pro-survival responses such as the engagement of cell-cycle checkpoints and DNA repair pathways and pro-death responses such as apoptosis [63, 64]. One reason for the huge interest in p53 is that it is the most commonly altered protein in human cancers [63, 65, 66]. Its central role in the DDR thus opens the door to exploiting molecular differences between normal and malignant cells for therapeutic benefit in the context of many forms of cancer therapy, including SRT. Understanding the roles of the wild-type and various mutant forms of p53 in the DDR will be critical in this context. Because many other proteins involved in the DDR (e.g., BRCA1/2) are also commonly disrupted in cancer cells, this could represent a general strategy for exploiting the very changes that cause cancer as an "Achilles heel" in developing new or improved therapeutics.

> *Questions and issues in this area include*: (1) how can we better exploit the molecular differences between tumors and normal tissues for therapeutic benefit in SRT; and (2) what specific DDR proteins can be targeted for inhibition for optimal therapeutic index in SRT?

Mechanisms of Cell Death: Recent Advances

The last 20 years has also witnessed a "sea change" in our understanding of how human cells lose their reproductive or "clonogenic" capacity (i.e., "die") following exposure to IR. Again, most of this understanding has emerged from studying acute HDR exposures, but we assume that the lessons learned will at least guide us towards asking the right questions relevant to the LDR exposures that characterize SRT. It is now apparent that cells can die post-IR by several different mechanisms (Table 21.2 [67–74]) depending on

Table 21.2 Characteristics of various modes of loss of clonogenic potential

Mode of cell death	Characteristics
Apoptosis	An energy-dependent genetically regulated form of "programmed cell death"
	Can be triggered by the "*intrinsic*/mitochondrial" pathway or by the *extrinsic*/death receptor pathway
	Mediated by the activation of a family of proteolytic enzymes known as caspases (cysteine *asp*artic acid-specific prote*ases*)
	Characterized by cytoplasmic shrinkage, chromatin/nuclear condensation, nonrandom degradation of the genomic DNA (ultimately to fragments of ~180 base pairs), membrane blebbing, and cell fragmentation to generate "apoptotic bodies" that are phagocytosed by macrophages
Premature senescence	Another genetically regulated response to genomic injury in which the cells stop dividing for extended periods but remain viable and metabolically active
	Cells exhibit enlarged/flattened morphology, increased granularity, and expression of the marker "senescence-associated β-galactosidase"
	Important molecular effectors include the cyclin-dependent kinase inhibitors $p21^{Waf1}$ (CDKN1A) and $p16^{INK4a}$
Autophagy	A genetically regulated conserved stress response whereby a cell essentially undergoes self-digestion [67]
	Occurs in some human tumor cell lines exposed to IR [68–70]
	Cells exit the cell cycle, shrink, auto-digest proteins and damaged organelles, and recycle fatty acids and amino acids
	Cells develop prominent cytoplasmic vacuoles that sequester mitochondria, ribosomes, and other organelles
	Does not appear to depend on caspases or p53
	Signaling through the mTOR (mammalian target of rapamycin) protein is an important regulator [71]
Mitotic catastrophe	The failure of a cell with a damaged genome to properly execute mitosis, likely because of aberrant chromosome segregation and cell fusion
	Could be a significant contributor to the loss of clonogenic potential in irradiated cell cultures [72, 73]
	Cells usually become enlarged and develop abnormal spindles, micronuclei, and de-condensed chromatin, often resulting in multinucleated/polyploid or "giant" cells
	May be especially relevant in p53-deficient solid tumors [74]
Necrosis	A passive form of cell death that is probably not subject to genetic regulation
	Typically occurs after relatively high doses of IR as a result of cells entering mitosis with a heavily damaged genome
	Involves progressive cell swelling, swelling of mitochondria, denaturation and coagulation of cytoplasmic proteins, random DNA degradation, and disintegration of the organelles and cell membrane

factors such as dose, cell type, genetic background, and local environmental cues such as those deriving from cell–cell and/or cell–matrix interactions [6, 71, 75, 76].

Since the first reports of apoptosis in the context of the cellular response to IR were published in the 1970s [77] it has taken center stage, often to the exclusion of alternative mechanisms. Indeed, PubMed now lists many thousands of papers on this subject. Because apoptosis represents a definitive, irreversible form of cell death that should not have later implications for tumor recurrence it is, clinically speaking, a highly desirable outcome. It is of considerable interest in the context of cancer therapeutics that the propensity of a cell to undergo apoptosis in response to cancer-therapeutic agents (the so-called "apoptotic threshold") is regulated both positively and negatively by a number of genes/gene products, many of which, such as BCL-2 and p53, are altered in many human cancers [78].

Whereas apoptosis has long been recognized as a major cell-death pathway, other modes of cell "death" such as stress-induced premature senescence (SIPS), autophagy, and mitotic catastrophe have not been fully characterized in terms of their contribution to therapeutic response and failure. SIPS, which has sometimes been referred to as terminal or irreversible growth arrest or more recently as accelerated/premature senescence [79, 80], is commonly seen in irradiated solid tumor-derived cell lines with wild-type p53 [81, 82], and it probably contributes to both normal tissue and tumor responses to XRT [74, 83–85]. Unlike in apoptosis, a tumor cell that has undergone SIPS is not necessarily eliminated from the organism; considering that these cells retain long-term metabolic activity, there is some concern about what might happen to them at later times.

Questions and issues in this area include: (1) is apoptosis the major contributor to SRT/LDR responses, or are other modes of cell death such as SIPS also important in this setting; and (2) is there a potential for using pharmacological modifiers, e.g., of the apoptotic threshold, in SRT, considering that apoptosis may be the preferred clinical outcome?

The Phenomenon of "Low Dose Hyper-Radiosensitivity-Increased Radioresistance"

During the 1990s the use of automated methods to construct clonogenic survival curves based on counting individual "dead" cells rather than surviving colonies (which is much less sensitive in the low-dose region) led to the astonishing observation that the single acute-dose survival curves for many human cell lines actually display an initial hypersensitive response to doses below ~0.25 Gy; when the dose approaches ~0.5 Gy the cells become increasingly radioresistant [86, 87]. Only above ~1 Gy does the surviving fraction decrease as predicted by the LQ equation. This phenomenon, which has been termed "low dose hyper-radiosensitivity-increased radioresistance" or HRS-IRR, was a radical departure from conventional thinking and contradicted the basic principles of all survival curve models developed to that point, so it naturally generated skepticism; however, it has largely been borne out in a range of model systems. For those cell lines that exhibit HRS, the LQ equation significantly under-predicts the level of cell killing at lower doses.

Of potential relevance from the therapy perspective, HRS seems to be more pronounced in tumor cells than normal cells [88, 89]. However, this is not universal, e.g., the MCF7 cell line that is widely used as an experimental model for human breast cancer does not show an HRS-IRR phenotype [90]. In vivo responses to XRT consistent with HRS have been reported in tumor xenograft models [91], tumors [92, 93] and metastatic tumor nodules [94] as well as normal skin [95–97] and salivary glands [87].

Mechanism of HRS-IRR

It is widely assumed that HRS-IRR must reflect differences in how efficiently cells activate the DDR network (Fig. 21.4) as a function of dose, i.e., that low doses in the HRS range either fail to or inefficiently trigger one or more critical radioprotective steps. Only above the threshold of ~0.25 Gy should such radioprotective mechanisms be fully triggered. So, is this expectation borne out experimentally, i.e., is there a cellular dose threshold for activating any of the major components of the DDR network that coincides with the transition from HRS to IRR? Some reports do indicate a more efficient repair of DSBs above the HRS-IRR threshold in various human cell lines (e.g., [98, 99]). Other studies report similar rates of γ-H2AX foci resolution above and below this threshold [100, 101]. As regards the BER pathway, one study did report a gradual dose-dependent increase in BER activity after γ-ray doses up to ~50 cGy in the M1/2 murine myeloid cell line expressing wild-type p53, with higher doses inhibiting BER activity [102]. BER activity in p53-deficient cells did not show this biphasic pattern, but instead increased progressively with dose.

The phenotypic data on the repair of DNA lesions are therefore equivocal. What about the activation of damage-sensor/signaling proteins such as ATM as a function of dose? In human fibroblasts, ATM autophosphorylation at serine-1981 (a marker for ATM activation) was observed after as little as 10 cGy and was saturated by ~40 cGy [32]. A similar dose response was seen for T98G glioma cells [103]. Such data suggest that ATM activation could be a key step in triggering radioprotective processes related to IRR [104]. However, very different patterns have been seen in other types of cells [103, 105], so this does not appear to be a general mechanism.

What about the activation of DDR components downstream of ATM? The phosphorylation of ATM substrates such as H2AX is typically a linear function of dose in various cell types regardless of whether or not they exhibit HRS [99]. Another key ATM substrate is the wild-type p53 protein; however, defining its dose–response is complicated because p53 activation and stabilization involves a variety of concomitant posttranslational modifications to the protein (including phosphorylation, acetylation and sumoylation) whose significance remains to be established (for a review, see ref. [99]). Whether the HRS-IRR phenotype per se is dependent on p53 status is ambiguous; thus, some cell lines with abrogated p53 have a diminished HRS-IRR

response [90], whereas in a panel of human tumor cell lines there was no clear association between p53 status and HRS [106].

The next DDR component of interest is the activation of cell-cycle checkpoints. It has been observed that HRS-IRR is itself cell-cycle phase dependent, occurring preferentially in a subset of cells in the G_2 phase [89, 104]. The early-G_2 checkpoint [62] may be a key mediator of the transition from the HRS to IRR states [89, 103, 107]. Cell lines that exhibit HRS have a threshold for activating this checkpoint at doses around 0.3 Gy, i.e., they do not activate the checkpoint after low doses and enter mitosis with unrepaired DNA damage and die [103]; cell types that lack HRS show no such threshold, the early-G_2 checkpoint instead being activated even by low doses [89].

Conventional Versus "Inverse" Dose-Rate Effects

From the SRT perspective, understanding the response of cells to LDR exposures is much more relevant than their response to low dose exposures delivered at HDR. As noted earlier, classical models lead us to expect that cell killing will decrease progressively with decreasing dose rate over the range of ~100 cGy/min down to ~1 cGy/min because of the repair of β-type sub-lesions and because of the compensatory effect of cell proliferation at even lower dose rates. A given dose of IR delivered by SRT should thus be less biologically effective than the same dose of XRT. It is therefore of great importance to note that several studies with human cell lines have reported findings that are at variance with this expectation. Specifically, for some cell types under some conditions cell killing has been observed to *increase* as the dose rate is lowered. Such "inverse dose-rate effects" were first reported by Mitchell et al. [108, 109]; for S3 HeLa human cervix cancer cells exposed to the same total dose, irradiation at a dose rate of 37 cGy/h was more cytotoxic than irradiation at 74 or 154 cGy/h (Fig. 21.5). Further examples of inverse dose-rate effects over certain dose ranges were subsequently reported for other cell types [110–115]; an example of such

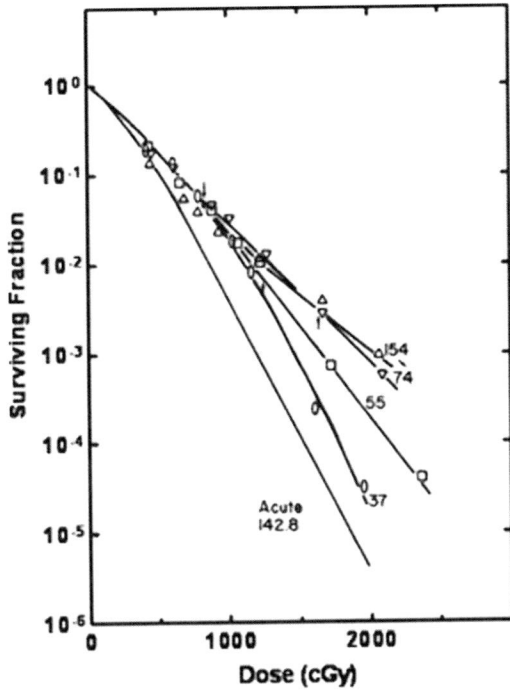

Fig. 21.5 An example of an inverse dose-rate effect for cell killing. Survival curves for log-phase S3 HeLa cells exposed to continuous irradiation at different dose rates. An inverse dose-rate effect is apparent at dose rates below 74 cGy/h, especially after higher total doses above ~7 Gy. The acute dose rate was 142.8 cGy/min. Adapted from Mitchell et al. [109], with permission

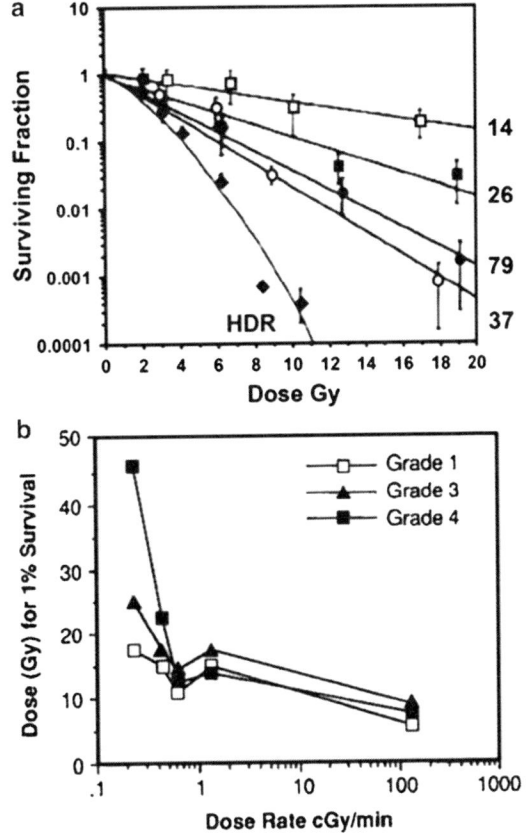

Fig. 21.6 (a) Survival curves for grade-4 human astrocytic tumor cell lines irradiated with ^{137}Cs γ-rays at HDR (78 Gy/h) and LDR (79, 37, 26, and 14 cGy/h). Note the inverse dose rate effect at a dose rate of 37 cGy/h (~0.62 cGy/min). (b) Dose required for 1 % cell survival vs. dose rate for grades 1, 3, and 4 astrocytic tumor cell lines. Note the inverse dose rate effect at 37 cGy/h (~0.62 cGy/min) in all cell types. From Schultz and Geard [112], with permission

behavior in astrocytic tumor cell lines [112] is shown in Fig. 21.6a.

Inverse dose-rate effects typically occur at dose rates below ~1 cGy/min and are more pronounced at higher doses. Effects vary from slight inversions in an otherwise overall sparing effect (e.g., [112]) to a major inversion that in some cases results in a radiosensitivity per unit dose for very LDRs that exceeds that seen after HDR exposure (e.g., [114, 115]). In addition to a differing cellular susceptibility to inverse dose rate effects per se (see below), these diverse patterns may reflect the varying contribution of proliferation to sparing at very-LDR, which will reflect both the doubling time for the particular cell line as well as the extent to which checkpoint activation occurs during the protracted LDR exposure. This scenario is seen for astrocytic tumor cell lines in Fig. 21.6b [112], where the obscuring effect of proliferation appears to take

effect at dose rates below ~0.5 cGy/min, i.e., just as the inverse dose-rate effect is beginning to be discriminated. Interestingly, there does appear to be a relationship between tumor grade and the impact of proliferation in this data set.

A role for G_2 synchronization in inverse dose-rate effects? Inverse dose-rate effects may reflect the ability of certain continuous LDR exposures to synchronize cells in G_2 phase via a persistent activation of the G_2/M checkpoint, coupled with the general radiosensitivity of cells in this phase of the cell cycle [13, 108–112, 116]. Such a mechanism was invoked to explain the effective tumor control obtained with protracted LDR radioimmunotherapy in patients with lymphoma and other tumors [117] as well as the sensitivity of preclinical tumor models to in vivo LDR exposures [16, 118]. However, G_2-synchronization may not be the only mechanism in play here. For example, the inverse dose-rate effect seen with mouse Bp8 ascites sarcoma cells in vivo was suggested to reflect a suboptimal activation of DNA repair pathways at LDR [119]. Furthermore, inverse dose-rate effects observed in some human prostate cancer cell lines did not correlate with G_2 synchronization [113].

A role for HRS-IRR in inverse dose-rate effects? The expectation here is that a particular LDR exposure might fail to trigger the radioprotective IRR response, analogous to the situation for single HDR exposures below ~0.3 Gy. In this case, cell types with a pronounced HRS phenotype should exhibit more dramatic inverse dose-rate effects. Indeed, three human glioma and prostate cancer cell lines that exhibited a clear HRS response also exhibited an inverse dose-rate

effect, with radiosensitivity increasing by ~4-fold when the dose rate was lowered from 100 cGy/h down to 2–5 cGy/h, with a dose rate of 2 cGy/h actually being more cytotoxic than an acute exposure ([114]; Fig. 21.7a). An HRS-negative glioma line showed no such effect. At 5 cGy/h the glioma cells did not accumulate in G_2 at any dose regardless of whether or nor they exhibited HRS, suggesting that G_2-synchronization was not responsible for the observed inverse dose-rate effect. This conclusion was supported by the clear inverse dose-rate effect seen in confluent glioma-cell cultures (Fig. 21.7b) where synchronization effects should not occur [114].

Dose-rate effect and activation of the DDR network. Although both G_2-synchronization and HRS may contribute to inverse dose-rate effects, their relative contribution is not clear at this time. As noted above, HRS appears to be related to an inability of low doses below the "induced repair" threshold to trigger a robust DDR response. If HRS is mechanistically related to inverse dose-rate effects, it would be logical to ask whether protracted LDR exposures typical of those used

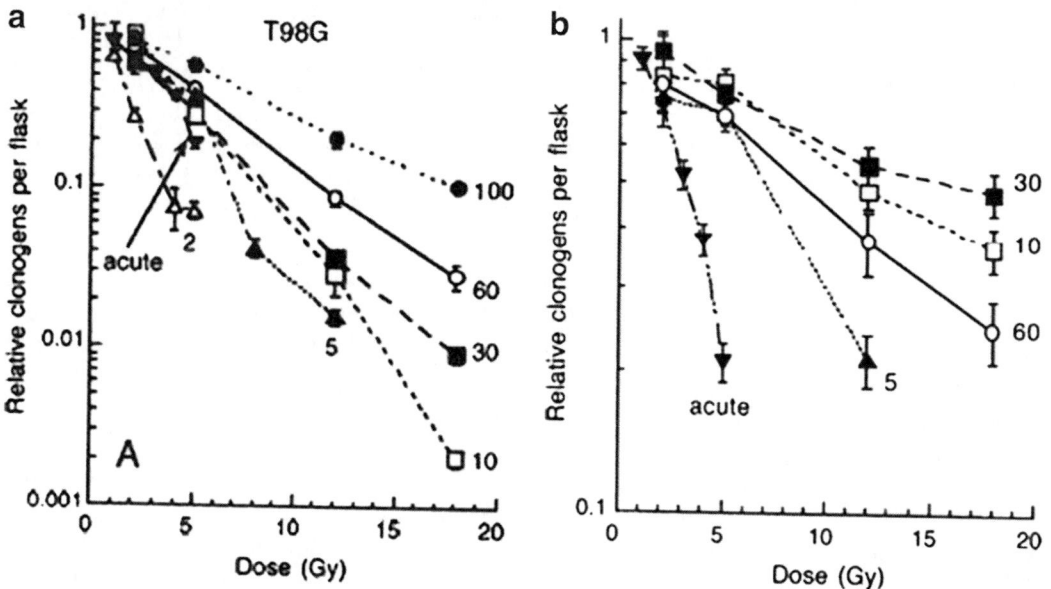

Fig. 21.7 Inverse dose-rate effect for cell killing in proliferating (**a**) and confluent (**b**) cultures of T98G human glioma cells exposed to ^{60}Co γ-rays at dose rates between 30 and 5 cGy/h. *Numbers* represent the dose rate in cGy/h. The acute dose rate was 33 Gy/h. From Mitchell et al. [114], with permission

Fig. 21.8 (a) Inverse dose-rate effect for cell killing in the RKO (colon) and DU145 (prostate) human cancer cell lines. Cells were exposed to a total dose of 2 Gy at either HDR (45 Gy/h; *solid bar*) or LDR (9.4 cGy/h; *striped bar*). (b) Corresponding data for H2AX phosphorylation at HDR and LDR. From Collis et al. [115], with permission

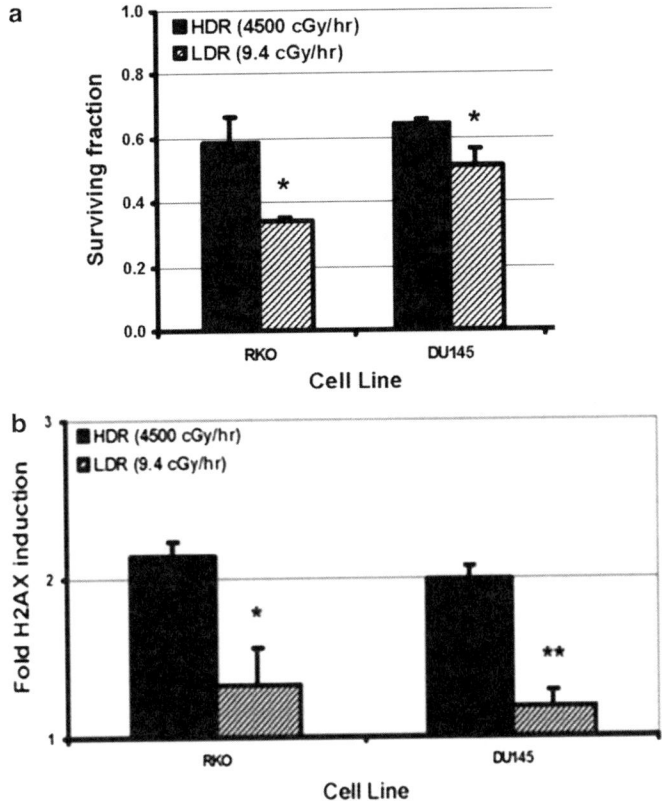

in SRT (which will result in transient low levels of DSBs that are being continuously induced and repaired) might similarly fail to trigger the full radioprotective DDR response in cell types that exhibit inverse dose-rate effects.

An important caveat here is that it is not trivial to decipher the molecular underpinnings of LDR effects because of the very long times needed to deliver the dose under conditions where the cells will be actively responding to DNA injury; however, some have tried. For example, several human tumor cell lines that showed a marked inverse dose-rate effect for cytotoxicity (Fig. 21.8a) showed greatly reduced markers of DDR activation—phosphorylation of ATM, NBS1, and H2AX (Fig. 21.8b)—following LDR exposure compared with HDR exposure [115]. In that study the HDR exposure at 45 Gy/h should induce ~1,800 DSBs/h, and the LDR exposure at 9.4 cGy/h should induce ~4 DSBs/h. Thus, the low levels of DSBs produced at LDR do appear to evade detection by the DDR to some extent. Similar observations have been

made using hTERT-immortalized human fibroblasts; whereas irradiation of these cells at HDR (1.8 Gy/min) resulted in significant phosphorylation of H2AX and p53, exposure at LDR (0.03 cGy/min) induced little phosphorylation of these proteins [120]. Levels of p53 phosphorylation in mouse cells similarly were not increased after continuous LDR exposures at 1.5 or 9 cGy/h [121]; in this case, though, the effect was attributed to degradation of the phosphorylated protein during the protracted (72 h) irradiation period, emphasizing the challenge in interpreting such findings.

Dose-rate effects for specific modes of cell death. What is the role, if any, of apoptosis in tumor responses to LDR exposures/SRT? The possibility that some tumors might readily undergo apoptosis after LDR exposures has often been suggested as a potential contributor to the effectiveness of SRT [11, 13, 116, 122]. Several experimental reports do indicate that LDR exposures are potent inducers of apoptosis, e.g., exposing human adenocarcinoma cells to doses of γ-rays as low as 2 Gy at LDR induced apoptosis very efficiently [12]. Protracted LDR exposure of HL60 human leukemia cells to 10 Gy of β radiation (^{188}Re) for 24 h (dose rate ~0.7 cGy/min) resulted in higher levels of apoptosis than were seen when the same dose was delivered at HDR over 0.5, 1, or 3 h [123]; thus, apoptosis was characterized by a modest inverse dose-rate effect in this system. As might be expected, such behavior is not seen with all cell types; e.g., ML-1 human myeloid tumor cells displayed a "conventional" dose-rate effect for apoptosis between 290 and 0.28 cGy/min [124]. Thus, apoptosis may be the preferred mode of cell death after LDR exposures in some but not all types of cells. Even for in vitro models, there is no information that we are aware of about the incidence of other modes of cell death such as SIPS, autophagy, and mitotic catastrophe at the LDRs typical of SRT.

Clinical implications. An obvious question is whether inverse dose-rate effects might be operative in SRT/LDR therapeutics. Such a scenario might help to explain the paradox outlined above as to why SRT sometimes exhibits antitumor efficacy after much lower estimated total absorbed doses to the tumor than those administered by XRT. As noted earlier, the average dose rate in SRT is typically ~10–40 cGy/h, so a considerable proportion of the dose to tumor (especially in the later stages) will be delivered at a rate below the "magic" 1 cGy/min, i.e., where inverse dose-rate effects are most in evidence.

Another important consideration is that components of the DDR network that are clearly at the center of LDR radiobiology are altered in some way in many types of cancer; this includes p53 and BRCA1/2. Furthermore, hypoxia arising in tumors (see above) can lead to the depletion of DSB repair factors such as BRCA1 [125] as well as selecting for certain p53 mutations [126]. It should not, therefore, be surprising if there are systematic differences in the way that tumors and normal tissues react to changing dose rate that might be exploitable for improving the therapeutic index in SRT. Details of the impact of such events will have to be clearly established if such information is to be exploitable in

the context of SRT (e.g., see Williams et al. [127] with respect to the effect of p53 status).

> *Questions and issues in this area include*: (1) what are the exact cellular parameters and mechanisms that give rise to inverse dose-rate effects for cell death; (2) are there different dose and dose-rate thresholds for activating the various modes of cell death; (3) how can cancer-associated molecular alterations in the DDR network (e.g., in p53) be exploited for therapeutic gain in SRT; and (4) might HRS-related effects play a role in the normal-tissue toxicity associated with SRT, a concern that has been expressed in the context of intensity-modulated radiation therapy (IMRT), where large volumes of normal tissue can receive a low dose of IR [128, 129]?

Crossfire Effects

The term "crossfire" describes the phenomenon where an ionizing particle that originated from a radionuclide taken up by one cell deposits its energy in a neighboring or distant cell. Such events depend predictably on the particle range, and they are inherent to and very important for efficacy in SRT protocols involving isotopes such as ^{131}I that emit β-particles that typically have a maximum range in tissue of several millimeters. Much of the dose from such radiopharmaceuticals is therefore delivered to the tumor by crossfire-type rather than direct cell-targeting events.

An illustration of crossfire in a model system is seen with the β-emitting radiopharmaceutical ^{131}I-mIBG [130, 131]. Glioma cells engineered to express the *NAT* gene were much more sensitive to the cytotoxic effects of ^{131}I-mIBG when exposed as multicellular spheroids rather than as monolayers; these observations are consistent with an additional cytotoxic effect due to crossfire killing from the β-particles in the 3-D system. Similar effects were recapitulated in a 3-D glioma spheroid model in which only a minority of the cells were *NAT*-positive; these effects were again attributed largely to crossfire events, albeit with a likely contribution from bystander effects (see below) [132].

Crossfire from β-emitters has positive implications for tumor control in SRT/radioimmunotherapy, especially in larger solid tumors where the distribution of the radiopharmaceutical (and thus of dose) may be heterogeneous. The down side for therapeutic index is that crossfire can also result in considerable dose to surrounding normal tissues.

Radiobiological Bystander Effects

Another phenomenon that could have major implications for SRT is the radiobiological "bystander effect" in which cells that are traversed by an ionizing particle can transmit signals to neighboring or distant non-irradiated cells. This results in manifestations of radiation injury (such as DNA damage, mutation, and death) in the cells that receive these signals. Bystander effects are considered to be "non-targeted" insofar as they do not result from an interaction between an ionizing particle track and the cellular DNA, and they should not be confused with the physical crossfire effects described in the previous section. Bystander effects are usually studied either by using a specialized microbeam irradiator that enables the dose to be targeted only to a sub-population of the cells in the test system, by allowing some type of communication between the irradiated and non-irradiated cells by mixing or coculturing, or by transferring the growth medium from irradiated cultures onto non-irradiated cultures. They are especially relevant after low doses, typically <0.2 Gy, although estimates vary [133, 134]. Bystander effects typically show a nonlinear dose response, being fully induced by low doses of IR, although it is not yet clear if every cell within a tissue is capable of responding to bystander signals. The mechanisms through which bystander signals generated by irradiated cells are communicated to non-irradiated cells have been reviewed elsewhere [134–137]. Important roles are indicated for cellular

stress pathways that normally respond to various environmental insults; key contributors are the mitogen-activated protein kinase (MAPK) signaling cascade, reactive oxygen/nitrogen species, gap-junction signaling, cytokines, and immune/inflammatory pathways.

As with HRS-IRR, early reports describing bystander effects generated considerable controversy [134]. In part, this was because they totally contradicted the basic dogma of classical radiobiology such as target theory and the belief that cell killing was the exclusive domain of damage to DNA in the context of ionizing particle tracks. The most important implication from the perspective of this chapter is that, for the LDR exposures typically delivered by SRT, the operation of bystander effects would result in more cell death than would be predicted using dosimetric estimates and conventional radiobiological models. (An important caveat here, and discussed below, is that some bystander effects may have a radioprotective function, but this is not the norm.) If such effects were to occur in vivo, they could have a huge impact on how we model therapeutic response to SRT and possibly help to explain why SRT is sometimes more efficacious than predicted from the absorbed dose to tumor (see above and ref. [134]). They could be therapeutically advantageous by helping overcome the anticipated negative impact of heterogeneous distribution of the radiopharmaceutical within the tumor [138]. However, there is no available information in regards to the specific role of bystander effects in clinical SRT at this time.

An early indication that radioactive small molecules might invoke bystander effects came from studies using mixed 3-D aggregates of non-labeled and ^{3}H-thymidine-labeled hamster cells [139, 140]. Because ^{3}H emits a short-range β-particle that causes ionization only of the labeled cells without significant crossfire, the observed killing of non-labeled cells was attributed to bystander signals deriving from the ^{3}H-labeled cells. There is some evidence that radiopharmaceuticals can also induce bystander effects in vivo in tumors. In particular, Kassis and his colleagues [138, 141, 142] looked for bystander effects involving LS174T human colorectal carcinoma

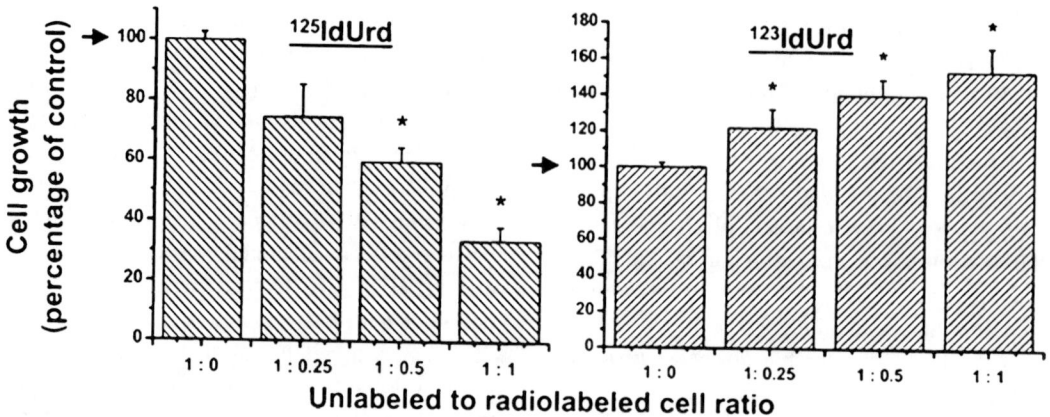

Fig. 21.9 In vitro bystander effect induced by [125]IdUrd- and [123]IdUrd-labeled LS174T cells. Unlabeled LS174T cells (0.4×10^6) were cocultured with varying numbers of lethally radioiodinated LS174T cells. Dead LS174T cells were added to bring the total number of cells to 0.8×10^6/ well. Growth of unlabeled LS174T cells on day 4 is shown as a percentage of control. *$P < 0.05$. From Kishikawa et al. [143], with permission

cells labeled with ^{125}I-deoxyuridine; this is a short-range Auger-electron emitting radiopharmaceutical that incorporates into DNA, where it causes highly localized ionization leading to a DSB that can kill the labeled cell without causing significant crossfire ionization of neighboring cells [138]. When ^{125}I-labeled cells were mixed with non-labeled tumor cells and subcutaneously co-injected into mice, the presence of ^{125}I-labeled cells greatly inhibited the growth of the resulting tumor. One likely interpretation of these findings is that bystander signals generated by the ^{125}I-labeled cells are transmitted to and kill the non-labeled cells. An interesting feature of these studies with Auger-electron emitters is that the in vivo bystander effect appeared to be almost fully activated at a relatively low ratio of radiolabeled to non-labeled cells, implying that it represents a binary "off-on" response capable of greatly amplifying the biological effects of the radiopharmaceutical [142]. However, there is much that still needs to be understood about bystander effects caused by Auger electrons; in particular, cells similarly labeled with [123]I (which has the same electron spectrum as ^{125}I) actually *stimulated* the growth of non-labeled LS174T cells [143]. The authors do note that there are differences between these agents, notably that ^{123}I has a much shorter half-life than ^{125}I such that the

dose rate for ^{123}I-labeled cells in these studies was >100-fold higher than that for ^{125}I-labeled cells. These authors [143] also found that [125]I-/^{123}I-deoxyuridine induced contradictory bystander effects in LS174T tumor cells in vitro based on coculturing and medium-transfer experiments; thus, cell proliferation was stimulated by [123]IdUrd but inhibited by [125]IdUrd, as shown in Fig. 21.9. Interesting mechanistic insight into these effects was provided by microarray data showing that the tissue inhibitor of matrix metalloproteinases 1 and 2 (TIMP1 and TIMP2) proteins, which are growth inhibitory, are selectively secreted by ^{125}I-labeled cells whereas angiogenin (which is growth stimulatory) is selectively secreted by ^{123}I-labeled cells.

Another series of experiments by Boyd and her associates looked at bystander effects caused by halogenated radiopharmaceuticals using the medium-transfer approach in a model system that combined gene therapy and targeted radionuclide therapy. Human tumor cells derived from glioma and transitional cell carcinoma of the bladder were transfected with the *NAT* gene and treated with the β-emitter ^{131}I-MIBG, the Auger-electron emitter ^{123}I-MIBG, or the α-emitter meta-[[211]At]-astatobenzylguanidine ([211]At-MABG) [144]. A strong bystander effect with each radiopharmaceutical at low activity was inferred from the cytotoxicity observed in non-irradiated cells exposed to growth medium from radiolabeled cells. These studies were extended to a 3-D glioma spheroid model containing differing ratios of *NAT*-positive and *NAT*-negative cells, where complete killing of all of the cells by the β-emitter ^{131}I-MIBG or the α-emitter [211]At-MABG was achieved even when only a small fraction (5 %) of the cells in a spheroid were *NAT* positive; given the greater effectiveness of the α-particle emitter and the relative lack of crossfire associated with [211]At α-emissions, it was concluded that radiobiological bystander effects represented a significant component of cell killing by the α-emitting agent [145, 146].

> *Questions and issues in this area include*: we clearly need a better understanding of the mechanistic basis of bystander signaling with different radiopharmaceuticals and isotopes and how it might be manipulated to therapeutic advantage. This includes: (1) the reasons for the lack of a dose response for bystander effects; (2) whether cells undergoing a bystander response invoke further bystander effects in their neighbors [147]; (3) whether there are differences in the generation of and response to bystander signals between and among normal and tumor cells [134]; (4) the impact of hypoxia on bystander signals; (5) the role of p53 in bystander signaling; and (6) the potential for using pharmacological modifiers of bystander effects (such as L-deprenyl and ondansetron) to improve therapeutic index in SRT [134].

Adaptive Responses

The term "adaptive response" refers to the phenomenon in which exposure of a cell population to a low or "priming" dose of IR results in increased resistance to a subsequent higher dose exposure. The second or "test" dose is typically given several hours after the priming dose. This effect was originally seen with human lymphocytes that were labeled with tritiated thymidine prior to a test X-ray exposure [148]. Many examples of adaptive responses have now been reported for various cell types, end points, and combinations of priming and test exposures [149–151]. Acceptance of this effect was slow, in part because it turns out that adaptive responses are probably not universal and even when they do occur they typically do so only within a window of priming doses around ~0.5–20 cGy [152]. Also, many studies have understandably focused on different types of tumor cells in which genetic or epigenetic factors important for adaptive responses may be altered; e.g., at least some adaptive responses to IR require wild-type p53 [153], although this has not been systematically studied.

Adaptive responses were anticipated to relate to the ability of the priming exposure to induce some type of radioprotective mechanism, such as DNA repair, but the generality of this view remains unclear. Thus, adaptive stimulation of the repair of some classes of DNA lesions was found in some studies (e.g., [154–156]) but not in others (e.g., [98]). Considering the above caveats relating to the dependence of adaptive responses on cell type and on the magnitude and timing of the priming and test doses, part of the controversy here is probably because not all of these DNA repair studies clearly established whether the model system actually exhibited a phenotypic adaptive response for cell killing.

Adaptive responses could play a role in SRT. Because LDR exposures might be regarded as a chronic priming exposure [116], any associated activation of an adaptive response in tumor cells could decrease the efficacy of SRT. Another setting in which adaptive responses might be operative is when a low diagnostic dose of a radiopharmaceutical is given to a patient for dosimetric purposes, followed by administration of a higher therapeutic dose of the SRT agent. This is sometimes done in radioimmunotherapy with Zevalin, where ^{111}In-labeled diagnostic antibody is followed by ^{90}Y-labeled therapeutic antibody [157].

Alternative Radionuclides with Potential Clinical Application

The most widely used radionuclides in SRT are β-particle emitters such as ^{131}I or ^{90}Y, and more recently ^{177}Lu because it has some favorable therapeutic characteristics [158]. The use of radionuclides such as ^{211}At and ^{212}Bi that emit α-particles which, unlike these β-particles, have a relatively short path length in tissue on the order of several cell diameters, is an area of active research for treating microscopic/disseminated tumors [159–161]. For example, the α-emitting radiopharmaceutical ^{211}At-MABG was ~1,000-fold more cytotoxic towards human neuroblastoma cells than its β-emitting counterpart [^{131}I]-mIBG, suggesting that it could be useful for treating micrometastatic disease [159]. The first phase-I trial of a ^{211}At-labeled therapeutic radiopharmaceutical in humans, which involves locoregional administration of an ^{211}At-labeled antibody that targets the extracellular matrix glycoprotein tenascin, was recently initiated for the treatment of recurrent brain tumors [162, 163]. Part of the rationale for expecting a therapeutic advantage from the use of α-particle emitters in SRT relates to the fact that cell killing by high-LET particles is not restricted by tumor hypoxia (see below). Other potential advantages of α-emitters have emerged from our improved understanding of LDR radiobiology, such as an expectation of significant bystander effects with limited crossfire and thus diminished normal tissue toxicity.

Isotopes such as ^{123}I, ^{125}I, and ^{111}In that emit Auger electrons have also generated clinical interest. Auger electrons are of low energy (~1 keV) and thus have a short range in tissue, typically only a few nanometers but at most several micrometers. They therefore deposit most of their dose close to their site of localization and thus target the cells in which they accumulate, with little crossfire dose. This could be useful clinically with radiopharmaceuticals that localize within the cell, such as with ^{125}I-deoxyuridine targeting to DNA (see above) or internalizing monoclonal antibodies [164, 165]. The dearth of crossfire events may explain the relatively low

normal-tissue toxicity associated with these agents [164]. Indeed, mIBG has been labeled with ^{125}I and ^{123}I, which should result in decreased crossfire and bone marrow toxicity. This contrasts, e.g., with the β-emitter ^{131}I-mIBG which is used for treating neuroblastoma but exhibits dose-limiting bone marrow toxicity that presumably results from crossfire ionization [166]. On the other hand, as noted earlier, bystander effects generated by Auger electron-emitting radiopharmaceuticals might enhance the therapeutic usefulness of these agents [138, 144]. Other Auger electron-emitting radionuclides such as ^{195m}Pt might also have some clinical potential because of their differing dose rates [141].

Hypoxia and SRT Responses

The development of regions of hypoxia (i.e., cells with low oxygenation status) within a tumor is a limitation to tumor control by external-beam XRT. This is partly because hypoxic cells are relatively (2.5–3 fold) resistant to acute single doses of IR [167] and because tumor hypoxia has other detrimental consequences, such as promoting tumor aggressiveness and metastasis [168]. Two distinct types of hypoxia are believed to occur in tumors [169]. "Chronic" hypoxia arises in cells located at the limits of the diffusion range of oxygen into the tissue, which typically begins at a distance of ~150 μm from an artery [167]. "Transient" hypoxia is a dynamic effect caused by an abnormal tumor vasculature; this leads to sluggish/irregular blood flow that fluctuates on a time scale of minutes to hours, such that regions of tumors adjacent to temporarily closed vessels may become hypoxic for short periods [169].

It was noted many years ago that the radioprotective effect of hypoxia may be less pronounced for LDR exposures that characterize SRT/radioimmunotherapy compared with the HDR exposures used in XRT [170]. Furthermore SRT, because of the continuous and protracted nature of the dose delivery to the tumor, might help to overcome the negative impact of both types of hypoxia on therapeutic outcome by optimally exploiting the reoxygenation of chronically hypoxic regions of tumors during therapy as well as offsetting the dynamic changes associated with transiently hypoxic regions of tumors. Because cellular radioresistance associated with hypoxia is less pronounced with high-LET particles [167], it is also anticipated that the use of radiopharmaceuticals that emit high-LET α-particles or Auger electrons should be more effective than β-emitting radiopharmaceuticals for the treatment of hypoxic tumors [13].

Heterogeneity and Fractionation of SRT

As noted above, the potential heterogeneity of radiopharmaceutical (and thus dose) distribution associated with single SRT treatments is a barrier to tumor control, especially in poorly vascularized tumors containing regions of hypoxia that the radiopharmaceutical may not easily access. As outlined earlier, the operation of crossfire and radiobiological bystander effects should help to overcome this problem. Another approach is to deliver SRT as a series of fractions [11]. Preclinical and clinical data suggest that fractionating radiolabeled antibodies and peptides can be advantageous and produce more uniform dose distributions [11, 171]. This approach has also shown clinical benefit with ^{131}I-mIBG therapy [172].

Future Directions

Enormous advances—sometimes paradigm-changing and controversial—have been made in our understanding of the radiobiological principles of SRT in recent years. Comprehending the relevance of this knowledge in the clinical setting represents an exciting opportunity and a significant challenge for the nuclear medicine community. Validating and quantifying the roles of bystander and inverse dose-rate effects in SRT in vivo would demand a reappraisal of our approach to assessing therapeutic response to SRT in the context of conventional dosimetry [138, 144]. One challenge may be the difficulty in developing unified criteria for tumor response and toxicity. Because

bystander, inverse dose-rate effects, and adaptive responses are not yet describable in the context of universal mechanisms, they might be difficult to exploit for clinical advantage until this knowledge is more complete [116].

Because of space limitations, we have not been able to review all active areas of research relevant to the biology of LDR effects. For example, immunological effects that occur in the context of LDR IR exposures could certainly contribute to the sometimes unexpected effectiveness of SRT [147]. Another important area is the application of patient-specific biomarkers to the prediction of tumor and normal tissue responses and thus to individualization of therapy [173]. Although biomarkers identified in the context of HDR exposures for XRT could prove useful in the context of SRT, biomarkers specifically useful for LDR therapeutics should also be sought. Because SRT is usually targeted to a specific type of cancer such as lymphomas or neuroendocrine tumors based on a tumor-associated target, the target itself also provides a biomarker of importance that can be assessed by molecular imaging, immunohistochemistry, or other methods. The XRT field has also been quick to embrace the latest systems biology and next-generation sequencing approaches to biomarker discovery through the successful establishment of several collaborative networks that link large numbers of biosamples to well-annotated clinical databases [173]; hopefully the near future will see similar initiatives in the SRT community to examine/identify biomarkers that appropriately reflect LDR radiobiology.

Finally, it has been reported in preclinical models that very-LDR IR exposures can increase the sensitivity of tumors to subsequent acute exposures to high doses of IR [174, 175]. Such observations raise the possibility of combining LDR IR exposures with XRT to exploit such radiosensitization.

Summary

The last 20 years has seen explosive growth in our understanding of the molecular underpinnings of the response of human cells and tissues to ionizing radiation and the application of this information to the treatment of cancer. Much of this information has been derived from studies using single or fractionated doses of radiation in the 1–10 Gy range delivered at a relatively HDR. The question is: how much can such studies inform us of the biological basis of targeted SRT where the dose is delivered to the tumor under conditions of nonuniform low and decaying dose rates? This chapter summarizes recent advances in our understanding of low-dose/LDR radiobiological mechanisms that might help us to understand the efficacy and limitations of SRT. These include the phenomena of inverse dose-rate effects, low dose hyper-radiosensitivity-increased radioresistance, radiobiological bystander effects, and adaptive responses, for which the underlying molecular mechanisms are a subject for intense debate and scientific investigation. Although these findings were often extremely controversial on their initial report, they raise important questions about conventional radiobiological models and their application to low dose/LDR ionizing radiation exposures that can only help the clinical practice of SRT to move forward by critically evaluating and utilizing this information to guide translational and clinical progress.

References

1. Withers HR. The four R's of radiotherapy. In: Lett JT, Adler H, editors. Advances in radiation biology, vol. 5. New York: Academic Press; 1975. p. 241–71.
2. Sisson JC, Wieland DM. Radiolabeled meta-iodobenzylguanidine: pharmacology and clinical studies. Amer J Physiol Imaging. 1986;1:96–103.
3. Wahl RL. Tositumomab and (131)I therapy in non-Hodgkin's lymphoma. J Nucl Med. 2005;46 Suppl 1:128S–40.
4. Borghaei H, Wallace SG, Schilder RJ. Factors associated with toxicity and response to yttrium 90-labeled ibritumomab tiuxetan in patients with indolent non-Hodgkin's lymphoma. Clin Lymphoma. 2004;5 Suppl 1:S16–21.
5. Larson SM, Krenning EP. A pragmatic perspective on molecular targeted radionuclide therapy. J Nucl Med. 2005;46 Suppl 1:1S–3.
6. Murray D, McEwan AJ. Radiobiology of systemic radiation therapy. Cancer Biother Radiopharm. 2007;22:1–23.
7. Flower MA, Fielding SL. Radiation dosimetry for 131I-mIBG therapy of neuroblastoma. Phys Med Biol. 1996;41:1933–40.
8. Brans B, Linden O, Giammarile F, Tennvall J, Punt C. Clinical applications of newer radionuclide therapies. Eur J Cancer. 2006;42:994–1003.
9. Goldenberg DM. Radioimmunotherapy. In: Freeman LM, editor. Nuclear medicine annual. Philadelphia: Lippincott Williams and Wilkins; 2001. p. 169–206.
10. McEwan AJ. Radioisotope therapy and clinical trial design: the need for consensus and innovation. J Nucl Med. 2002;43:87–8.
11. DeNardo GL, Schlom J, Buchsbaum DJ, Meredith RF, O'Donoghue JA, Sgouros G, et al. Rationales, evidence, and design considerations for fractionated radioimmunotherapy. Cancer. 2002;94 Suppl 4:1332–48.
12. Mirzaie-Joniani H, Eriksson D, Sheikholvaezin A, Johansson A, Löfroth PO, Johansson L, et al. Apoptosis induced by low-dose and low-dose-rate radiation. Cancer. 2002;94 Suppl 4:1210–4.
13. Dixon KL. The radiation biology of radioimmunotherapy. Nucl Med Commun. 2003;24:951–7.
14. Blake GM, Zivanovic MA, Blaquiere RM, Fine DR, McEwan AJ, Ackery DM. Strontium-89 therapy: measurement of absorbed dose to skeletal metastases. J Nucl Med. 1988;29:549–57.
15. Koral KF, Francis IR, Kroll S, Zasadny KR, Kaminski MS, Wahl RL. Volume reduction versus radiation dose for tumors in previously untreated lymphoma patients who received iodine-131 tositumomab therapy. Conjugate views compared with a hybrid method. Cancer. 2002;94 Suppl 4:1258–63.
16. Knox SJ, Sutherland W, Goris ML. Correlation of tumor sensitivity to low-dose-rate irradiation with G2/M-phase block and other radiobiological parameters. Radiat Res. 1993;135:24–31.
17. Dale R, Carabe-Fernandez A. The radiobiology of conventional radiotherapy and its application to radionuclide therapy. Cancer Biother Radiopharm. 2005;20:47–51.
18. Kassis AI, Adelstein SJ. Radiobiologic principles in radionuclide therapy. J Nucl Med. 2005;46 Suppl 1:4S–12.
19. Kennel SJ, Welch MJ. DOE's role in radiopharmaceutical technology research and development for targeted radionuclide therapy. Workshop summary; 2003. Cited in reference.
20. Alper T. Cellular radiobiology. Cambridge, UK: Cambridge University Press; 1979.
21. Steel GG. The dose rate effect: brachytherapy and targeted radiotherapy. In: Steel GG, editor. Basic clinical radiobiology. 3rd ed. London: Hodder Arnold; 2002. p. 192–204.
22. Bedford JS, Mitchell JB. Dose-rate effects in synchronous mammalian cells in culture. Radiat Res. 1973;54:316–27.
23. Travis EL. Primer of medical radiobiology. 2nd ed. Chicago, IL: Year Book Medical Publishers; 1989.
24. Travis EL, Peters LJ, McNeill J, Thames HD, Karolis C. Effect of dose-rate on total-body irradiation: lethal-

ity and pathologic findings. Radiother Oncol. 1985; 4:341–51.

25. Polishchuk AL, Dubois SG, Haas-Kogan D, Hawkins R, Matthay KK. Response, survival, and toxicity after iodine-131-metaiodobenzylguanidine therapy for neuroblastoma in preadolescents, adolescents, and adults. Cancer. 2011;117:4286–93.

26. Jackson SP. Sensing and repairing DNA double-strand breaks. Carcinogenesis. 2002;23:687–96.

27. Kurz EU, Lees-Miller SP. DNA damage induced activation of ATM and ATM-dependent signaling pathways. DNA Repair. 2004;3:889–900.

28. Jackson SP, Bartek J. The DNA-damage response in human biology and disease. Nature. 2009;461: 1071–8.

29. Ward JF. Complexity of damage produced by ionizing radiation. Cold Spring Harb Symp Quant Biol. 2000;65:377–82.

30. Georgakilas AG. Processing of DNA damage clusters in human cells: current status of knowledge. Mol Biosyst. 2008;4:30–5.

31. Shiloh Y. ATM: ready, set, go. Cell Cycle. 2003; 2:116–7.

32. Bakkenist CJ, Kastan MB. DNA damage activates ATM through intermolecular autophosphorylation and dimer dissociation. Nature. 2003;421:499–506.

33. Uziel T, Lerenthal Y, Moyal L, Andegeko Y, Mittelman L, Shiloh Y. Requirement of the MRN complex for ATM activation by DNA damage. EMBO J. 2003;22:5612–21.

34. Lee JH, Paull TT. Direct activation of the ATM protein kinase by the Mre11/Rad50/Nbs1 complex. Science. 2004;304:93–6.

35. Sun Y, Jiang X, Chen S, Fernandes N, Price BD. A role for the Tip60 histone acetyltransferase in the acetylation and activation of ATM. Proc Natl Acad Sci U S A. 2005;102:13182–7.

36. Niida H, Nakanishi M. DNA damage checkpoints in mammals. Mutagenesis. 2006;21:3–9.

37. Bartek J, Lukas J. Chk1 and Chk2 kinases in checkpoint control and cancer. Cancer Cell. 2003;3:421–9.

38. Matsuoka S, Ballif BA, Smogorzewska A, McDonald III ER, Hurov KE, Luo J, et al. ATM and ATR substrate analysis reveals extensive protein networks responsive to DNA damage. Science. 2007; 316(5828):1160–6.

39. Paull TT, Rogakou EP, Yamazaki V, Kirchgessner CU, Gellert M, Bonner WM. A critical role for histone H2AX in recruitment of repair factors to nuclear foci after DNA damage. Curr Biol. 2000;10: 886–95.

40. Löbrich M, Shibata A, Beucher A, Fisher A, Ensminger M, Goodarzi AA, et al. γH2AX foci analysis for monitoring DNA double-strand break repair: strengths, limitations and optimization. Cell Cycle. 2010; 9:662–9.

41. Pilch DR, Sedelnikova OA, Redon C, Celeste A, Nussenzweig A, Bonner WM. Characteristics of γ-H2AX foci at DNA double-strand breaks sites. Biochem Cell Biol. 2003;81:123–9.

42. Qvarnstrom OF, Simonsson M, Johansson KA, Nyman J, Turesson I. DNA double strand break quantification in skin biopsies. Radiother Oncol. 2004;72:311–7.

43. Simonsson M, Qvarnström F, Nyman J, Johansson KA, Garmo H, Turesson I. Low-dose hypersensitive γH2AX response and infrequent apoptosis in epidermis from radiotherapy patients. Radiother Oncol. 2008;88:388–97.

44. Lobrich M, Rief N, Kuhne M, Heckmann M, Fleckenstein J, Rübe C, et al. In vivo formation and repair of DNA double-strand breaks after computed tomography examinations. Proc Natl Acad Sci U S A. 2005;102:8984–9.

45. Rothkamm K, Balroop S, Shekhdar J, Fernie P, Goh V. Leukocyte DNA damage after multi-detector row CT: a quantitative biomarker of low-level radiation exposure. Radiology. 2007;242:244–51.

46. Kuefner MA, Grudzenski S, Schwab SA, Wiederseiner M, Heckmann M, Bautz W, et al. DNA double-strand breaks and their repair in blood lymphocytes of patients undergoing angiographic procedures. Invest Radiol. 2009;44:440–6.

47. Valerie K, Povirk LF. Regulation and mechanisms of mammalian double-strand break repair. Oncogene. 2003;22:5792–812.

48. Lieber MR. The mechanism of double-strand DNA break repair by the nonhomologous DNA end-joining pathway. Annu Rev Biochem. 2010;79:181–211.

49. Cromie GA, Connelly JC, Leach DR. Recombination at double-strand breaks and DNA ends: conserved mechanisms from phage to humans. Mol Cell. 2001;8:1163–74.

50. Weterings E, Chen DJ. The endless tale of nonhomologous end-joining. Cell Res. 2008;18:114–24.

51. Paull TT, Gellert M. A mechanistic basis for Mre11-directed DNA joining at microhomologies. Proc Natl Acad Sci U S A. 2000;97:6409–14.

52. Li X, Heyer WD. Homologous recombination in DNA repair and DNA damage tolerance. Cell Res. 2008;18:99–113.

53. Huen MS, Sy SM, Chen J. BRCA1 and its toolbox for the maintenance of genome integrity. Nat Rev Mol Cell Biol. 2010;11:138–48.

54. Thorslund T, West SC. BRCA2: a universal recombinase regulator. Oncogene. 2007;26:7720–30.

55. Almeida KH, Sobol RW. A unified view of base excision repair: lesion-dependent protein complexes regulated by post-translational modification. DNA Repair (Amst). 2007;6:695–711.

56. Friedberg EC, Walker GC, Siede W, Wood RD, Schultz RA, Ellenberger T. DNA repair and mutagenesis. 2nd ed. Washington, DC: ASM Press; 2006.

57. Chalmers AJ, Lakshman M, Chan N, Bristow RG. Poly(ADP-ribose) polymerase inhibition as a model for synthetic lethality in developing radiation oncology targets. Semin Radiat Oncol. 2010;20:274–81.

58. Chalmers A, Johnston P, Woodcock M, Joiner M, Marples B. PARP-1, PARP-2, and the cellular

response to low doses of ionizing radiation. Int J Radiat Oncol Biol Phys. 2004;58:410–9.

59. Kastan MB, Bartek J. Cell-cycle checkpoints and cancer. Nature. 2004;432(7015):316–23.

60. Willis N, Rhind N. Regulation of DNA replication by the S-phase DNA damage checkpoint. Cell Div. 2009;4:13.

61. Taylor WR, Stark GR. Regulation of the G2/M transition by p53. Oncogene. 2001;20:1803–15.

62. Xu B, Kim ST, Lim DS, Kastan MB. Two molecularly distinct G(2)/M checkpoints are induced by ionizing irradiation. Mol Cell Biol. 2002;22:1049–59.

63. Sengupta S, Harris CC. p53: traffic cop at the crossroads of DNA repair and recombination. Nat Rev Mol Cell Biol. 2005;6:44–55.

64. Murray D, Mirzayans R. Role of p53 in the repair of ionizing radiation-induced DNA damage. In: Landseer BR, editor. New research on DNA repair. Hauppauge, NY: Nova; 2007. p. 325–73.

65. Olivier M, Hussain SP, Caron de Fromentel C, Hainaut P, Harris CC. TP53 mutation spectra and load: a tool for generating hypotheses on the etiology of cancer. IARC Sci Publ. 2004;157:247–70.

66. Lane DP. p53 from pathway to therapy. Carcinogenesis. 2004;25:1077–81.

67. Hait WN, Jin S, Yang JM. A matter of life or death (or both): understanding autophagy in cancer. Clin Cancer Res. 2006;12:1961–5.

68. Ito H, Daido S, Kanzawa T, Kondo S, Kondo Y. Radiation-induced autophagy is associated with LC3 and its inhibition sensitizes malignant glioma cells. Int J Oncol. 2005;26:1401–10.

69. Daido S, Yamamoto A, Fujiwara K, Sawaya R, Kondo S, Kondo Y. Inhibition of the DNA-dependent protein kinase catalytic subunit radiosensitizes malignant glioma cells by inducing autophagy. Cancer Res. 2005;65:4368–75.

70. Paglin S, Yahalom J. Pathways that regulate autophagy and their role in mediating tumor response to treatment. Autophagy. 2006;2:291–3.

71. Brown JM, Attardi LD. The role of apoptosis in cancer development and treatment response. Nat Rev Cancer. 2005;5:231–7.

72. Jonathan EC, Bernhard EJ, McKenna WG. How does radiation kill cells? Curr Opin Chem Biol. 1999;3:77–83.

73. Brown JM, Wouters BG. Apoptosis: mediator or mode of cell killing by anticancer agents? Drug Resist Updat. 2001;4:135–6.

74. Eriksson D, Stigbrand T. Radiation-induced cell death mechanisms. Tumour Biol. 2010;31:363–72.

75. Abend M. Reasons to reconsider the significance of apoptosis for cancer therapy. Int J Radiat Biol. 2003;79:927–41.

76. Okada H, Mak TW. Pathways of apoptotic and non-apoptotic death in tumour cells. Nat Rev Cancer. 2004;4:592–603.

77. Wyllie AH, Kerr JF, Currie AR. Cell death: the significance of apoptosis. Int Rev Cytol. 1980;68:251–306.

78. McGill G, Fisher DE. Apoptosis in tumorigenesis and cancer therapy. Front Biosci. 1997;2:d353–79.

79. Roninson JB. Tumor cell senescence in cancer treatment. Cancer Res. 2003;63:2705–15.

80. Shay JW, Roninson IB. Hallmarks of senescence in carcinogenesis and cancer therapy. Oncogene. 2004;23:2919–33.

81. Chang BD, Broude EV, Dokmanovic M, Zhu H, Ruth A, Xuan Y, et al. A senescence-like phenotype distinguishes tumor cells that undergo terminal proliferation arrest after exposure to anticancer agents. Cancer Res. 1999;59:3761–7.

82. Mirzayans R, Scott A, Cameron M, Murray D. Induction of accelerated senescence by γ radiation in human solid tumor-derived cell lines expressing wild-type TP53. Radiat Res. 2005;163:53–62.

83. Suzuki M, Boothman DA. Stress-induced premature senescence (SIPS) — influence of SIPS on radiotherapy. J Radiat Res (Tokyo). 2008;49:105–12.

84. Gewirtz DA, Holt SE, Elmore LW. Accelerated senescence: an emerging role in tumor cell response to chemotherapy and radiation. Biochem Pharmacol. 2008;76:947–57.

85. Bromfield GP, Meng A, Warde P, Bristow RG. Cell death in irradiated prostate epithelial cells: role of apoptotic and clonogenic cell kill. Prostate Cancer Prostatic Dis. 2003;6:73–85.

86. Marples B, Lambin P, Skov KA, Joiner MC. Low dose hyper-radiosensitivity and increased radioresistance in mammalian cells. Int J Radiat Biol. 1997;71:721–35.

87. Joiner MC, Marples B, Lambin P, Short SC, Turesson I. Low-dose hypersensitivity: current status and possible mechanisms. Int J Radiat Oncol Biol Phys. 2001;49:379–89.

88. Marples B, Joiner MC. The response of Chinese hamster V79 cells to low radiation doses: evidence of enhanced sensitivity of the whole cell population. Radiat Res. 1993;133:41–51.

89. Marples B, Wouters BG, Collis SJ, Chalmers AJ, Joiner MC. Low-dose hyper-radiosensitivity: a consequence of ineffective cell cycle arrest of radiation-damaged G2-phase cells. Radiat Res. 2004;161:247–55.

90. Enns L, Bogen KT, Wizniak J, Murtha AD, Weinfeld M. Low-dose radiation hypersensitivity is associated with p53-dependent apoptosis. Mol Cancer Res. 2004;2:557–66.

91. Spring PM, Arnold SM, Shajahan S, Brown B, Dey S, Lele SM, et al. Low dose fractionated radiation potentiates the effects of taxotere in nude mice xenografts of squamous cell carcinoma of head and neck. Cell Cycle. 2004;3:479–85.

92. Pulkkanen K, Lahtinen T, Lehtimäki A, Joiner M, Kataja V. Effective palliation without normal tissue toxicity using low-dose ultrafractionated re-irradiation for tumor recurrence after radical or adjuvant radiotherapy. Acta Oncol. 2007;46:1037–41.

93. Arnold SM, Regine WF, Ahmed MM, Valentino J, Spring P, Kudrimoti M, et al. Low-dose fractionated radiation as a chemopotentiator of neoadjuvant

paclitaxel and carboplatin for locally advanced squamous cell carcinoma of the head and neck: results of a new treatment paradigm. Int J Radiat Oncol Biol Phys. 2004;58:1411–7.

94. Harney J, Short SC, Shah N, Joiner M, Saunders MI. Low dose hyper-radiosensitivity in metastatic tumors. Int J Radiat Oncol Biol Phys. 2004;59:1190–5.

95. Turesson I, Joiner MC. Clinical evidence of hypersensitivity to low doses in radiotherapy. Radiother Oncol. 1996;40:1–3.

96. Hamilton CS, Denham JW, O'Brien M, Ostwald P, Kron T, Wright S, et al. Underprediction of human skin erythema at low doses per fraction by the linear quadratic model. Radiother Oncol. 1996;40:23–30.

97. Harney J, Shah N, Short S, Daley F, Groom N, Wilson GD, et al. The evaluation of low dose hyper-radiosensitivity in normal human skin. Radiother Oncol. 2004;70:319–29.

98. Murray D, Wang JYJ, Mirzayans R. DNA repair after low doses of ionizing radiation. Int J Low Radiat. 2006;3:255–72.

99. Murray D, Weinfeld M. Radiation biology of targeted radiotherapy. In: Reilly RM, editor. Monoclonal antibody and peptide-targeted radiotherapy of malignancies. Hoboken, NJ: Wiley; 2010. p. 419–71.

100. Wykes SM, Piasentin E, Joiner MC, Wilson GD, Marples B. Low-dose hyper-radiosensitivity is not caused by a failure to recognize DNA double-strand breaks. Radiat Res. 2006;165:516–24.

101. Short SC, Bourne S, Martindale C, Woodcock M, Jackson SP. DNA damage responses at low radiation doses. Radiat Res. 2005;164:292–302.

102. Offer H, Erez N, Zurer I, Tang X, Milyavsky M, Goldfinger N, et al. The onset of p53-dependent DNA repair or apoptosis is determined by the level of accumulated damaged DNA. Carcinogenesis. 2002;23:1025–32.

103. Krueger SA, Collis SJ, Joiner MC, Wilson GD, Marples B. Transition in survival from low-dose hyper-radiosensitivity to increased radioresistance is independent of activation of ATM Ser 1981 activity. Int J Radiat Oncol Biol Phys. 2007;69:1262–71.

104. Marples B. Is low-dose hyper-radiosensitivity a measure of G2-phase cell radiosensitivity? Cancer Metastasis Rev. 2004;23:197–207.

105. Buscemi G, Perego P, Carenini N, Nakanishi M, Chessa L, Chen J, et al. Activation of ATM and Chk2 kinases in relation to the amount of DNA strand breaks. Oncogene. 2004;23:7691–700.

106. Chandna S, Dwarakanath BS, Khaitan D, Mathew TL, Jain V. Low-dose radiation hypersensitivity in human tumor cell lines: effects of cell-cell contact and nutritional deprivation. Radiat Res. 2002;157:516–25.

107. Marples B, Collis SJ. Low-dose hyper-radiosensitivity: past, present, and future. Int J Radiat Oncol Biol Phys. 2008;70:1310–8.

108. Mitchell JB, Bedford JS, Bailey SM. Dose-rate effects on the cell cycle and survival of S3 HeLa and V79 cells. Radiat Res. 1979;79:520–6.

109. Mitchell JB, Bedford JS, Bailey SM. Dose-rate effects in mammalian cells in culture III. Comparison of cell killing and cell proliferation during continuous irradiation for six different cell lines. Radiat Res. 1979;79:537–51.

110. Furre T, Koritzinsky M, Olsen DR, Pettersen EO. Inverse dose-rate effect due to pre-mitotic accumulation during continuous low dose-rate irradiation of cervix carcinoma cells. Int J Radiat Biol. 1999;75:699–707.

111. Marin LA, Smith CE, Langston MY, Quashie D, Dillehay LE. Response of glioblastoma cell lines to low dose rate irradiation. Int J Radiat Oncol Biol Phys. 1991;21:397–402.

112. Schultz CJ, Geard CR. Radioresponse of human astrocytic tumors across grade as a function of acute and chronic irradiation. Int J Radiat Oncol Biol Phys. 1990;19:1397–403.

113. DeWeese TL, Shipman JM, Dillehay LE, Nelson WG. Sensitivity of human prostatic carcinoma cell lines to low dose rate radiation exposure. J Urol. 1998;159:591–8.

114. Mitchell CR, Folkard M, Joiner MC. Effects of exposure to low-dose-rate (60)Co gamma rays on human tumor cells in vitro. Radiat Res. 2002;158:311–8.

115. Collis SJ, Schwaninger JM, Ntambi AJ, Keller TW, Nelson WG, Dillehay LE, et al. Evasion of early cellular response mechanisms following low level radiation-induced DNA damage. J Biol Chem. 2004;279:49624–32.

116. Murtha AD. Review of low-dose-rate radiobiology for clinicians. Semin Radiat Oncol. 2000;10:133–8.

117. Ning S, Knox SJ. G2/M-phase arrest and death by apoptosis of HL60 cells irradiated with exponentially decreasing low-dose-rate gamma radiation. Radiat Res. 1999;151:659–69.

118. van Oostrum IE, Erkens-Schulze S, Petterson M, Wils IS, Rutgers DH. The relationship between radiosensitivity and cell kinetic effects after low- and high-dose-rate irradiation in five human tumors in nude mice. Radiat Res. 1990;122:252–61.

119. Cao S, Skog S, Tribukait B. Comparison between protracted and conventional dose rates of irradiation on the growth of the Bp8 mouse ascites sarcoma. Acta Radiol Oncol. 1983;22:35–47.

120. Ishizaki K, Hayashi Y, Nakamura H, Yasui Y, Komatsu K, Tachibana A. No induction of p53 phosphorylation and few focus formation of phosphorylated H2AX suggest efficient repair of DNA damage during chronic low-dose-rate irradiation in human cells. J Radiat Res (Tokyo). 2004;45:521–5.

121. Sugihara T, Murano H, Tanaka K, Oghiso Y. Inverse dose-rate-effects on the expressions of extra-cellular matrix-related genes in low-dose-rate gamma-ray irradiated murine cells. J Radiat Res (Tokyo). 2008;49:231–40.

122. Lennon SV, Martin SJ, Cotter TG. Dose-dependent induction of apoptosis in human tumour cell lines by widely diverging stimuli. Cell Prolif. 1991;24:203–14.

123. Friesen C, Lubatschofski A, Kotzerke J, Buchmann I, Reske SN, Debatin KM. Beta-irradiation used for systemic radioimmunotherapy induces apoptosis and activates apoptosis pathways in leukaemia cells. Eur J Nucl Med Mol Imaging. 2003;30:1251–61.

124. Amundson SA, Lee RA, Koch-Paiz CA, Bittner ML, Meltzer P, Trent JM, et al. Differential responses of stress genes to low dose-rate gamma irradiation. Mol Cancer Res. 2003;1:445–52.

125. Bindra RS, Gibson SL, Meng A, Westermark U, Jasin M, Pierce AJ, et al. Hypoxia-induced down-regulation of BRCA1 expression by E2Fs. Cancer Res. 2005;65:11597–604.

126. Graeber TG, Osmanian C, Jacks T, Housman DE, Koch CJ, Lowe SW, et al. Hypoxia-mediated selection of cells with diminished apoptotic potential in solid tumours. Nature. 1996;379(6560):88–91.

127. Williams JA, Zhang Y, Zhou H, Gridley DS, Koch CJ, Slater JM, et al. Overview of radiosensitivity of human tumor cells to low-dose-rate irradiation. Int J Radiat Oncol Biol Phys. 2008;72:909–17.

128. Honoré HB, Bentzen SM. A modelling study of the potential influence of low dose hypersensitivity on radiation treatment planning. Radiother Oncol. 2006;79:115–21.

129. Welsh JS, Limmer JP, Howard SP, Diamond D, Harari PM, Tome W. Precautions in the use of intensity-modulated radiation therapy. Technol Cancer Res Treat. 2005;4:203–10.

130. Boyd M, Cunningham SH, Brown MM, Mairs RJ, Wheldon TE. Noradrenaline transporter gene transfer for radiation cell kill by 131I meta-iodobenzylguanidine. Gene Ther. 1999;6:1147–52.

131. Boyd M, Mairs RJ, Cunningham SH, Mairs SC, McCluskey A, Livingstone A, et al. A gene therapy/targeted radiotherapy strategy for radiation cell kill by [131I]meta-iodobenzylguanidine. J Gene Med. 2001;3:165–72.

132. Boyd M, Mairs SC, Stevenson K, Livingstone A, Clark AM, Ross SC, et al. Transfectant mosaic spheroids: a new model for evaluation of tumour cell killing in targeted radiotherapy and experimental gene therapy. J Gene Med. 2002;4:567–76.

133. Prise KM, Schettino G, Vojnovic B, Belyakov O, Shao C. Microbeam studies of the bystander response. J Radiat Res (Tokyo). 2009;50(Suppl A):A1–6.

134. Mothersill C, Seymour CB. The bystander effect in targeted radiotherapy. In: Reilly RM, editor. Monoclonal antibody and peptide-targeted radiotherapy of malignancies. Hoboken, NJ: Wiley; 2010. p. 507–25.

135. Hei TK, Zhou H, Ivanov VN, Hong M, Lieberman HB, Brenner DJ, et al. Mechanism of radiation-induced bystander effects: a unifying model. J Pharm Pharmacol. 2008;60:943–50.

136. Hei TK, Zhou H, Chai Y, Ponnaiya B, Ivanov VN. Radiation induced non-targeted response: mechanism and potential clinical implications. Curr Mol Pharmacol. 2011;4:96–105.

137. Mothersill C, Seymour CB, Joiner MC. Relationship between radiation-induced low-dose hypersensitivity and the bystander effect. Radiat Res. 2002;157:526–32.

138. Xue LY, Butler NJ, Makrigiorgos GM, Adelstein SJ, Kassis AI. Bystander effect produced by radiolabeled tumor cells in vivo. Proc Natl Acad Sci U S A. 2002;99:13765–70.

139. Bishayee A, Rao DV, Howell RW. Evidence for pronounced bystander effects caused by nonuniform distributions of radioactivity using a novel three-dimensional tissue culture model. Radiat Res. 1999;152:88–97.

140. Bishayee A, Hill HZ, Stein D, Rao DV, Howell RW. Free radical-initiated and gap junction-mediated bystander effect due to nonuniform distribution of incorporated radioactivity in a three-dimensional tissue culture model. Radiat Res. 2001;155:335–44.

141. Bodei L, Kassis AI, Adelstein SJ, Mariani G. Radionuclide therapy with iodine-125 and other auger-electron-emitting radionuclides: experimental models and clinical applications. Cancer Biother Radiopharm. 2003;18:861–77.

142. Kassis AI. In vivo validation of the bystander effect. Hum Exp Toxicol. 2004;23:71–3.

143. Kishikawa H, Wang K, Adelstein SJ, Kassis AI. Inhibitory and stimulatory bystander effects are differentially induced by Iodine-125 and Iodine-123. Radiat Res. 2006;165:688–94.

144. Boyd M, Ross SC, Dorrens J, Fullerton NE, Tan KW, Zalutsky MR, et al. Radiation-induced biologic bystander effect elicited in vitro by targeted radiopharmaceuticals labeled with alpha-, beta-, and auger electron-emitting radionuclides. J Nucl Med. 2006;47:1007–15.

145. Boyd M, Mairs RJ, Keith WN, Ross SC, Welsh P, Akabani G, et al. An efficient targeted radiotherapy/gene therapy strategy utilising human telomerase promoters and radioastatine and harnessing radiation-mediated bystander effects. J Gene Med. 2004;6:937–47.

146. Boyd M, Sorensen A, McCluskey AG, Mairs RJ. Radiation quality-dependent bystander effects elicited by targeted radionuclides. J Pharm Pharmacol. 2008;60:951–8.

147. Sgouros G, Knox SJ, Joiner MC, Morgan WF, Kassis AI. MIRD continuing education: bystander and low dose-rate effects: are these relevant to radionuclide therapy? J Nucl Med. 2007;48:1683–91.

148. Olivieri G, Bodycote J, Wolff S. Adaptive response of human lymphocytes to low concentrations of radioactive thymidine. Science. 1984;223:594–7.

149. Ikushima T. Chromosomal responses to ionizing radiation reminiscent of an adaptive response in cultured Chinese hamster cells. Mutat Res. 1987;180:215–21.

150. Wolff S. The adaptive response in radiobiology: evolving insights and implications. Environ Health Perspect. 1998;106 Suppl 1:277–83.

151. Upton AC. Radiation hormesis: data and interpretations. Crit Rev Toxicol. 2001;31:681–95.

152. Preston RJ. Radiation biology: concepts for radiation protection. Health Phys. 2004;87:3–14.

153. Sasaki MS, Ejima Y, Tachibana A, Yamada T, Ishizaki K, Shimizu T, et al. DNA damage response pathway in radioadaptive response. Mutat Res. 2002;504:101–18.

154. Le XC, Xing JZ, Lee J, Leadon SA, Weinfeld M. Inducible repair of thymine glycol detected by an ultrasensitive assay for DNA damage. Science. 1998;280:1066–9.

155. Ikushima T, Aritomi H, Morisita J. Radioadaptive response: efficient repair of radiation-induced DNA damage in adapted cells. Mutat Res. 1996;358:193–8.

156. Tachibana A. Genetic and physiological regulation of non-homologous end-joining in mammalian cells. Adv Biophys. 2004;38:21–44.

157. Otte A. Diagnostic imaging prior to 90Y-ibritumomab tiuxetan (Zevalin) treatment in follicular non-Hodgkin's lymphoma. Hell J Nucl Med. 2008;11:12–5.

158. Kwekkeboom DJ, Bakker WH, Kooij PP, Konijnenberg MW, Srinivasan A, Erion JL, et al. [177Lu-DOTAOTyr3]octreotate: comparison with [111In-DTPAo]octreotide in patients. Eur J Nucl Med. 2001;28:1319–25.

159. Vaidyanathan G, Zalutsky MR. Targeted therapy using alpha emitters. Phys Med Biol. 1996;41:1915–31.

160. Zalutsky MR, Bigner DD. Radioimmunotherapy with alpha-particle emitting radioimmunoconjugates. Acta Oncol. 1996;35:373–9.

161. Zalutsky MR. Targeted alpha-particle therapy of microscopic disease: providing a further rationale for clinical investigation. J Nucl Med. 2006;47:1238–40.

162. Zalutsky MR, Reardon DA, Akabani G, Coleman RE, Friedman AH, Friedman HS, et al. Clinical experience with alpha-particle emitting 211At: treatment of recurrent brain tumor patients with 211At-labeled chimeric antitenascin monoclonal antibody 81C6. J Nucl Med. 2008;49:30–8.

163. Zalutsky MR, Reardon DA, Bigner DD. Targeted radiotherapy of central nervous system malignancies. In: Reilly RM, editor. Monoclonal antibody and peptide-targeted radiotherapy of malignancies. Hoboken, NJ: Wiley; 2010. p. 139–67.

164. Behr TM, Behe M, Lohr M, Sgouros G, Angerstein C, Wehrmann E, et al. Therapeutic advantages of Auger electron- over beta-emitting radiometals or radioiodine when conjugated to internalizing antibodies. Eur J Nucl Med. 2000;27:753–65.

165. Capello A, Krenning EP, Breeman WA, Bernard BF, de Jong M. Peptide receptor radionuclide therapy in vitro using [111In-DTPA0]octreotide. J Nucl Med. 2003;44:98–104.

166. Reilly RM, Kassis A. Targeted Auger electron radiotherapy of malignancies. In: Reilly RM, editor. Monoclonal antibody and peptide-targeted radiotherapy of malignancies. Hoboken, NJ: Wiley; 2010. p. 289–348.

167. Hall EJ. Radiobiology for the radiologist. 5th ed. Philadelphia, PA: Lippincott Williams and Wilkins; 2000.

168. Chan DA, Giaccia AJ. Hypoxia, gene expression, and metastasis. Cancer Metastasis Rev. 2007;26:333–9.

169. Brown JM. Exploiting the hypoxic cancer cell: mechanisms and therapeutic strategies. Mol Med Today. 2000;6:157–62.

170. Ling CC, Spiro IJ, Mitchell J, Stickler R. The variation of OER with dose rate. Int J Radiat Oncol Biol Phys. 1985;11:1367–73.

171. Teunissen JJ, Kwekkeboom DJ, de Jong M, Esser JP, Valkema R, Krenning EP. Endocrine tumours of the gastrointestinal tract. Peptide receptor radionuclide therapy. Best Pract Res Clin Gastroenterol. 2005;19:595–616.

172. Buscombe JR, Cwikla JB, Caplin ME, Hilson AJ. Long-term efficacy of low activity meta-[131I]iodobenzylguanidine therapy in patients with disseminated neuroendocrine tumours depends on initial response. Nucl Med Commun. 2005;26:969–76.

173. Parliament MB, Murray D. Single nucleotide polymorphisms of DNA repair genes as predictors of radioresponse. Semin Radiat Oncol. 2010;20:232–40.

174. Gridley DS, Williams JR, Slater JM. Low-dose/low-dose rate radiation: a feasible strategy to improve cancer radiotherapy? Cancer Ther. 2005;3:105–30.

175. Williams JA, Williams JR, Yuan X, Dillehay LE. Protracted exposure radiosensitization of experimental human malignant glioma. Radiat Oncol Investig. 1998;6:255–63.

Release Criteria and Other Radiation Safety Considerations for Radionuclide Therapy

22

Pat B. Zanzonico

Introduction

Historically, nuclear medicine has been largely a diagnostic specialty, utilizing relatively low administered activities to obtain important diagnostic information whose benefits far outweigh the small potential risk associated with the attendant low normal-tissue radiation doses to the patient. Doses and risks to members of the patient's household and other individuals encountering the patient are, of course, far lower — to the point that medical confinement of and other regulatory restrictions on diagnostic nuclear medicine patients are entirely unnecessary. However, by incorporation of appropriate radionuclides in appropriately large amounts into target tissue-avid radiopharmaceuticals, a sufficiently high radiation dose may be delivered to produce a therapeutic response in tumor or other target tissues. And radionuclide therapy — most notably, radioiodine treatment of thyroid diseases such as hyperthyroidism and differentiated thyroid cancer — has long proven to be effective and safe for patients and for individuals around the patient. With the approval of the Texas State Department of Health, for example, Allen and Zelenski pro-

spectively treated 430 home-bound outpatients over 30 years with 30–400 mCi of iodine-131 and reported that there was no demonstrable health hazard to family members or the general public [1]. Nonetheless, concerns persist regarding stochastic radiogenic risks (i.e., carcinogenesis and germ cell mutagenesis) to individuals incidentally irradiated by radionuclide-treated patients. Such concerns have led governmental authorities worldwide to establish regulatory criteria for the release of radionuclide therapy patients from medical confinement, until 1997 1,110 MBq (30 mCi) of iodine-131 (^{131}I) in the United States but as low as 74 MBq (2 mCi) in some European countries [2–7]. To optimize clinical efficacy, cost-effectiveness, and accessibility to ^{131}I and other radionuclide therapies and their benefits, such regulations must be based on sound dosimetric and radiobiologic principles and available relevant data. In the 1990s, major regulatory changes were implemented in the United States by the Nuclear Regulatory Commission (NRC) regarding release from medical confinement of patients who have received therapeutic amounts of radioactivity [6, 7]. Most notably, release may now be based on the projected effective dose equivalent to individuals exposed to radioactive patients rather than retained activity, thus allowing consideration of patient-specific kinetic and dosimetric data and other patient-specific factors.

New forms of radionuclide therapy continue to be developed and are being used more widely [8]. These therapies include palliation of bone

P.B. Zanzonico, Ph.D. (✉)
Department of Medical Physics,
Memorial Sloan-Kettering Cancer Center,
1275 York Avenue, New York, NY 10021, USA
e-mail: zanzonip@mskcc.org

C. Aktolun and S.J. Goldsmith (eds.), *Nuclear Medicine Therapy: Principles and Clinical Applications*,
DOI 10.1007/978-1-4614-4021-5_22, © Springer Science+Business Media New York 2013

pain resulting from skeletal metastases using bone-seeking radiopharmaceuticals, radioimmunotherapy of cancer using radiolabeled antibodies and antibody fragments, and radiolabeled peptides targeting growth factor receptors over-expressed on various cancers. Clinical as well as regulatory developments, then, warrant a review of release criteria and other radiation safety considerations for radionuclide.

Administration of Radionuclide Therapy

Therapeutic amounts of radioactivity must be stored, transported, and administered with the use of sufficient shielding so as to maintain personnel exposures as low as reasonably achievable (ALARA). For orally administered therapeutic radiopharmaceuticals such as ^{131}I-sodium iodide, the activity may be administered in liquid form with the activity provided in a shielded, spill-proof container with a port, or opening, for the patient to ingest the material (typically through a straw), a vent to draw in air as the patient draws up and ingests the activity-containing liquid, and a port for one or more rinses of the container. Alternatively, and perhaps more commonly, therapeutic activities of ^{131}I-iodide may be provided in the form of one or more capsules in a shielded container. The capsules are then transferred individually to a plastic cup using long-handled tongs; the patient then picks up the cup, swallows the capsule(s), and drinks sufficient amounts of water to ensure that each capsule is swallowed completely and not, for example, lodged in his or her esophagus. For intravenous use of therapeutic radiopharmaceuticals administered by bolus injection, the activity-containing syringe should be placed within a syringe shield with a transparent window that allows visual monitoring of the injectate. The use of an in-dwelling venous catheter is advisable in such cases. For a pure β-particle emitting radionuclide, a plastic syringe shield minimizes the production of *bremsstrahlung* and should be sufficient to reduce hand exposure. For intravenous therapeutic radiopharmaceuticals administered by "slow," or drip, infusion, the

activity-containing container, typically an intravenous bag, should be placed within a suitable shield. For high-energy photons, such shields will typically be made of lead. Intravenous administrations involving the use of infusion pumps will generally require lead shielding for the pump-mounted syringe. As with all aspects of radionuclide therapy, the input of the radiation safety officer (RSO)[1] in such determinations is critical.

Syringes, burettes, cups, tubing, and other materials used in parenteral administration should be flushed/rinsed with isotonic saline (or other physiologic buffer). The use of water rinses may be sufficient for oral administration to achieve complete or near-complete administration of the prescribed activity to the patient. All contaminated items from the administration procedure should be labeled with the radionuclide, the date, and a radiation precaution sticker and held for complete decay in storage in an appropriately shielded and secure area.

Immediately prior to administration of any therapeutic radiopharmaceutical, the identity of the radionuclide and the radiopharmaceutical, the total activity, and the date and time of calibration should be cross-verified between the requisition form and the radiopharmaceutical label. The administered activity should be verified by assay in a dose calibrator to insure that the total activity does not deviate from that prescribed by more than 5 %. After administration of the therapeutic radiopharmaceutical, the residual activity in the syringe, cups, tubing, and other materials used in the administration should be assayed so that the net activity actually administered can be calculated.

To avoid administration of a therapeutic radiopharmaceutical to the wrong patient, the identity of the patient should be verified verbally with the patient and checked independently by inspection of the patient's hospital wristband and medical record (i.e., chart) or, in the case of outpatient therapy, the patient's driver's license or other photo identification. In no case should a

---

[1] Here and throughout the current chapter, the term, "radiation safety officer (RSO)," refers to the RSO himself and his staff or other designee(s).

radiopharmaceutical be administered to a patient whose identity cannot be definitively verified at the time of administration.

Radiation Precautions for Inpatient Radionuclide Therapy

A patient receiving a therapeutic administration of a radionuclide on an inpatient basis must be placed in a private hospital room with a private toilet and sink. The treating physician should arrange with the hospital's admitting office for the room to be available immediately prior to administration and for the duration of the admission and should provide the RSO with the date of the treatment, the radionuclide, the radiopharmaceutical, and the prescribed administered activity as far in advance as possible. The use of disposable plastic-backed absorbent pads taped in place in areas of the patient's room most likely to be contaminated, such as the floor around the toilet and bathroom sink, is generally recommended. Corner rooms are preferable for radionuclide therapy patients, as the number of potentially exposed individuals in adjoining rooms and passing in the corridor is minimized. The RSO should survey the closest rooms and public areas in the floors immediately above and below the patient's room as well as any adjoining rooms and public areas on the same floor to verify that exposure rates are within institutional and regulatory limits (typically, 0.05 mSv/h (5 mR/h) or less). The use of portable shielding in patient's rooms for reducing the dose to medical staff caring for the patient and visitors may be necessary. Generally, there is no need to isolate or otherwise limit access to patients who have received radionuclide therapy with a pure β-ray-emitter such as strontium-89 (^{89}Sr) or yttrium-90 (^{90}Y). Standard universal precautions should be used with all radionuclide therapy patients, however.

To minimize exposure of personnel, it is generally recommended that radionuclide therapy patients not be housed together in one area or treated at one time but dispersed spatially and temporally (if clinically and logistically possible). However, in institutions, which have many such patients, such dispersal may be undesirable and it may be preferable to concentrate them in designated areas under the care of specially trained, experienced personnel. Nurses, physicians, and other healthcare personnel are to perform all routine duties, including those requiring direct patient contact, in a normal manner but should avoid lingering near the patient unnecessarily. Pregnant women should not be responsible for the routine care of patients receiving therapeutic amounts of radioactivity, however. Patients should be apprised in advance of the necessity for personnel to minimize contact, so that this precaution will not be misinterpreted as a lack of concern. To the extent possible, any verbal communication with the patients should be conducted from a distance (e.g., from the doorway of the patient's room). Housekeeping, food service, and other ancillary personnel should likewise perform all essential routine tasks expeditiously and should avoid entering the patient's room for any nonessential tasks. Such personnel should not enter the patient's room without first conferring with the nursing staff on the patient's floor. Personnel caring for such a patient or otherwise entering his or her room should observe universal precautions and thoroughly wash their hands after leaving the patient's room. In some cases, persons entering the room of a patient may need to don protective clothing before entering and, when exiting, to leave such clothing in designated waste receptacles in or immediately outside the room.

Inpatients may have visitors during the period that radiation precautions are in effect, excluding children less than 18 years of age and pregnant and nursing women. Limitations on visiting time will be established by the RSO in consultation with the treating physician and may depend on the patient's medical condition as well as the radiopharmaceutical therapy. Visitors should first report to the nursing station for instructions.

Prior to administration of the therapeutic radionuclide, all radiation safety precautions must be explained to the patient (including the anticipated duration of radiation precautions) prior to admission to the hospital so that any questions and concerns can be addressed in advance of the treatment. To avoid or at least minimize any anxiety, the patient should clearly understand the necessity to stay in his/her room and limitations on staff contact and on the duration of visits. Measurement of the anterior exposure rates (e.g., in mR/h) at the surface of and 1 m from the upright patient and at the level of his or her umbilicus should be made using a calibrated (in exposure rate units such as mR/h) radiation monitor, such as a portable ionization chamber. This initial measurement should be performed within 1 h of administration of the radiopharmaceutical therapy and prior to any post-therapy excretion by the patient. Each day following administration of the therapeutic radionuclide, the RSO resurveys the patient and the measured exposure rates used to determine the retained activity in the patient, $A(t)$, at time t post-administration:

$$A(t) = A(0)\frac{\dot{X}(t)}{\dot{X}(0)} \qquad (22.1)$$

where $A(0)$ is the activity administered to the patient (i.e., the patient's retained activity at time $t=0$), $\dot{X}(0)$ is the measured exposure rate immediately following the administration (i.e., at time $t=0$), and $\dot{X}(t)$ is the measured exposure rate at time t post-administration. The patient exposure rate or retained activity may be used to determine if the patient can be released from medical confinement if based on exposure rate or retained activity, respectively, and in formulating post-release radiation instructions, if any. A "Radiation Precautions" sign should be posted on the door to the patient's room and a "Radioactive Precautions" wristband placed on the patient. A signed and dated copy of the radiation safety precautions should be placed in the patient's medical record. The RSO should provide a plastic-lined container for the patient's room for short-term disposal/storage of all disposable items used by the patient, with food and beverages provided with disposable trays, cups, utensils, etc. The patient may use the toilet and dispose of urine and feces as usual, flushing the toilet several times after each use. Although a common practice in certain countries, collection and holding of patient excrement is not required in the United States and is not advised. Disposal in the sewer system, rather

than sequestration in on-site holding tanks, widely disperses and dilutes radioactive waste to the point that significant exposures are highly unlikely. The patient's linen and gowns may also be contaminated and should be held for assay by the RSO before being placed in the facility laundry. Removal of contaminated non-disposable items (e.g., linens and bedding) from the patient's room should be done on a daily basis.

Upon discharge of the patient, the RSO removes all remaining trash and contaminated items from the patient's hospital room, placing them in plastic bags and using separate bags for disposable and for any remaining non-disposable items. All radioactively contaminated items should be placed in plastic bags labeled with radiation precaution stickers and with the radionuclide, date and time, and held for complete decay-in-storage in an appropriately shielded and secure area. All waste and other items being held for decay in storage should be re-assayed periodically. Once the measured count or exposure rates are no greater than a specified threshold value (typically twice the background value), trash and non-disposable items may be handled as "nonradioactive." The patient's room must be surveyed and checked for removable contamination. Initially, this check can be performed using a hand-held survey meter, such as a Geiger counter or scintillation survey meter. These checks can be followed as necessary with "wipe testing." When the applicable criteria for removable radioactive contamination are satisfied (again, typically values no greater than twice background), the medical facility should be informed that the room is available for general patient use.

A list of names and "24×7" contact numbers of individuals (e.g., the RSO and nuclear medicine resident or fellow on-call) to contact in the event of a radiation emergency must be available to hospital personnel caring for radionuclide therapy patients. In the event of a large-volume spill of blood, urine, or vomitus, personnel should contain the spill by covering it with plastic-backed absorbent pads and immediately contact the RSO for further instructions. Minor spills can be managed by nursing personnel, wearing disposable gloves and disposing of paper toweling and any other contaminated items in the plastic-lined trash container or, for very minor spills wiped with flushable paper toweling, in the toilet in the patient's room.

Release Criteria and Post-release Precautions for Outpatient Radionuclide Therapy

Historically, the United States Nuclear Regulatory Commission (NRC) and Agreement States required patients receiving radionuclide therapy to remain hospitalized until the retained activity in the patient was less than 1,110 MBq (30 mCi) or the dose rate at 1 m from the patient was less than 0.05 mSv/h (5 mrem/h) [4].[2] The NRC amended its regulations concerning radionuclide therapy patients through the issuance of new rules [6, 7] that appeared in the Federal Register on January 29, 1997. The new NRC regulations, revised 10CFR 35.75 effective May 1997, allow for the release from medical confinement of patients if the expected total effective dose equivalent (TEDE) to individuals exposed to the patient is not likely to exceed 5 mSv (500 mrem). A prior regulatory analysis of replacing the traditional activity- and dose rate-based release criteria with the new dose-based criterion concluded that the proposed regulation would result in shorter hospitalization of patients, reduced health care costs and possibly a positive impact on the psychological well-being of patients and their families [9].

Guidance to licensees on determining when patients may be released based on the new criteria, when written instructions on post-release radiation precautions must be provided, and when records related to the release of the patient must be maintained are provided in NRC Regulatory Guide 8.39 [6]. A licensee may release from his control any patient administered (diagnostic or

therapeutic) radiopharmaceuticals (or therapeutically implanted with sealed radioactive sources) if the TEDE to any individual from exposure to the patient after release is not likely to exceed 5 mSv (500 mrem). Compliance with this dose limit may be demonstrated using either (a) a default table in Regulatory Guide 8.39 for activity (e.g., less than 1,221 MBq (33 mCi) of ^{131}I retained by the patient) or dose rate (e.g., less than 7 mrem/h at 1 m from an ^{131}I-containing patient) or (b) patient-specific kinetic data using effective half-times or residence times, dose rate measurements, and a patient-specific projected dose calculation [6]. An important assumption in the application of method (b), the patient-specific projected dose calculation, is that the only significant contribution to the dose received by individuals around the patient is the external dose, that is, internalization of activity and the resulting internal dose are insignificant. The use of method (b) will generally result in patients being released with substantially higher activities than would method (a). Importantly, in basing release on patient-specific information (method (b)), the NRC regulations allow for representative kinetic data such as effective half-times or residence times for a particular population of patients (e.g., hyperthyroid patients) to be applied to an individual patient in that population, thus obviating the need in certain cases for the measurement of kinetic data on an individual patient basis.

The revised NRC regulations require that the licensee provide written instructions to the released patient regarding radiation precautions to maintain the doses to others as low as reasonably achievable if the doses are likely to exceed 1 mSv (100 mrem) [6]. In the case of ^{131}I, for example, such written instructions must be provided if the activity retained at release is greater than 259 MBq (7 mCi), the dose rate at 1 m at release is greater than 0.02 mSv/h (2 mrem/h), or a patient-specific dose calculation for release is performed [6]. Post-release radiation safety instructions to the patient should address maintenance of distance from other persons, separate sleeping arrangements, minimizing time spent in public places including public transportation

---

[2] The terms "dose rate" (in mSv/h or mrem/h) is actually the dose equivalent rate. For x- and γ-rays, the type of radiation to which individuals around a radionuclide therapy patients are potentially exposed, the absorbed dose (rate) and dose-equivalent (rate) as well as the exposure (rate) are very nearly numerically equal and are used interchangeably in the in the current chapter.

facilities such as buses, trains, and planes, and measures to reduce environmental contamination. In the case of nursing mothers, recommendations on discontinuation of breast-feeding should be included as well. Information on the duration of post-release radiation precautions must also be provided. These considerations are discussed further below.

In deciding whether a radionuclide therapy patient may be treated on an outpatient basis or requires medical confinement pursuant to the NRC's amended rules, the treating physician in consultation with the RSO must reasonably determine that the patient is willing and is physically and mentally able to comply with appropriate radiation safety precautions at home after release. Importantly, if a determination is made that the patient is unwilling and/or unable to comply with such precautions and would therefore pose an unreasonable radiation hazard to the staff of the medical facility if hospitalization were warranted or others if outpatient therapy were considered, radiopharmaceutical therapy may be withheld altogether and alternative treatments considered. If the treating physician determines that a patient be safely treated with appropriate and reasonable medical supervision while hospitalized, treatment may proceed on an inpatient basis. For an incontinent patient, for example, hospitalization and urinary catheterization may be required to insure safe collection and disposal of radioactively contaminated urine. Determining the proprietary of outpatient radionuclide therapy must also include consideration of: the type of dwelling (e.g., house, apartment, nursing home, etc.); presence in the household of pregnant or breast-feeding women; the age, gender, and relationship to the patient of each household member; sleeping arrangements and sleeping partner information (e.g., age, pregnancy, etc.); workplace and school information and schedule; post-treatment transportation from the hospital to home; and, as noted, the physical and mental capacity of the patient to comprehend and follow post-release precautions.

A generally applicable algorithm for implementation of method (b) for the determination of the time of release and the duration of post-release radiation precautions following radionuclide therapy based on patient-specific information and derived from prevailing recommendations for maximum permissible TEDEs promulgated by the National Council on Radiation Protection and Measurements [10, 11], 5 mSv (500 mrem) to nonpregnant adult family members and 1 mSv (100 mrem) to pregnant women, children, and members of the general public, was published in NCRP Report 155 [12]. This algorithm was originally published by Zanzonico et al. [13], generalizing and extending the algorithm developed by Gates et al. [14] and Siegel [15] for therapy of non-Hodgkin's B-cell lymphoma with ^{131}I-labeled anti-B1 monoclonal antibody, which exhibits monoexponential total-body kinetics, to multiexponential total-body kinetics. It requires dose rate measurements immediately post-administration of the therapeutic activity at 0.3 m to estimate TEDEs to the sleeping partner of the patient and to a child held by the patient and at 1 m to estimate TEDEs to members of the general public and of the patient's family and derivation of the total-body kinetics of the therapeutic radiopharmaceutical (either from serial total-body activity measurements of the patient or published total-body kinetic data for the radiopharmaceutical).

Important in the estimation of external absorbed dose are two interrelated parameters, the "exposure factor" (also known as the "occupancy factor") [6, 16] and the "index distance" [12]. The exposure factor, $E(r_j)$, at an index distance, r_j, from a radioactive patient is the fraction of time an individual spends at the index distance, r_j, from the patient such that $\sum_{j=1}^{m} E(r_j) = 1$. Consistent with previous regulatory practice, the index distance for everyday activities is set at 1 m. The mean index distance between sleeping partners and between a child and an individual holding the child is set at 0.3 m. Although difficult to establish precisely and somewhat arbitrary, the foregoing index distances appear to be consistent with the limited anthropological data available [15, 17, 18]. The current algorithm is not dependent on any specific values of exposure factors and index distances, however, and the recommended default values of these parameters (Table 22.1) may be modified as deemed appropriate.

Table 22.1 Parameter values for the application of dose-based release criteria and estimation of the duration of post-release radiation precautions, including recommended default values of index distances r_j and exposure factors $E(r_j)$ and regulatory and recommended maximum permissible doses MPEDEs for different cohorts of potentially exposed individuals around a radionuclide therapy patient

Cohort	Index distance, r_j (m)	Exposure factor, $E(r_j)$	NRC regulation mSv	NRC regulation mrem	NCRP recommendation mSV	NCRP recommendation mrem
Family members						
Non-sleeping partner						
Non-pregnant adult/older child	1.0	0.25	5	500	5	500
Pregnant woman	1.0	0.25	5	500	1	100
Baby/younger child[a]	0.30	0.20	5	500	1	100
Sleeping partner						
Non-pregnant adult	0.30	0.33	5	500	5	500
Pregnant woman	0.30	0.33	5	500	1	100
Individuals other than family members						
Co-worker	1.0	0.25	5	500	5	500
Miscellaneous	1.0	0.25	5	500	5	500

The maximum permissible dose, MPEDE columns span NRC regulation (mSv, mrem) and NCRP recommendation (mSV, mrem).

[a]A "baby/younger child," in the current context, is a child young enough to be held for an extended period of time on a daily basis by a parent or other caregiver

As presented in Zanzonico et al. [13] and NCRP Report 155 [12], the duration of medical confinement (i.e., the time (day) of release post-treatment, $(t_{release})_{MPEDE}$) may be derived based on the maximum permissible total effective dose equivalent (MPEDE = 5 mSv (500 mrem)), $TEDE_{MPEDE}$, from a radionuclide therapy patient using the following equation:

$$TEDE_{MPEDE} = 34.6 \sum_{j=1}^{m} E(r_j) \dot{X}(r_j,0) \sum_{i=1}^{n} T(e_i) F_i e^{-0.693(t_{release})_{MPEDE}/T_{e_i}} \quad (22.2)$$

where $E(r_j)$ = the exposure factor at index distance $r_j = 1$ m,

$\dot{X}(r_j,0)$ = the exposure rate measured at $r_j = 1$ m from the patient immediately following therapeutic radionuclide administration,

T_{e_i} = the effective half-life (day) of exponential component i of the time-dependent exposure rate at $r_j = 1$ m from the patient,

= the effective half-life (day) of exponential component i of the time-dependent total-body activity in the patient,

$$\frac{T_p T_{b_i}}{T_p + T_{b_i}} \quad (22.3)$$

T_p = the physical half-life (day) of the therapeutic radionuclide,

T_{b_i} = the biological half-life (day) of exponential component i of the total-body activity in the patient,

and F_i = the zero-time intercept of exponential component i of the total-body activity in the patient expressed as a fraction of the administered activity such that $\sum_{i=1}^{n} F_i = 1$.

Implicit in (22.2) is the assumption that the only significant contribution to the dose received by individuals around the patient is the external dose, as noted above.

Equation (22.2) cannot be solved analytically for the parameter $(t_{release})_{MPEDE}$, that is, to provide an explicit formula for the parameter $t_{release}$ for a multi-exponential total-body time-activity function [19].

However, the time post-administration of release of the patient from medical confinement, $(t_{release})_{MPEDE}$, may be determined "iteratively" from (22.2); the duration of various post-release precautions (see below) may also be determined "iteratively" using equations mathematically analogous to (22.2). If the TEDE (1 m), at a distance of 1 m from the radionuclide therapy patient as given by (22.2) does *not* exceed the MPEDE of 0.5 cSv (0.5 rem) [10] for time $t=0$ the patient may be released immediately after administration of the therapeutic radiopharmaceutical, that is, no medical confinement is required. If, however, TEDE (1 m) at an index distance of 1 m from the radionuclide therapy or brachytherapy patient as given by (22.2) does exceed the MPEDE of 0.5 cSv (0.5 rem) for $t=0$, possible values of the time post-administration of release of the patient from medical confinement, $(t_{release})_{0.5\ cSv}$, may be substituted into the right side of the equation (22.2). Thus, beginning with a time of 1 day and substituting time values in 1-day increments, the earliest time value (1, 2, 3 days,…) which yields a value on the right side of the equation (22.2) equal to or less than the MPEDE is the time post-administration of release of the patient from medical confinement, $(t_{release})_{MPEDE}$. Similarly, the duration in terms of times post-administration of post-release radiation precautions—specifically, *not* working, avoiding pregnant women and children, *not* holding children, and sleeping partners sleeping apart—may also be determined using (22.2) by substituting the MPEDEs of the respective cohorts and the corresponding index distances, r_j, exposure factors, $E(r_j)$, and measured zero-time exposure rates, $\dot{X}(r_j,0)$. For determining the duration of not holding children and of not sleeping with one's sleeping partner, the dose contribution to a child and to the patient's sleeping partner from other daily activities (i.e., at an index distance of 1 m) must be added to that from the patient actually holding the child and sleeping with his or her partner (i.e., at an index distance of 0.3 m), respectively. Depending on the cohort(s) of interest, which in turn depends upon the household circumstances of the individual patient, the pertinent values of the maximum permissible

effective dose equivalents, the index distances, r_j, and the exposure factors, $E(r_j)$ will vary. As noted, a compilation of exposure factors and associated index distances assumed for different cohorts of individuals and for different activities are presented in Table 22.1. When not specifically in the company of the radioactive patient, an individual will be at distances well beyond the index distance of 1 m. Because of the rapid decrease in exposure rate with distance from the patient, for distances other than and farther from the radioactive patient than the specified index distances, the exposure rates may be considered negligibly small. Accordingly, in practice, distances other than specified index distances and the associated occupancy factors are not explicitly considered and therefore $\sum_{j=1}^{m} E(r_j)$ will not be equal to 1.

Currently in the United States, the regulatory maximum permissible dose is the same, 5 mSv (500 mrem), for all exposed or potentially exposed cohorts, including pregnant women and children as well as nonpregnant adults [6, 7] The NCRP and other advisory bodies, however, recommend a lower dose limit, 1 mSv (100 mrem), for pregnant women and children [3, 11, 12]. If one chooses to follow the lower 1 mSv (100 mrem) dose limit for these cohorts, the duration of certain post-release precautions (such as not holding a child and not sleeping with one's pregnant partner) may be much longer—up to ~1 month—than one might expect (Table 22.2). However, if a patient treated on an outpatient basis were not to return home immediately post-treatment but rather stay at a hotel or with another relative for 1 or 2 days before returning home, the duration of these post-release precautions would be shortened considerably for both the 1-mSv (100-mrem) and 5-mSv (500-mrem) dose limits. This is because the dose that otherwise would have been delivered to members of the patient's household over that first 1 or 2 days post-treatment, when the patient is most radioactive, would be eliminated. Predictably, the duration of post-release precautions would be much shorter for the 5-mSv (500-mrem) dose limit than for the 1-mSv (100-mrem) dose limit in all cases.

Table 22.2 Time to release and duration of post-release radiation safety restrictions for a hypothetical metastatic thyroid cancer patient treated post-thyroidectomy with 5,250 (175 mCi) of 131I-iodide

Time to release post-administration (days)	Duration of restriction (days) once patient returns home				
	Not sleeping with sleeping partner			Not holding child	
	If sleeping partner not pregnant	If sleeping partner pregnant		5-mSv dose limit	1-mSv dose limit
		5-mSv dose limit	1-mSv dose limit		
0	4	4	35	1	32
	2	1	19	0	15
	0	0	16	0	14

It was assumed that the total-body time-activity function was bi-exponential, with 95 % of the activity eliminated with an effective half-time of 0.32 day and 5 % of the activity eliminated with an effective half-time of 5.2 day. The assumed exposure rates immediately post-administration were 18 and 210 mR/h at the index distances of 1.0 and 0.3 m, respectively. The foregoing exposure rates were estimated by modeling the patient as a point source (and therefore assuming the exposure rate decreases as the inverse of the square of the distance from the patient), using the exposure rate constant for ^{131}I (2.23 R-cm^2/h-mCi), and assuming 0.6 of the x- and γ-rays emitted by the patient escape (i.e., are not attenuated). The exposure factors were those give in Table 22.1. For individuals other than the patient's sleeping partner and a child held by the patient, the projected TEDE at 1 m was 90 mrem, well-below the maximum permissible TEDE of 500 mrem. Therefore, this patient did not require medical confinement, that is, the time to release post-administration was 0 day. Three possible scenarios were evaluated in terms of determining the duration of post-release radiation safety restriction, specifically, the patient not sleeping with his or her sleeping partner and not holding children: the patient returns home immediately (i.e., 0 day) post-treatment, 1 day post-treatment, or 2 days post-treatment. In the latter two scenarios, the patient may, for example, choose to stay at a hotel or with another relative for 1 or 2 days before returning home. The duration of the post-release restrictions was also evaluated for both a 5-mSv (500-mrem) and 1-mSv (100-mrem) dose limit. The former is the current regulatory limit in the United States for all individuals; the latter is the limit recommended by the NCRP and other advisory bodies for pregnant women and children.

It is quite straightforward to iteratively determine the time of release post-treatment and the duration of post-release precautions using a computerized spreadsheet and such a spreadsheet (EXCEL (Microsoft Corp, Redmond, WA)) was developed in conjunction with NCRP Report 155 [12] and is available upon request from the NCRP.[3] In addition to the specific post-release precautions specified above (not working, avoiding pregnant women and children, not holding children, and sleeping partners sleeping apart), radionuclide therapy patients should observe the following precautions upon release following treatment.

- To the extent practical, radionuclide therapy patients should remain some distance from other individuals.

- After using the toilet, patients should flush twice and, as usual, wash their hands, using, if possible, flushable paper towels to dry their hands and flushing the paper toweling down the toilet.

- Patients should otherwise observe good personal hygiene and may shower, bathe, shave, etc., as they would normally would, rinsing the shower stall, tub, or sink thoroughly after use.

- Patients should wipe up any spills of urine, saliva, and/or mucus with flushable paper toweling, disposing of the paper toweling in the toilet, and flushing the toilet two times.

- Patients should use non-disposable plates, bowls, spoons, knives, forks, and cups and, if possible, wash their own tableware, using a separate sponge from that used by the rest of the household and rinsing the sink thoroughly and wiping the fixtures with disposable paper toweling after use. If dishwasher is used, the

[3] On behalf of the NCRP, the author of this chapter will provide this EXCEL file upon request.

patient's tableware should be cleaned separately from those of the rest of your household.

- Patients should store and launder their soiled/used clothing and bed linens separately from those of the rest of your household, running the rinse cycle two times at the completion of machine laundering.
- Patients should not share food or drinks with anyone.
- After using the telephone, patients should wipe the receiver (especially the mouth piece) with disposable paper toweling.

While difficult to generalize, observing the foregoing precautions for 5–7 days post-treatment is not unreasonable in most cases.

Release of Radionuclide Therapy Patients to Hotels

Some patients treated with radionuclides on an outpatient basis are spending the first one to several days post-treatment at hotels rather than return home in order to minimize radiation exposure to members of their household. This has precipitated considerable controversy and calls for regulatory prohibition of this practice [20]. This is based on concern that hotel staff (especially housekeeping staff cleaning such a patient's guest room) and guests would unknowingly receive "excessive" radiation doses, both from direct irradiation by the patients and from radioactive contamination from the patient (on bathroom and other surfaces, soiled linens, etc.). The scope of this practice and the severity of the associated radiation hazard remain ill-defined at this point, as does the need for any restriction on this practice. Importantly, however, the criteria for releasability of radionuclide therapy patients to a hotel should be no less stringent than those for release to home, that is, patients should be intellectually and physically capable of understanding and complying with post-release radiation precautions and of practicing sound personal hygiene and should not be incontinent. Thus, the likelihood of a major radioactive contamination of the patient's living space (e.g., from urine) should be minimal. Likewise, based on standard instructions to patients to minimize or

avoid close-distance interactions with other individuals, direct-exposure doses should be minimal as well.

The NRC's Advisory Committee on Medical uses of Isotopes (ACMUI) recently reported its technical analysis on the release of radionuclide therapy patients to hotels [21], adapting the dose-calculation algorithm in NCRP Report No 155 [12] (described above) to hotel workers and guests using the appropriate index distances and occupancy factors. Housekeeping staff in hotels presumably following basic occupational hygiene practices such as wearing water-proof gloves should not have any direct physical contact with guests, so the risk of internalization of radioactivity from a patient or items in a patient's hotel room (on linens, towels, etc.,) should be no greater than that to a member of the patient's household at home, which is considered negligibly low. Hotel housekeeping staff typically service 16 rooms per shift and spend up to 30 min servicing each room, according to the Canadian Centre for Occupational Health and Safety (www.ccohs.ca), corresponding to an occupancy factor of up to 0.5 h/24 h = 0.021. For dose calculation purposes, one could conservatively assume that 20 % of the activity in a patient at a given time point post-administration was at a distance of 0.3 m from a hotel worker for 20 min each day; this assumption implies that 20 % of the remaining patient activity was urinated or otherwise discharged onto towels, bed linens, etc., and those soiled, radioactively contaminated items were then held by the housekeeper for 20 min while he or she serviced the patient's room. One could apply the same conservative assumptions to hotel laundry staff and thereby calculate the same dose to members of that staff from handling of contaminated linens. (As such staff generally do not have direct interactions with guests themselves, that would represent the total dose to the laundry staff.) Since hotel guests are typically *not* present when their rooms are being cleaned or otherwise serviced, there should be no additional occupancy factor for housekeeping staff with respect to the patient. However, one can conservatively assume that a patient will stand or sit at a distance of 1 m from a hotel housekeeper for 2 h per day, yielding an

Table 22.3 Radiation doses to hotel workers and guests for a hypothetical hyperthyroid patient and a hypothetical metastatic thyroid cancer patient treated post-thyroidec-tomy with 1,110 MBq (30 mCi) and 5,250 MBq (175 mCi) of 131I-iodide, respectively

		Hyperthyroid patient			Cancer patient		
Duration of hotel stay (days)		1	2	3	1	2	3
Hotel housekeeper	mSv	0.12	0.22	0.31	0.35	0.43	0.47
	mrem	12	22	31	35	43	47
Hotel laundry worker	mSv	0.059	0.11	0.15	0.16	0.19	0.21
	mrem	5.9	11	15	16	19	21
Hotel guest in room adjoining that of patient	mSv	0.13	0.24	0.33	0.40	0.48	0.53
	mrem	13	24	33	40	48	53
Hotel worker other than housekeeper or laundry worker or hotel guest in room other than one adjoining that of patient	mSv	0.064	0.12	0.16	0.20	0.24	0.26
	mrem	6.4	12	16	20	24	26

It was assumed that the total-body time-activity functions were bi-exponential for both hyperthyroid and thyroid cancer patients. For hyperthyroid patients, it is assumed that 20 % of the activity is eliminated with an effective half-time of 0.32 day and 80 % of the activity eliminated with an effective half-time of 5.2 days. For thyroid cancer patients, it is assumed that 95 % of the activity is eliminated with an effective half-time of 0.32 day and 5 % of the activity eliminated with an effective half-time of 5.2 days. The assumed exposure rates immediately post-administration were 4 and 43 mR/h for the hyperthyroid patient and 23 and 253 mR/h for the thyroid cancer patient at the index distances of 1.0 and 0.3 m, respectively. The foregoing exposure rates were estimated by modeling the patient and soiled items as point sources (and therefore assuming the exposure rate decreases as the inverse of the square of the distance from the patient), using the exposure rate constant for ^{131}I (2.23 R-cm^2/h-mCi), and assuming 0.6 and 1.0 of the x- and γ-rays emitted by the patient and the soiled items escape (i.e., are not attenuated), respectively. It was further assumed that walls between rooms provided no shielding. See text for additional assumptions

occupancy factor at 1 m of 2 h/24 h=0.083. One then could calculate the additional dose contribution to a hotel housekeeper from this direct patient exposure. The total dose to a hotel housekeeper would then be the sum of the dose contributions from handling contaminated items and from the direct exposure.

For estimation of the direct-exposure dose to a hotel guest in a room adjoining that of the patient, the area of a hotel room may be assumed to be at least 27 m^2 (i.e., 5.2×5.2 m=17×17 ft). A reasonably conservative "index position" for a hotel guest in his or her room is 1/3 of the room length from a wall shared with the adjoining room, yielding an index distance of (1/3×5.2 m)+(1/3 ×5.2 m)=3.5 m, with an occupancy factor of 10 h/24 h=0.42, assuming that a hotel guest occupies his or her room at this index position for 10 h out of every day. The dose to hotel guests other than those in rooms adjoining that of the patient may be estimated by conservatively assuming that a patient will stand or sit at a distance of 1 m from another hotel guest for 2 h per day, yielding an occupancy factor at 1 m of 3 h/24 h=0.083. One can then calculate the dose to other hotel guests—that is, hotel guests other than those in rooms adjoining that of the patient— from this direct patient exposure (e.g., in the hotel lobby, restaurant, etc.). The total dose to a hotel guest in a room adjoining that of the patient would be the sum of the dose contributions from the direct exposure while that guest is in his or her room and that from the direct patient exposure elsewhere.

Based on the foregoing considerations, the hypothetical doses to hotel workers and guests have been calculated for patients receiving 1,110 MBq (30 mCi) or 5,250 MBq (175 mCi) of ^{131}I for the treatment of hyperthyroidism or thyroid cancer, respectively (Table 22.3). The highest doses were received by the hotel housekeeper servicing the patient's room and the guest staying in the room adjoining that of the patient, 0.47 mSv (47 mrem) and 0.53 mSv (53 mrem), respectively, for a 3-day stay by a thyroid cancer patient who received 5,250 MBq (175 mCi) of ^{131}I. Despite the conservative assumptions used, all doses are at or below the 1-mSv (100-mrem) annual dose limit for the general population and well below the 5-mSv (500-mrem) dose limit for nonoccupationally exposed individuals. Therefore, the release of radionuclide therapy patients to a hotel should generally be permissible under the same conditions for which release to the patient's home would be.

Travel by Radionuclide Therapy Patients

An important practical issue for radionuclide therapy patients is possible restrictions on travel, as this will typically involve exposure by the patient of one or more individuals at relatively close distances in a confined space such as an automobile or plane. Various authors have reported dose rates at 0.1–1 m from ^{131}I-treated hyperthyroid and thyroid cancer patients immediately post-administration [17, 22–28]. While difficult to succinctly summarize these data, traveling with a patient for up to several hours following administration of ^{131}I is unlikely to result in a dose in excess of 1 mSv (100 mrem) at a distance 0.3 m or further from a patient who received an activity of the order of 370 MBq (10 mCi) or at a distance 1 m or further from a patient who received an activity of the order of 3,700 MBq (100 mCi). Thus, use of public transportation by radioiodine-treated hyperthyroid patients is permissible immediately post-treatment [3, 12]. In the case of administered activities of the order of 3,700 MBq (100 mCi), however, and at distances from the patient of 0.3 m or less, a dose in excess of 5 mSv (500 mrem) may be accrued over 1 h. Thus, travel for up to several hours immediately post-treatment in a private automobile large enough for a patient to maintain a distance of 1 m or greater from the other occupant(s) is generally permissible for thyroid cancer patients as well as hyperthyroid patients [3, 12]. On the other hand, thyroid cancer patients receiving of the order of 3,700 MBq (100 mCi) should avoid using publication transportation for the first 24 h following the therapy administration [3, 12]. However, a case-by-case analysis is recommended to determine the actual travel restrictions for each patient, especially for longer trips and/or for travel by public bus or train,

commercial airliner, or other conveyance in which travelers may be crowded together.

Radionuclide therapy patients will likely trigger radiation detection systems in place for security purposes at bridges, tunnels, train stations, airports, and elsewhere, and this may persist for weeks to months following treatment [3]. Each such patient should be apprised of this likelihood and provided with documentation (perhaps in the form of a "wallet card") to present to the authorities, identifying the individual as having received a therapeutic amount of radioactivity and specifying the radionuclide, the date of administration, the activity administered, the hospital which administered the activity, and an individual to be contacted for further information.

Dosimetric Studies of Individuals Exposed to Radionuclide Therapy Patients

Over the years, a number of investigators have evaluated the radiation exposure to medical personnel, members of the patient's household, and members of the general public who come in contact with radionuclide-treated patients in the immediate post-treatment period; predictably, most of these studies involved hyperthyroid or thyroid cancer patients treated with radioiodine [17, 22–24, 27–43]. This has been done in several different ways: serial measurements using a survey meter (such as a Geiger counter) of the dose rate at discrete distances from treated patients; measurement of the integral, or total, dose using thermoluminescent dosimeters (TLDs) worn continuously by members of the patient's household; and serial measurements using an uptake probe of the ^{131}I activity in the thyroid of members of the patient's household and calculation of their resulting thyroid doses. The first two methods evaluate the external radiation hazard only, with the TLD-based measurement of external dose, rather than discrete dose rates, being more realistic and presumably more accurate. The third method evaluates the environmental contamination hazard only. Of course, the overall hazard is a combination of both the external and internal radiation hazards.

For hyperthyroid patients [27, 32, 44] treated with 370 MBq (10 mCi) of ^{131}I, the measured dose rates are uniformly less than 0.05 Sv/h (5 mrem/h) at a distance of 0.5 m or greater immediately post-treatment, with dose rates at 1 day post-administration of 0.09, 0.02, and 0.01 mSv/h (9, 2, and 1 mrem/h) at 0.1, 0.6, and 1 m, respectively. Consistent with the long biological half-life in the thyroid gland and therefore the total body, however, the dose rates from ^{131}I-treated hyperthyroid patients decrease only slowly (i.e., with an effective half-life nearly equivalent to the 8-day physical half-life of ^{131}I). For thyroid cancer patients [28, 42, 45] treated with 5,550 MBq (150) mCi of ^{131}I, the dose rates are predictably much higher, 0.9, 0.2, and 0.05 mSv/h (90, 20, and 5 mrem/h) at 0.1, 0.3, and 1 m, respectively, immediately post-treatment. The dose rates at 1 day post-administration are 4, 0.16–1, 0.7, 0.05–0.4 mSv/h (400, 16–100, 70, and 5–40 mrem/h) at 0.1, 0.3, 0.6, and 1 m, respectively. Consistent with the short biological half-life in the total body of radioiodine in athyreotic patients, the dose rates from ^{131}I-treated thyroid cancer patients decrease rapidly (i.e., with a half-time of ~1 day). The foregoing distance- and time-dependent dose rates suggest that medical personnel providing routine care to radioiodine-treated patients will generally not exceed or even approach the annual maximum permissible dose of 0.05 mSv (5 rem) for occupationally exposed individuals in the United States. Even in the extreme, and unlikely, event of major surgery (4 h in duration) immediately post-administration of radioiodine, the hypothetical doses to surgical personnel would be 0.5 and 40 mSv (50 and 4,000 rem) from hyperthyroid (370 MBq (10 mCi)) and thyroid cancer (1,550 MBq (150 mCi)) patients, respectively. Further, in a study over 1–4 months of 62 nurses caring for hospitalized ^{131}I-treated patients, Castronovo [45] found that 97 % received a dose of less than 0.1 mSv (10 mrem), the minimum detectable using a film badge, and all received a dose of less than 0.2 mSv (20 mrem).

Dosimetric studies of individuals exposed to ^{131}I-treated patients also demonstrate the relatively small dose contribution (consistently less than 10 %) of internalized radioiodine [3, 6, 33, 38], consistent with the assumption in NCRP Report 155 [12] and NRC Regulatory Guide 8.39 [6] that this contribution may be ignored in the implementation of dose-based release criteria. A common rule of thumb is to assume that no more than one millionth of unsealed activity being "handled" will be internalized by an individual handling the activity [3]. Thomson and Harding [46] nonetheless cautioned that internalization of radioiodine by babies and small children potentially could result in significant thyroid doses. Potential sources (with the activity concentration expressed as percent of the administered activity per milliliter, %/mL) of such environmental contamination from radioiodine-treated patients are [47]: saliva (~0.1 %/mL), from iodide concentrated by and secreted from the salivary glands; urine (~0.01 %/mL), from renally excreted iodide; blood (~0.001 %/mL), from circulating inorganic iodide and protein-bound iodine; feces (<0.001 %/g), from iodide excreted from the gut; perspiration (~0.0001 %/mL), from iodide in the extracellular fluid; and exhaled air (at a rate of ~0.0001 %/h), from iodide converted to volatile iodine (I_2) [47–51]. Based on sampling of room air, room surfaces, patients' exhaled breadth, skin, and saliva, and gloves used by the hospital staff for hospitalized ^{131}I-treated thyroid cancer patients, Ibis et al. [50] found significant activity levels in all samples through 48 h and generally peaking at 24 h post-administration. Importantly, however, assay of thyroid activity among hospital staff at 2 day post-administration showed no significant uptake, demonstrating the effectiveness of appropriate radiation safety precautions. These findings are consistent with the low thyroid doses reported among family members of radioiodine-treated thyroid patients, including children, compared to the external dose.

In a study measuring doses to family members from released ^{131}I-treated hyperthyroid patients, Barrington et al. [52] found that 89 % of all children received less than 1 mSv (100 mrem). However, 35 % of younger children (age 3 years or younger) received more than 1 mSv (100 mrem), suggesting the need for special precautions for younger children. A study by Mathieu et al. [40] indicated that, when children stayed away from home for the first 8 days following therapy, the median doses they received over the following 2 weeks were 0.08 and 0.13 mSv (8 and 12 mrem) from thyroid cancer and hyperthyroid patients, respectively. Some authors have therefore recommended that for families with young children a short hospital stay may be preferable to returning home immediately post-treatment [53].

Miller [35] and Thomson et al. [32, 44] found that 88 % and 84 %, respectively, of the external dose to the spouses of ^{131}I-treated hyperthyroid patients was accrued while sleeping together and/ or during sexual intimacy. Moreover, Thomson et al. [32, 44] found that separate sleeping arrangements reduced the external total-body dose equivalent accrued at night by 85 %. Wasserman and Klopper [54] deduced that maintaining separate sleeping arrangements for 14 days would reduce the external total body dose equivalent to the spouse by nearly 50 %. Thus, separate sleeping arrangements are a particularly effective radiation precaution.

Based on an analysis of the foregoing literature (unpublished), the median hypothetical retained activities at discharge achieving compliance with the MPEDE of 5 mSv (500 mrem) were as much as 2,640 MBq (71.3 mCi) and 11,000 MBq (298 mCi) for ^{131}I therapy of hyperthyroidism and thyroid cancer, respectively, substantially greater than the 1,110-MBq (30-mCi) retained-activity limit previously in effect in the United States and much greater than the even lower retained-activity limits still in effect elsewhere. Consistent with this finding, the analysis of Siegel [15] of over 50 non-Hodgkin's B-cell lymphoma patients treated with 1,850–5,660 MB (50–153 mCi) of ^{131}I-labeled anti-B1 monoclonal antibody found that all such patients would have been treatable on an outpatient basis without exceeding the MPEDE of 5 mSv (500 mrem).

Summary and Conclusions

Radionuclide therapy, over many years of use, has proven effective for patients and safe for other individuals as well as for the patients themselves. Nonetheless, the potential remains for radiation exposures exceeding regulatory limits

to personnel treating and caring for the patient, members of the patient's household, and others. Reasonably straightforward, practical precautions can maintain doses to such individuals well below such limits. Of course, detectable levels of radiation and radioactivity do not correspond, necessarily, to hazardous levels, and it is impossible to reduce ambient radiation and environmental radioactivity associated with radionuclide therapy patients to undetectably low levels. Importantly, however, it is *not* necessary to do so in order to ensure the safety of individuals encountering or in the vicinity of radionuclide-therapy patients.

Current radiation dose-based (versus prior activity-based) release criteria for radionuclide therapy patients are predicated on the following considerations.

• Dose-based release criteria generally allow radionuclide therapy to be performed on an outpatient basis, and there are tangible medical, psychological, and logistical (including but not limited to financial) advantages associated with outpatient radionuclide therapy.

• Dose-based release criteria are more scientifically rigorous than activity-based criteria and better protect public safety by basing patient releasability on the quantity, dose, *directly* related to potential radiation hazard rather than on a quantity, activity, *indirectly* related to this potential hazard.[4]

• Implicit in outpatient radionuclide therapy is that patients are capable, intellectually and physically, of understanding and complying

---

[4] In the case of radioiodine treatment of thyroid cancer, for example, the administered radioiodine is rapidly excreted (with a whole-body biological half-time of only ~2 days or less). In treating hyperthyroidism, however, 25–50 % of the radioiodine localizes in the thyroid, and that activity is cleared from the gland (and, in turn, the body) much more slowly, with half-times of ~20 days or longer. Accordingly, the retained activity from the much higher activity (typically greater than 100 mCi) administered to the thyroid cancer patient is rapidly reduced to a lower activity than that retained by the hyperthyroid patient (who typically receive only 10 mCi). Thus, higher dose-rate irradiation of individuals around the patient persists considerably longer in the case of hyperthyroidism than of thyroid cancer, despite the much larger activities used to treat the latter.

with post-release radiation precautions. This determination, as well as all of other aspects of the suitability of a patient for outpatient therapy (including his or her home situation), must be made by the attending physician in conjunction with the radiation safety office.

With patient-specific dosimetric analyses, outpatient radionuclide therapy can be performed safely and well within prevailing regulatory dose limits

References

1. Allen H, Zelenski J. 430 Non-hospitalized thyroid cancer patients treated with single doses of 40–400 mCi (abstract). J Nucl Med. 1992;33:784.
2. Beckers C. Regulations and policies in radiodine 131I therapy in Europe. Thyroid. 1997;7:221–4.
3. IAEA. Release of patients after radionuclide therapy. Safety Report Series 63. Vienna, Austria: International Atomic Energy Agency (IAEA); 2009.
4. Vetter RJ. Regulations for radioiodine therapy in the United States: current status and the process of change. Thyroid. 1997;7:209–11.
5. ICRP. Release of patients after radionuclide therapy with unsealed radionuclides. International Commission on Radiological Protection (ICRP) publication 94. Oxford: Elsevier; 2004.
6. NRC. Release of individuals administered radioactive material, Nuclear Regulatory Commission (NRC) Regulatory Guide 8.39. Washington, DC: USNRC; 1996.
7. NRC. Criteria for the release of individuals administered radioactive material, Nuclear Regulatory Commission (NRC). Washington, DC: USNRC; 1997.
8. Speer T, editor. Targeted radionuclide therapy. Philadelphia, PA: Lippincott Williams & Wilkins; 2011.
9. Schneider S, McGuire S. Regulatory analysis on criteria for the release of patients administered radioactive material, NUREG-1492. Washington, DC: US Nuclear Regulatory Commission; 1996.
10. NCRP. Limitation of exposure to ionizing radiation, NCRP Report No 116. Bethesda, MD: National Council on Radiation Protection and Measurement (NCRP); 1993
11. NCRP. Dose limits for individuals who receive exposure from radionuclide therapy patients, NCRP Commentary No 11. Bethesda, MD: National Council on Radiation Protection and Measurement (NCRP); 1995.
12. NCRP. Management of radionuclide therapy patients. National Council on Radiation Protection and Measurements (NCRP) Report 155. Bethesda, MD: National Council on Radiation Protection and Measurements (NCRP); 2007.
13. Zanzonico PB, Siegel JA, St Germain J. A generalized algorithm for determining the time of release and the duration of post-release radiation precautions following radionuclide therapy. Health Phys. 2000;78(6):648–59. Epub 2000/06/01. PubMed PMID: 10832924.
14. Gates VL, Carey JE, Siegel JA, Kaminski MS, Wahl RL. Nonmyeloablative iodine-131 anti-B1 radioimmunotherapy as outpatient therapy. J Nucl Med. 1998;39(7):1230–6.
15. Siegel JA. Revised nuclear regulatory commission regulations for release of patients administered radioactive materials: outpatient iodine-131 anti- B1 therapy. J Nucl Med. 1998;39(8 Suppl):28S–33.
16. NCRP. Precautions in the management of patients who have received therapeutic amounts of radionuclides, NCRP Report No 37. Bethesda, MD: National Council on Radiation Protection and Measurement (NCRP); 1970.
17. Culver C, Dworkin H. Radiation safety considerations for post-iodine-131 hyperthyroid therapy. J Nucl Med. 1991;32:169–73.
18. Hall E. The hidden dimension. New York: Doubleday Comp Inc; 1966.
19. Cormack J, Shearer J. Calculation of radiation exposures from patients to whom radioactive materials have been administered. Phys Med Biol. 1998;43: 501–16.
20. Markey E. Radioactive roulette: how the nuclear regulatory commission's cancer patient radiation rules gamble with public health and safety. Washington, DC: US House of Representatives; March 18, 2010.
21. ACMUI. Patient Release Report. Advsiory Committee on the medical uses of isotopes (ACMUI), Rockville, MD: Nuclear Regulatory Commission, 2010; December 13, 2010.
22. Barrington S, Kettle A, Mountford P, Thomas W, Batchelor S, Burrell D, et al. Radiation exposure of families of thyrotoxic patients treated with radioiodine (abstract). Thyroid. 1997;7:305.
23. Barrington S, Kettle A, O'Doherty M, Wells C, Somer E, Coakley A. Radiation dose rates from patients receiving iodine-131 therapy for carcinoma of the thyroid. Eur J Nucl Med. 1996;23:123–30.
24. Culver C, Dworkin H. Radiation safety considerations for post-iodine-131 thyroid cancer therapy. J Nucl Med. 1992;33:1402–5.
25. Gunesekara R, Thomson W, Harding L. Use of public transport by 131I therapy patients (abstract). Nucl Med Commun. 1996;17:275.
26. Leslie WD, Havelock J, Palser R, Abrams DN. Large-body radiation doses following radioiodine therapy. Nucl Med Commun. 2002;23(11):1091–7. Epub 2002/11/02. doi:10.1097/01.mnm.0000040971.43128. cd. PubMed PMID: 12411838.
27. O'Doherty M, Kettle A, Eustance C, Mountford P, Coakley A. Radiation dose rates from adult patients

receiving I131 therapy for thyrotoxicosis. Nucl Med Commun. 1993;14:160–8.

28. Pochin E, Kermode J. Protection problems in radionuclide therapy: the patient as a gamma radiation source. Br J Radiol. 1975;48:299–305.

29. Kettle A, Barrington S, O'Doherty M. Radiation dose rates from post 131I therapy and advice to patients on discharge from hospital (letter). Health Phys. 1997; 72:711.

30. Mountford PJ, O'Doherty MJ, Forge NI, Jeffries A, Coakley AJ. Radiation dose rates from adult patients undergoing nuclear medicine investigations. Nucl Med Commun. 1991;12(9):767–77.

31. Grigsby PW, Siegel BA, Baker S, Eichling JO. Radiation exposure from outpatient radioactive iodine (131I) therapy for thyroid carcinoma. JAMA. 2000;283(17):2272–4. Epub 2000/05/12. PubMed PMID: 10807387.

32. Thomson W, Mills A, Smith N, Mostafa A, Notghi A, Harding LK. Radiation doses to patients' relatives: day and night components and their significance in terms of ICRP 60 (abstract). Eur J Nucl Med. 1993; 20:993.

33. Buchan R, Brindle J. Radioiodine therapy to outpatients: the contamination hazard. Br J Radiol. 1970;43:479–82.

34. Buchan R, Brindle J. Radioiodine therapy to out-patients: the radiation hazard. Br J Radiol. 1971;44:973–5.

35. Miller K. External radiation doses in a household from a patient receiving a therapeutic amount of 131I. New York, NY: Environmental Measurements Laboratory, Report No.: EML-547;1992.

36. Harbert J, Wells N. Radiation exposure of the family of radioactive patients. J Nucl Med. 1974;15:887–8.

37. Plato P, Jacobson A, Homann S. In vivo thyroid monitoring for iodine-131 in the environment. Int J Appl Radiat Isot. 1976;27:539–45.

38. Jacobsen A, Plato P, Toeroek D. Contamination of the home environment by patients treated with iodine-131: initial results. Am J Public Health. 1978; 68:228–30.

39. Mathieu I, Caussin J, Smeesters P, Wambersie A, Beckers C. Doses in family members after 131I treatment. Lancet. 1997;345:1074–5.

40. Mathieu I, Caussin J, Smeesters P, Wambersie A, Beckers C. Recommended restrictions after 131I therapy: measured values in family members. Health Phys. 1999;76:129–36.

41. Hilditch T, Connell J, Davies D, Watson W, Alexander W. Radiological protection guidance for radioactive patients—new data for therapeutic I131. Nucl Med Commun. 1991;12:485–95.

42. Mohammadi H, Saghari M. Hospital discharge policy in thyroid cancer patients treated with 131I: the effect of changing from fixed time to exposure rate threshold. Health Phys. 1997;72:476–80.

43. Patients leaving hospital after administration of radioactive substances. Working Party of the Radiation Protection Committee of the British Institute of Radiology. Br J Radiol. 1999;72(854):121–5. Epub 1999/06/12. PubMed PMID: 10365059.

44. Thomson W, Mills A, Smith N, Mostafa A, Notghi A, Harding L. Day and night radiation doses to patients' relatives: Implications of ICRP 60 (abstract). Nucl Med Commun. 1993;14:275.

45. Castronovo Jr FP, Beh RA, Veilleux NM. Dosimetric considerations while attending hospitalized I-131 therapy patients. J Nucl Med. 1982;10:157–60.

46. Thomson W, Harding L. Radiation protection issues associated with nuclear medicine out-patients. Nucl Med Commun. 1995;16:879–92.

47. Nishizawa K, Ohara K, Oshima M, Maekoshi H, Orito T, Watanabe T. Monitoring of excretions and used materials of patients treated with I131. Health Phys. 1980;38:467–81.

48. Browning E, Banerjee K, Reisinger W. Airborne concentration of I-131 in a nuclear medicine laboratory. J Nucl Med. 1978;19:1078–81.

49. Goble J, Wagner W. Volatilization during iodine therapies: assessing the hazard (abstract). Health Phys. 1978;35:911.

50. Ibis E, Wilson C, Collier B, Arkansel G, Isitman A, Yoss R. Iodine-131 contamination from thyroid cancer patients. J Nucl Med. 1992;33:2110–5.

51. Knight M, Burr J, Blair D, Eddy M, Oresnick L, Rosen J. Airborne release of 131I associated with patient therapy (abstract). Health Phys. 1978;35:911.

52. Barrington SF, O'Doherty MJ, Kettle AG, Thomson WH, Mountford PJ, Burrell DN, et al. Radiation exposure of the families of outpatients treated with radioiodine (iodine-131) for hyperthyroidism. Eur J Nucl Med. 1999;26(7):686–92. Epub 1999/07/10. PubMed PMID: 10398815.

53. Reiners C, Lassmann M. Radioiodine (131I) treatment of hyperthyroidism: radiation protection and quality assurance. Eur J Nucl Med. 1999;26(7):683–5. Epub 1999/07/10. PubMed PMID: 10398814.

54. Wasserman H, Klopper J. Analysis of radiation doses received by the public from 131I treatment of thyrotoxic outpatients. Nucl Med Commun. 1993;14:756–60.

Challenges Associated with Radionuclide Therapy and Need for Interdepartmental Collaboration

23

Cumali Aktolun

Introduction

Diagnostic procedures and radionuclide therapy are the main clinical functions of Nuclear Medicine Physicians. As an imaging physician, like a diagnostic radiologist, the nuclear medicine specialist deals with various diagnostic procedures including radionuclide imaging, bone mineral densitometry, radionuclide uptake studies, blood volume measurement, and breath tests. As a treating physician, s/he deals with various therapeutic procedures for patients referred by Endocrinologists, Oncologists, Hematologists, Hepatologists, Urologists, Rheumatologists, and Surgeons, among others.

Challenges

While diagnostic procedures require specific nuclear medicine knowledge, expertise and skills, radionuclide therapy further requires knowledge and skills in other disciplines including Oncology, Endocrinology, Hematology, Hepatology, Immunology, Urology, and Rheumatology. Most importantly, the Nuclear Medicine therapy physician is involved in the *healing process* directly,

which is not a usual requirement for diagnostic procedures.

Currently, except for radioiodine therapy of thyroid cancers, most of the radionuclide therapy methods are offered to the patients after trying all available non-Nuclear Medicine treatment techniques before the patient is referred for Nuclear Medicine therapy as a *final tool* with limited therapeutic expectations. Patients are usually referred for "symptom palliation" instead of "cure." The patients are therefore at an advanced stage with considerable side-effects and complications of previous nonradionuclide treatments and comorbidities. This situation creates further challenges for the Nuclear Medicine physician as the radionuclide therapy method itself may be also associated with significant side-effects including renal, hepatic, and hematological toxicities.

High dose rate radiation as delivered by external beam radiation therapy has different effects on tumor cells from the effects of persistent, low dose rate radiation delivered through radionuclide therapy see Chap. 21. Nuclear Medicine Physicians should be aware of the scientific details of the biological effects of low dose rate radiation on healthy and tumor cells.

Also, reducing side-effects and increasing the total amount of radioactivity is proven to be possible by using fractionation of the total dose into multiple cycles, which require a continuous monitoring and follow-up of the patients being treated. A way of augmentation of the cell-kill effects of radionuclide therapy is the combination of radionuclide therapy with classical chemotherapeutic

C. Aktolun, M.D., M.Sc. (✉)
Tirocenter Nuclear Medicine Center, Istanbul, Turkey
e-mail: aktolun@aktolun.com

C. Aktolun and S.J. Goldsmith (eds.), *Nuclear Medicine Therapy: Principles and Clinical Applications*,
DOI 10.1007/978-1-4614-4021-5_23, © Springer Science+Business Media New York 2013

agents, bio-therapeutic agents, or radiosensitizers. This approach also creates the opportunity of lowering the radionuclide dose and brings further responsibility to the Nuclear Medicine physician of the awareness of the scientific background of these non-nuclear agents and the collaboration with Medical Oncologists.

Radioimmunotherapy, an efficient targeted model of radionuclide therapy may be associated with immunological reactions in patients after treatment. These reactions may result in serious clinical side-effects and symptoms, and also decrease the efficacy of radioimmuntherapy. These side-effects need to be addressed to prevent patients from life-threatening risks and to avoid the negative effects on the efficacy of radioimuno-therapy requiring knowledge of Immunology and collaboration with Immunologists. This is in addition to the requirement of having sufficient knowledge in Immunology during the process of developing these radioimmunotherapeutic agents.

Procedure related follow-up is not a common function for nuclear medicine specialists after diagnostic procedures but it is an important task after radionuclide therapy to assess the therapeutic response and repeat the therapeutic procedures as needed. This requires a *continuous relationship* with the patients, not usually associated with diagnostic procedures.

Also, depending on the therapeutic procedures and local regulations, some of the therapeutic procedures require hospitalization of the patients; hence the need for in-patient care. Currently, standard curriculum of Nuclear Medicine training does not include in-patient clinical care sufficiently.

It is likely that the therapeutic function of Nuclear Medicine will expand rapidly. Every nuclear medicine physician will unavoidably be involved in therapy of various malignant and benign diseases at sometime. An additional challenge is that the referrals may come from various departments reflecting diverse clinical problems. The Nuclear Medicine physician can treat a patient with prostate cancer referred from Urology on one day, and another patient with non-Hodgkin's lymphoma referred from Hematology on another day or a patient with liver tumor (a malignant disease) in the morning referred from Hepatology and another

patient with osteoarthritis (a benign disease) referred from Rheumatology in the afternoon.

A detailed history written by the requesting physician is usually sufficient for reporting the diagnostic procedures. For therapeutic procedures, the Nuclear Medicine physician himself must take a detailed history, perform a physical examination on the patient, and order new tests if necessary before the radionuclide treatment. S/He decides on and performs therapy-related additional nuclear medicine imaging procedures before radionuclide therapy. For example, before the radionuclide therapy of liver tumors with Y-90 labeled microspheres, a Tc-99m MAA scintigraphy including SPECT or SPECT/CT is necessary for the assessment of liver tumor perfusion and scoring of the lung shunt.

In addition, the Nuclear Medicine physician has the responsibility to assess the success of the therapy with Nuclear Medicine procedures. For example, following treatment of a patient with a neuroendocrine tumor with a high dose of lutetium-177 DOTATATE, gamma camera imaging of the gamma photon component of Lu-177 or alternately PET/CT using gallium-68 DOTATOC is performed to assess the therapeutic response during follow-up visits.

Therapy requires involvement of the Nuclear Medicine physician at the very early stages including the decision making process for eligibility, patient selection, and indication. Actually, this is the most important stage for the success of the therapeutic procedure. It involves attending a joint meeting with the referring physician(s) and/or surgeon(s). This can be repeated in some patients who require further examinations before making a final eligibility decision for radionuclide therapy. In order to survive in these meetings, Nuclear Medicine physicians should be equipped with sufficient knowledge in that particular field.

Compared to therapeutic procedures, the amount of activity used and the radiation absorbed dose in diagnostic imaging in Nuclear Medicine is low, and usually not associated with radiation toxicity. With radionuclide therapy, however, one of the most important concerns is the serious, sometimes life-threatening radiation toxicity associated with the administration of large dose of radioactive therapeutic agent. Actually, it is the most important feature limiting the success of the radionuclide therapy. Nuclear Medicine physician should be aware of these toxicities and the measures to avoid them and means to treat them. For example, coinfusion of amino acids is performed by the treating Nuclear Medicine physicians to minimize the effect of radiotoxicity on the kidneys of lutetium-177 DOTATATE in the treatment of neuroendocrine tumors. The choice of amino acid, time to initiate, and the speed of this infusion and amount of amino acids are all within Nuclear Medicine physicians' responsibility. Close follow-up of liver and bone marrow function is necessary also during the decision for planning additional cycles of radionuclide therapy in these patients.

Not all tumors treated with radionuclides are slow growing neoplasms like thyroid cancers. Neuroendocrine tumors are differentiated neoplasms and although often slow growing, they may become aggressive and very symptomatic. Furthermore, radionuclide therapy of pheochromacytoma may result in the release of large amounts of catecholamines. Radionuclide therapy regimens should therefore also include measures and medications controlling and relieving these symptoms and the physiologic consequences of the release of these metabolically active substances. Most of the other tumors treated with radionuclides are at an advanced stage requiring comprehensive clinical knowledge and skills to deal with associated health problems.

The end-result of treatment is not limited to failure, palliation, or cure of cancer. "Disease stabilization" is now an accepted "end-result" of anticancer treatment. The patient lives with his disease, recurrences may occur but the survival is almost equal to the life-span of healthy people. This concept is best defined in patients with well differentiated thyroid cancer. Radiopeptide therapy of neuroendocrine tumors is expected to give the same opportunity to the patients with this disease in future.

Cancer causes decrease in performance of patients, and therapy associated risks increase when a patient with poor performance score is treated. Also, killing cancer cells by any anticancer treatment modality is associated with serious side-effects and toxicities which may negatively affect the patient's quality of life. Therapeutic Nuclear Medicine physician has to take these concepts into consideration and objectively assess and score physical and psychological performances before deciding on the feasibility of radionuclide therapy, the dose of radionuclide to be administered, and the number of cycles of radionuclide therapy in each patient.

Once the decision is made to proceed with radionuclide therapy, the role of the Nuclear Medicine physician becomes more important by taking over the *primary* responsibility of the patient, at least temporarily during the period involving assessment, administration of the therapeutic radionuclide, and immediate follow-up.

Patient preparation is vital for the success of radionuclide therapy. This is particularly important for thyroid carcinomas and neuroendocrine tumors. Patient preparation aims to augment the therapeutic effect and minimize the side-effects.

Teamwork: Requirement for Interdepartmental Collaboration

Radionuclide therapy requires interdepartmental collaboration at every stage and involves at least two different medical disciplines for a single therapeutic intervention (viz. Departments of Rheumatology and Nuclear Medicine for radiosynovectomy). It may, however, sometimes be necessary for as many as six departments to collaborate as needed in the radiolabeled microsphere therapy of liver tumors: Hepatology, Medical Oncology, Radiation Oncology, Surgery, Interventional Radiology, and Nuclear Medicine. Each discipline brings its expertise and skills to the table (Fig. 23.1).

The collaboration starts at the initial decision making stage (i.e., patient selection and indication). The Nuclear Medicine physician should get involved in the process from the beginning, and

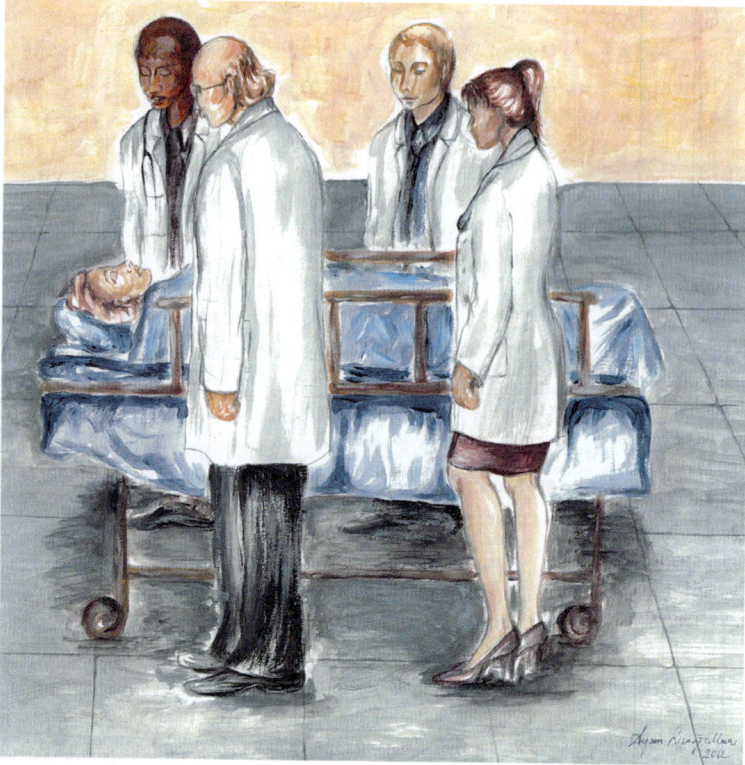

Fig. 23.1 Teamwork. Courtesy, Miss Asun Kisaogullari

propose additional Nuclear Medicine tests if s/he needs further information or a more comprehensive pretreatment workup. At this stage, the details of radionuclide therapy, potential benefits, limitations, possible side-effects, and contraindications should be shared with the other members of the therapy team.

Once the decision for radionuclide therapy is made, the Nuclear Medicine physician has the patient's primary clinical responsibility. The therapeutic procedure should be explained in plain language to the patient and his/her relative or guardian before proceeding to the treatment process.

Careful planning within the Nuclear Medicine department is vital for therapeutic success. This planning includes staffing, logistics of therapeutic agent, and availability of therapy facility.

Radionuclide therapy is associated with new opportunities for the specialty of Nuclear Medicine but it also is associated with several

Table 23.1 Challenges for nuclear medicine therapy physician

Primary responsibility of the patient
Direct involvement in healing process
Side-effects and complications resulting from other previous treatments
Continuous relation with the patient
In-patient care requirement for some patients
Involvement in both benign and malignant disease at the same time
Associated radiation toxicity
Need for knowledge in other disciplines

challenges (Table 23.1). Some of these challenges are new for Nuclear Medicine physicians.

Comorbidities should be noted and properly addressed before actual radionuclide treatment. This may require collaboration with additional departments (e.g., the patient may have paraneoplastic syndrome which requires the intervention of more than one discipline).

The medications that the patient is receiving may interfere with radionuclide therapy. Some medications directly affect therapeutic success while other may augment the side-effects of therapy, requiring collaboration with other relevant department for replacing these medications if necessary.

The therapeutic procedure may be performed at the Nuclear Medicine department by a Nuclear Medicine physician only (e.g., lutetium-177 DOTATATE therapy of neuroendocrine tumors) or is performed in the Radiology intervention room by a Nuclear Medicine Physician and an Interventional Radiologist jointly (e.g., yttrium-90 microsphere therapy of liver tumors) requiring close interdepartmental collaboration. It may even be necessary for the surgeon to actively join the therapeutic process (avidin-biotin pretargeting) in the surgical theater of the radionuclide therapy of breast carcinomas as described in Chap. 10. The radionuclide may sometimes be administered for local irradiation of brain tumors through a subcutaneous pump in an intensive care unit or another department as described in Chap. 7.

Possible Conflicts and Conflict Management

Contrary to diagnostic procedures, radionuclide therapy is definitely a team at work. The role of the treating Nuclear Medicine physician is neither defined nor universally standardized. This may cause frictions and conflicts. Each and every member of the therapy team has a vital role in the process. Undermining the role of one of the other participants is a common mistake that could contribute to treatment failure. The Nuclear Medicine physician should not be seen as the "*radiation delivery specialist*." Radionuclide therapy emphasizes the "*clinical physician*" role of the Nuclear Medicine specialist. To fulfill this role efficiently, the Nuclear Medicine physician should be equipped with the necessary knowledge and skills.

Interdepartmental competition is a common source of conflict and destructive to team spirit. This competition may be due to over-motiva-tion, which leads to trying to dominate the team or an unwillingness to share the rewards of a successful therapeutic result within a team.

Also, lack of open dialogue is another cause that results in delay and conflict. Misunderstanding which results from poor communication always causes a hostile environment. Briefing of the team members at every major steps and sharing the details of side-effects and complications immediately with the team is useful to avoid conflicts resulting from misunderstanding and rumors.

Strict hierarchical structure may also result in conflicts in some hospitals. Currently, in most departments, there is usually a physician in charge of therapeutic procedures. This physician is expected to have knowledge and skill necessary for therapy and perform the procedure independently. Some departments have a strict order of hierarchy which may prevent this physician from performing his/her role freely.

Poor planning and lack of coordination complicate the procedure and cause friction among the members of the team. The responsibility of failure due to poor planning is not usually assumed by any member.

Hostile atmosphere among the members of the team should be clearly eliminated. Interdepartmental conflict is the only problem that guarantees failure of radionuclide therapy, and thus should be absolutely avoided.

Causes for Interdepartmental Conflict

- Undermining other party's role
- Interdepartmental competition
- Poor communication
- Strict hierarchical structure
- Poor planning
- Lack of coordination

Priority should be given to the prevention of interdepartmental conflicts. If it cannot be prevented, conflicts should be professionally managed.

Clear role definition for each member of the team, involving all parties in the whole process, efficient communication, sharing benefits and merits of success, proper pretreatment preparation, negotiation and conflict resolution skills, and accountability for failure are essential for a harmonious interdepartmental collaboration [1–6]. Collaboration in a teamwork spirit is the only remedy for the resolution of interdepartmental conflicts.

Conclusion

Radionuclide therapy is associated with new opportunities as well as challenges. It brings significant responsibilities and active involvement of Nuclear Medicine physician in the whole process. Interdepartmental collaboration is vital for success. Conflicts do arise and should be professionally managed with team spirit.

Conflict Prevention and Resolution

- Clear role definition for each member of the team
- Involving all parties in the whole process
- Efficient communication
- Sharing benefits and merits of success
- Proper pretreatment preparation and coordination
- Negotiation and conflict resolution skills
- Accountability for failure

References

1. Barnett E. Managing conflicts in system development. Hosp Mater Manage Q. 1997;18:1–6.
2. Pape T. A systems approach to resolving O.R. conflict. AORN J. 1999;69:551–3; 556–7; 560–6.
3. Mellick LB. Special report: resolving conflicts. What to do about tension with other departments. ED Manag. 1999;11:142–4.
4. Stewart S. Tearing down the walls between O.R. and S.P.D. Can Oper Room Nurs J. 2004;22:7–8; 10; 15.
5. Otero HJ, Nallamshetty L, Rybicki FJ. Interdepartmental conflict management and negotiation in cardiovascular imaging. J Am Coll Radiol. 2008;5:834–41.
6. DeAngelis C. Facts and frictions: conflicts of interest in medical research. Methodist Debakey Cardiovasc J. 2011;7:24–7.

Index

C. Aktolun and S.J. Goldsmith (eds.), *Nuclear Medicine Therapy: Principles and Clinical Applications*,
DOI 10.1007/978-1-4614-4021-5, © Springer Science+Business Media New York 2013

Printed by Publishers' Graphics LLC
CIMO20130408.15.01.13